Clinical Laboratory Science Review

Third Edition

Clinical Laboratory Science Review

Third Edition

ROBERT R. HARR, MS, MT (ASCP)

Chair, Department of Public and Allied Health
Bowling Green State University
Bowling Green, Ohio

F. A. DAVIS COMPANY · Philadelphia

F. A. Davis Company
1915 Arch Street
Philadelphia, PA 19103
www.fadavis.com

Printed in the United States of America

Last digit indicates print number: 10 9 8 7

Acquisitions Editor: Christa Fratantoro
Manager, Content Development: Deborah Thorp
Developmental Editor: Melissa Reed
Art and Design Manager: Carolyn O'Brien

As new scientific information becomes available through basic and clinical research, recommended treatments
and drug therapies undergo changes. The author(s) and publisher have done everything possible to make this
book accurate, up to date, and in accord with accepted standards at the time of publication. The author(s),
editors, and publisher are not responsible for errors or omissions or for consequences from application of the
book, and make no warranty, expressed or implied, in regard to the contents of the book. Any practice
described in this book should be applied by the reader in accordance with professional standards of care used
in regard to the unique circumstances that may apply in each situation. The reader is advised always to check
product information (package inserts) for changes and new information regarding dose and contraindications
before administering any drug. Caution is especially urged when using new or infrequently ordered drugs.

ISBN 10: 0-8036-1373-3
ISBN 13: 978-0-8036-1373-7

Library of Congress Cataloging-in-Publication Data

Clinical laboratory science review / [edited by] Robert R. Harr. —3rd ed.
        p. ; cm.
    Includes bibliographical references.
    ISBN-13: 978-0-8036-1373-7
    ISBN-10: 0-8036-1373-3
  1. Medical laboratory technology—Examinations, questions, etc. I. Harr,
Robert R.
    [DNLM: 1. Laboratory Techniques and Procedures—Examination Questions.   2.
Chemistry, Clinical—methods—Examination Questions.   3. Technology,
Medical—Examination Questions. QY 18.2 C6415 2007]
    RB38.25.C574 2007
    616.07'5076—dc22   2006031808

The primary purpose of the *Clinical Laboratory Science Review* is to assist candidates who are preparing for certification or licensure examinations in clinical laboratory science. This review can also be used by those who wish to update their medical laboratory knowledge and renew their theoretical skills. In addition, educators in clinical laboratory science and medical technology programs may wish to recommend this review as a study guide for their students in various courses.

The *Clinical Laboratory Science Review* is designed to facilitate learning. Unlike other review books, the questions create a progression of related content. Explanations accompanying each question expand upon the content. The book includes more than 1500 multiple choice questions grouped into ten content areas. Questions appear together with answers, short explanations, test item classifications, and taxonomy levels. The questions of each section comprise a thorough review of the discipline and are ordered to facilitate the coherent understanding of the subject. Mock certification examinations can be created using the accompanying CD to provide additional practice. Regardless of certification examination format or sponsor, the *Clinical Laboratory Science Review* provides a rapid and efficient review and self-assessment for both generalist and categorical exams at both the CLT/MLT and CLS/MT levels.

The review begins with the Introduction section, which includes information on the design of the questions, use of this book to prepare for an examination, and test-taking skills. The introductory section is followed by questions arranged within the ten major content areas. Each section contains a list of references, which are also recommended for further review. A comprehensive certification examination is given at the end of the question sections using questions selected from the book. This examination will help the students to determine their levels of retention and learning from the book. The CD contains a database with over 800 questions different from those in the book, including over 200 images with accompanying questions. Students can use the CD program engine to create customized examinations for specific subjects or examinations based upon difficulty.

The materials in the *Clinical Laboratory Science Review* were prepared by educators and clinical experts who have received national recognition for their accomplishments in clinical laboratory science. Materials from recent developments in practice as well as major textbooks were used in formulating these questions. Peer review of the questions was performed as part of the publication process. Many new questions have been added in the new edition. The *CLS Review* has been designed as an individual guidebook for measuring personal knowledge and test-taking skills. It should prove to be a valuable tool for ensuring the success of the student preparing for a national certification examination, course examinations, or licensure, and for the practitioner updating theoretical skills.

Robert R. Harr

REVIEWERS

Carol E. Becker, MS, MT(ASCP), CLS(NCA)
Program Director
Clinical Laboratory Sciences
OSF Saint Francis Medical Center
Peoria, Illinois

Bruce Brown, MS, EdD, MT(ASCP), SM(NRM)
Associate Professor
Clinical Laboratory Sciences
Marshall University
Huntington, West Virginia

Stephen M. Johnson, MS, MT(ASCP)
Program Director
Medical Terminology
St. Vincent Health Center
Erie, Pennsylvania

Janet B. Martin, MLT/MT, CLT/CLS, BA, MEd
Associate Professor/Director
Medical Laboratory Technology
Amarillo College
Amarillo, Texas

Teresa S. Nadder, PhD, MT(ASCP), CLS(NCA)
Associate Professor
Clinical Laboratory Sciences
Virginia Commonwealth University
Richmond, Virginia

Camellia St. John, MEd, MT(ASCP)SBB
Associate Professor
Clinical Laboratory Sciences
School of Allied Health
University of Texas – Galveston
Galveston, Texas

Carol A. Watkins, MT(ASCP), MBA
Associate Professor/Program Director
Fundamental and Applied Sciences
Wayne State University
Detroit, Michigan

CONTRIBUTORS

Denise M. Harmening, PhD, MT(ASCP), CLS(NCA)
Professor
Department of Medical and Research Technology
School of Medicine
University of Maryland at Baltimore
Baltimore, Maryland
   Chapter 1 Hematology

Betty Ciesla, MS, MT(ASCP)SH
Faculty
Medical Technology Program
Morgan State University
Baltimore, Maryland
   Chapter 1 Hematology

Barbara Caldwell, BS, MT(ASCP)SH
Assistant Professor
Department of Medical and Research Technology
School of Medicine
University of Maryland at Baltimore
Baltimore, Maryland
   Chapter 1 Hematology

Mitra Taghizadeh, MS, MT(ASCP)
Assistant Professor
Department of Medical and Research Technology
School of Medicine
University of Maryland at Baltimore
Baltimore, Maryland
   Chapter 1 Hematology
   Chapter 2 Hemostasis

Thomas S. Alexander, Ph.D. D(ABMLI)
Immunologist
Summa Health System
Department of Pathology and Laboratory Medicine
Akron, Ohio
   Chapter 3 Immunology

Virginia C. Hughes, MS, MT(ASCP)SBB, CLS(NCA)I
Assistant Professor
Division of Clinical Laboratory Sciences
Auburn University Montgomery
Montgomery, Alabama
   Chapter 4 Immunohematology

Robert R. Harr, MS, MT(ASCP)
Associate Professor and Chair
Public and Allied Health
Bowling Green State University
Bowling Green, Ohio
   Chapter 5 Clinical Chemistry
   Chapter 6 Urinalysis and Body Fluids
   Chapter 8 Molecular Diagnostics
   Chapter 10 Photomicrographs and Color Plates

Pamella Phillips, MEd, MT(ASCP)SM
Education Coordinator, Program in Medical Technology
Public and Allied Health
Bowling Green State University
Bowling Green, Ohio
   Chapter 7 Microbiology
   Chapter 9 Education and Management

Lynn Shore Garcia, MS F(AAM), CLS(NCA)
Director
LSC & Associates
Santa Monica, California
   Chapter 7, Unit 11 Parasitology

CONTENTS

Preface   v

Reviewers   vii

Contributors   ix

Introduction   xv
   Design of Questions   xv
   Prepare for Your Certification Examination   xvi
   Test-Taking Skills   xvii

CHAPTER **1**   **HEMATOLOGY**   **1**

1.1   *Basic Hematology Concepts/Laboratory Procedures   3*
1.2   *Normocytic/Normochromic Anemias   9*
1.3   *Hypochromic/Microcytic Anemias   14*
1.4   *Macrocytic/Normochromic Anemias   16*
1.5   *Qualitative/Quantitative WBC Disorders   18*
1.6   *Acute Leukemias   21*
1.7   *Lymphoproliferative/Myeloproliferative Disorders   25*
1.8   *Hematology Problem Solving   29*

CHAPTER **2**   **HEMOSTASIS**   **39**

2.1   *Coagulation/Fibrinolytic Systems   41*
2.2   *Platelet/Vascular Disorders   45*
2.3   *Coagulation System Disorders   49*
2.4   *Inhibitors, Thrombotic Disorders, and Anticoagulant Drugs   53*
2.5   *Problem Solving in Hemostasis   60*

CHAPTER **3**   **IMMUNOLOGY**   **69**

3.1   *Basic Principles of Immunology   71*
3.2   *Immunological Procedures   77*
3.3   *Infectious Diseases   82*
3.4   *Autoimmune Diseases   93*
3.5   *Hypersensitivity   96*
3.6   *Immunoglobulins, Complement, and Cellular Testing   99*
3.7   *Tumor Testing and Transplantation   102*
3.8   *Immunology Problem Solving   105*

CHAPTER 4 · IMMUNOHEMATOLOGY 113

4.1   Genetics and Immunology of Blood Groups   115
4.2   ABO Blood Group System   118
4.3   Rh Blood Group System   122
4.4   Testing for Antibodies   126
4.5   Compatibility Testing   131
4.6   Transfusion Reactions   136
4.7   Components   138
4.8   Donors   143
4.9   Hemolytic Disease of the Newborn   147
4.10 Serological Testing of Blood Products   151
4.11 Immunohematology Problem Solving   153

CHAPTER 5 · CLINICAL CHEMISTRY 159

5.1   Instrumentation   161
5.2   Blood Gases, pH, and Electrolytes   175
5.3   Glucose, Hemoglobin, Iron, and Bilirubin   189
5.4   Calculations, Quality Control, and Statistics   203
5.5   Creatinine, BUN, Ammonia, Amino Acids, and Uric Acid   217
5.6   Proteins, Electrophoresis, and Lipids   225
5.7   Enzymes and Cardiac Markers   242
5.8   Clinical Endocrinology   261
5.9   Toxicology and Therapeutic Drug Monitoring   273
5.10 Tumor Markers   282
5.11 Clinical Chemistry Problem Solving   289

CHAPTER 6 · URINALYSIS AND BODY FLUIDS 305

6.1   Routine Physical and Biochemical Urine Tests   307
6.2   Urine Microscopy and Clinical Correlations   320
6.3   Cerebrospinal, Serous, and Synovial Fluids   330
6.4   Amniotic, Gastrointestinal, and Seminal Fluids   340
6.5   Body Fluids Problem Solving   350

CHAPTER 7 · MICROBIOLOGY 357

7.1   Specimen Collection, Media, and Methods   359
7.2   Enterobacteriaceae   364
7.3   Nonfermentative Bacilli   375
7.4   Miscellaneous and Fastidious Gram-Negative Rods   380

7.5   *Gram-Positive and Gram-Negative Cocci   387*

7.6   *Aerobic Gram-Positive Rods, Spirochetes, Mycoplasmas and Ureaplasmas, and Chlamydia   397*

7.7   *Anaerobic Bacteria   401*

7.8   *Mycobacteria   406*

7.9   *Mycology   412*

7.10   *Virology   421*

7.11   *Parasitology   427*

7.12   *Problem Solving in Microbiology and Parasitology   439*

CHAPTER **8**   **MOLECULAR DIAGNOSTICS**   **455**

8.1   *Molecular Methods   457*

8.2   *Molecular Diagnostics   469*

CHAPTER **9**   **EDUCATION AND MANAGEMENT**   **479**

CHAPTER **10**   **PHOTOMICROGRAPHS AND COLOR PLATES**   **489**

CHAPTER **11**   **SAMPLE CERTIFICATION (SELF-ASSESSMENT) EXAMINATION**   **501**

11.1   *ANSWER KEY   512*

The *Clinical Laboratory Science Review* has been designed to provide a challenging personal assessment of practical and theoretical knowledge needed by clinical laboratory scientists. The *Clinical Laboratory Science Review* will help you identify strengths, weaknesses, and gaps in your knowledge base. Because taxonomy level is a part of the assessment, you will also be able to concentrate on the type of question that causes the most difficulty. The suggested approach to maximizing use of the *Clinical Laboratory Science Review* is to read the explanation that follows each question thoroughly, regardless of whether you answered it correctly or not. Highlight the content you did not know, and study it until you have committed it to memory.

This *Clinical Laboratory Science Review* was developed as a tool to facilitate both self-assessment and new learning. The units are arranged in a logical sequence corresponding to the organization of a textbook and follow the pattern of presentation used in clinical laboratory science lectures. The questions within a unit are related and can be used by students as they progress through their courses in order to improve understanding. The sections are comprehensive and suitable for all certification levels, although some questions may be more appropriate for one certification level than another. The *Clinical Laboratory Science Review* is intended to supplement courses in the curriculum and assist technologists and technicians who are re-entering the laboratory. In addition, it is designed to improve performance on generalist, categorical, and specialist certification examinations.

Design of Questions

Test questions used in certification examinations are multiple choice. Each consists of a question, incomplete statement, or problem to be solved called the stem and four alternative responses. One of the alternatives is the correct response and the remaining three are incorrect (these may be wrong, incomplete, partially correct, or less correct than the most appropriate response). Incorrect alternatives that appear plausible are called distractors. The difficulty of a question is determined by how close the distractors are to the correct response. Some questions were written for assessment of your knowledge and others for learning. For pedagogic reasons, the latter may contain an "all of the above" alternative. This makes such questions into three true or false statements that are related by the subject (stem) of the question. If you are reasonably sure that two of the responses are true, then the correct response must be "all of the above." For this reason such questions are used rarely if at all on certification examinations. Questions involving combinations of statements (multiple, multiple choice) are not used on certification examinations or in this book.

All of the questions in this book are multiple choice. Each question is followed by the correct answer, a brief explanation, and a test item classification. The test item classification consists of the subject category, task, and taxonomy level of the question. A question in Blood Banking, for example, which asks for an interpretation of an ABO problem, may have a test item classification, "Blood Bank/Evaluate laboratory data to recognize problems/ABO discrepancy/3." The test item classification places the question in the major category of blood banking; the question asks for an evaluation of data; the subcategory is ABO discrepancy; and the taxonomy level classifies the question as problem solving. Taxonomy level 1 questions address recall of information. Taxonomy 2 questions require calculation, correlation, comprehension, or relation. Taxonomy 3 questions require problem solving, interpretation, or decision-making.

This question design allows you to compute a score, which helps you to identify strengths and weaknesses in various content areas and tasks. You may then focus study time on a particular content area or on practicing with questions of a specific taxonomy level. For example, if several mycology questions are answered incorrectly, extra time should be devoted to studying this content area. If, however, several recall questions (taxonomy 1 level) are missed over several different content areas such as hematology, chemistry, and immunology, then repetitive review is indicated for all of these sections. Poor performance with questions that require mathematical solutions (taxonomy 2 level) requires you to review formulas used for laboratory calculations and to practice solving them. If interpretation or problem solving (taxonomy 3 level) is identified as a weakness, then the best approach is to study the explanation that follows each question in order to understand the logic or reasoning behind the answer.

Because the answers and explanations appear on the same page as the questions, it is recommended that you use a folded piece of paper or cardboard to cover the answers while answering the questions. When you have answered a question, slide the cover down the page to reveal the answer and explanation.

Prepare for Your Certification Examination

Ideally, an examination score should reflect your knowledge of the content without the influence of other variables. However, variables such as stress, wellness, self-confidence, emotional state, and alertness all influence performance. In addition, examination skills often factor into examination scores and can be decisive. A single question answered correctly can make the difference between passing or failing, the only two meaningful scores for a certification examination.

Certification examinations are usually delivered by computer. There are two types of computer-based examinations, traditional and adaptive. Traditional examinations are of fixed length and content. Therefore, everyone taking the examination does so at the same time and receives the same set of questions. Computer adaptive examinations may be fixed or variable in length, but every one is different because the difficulty of the next question is determined by whether you answer the current question correctly. Since the difficulty of the questions answered correctly and not the number of questions answered correctly determines passing or failing, you should always give your best answer the first time. Although every examinee's question set is different, all questions come from a common database, and therefore there is some overlap between the questions used. The examination is constructed so that the number of questions in each category (e.g., hematology) are within the specifications published for the examination; however the distribution of questions within a category will vary more than for a traditional examination. Certification examinations are criterion referenced. This means that examination performance is scored passing or failing independently of the performance of other candidates taking the examination. The minimum passing score for certification examinations is normalized in order to minimize the variance between examinations. However, the minimum passing score usually falls within the range of 65% to 70% correct responses. A score below 65% on any content area in the *Clinical Laboratory Science Review* is a strong indicator that you have not mastered the material in this area and that further study is required.

Preparation for a certification examination requires a study plan. Begin with a review of the examination content outline that is made available by the certification agency. For example, if 20% of the examination is Microbiology but only 2% is Laboratory Management, you should spend significantly more time studying the former. Within each content area there are subcategories (e.g., Bacteriology and Parasitology under Microbiology). If 60% of the Microbiology content is Bacteriology and only 10% is Parasitology, then devote significantly more time to studying the former.

Allow yourself sufficient time prior to the examination to review each major content area no less than three times. Begin studying your strongest subject, then progress to your weakest. Study your class notes first, then use this review book to test your knowledge of the respective content area. Devote time to reading the explanation for each question, regardless of whether you answered it correctly or not. Highlight information you did not know and review it before taking the tests in this book a second time. Rarely, will you encounter any of the same questions on your certification examination; however, you are likely to encounter variants of the questions, and the explanations will help prepare you to answer these correctly. When finished with the second round, take the comprehensive examination included with this book. Evaluate your performance by both subject and taxonomy. If you score lower in Clinical Chemistry, devote more time to it in your third round of study. If you are weakest in recall type questions, make note cards with charts and tables, and study them regularly until the information on them is committed to memory. Note your progress from the first to the second round. If your progress is significant, use the same approach on the third round. If not, devote more time to the respective content area. Plan your final round so that you end with your weakest subject. Finally, take the examinations on the CD included with this book. These questions are all different than those in the book. Devote more study time to your weakest areas.

Test-Taking Skills

Before the Examination

First, make a study plan such as the one suggested above. You cannot expect to review all of this material in only a few days. Allow yourself at least one month to study all areas completely and carefully. Set aside an allotted time period of at least one hour each day when you are alert and can stay focused.

Assemble all of your study materials before you begin your review. Searching for old notes or textbooks may become time consuming and frustrating. You may have a tendency to "give up" looking for needed materials if you do not have them readily available. A major content area, therefore, may be neglected or unstudied.

Provide a study environment. Choose a quiet, comfortable area for your study. Find a place where you will not be distracted or disturbed. Simulate test conditions. Regardless of your study plan, some portion of the review process, for example, the mock examination, should be taken under simulated test conditions. Examinations should be timed, uninterrupted, and designed to observe other realistic testing practices.

A few days before the examination, read through the instructions sent to you by the certification agency. Some types of calculators may be prohibited and you should know what you can and cannot bring with you. Make your travel arrangements and familiarize yourself with directions to the site. Finally, go to sleep early the night before the examination, and leave yourself extra time if you have to travel a long distance to the examination site.

On Examination Day

Eat properly and, if possible, engage in some light physical activity such as walking prior to leaving for the examination. Dress comfortably; layered clothing may provide some alternatives if the examination room is too hot or too cold.

Wear a watch so that you can keep track of time. Do not take notes or books with you. If you have not prepared prior to the examination day, you won't succeed by trying to cram last-minute facts. If you become anxious before or during the examination, close your eyes and breathe deeply for a few seconds. Perhaps focus on a special activity that you may have planned as a reward for yourself after the examination.

Have confidence in your abilities. At this point, you have successfully completed a rigorous course of classroom and clinical training and the examination represents merely the last step in this long process. Tell yourself that you have adequately practiced and prepared for the examination and that you are ready.

During the Examination

Read all directions. Make sure you understand how to take the examination. Read the questions carefully and note key words. Accept the question as you first read it; do not read your own thoughts into the question and do not look for hidden meanings.

Quickly look at all of the answers. Next, carefully read all choices. You may wish to mentally place a T for true or an F for false beside each alternative or to reject outright obviously wrong choices. Select your first choice and do not change your answer. Answer all of the questions. There is no penalty for guessing on certification examinations. Always answer to the best of your ability the first time. A computer adapted examination selects the next question based upon your previous answer.

Apply a few simple rules to those questions you cannot answer. Consistently choose the same letter on those questions. "B" is the most common correct answer. Choose one of the longest answers. Pick items that are more specific or detailed than the others.

Do not overlook words such as *not, never, always, most, least, best, worst, except*. Statements that contain unqualified absolutes (*always, never*) are usually incorrect. In contrast, alternatives that are worded to contain exceptions (*usually, generally*) are often true. Do not panic if you do not know an answer. Continue the test and do not allow anxiety to make you forget items that you know.

Work steadily and do not spend too much time on questions you do not know; keep an eye on the time. Try to pace yourself so that sufficient time remains after completing the test to review all of your answers. Do not change your original answer unless you are certain that you made a mistake when you answered the question initially.

CHAPTER **1**

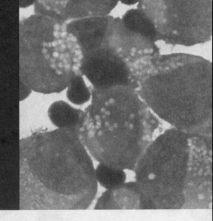

Hematology

1.1   BASIC HEMATOLOGY CONCEPTS/LABORATORY PROCEDURES

1.2   NORMOCYTIC/NORMOCHROMIC ANEMIAS

1.3   HYPOCHROMIC/MICROCYTIC ANEMIAS

1.4   MACROCYTIC/NORMOCHROMIC ANEMIAS

1.5   QUALITATIVE/QUANTITATIVE WHITE BLOOD CELL DISORDERS

1.6   ACUTE LEUKEMIAS

1.7   LYMPHOPROLIFERATIVE/MYELOPROLIFERATIVE DISORDERS

1.8   HEMATOLOGY PROBLEM SOLVING

1. Insufficient centrifugation will result in:
   A. A false increase in hematocrit (Hct) value
   B. A false decrease in Hct value
   C. No effect on Hct value
   D. All of the above, depending on the patient

   Hematology/Apply principles of basic laboratory procedures/Microscopic morphology/Differential/2

2. Erythrocytes that vary in size from the normal 6–8 μm are described as exhibiting:
   A. Anisocytosis
   B. Hypochromia
   C. Poikilocytosis
   D. Pleocytosis

   Hematology/Apply knowledge of fundamental biological characteristics/Microscopic morphology/RBCs/1

3. Which of the following is the preferable site for bone marrow aspiration and biopsy in an adult?
   A. Iliac crest
   B. Sternum
   C. Tibia
   D. Spinous processes of a vertebra

   Hematology/Apply knowledge of fundamental biological characteristics/Bone marrow/1

4. Mean cell volume (MCV) is calculated using the following formula:
   A. $(Hgb \div RBC) \times 10$
   B. $(Hct \div RBC) \times 10$
   C. $(Hct \div Hgb) \times 100$
   D. $(Hgb \div RBC) \times 100$

   Hematology/Calculate/RBC Indices/2

5. What term describes the change in shape of erythrocytes seen on a Wright's-stained peripheral blood smear?
   A. Poikilocytosis
   B. Anisocytosis
   C. Hypochromia
   D. Polychromasia

   Hematology/Apply knowledge of fundamental biological characteristics/Microscopic morphology/RBCs/1

Answers to Questions 1–5

1. **A** Insufficient centrifugation does not pack down the red blood cells; therefore, the Hct, which is the volume of packed cells, will increase.

2. **A** A mature erythrocyte is approximately 7 μm in diameter. Variation in normal size is denoted by the term *anisocytosis*. *Hypochromia* is a term that indicates increased central pallor in erythrocytes, and *poikilocytosis* denotes variation in red cell shape.

3. **A** The iliac crest is the most frequently used site for bone marrow aspiration and biopsy. This site is the safest and most easily accessible, with the bone just beneath the skin, and neither blood vessels nor nerves are in the vicinity.

4. **B** MCV is the average "volume" of the red cells. This is obtained by dividing the Hct or packed cell volume (PCV) by the red blood cell (RBC) count in millions per microliter of blood and multiplying by 10. The MCV is expressed in cubic microns (μm^3) or femtoliters (fL).

5. **A** Variation in shape of the erythrocytes on a peripheral blood smear is poikilocytosis. Anisocytosis refers to a change in size. Hypochromia is an increase in central pallor in erythrocytes. Polychromasia describes the bluish tinge of the immature erythrocytes (reticulocytes) circulating in the peripheral blood.

6. Calculate the mean cell hemoglobin concentration (MCHC) using the following values:

Hgb: 15 g/dL (150 g/L); RBC: $4.50 \times 10^6/\mu L$ ($4.50 \times 10^{12}/L$); Hct: 47 mL/dL (0.47).

A. 9.5% (.095)
B. 10.4% (.104)
C. 31.9% (.319)
D. 33.3% (.333)

Hematology/Calculate/RBC Indices/2

7. A manual white blood cell (WBC) count was performed. A total of 36 cells were counted in all 9-mm² squares of a Neubauer-ruled hemacytometer. A 1:10 dilution was used. What is the WBC count?

A. $0.4 \times 10^9/L$
B. $2.5 \times 10^9/L$
C. $4.0 \times 10^9/L$
D. $8.0 \times 10^9/L$

Hematology/Calculate/Manual WBC/2

8. When an erythrocyte containing iron granules is stained with Prussian blue, the cell is called a:

A. Spherocyte
B. Leptocyte
C. Schistocyte
D. Siderocyte

Hematology/Apply knowledge of fundamental biological characteristics/RBCs Microscopic morphology/Stain/1

9. A 7.0-mL etheylenediaminetetraacetic acid (EDTA) tube is received in the laboratory containing only 2.0 mL of blood. If the laboratory is using manual techniques, which of the following tests will most likely be erroneous?

A. RBC count
B. Hemoglobin (Hgb)
C. Hct
D. WBC count

Hematology/Apply knowledge to identify sources of error/Specimen collection and handling/Hematocrit/2

10. A 1:200 dilution of a patient's sample was made and 336 red cells were counted in an area of 0.2 mm². What is the RBC count?

A. $1.68 \times 10^{12}/L$
B. $3.36 \times 10^{12}/L$
C. $4.47 \times 10^{12}/L$
D. $6.66 \times 10^{12}/L$

Hematology/Calculate/Manual RBCs/2

11. What phagocytic cells produce lysozymes that are bacteriocidal?

A. Eosinophils
B. Lymphocytes
C. Platelets
D. Neutrophils

Hematology/Apply knowledge of fundamental biological characteristics/Leukocytes/1

12. If a patient has a reticulocyte count of 7% and an Hct of 20%, what is the corrected reticulocyte count?

A. 1.4%
B. 3.1%
C. 3.5%
D. 14%

Hematology/Apply principles of basic laboratory procedures/Calculate/Reticulocyte/2

Answers to Questions 6–12

6. **C** MCHC is the average concentration of Hgb in red cells expressed in percent. It expresses the ratio of the weight of Hgb to the volume of erythrocytes and is calculated by dividing Hgb by the Hct, and then multiplying by 100. A decreased MCHC indicates that cells are hypochromic. In this example $(15 \div 47) \times 100 = 31.9\%$.

7. **A** The formula used for calculating manual cell counts using a hemocytometer is: Number of cells counted × dilution factor × depth factor (10) divided by the area. In this example, $36 \times 10 \times 10 = 3600 \div 9 = 400/mm^3$ or $0.4 \times 10^9/L$.

8. **D** Siderocytes are red cells containing iron granules and are visible when stained with Prussian blue.

9. **C** Excessive anticoagulant causes shrinkage of cells; thus the Hct will be affected. RBC and WBC counts remain the same, as does the Hgb content.

10. **B** RBC count = number of cells counted × dilution factor × depth factor (10), divided by the area. In this example, $336 \times 200 \times 10 = 672,000 \div 0.2 = 3.36 \times 10^6/mm^3 = 3.36 \times 10^{12}/L$.

11. **D** Neutrophils are highly phagocytic and release lysozymes, peroxidase, and pyrogenic proteins. Eosinophils migrate to sites where there is an allergic reaction or parasitic infestation, releasing peroxidase, pyrogens, and other enzymes, including an oxidase that neutralizes histamine. They are poorly phagocytic and do not release lysozyme.

12. **B** In anemic states the reticulocyte percentage is not a true measure of reticulocyte production. The following formula must be applied to calculate the corrected (for anemia) reticulocyte count. Corrected reticulocyte count = reticulocytes (%) × Hct ÷ 45, the average normal Hct. In this case, $7 \times (20 \div 45) = 3.1$.

13. A decreased osmotic fragility test would be associated with which of the following conditions?
   A. Sickle cell anemia
   B. Hereditary spherocytosis
   C. Hemolytic disease of the newborn
   D. Acquired hemolytic anemia

Hematology/Apply principles of basic laboratory procedures/RBCs/Osmotic fragility/2

14. What effect would using a buffer at pH 6.0 have on a Wright's-stained smear?
   A. Red cells would be stained too pink
   B. White cell cytoplasm would be stained too blue
   C. Red cells would be stained too blue
   D. Red cells would lyse on the slide

Hematology/Evaluate laboratory data to recognize problems/Microscopic morphology/Stain/2

15. Which of the following erythrocyte inclusions *can* be visualized with supravital stain but *cannot* be detected on a Wright's-stained blood smear?
   A. Basophilic stippling
   B. Heinz bodies
   C. Howell-Jolly bodies
   D. Siderotic granules

Hematology/Apply principles of basic laboratory procedures/Microscopic morphology/RBC inclusions/2

16. A falsely elevated Hct is obtained. Which of the following *calculated* values will *not* be affected?
   A. MCV
   B. MCH
   C. MCHC
   D. Red cell distribution width (RDW)

Hematology/Evaluate sources of error/Microhematocrit/2

17. A Miller disk is an ocular device used to facilitate counting of:
   A. Platelets
   B. Reticulocytes
   C. Sickle cells
   D. Nucleated red blood cells (NRBCs)

Hematology/Apply knowledge of standard operating procedures/Reticulocytes/1

18. SITUATION: RBC indices obtained on a patient are as follows: MCV 88 μm^3 (fL); MCH 30 pg; MCHC 34% (.340). The RBCs on the peripheral smear would appear:
   A. Microcytic, hypochromic
   B. Microcytic, normochromic
   C. Normocytic, normochromic
   D. Normocytic, hypochromic

Hematology/Evaluate laboratory data to recognize health and disease states/RBC Indices/2

13. **A** Osmotic fragility is decreased when numerous sickle cells and target cells are present and is increased in the presence of spherocytes. Spherocytes are a prominent feature of hereditary spherocytosis (HS), hemolytic disease of the newborn, and acquired hemolytic anemia. The osmotic fragility test is increased in the presence of spherocytes, whereas this test is decreased when sickle cells, target cells, and other poikilocytes are present.

14. **A** The pH of the buffer is critical in Romanowsky stains. When the pH is too low (<6.4), the red cells take up more acid dye (eosin), becoming too pink. Leukocytes also show poor nuclear detail when the pH is decreased.

15. **B** Heinz bodies are irregular, refractile, purple inclusions that are not visible with Wright's stain but show up with supravital staining. The other three inclusions can be detected with Wright's stain.

16. **B** The MCH = Hgb × 10/RBC count and is not affected by the Hct. The MCV = Hct × 10/RBC count, and MCHC = Hgb × 100/Hct; therefore, an erroneous Hct will affect these parameters. Centrifugal force for microhematocrit determination should be 12,000 g for 5 min in order to avoid error caused by trapped plasma. The red cell distribution width (RDW) is calculated by electronic cell counters and reflects the variance in the size of the red cell population. Electronic cell counters calculate Hct from the MCV and RBC count. Therefore, the RDW would be affected by an erroneous MCV.

17. **B** The traditional reticulocyte count involves the counting of 1000 RBCs. The Miller disk is a reticle (grid) that is placed in the eyepiece of the microscope and divides the field into two squares, one being nine times larger in size than the other. Reticulocytes are enumerated in both the squares as the red cells are counted in the smaller one.

18. **C** The MCV, MCH, and MCHC are all within the reference interval (normal range); hence, the erythrocytes should be of normal size and should reflect normal concentrations of Hgb; therefore, the anemia is normocytic normochromic.

19. All of the following factors may influence the erythrocyte sedimentation rate (ESR) *except:*
  A. Blood drawn into a sodium citrate tube
  B. Anisocytosis, poikilocytosis
  C. Plasma proteins
  D. Caliber of the tube

Hematology/Apply principles of basic laboratory procedures/ESR/2

20. What staining method is used most frequently to stain and count reticulocytes?
  A. Immunofluorescence
  B. Supravital staining
  C. Romanowsky staining
  D. Cytochemical staining

Hematology/Apply knowledge of standard operating procedures/Reticulocytes/1

21. The Coulter principle for counting of cells is based upon the fact that:
  A. Isotonic solutions conduct electricity better than cells do
  B. Conductivity varies proportionally to the number of cells
  C. Cells conduct electricity better than saline does
  D. Isotonic solutions cannot conduct electricity

Hematology/Apply principles of basic laboratory procedures/Instrumentation/Cell counter/2

22. A correction is necessary for WBC counts when nucleated RBCs are seen on the peripheral smear because:
  A. The WBC count would be falsely lower
  B. The RBC count is too low
  C. Nucleated RBCs are counted as leukocytes
  D. Nucleated RBCs are confused with giant platelets

Hematology/Evaluate laboratory data to take corrective action according to predetermined criteria/Leukocytes/2

23. Using a Coulter counter analyzer, an increased RDW should correlate with:
  A. Spherocytosis
  B. Anisocytosis
  C. Leukocytosis
  D. Presence of NRBCs

Hematology/Correlate laboratory data with other laboratory data to assess test results/RBC Microscopic morphology/2

24. Given the following values, which set of red blood cell indices suggests spherocytosis?
  A. MCV 76 μm^3 MCH 19.9 pg   MCHC 28.5%
  B. MCV 90 μm^3 MCH 30.5 pg   MCHC 32.5%
  C. MCV 80 μm^3 MCH 36.5 pg   MCHC 39.0%
  D. MCV 81 μm^3 MCH 29.0 pg   MCHC 34.8%

Hematology/Evaluate laboratory data to recognize health and disease states/RBC Indices/3

25. Which of the following statistical terms reflects the best index of precision?
  A. Mean
  B. Median
  C. Coefficient of variation
  D. Standard deviation

Hematology/Correlate laboratory data with other laboratory data to assess test results/QC/Statistics/3

Answers to Questions 19–25

19. **A** EDTA and sodium citrate can be used without any effect on the ESR. Anisocytosis and poikilocytosis may impede rouleaux formation, thus causing a low ESR. Plasma proteins, especially fibrinogen and immunoglobulins, enhance rouleaux, increasing the ESR. Reference ranges must be established for different caliber tubes.

20. **B** The reticulum within the reticulocytes consists of ribonucleic acid (RNA), which cannot be stained with Wright's stain. Supravital staining with new methylene blue is used to identify the reticulocytes.

21. **A** Coulter cell counters use the principle of electrical impedance. Two electrodes suspended in isotonic solutions are separated by a glass tube having a small aperture. A vacuum is applied, and as a cell passes through the aperture it impedes the flow of current and generates a voltage pulse.

22. **C** The automated hematology analyzers enumerate all nucleated cells. NRBCs are counted along with WBCs, falsely elevating the WBC count. To correct the WBC count, determine the number of NRBCs per 100 WBCs. Corrected WBC count = (uncorrected WBC count ÷ [NRBC's + 100]) × 100.

23. **B** The Coulter counter's RDW parameter correlates with the degree of anisocytosis seen on the morphological examination. The reference range is 11.5%–14.5%.

24. **C** Spherocytes have a decreased cell diameter and volume, which results in loss of central pallor and discoid shape. The index most affected is the MCHC, usually being in excess of 36%.

25. **C** Standard deviation(s) describes the distribution of a sample of observations. It depends upon both the mean (average value) and dispersion of results and is most influenced by reproducibility or precision. Because s is influenced by the mean and expressed as a percentage of the mean, the coefficient of variation ([s ÷ mean] × 100) can be used to compare precision of tests with different means (e.g., WBC and RBC counts or low vs high controls).

26. Which of the following is considered a normal hemoglobin?
    A. Carboxyhemoglobin
    B. Methemoglobin
    C. Sulfhemoglobin
    D. Deoxyhemoglobin

*Hematology/Apply knowledge of fundamental biological
characteristics/Hemoglobin/1*

27. Which condition will shift the oxyhemoglobin dissociation curve to the right?
    A. Acidosis
    B. Alkalosis
    C. Multiple blood transfusions
    D. Increased quantities of hemoglobin S or C

*Hematology/Correlate laboratory data with other labo-
ratory data to assess test results/RBC/Metabolism/2*

28. What is the major type of leukocyte seen in the
peripheral smear of a patient with aplastic anemia?
    A. Segmented neutrophil
    B. Lymphocyte
    C. Monocyte
    D. Eosinophil

*Hematology/Correlate clinical and laboratory data/
Leukocyte/Aplastic anemia/1*

29. What is the normal WBC differential lymphocyte percentage (range) in the adult population?
    A. 20%–50%
    B. 10%–20%
    C. 5%–10%
    D. 50%–70%

*Hematology/Correlate basic laboratory
values/Differentials/1*

30. In which age group would 60% lymphocytes be a normal finding?
    A. 40–60 years
    B. 11–15 years
    C. 6 months–2 years
    D. 4–6 years

Hematology/Evaluate laboratory data/Differentials/2

31. Which of the following results on an automated differential suggests that a peripheral smear should be
reviewed manually?
    A. Segs = 70%
    B. Band = 6%
    C. Mono = 15%
    D. Eos = 2%

Hematology/Correlate laboratorydata/Instrumentation/2

32. In which stage of erythrocytic maturation does Hgb
formation begin?
    A. Reticulocyte
    B. Pronormoblast

C. Basophilic normoblast
D. Polychromatic normoblast

*Hematology/Apply knowledge of fundamental biological
characteristic/Microscopic morphology/1*

26. **D** Deoxyhemoglobin is the physiological Hgb
that results from the unloading of oxygen by
Hgb. This is accompanied by the widening of the
space between β–chains and the binding of 2,3-
diphosphoglycerate (2,3-DPG) on a mole-for-
mole basis.

27. **A** Acidosis is associated with a shift to the right of
the oxyhemoglobin dissociation curve and, therefore, increased oxygen release (decreased affinity of
Hgb for oxygen). Alkalosis does the opposite.
Multiple blood transfusions shift the curve to the
left because the transfused blood is low in 2,3-DPG.
Hgb S and Hgb C do not change the affinity of oxygen for hemoglobin; however, many hemoglobinopathies do. For example, Hgb Kansas causes a
right shift and Hgb Chesapeake causes a left shift of
the oxyhemoglobin dissociation curve.

28. **B** Lymphocytes constitute the majority of the
nucleated cells seen. The bone marrow in aplastic
anemia is spotty with patches of normal cellularity.
Absolute granulocytopenia is usually present; however, lymphocyte production is less affected.

29. **A** The normal adult percentage of lymphocytes in a
white cell differential is between 20% and 50%. This
range is higher in the pediatric population.

30. **C** There is a relative neutropenia in children from
ages 4 months to 4 years of age. Because of this, the
percentage of lymphocytes is increased in this population. This is commonly referred to as a reversal
in the normal differential percentage (or inverted
differential).

31. **C** A relative monocyte count of 15% is abnormal,
given that the baseline monocyte count in a normal
differential is between 1% and 8%. An increased
monocyte count may signal a myeloproliferative
process such a chronic myelomonocytic leukemia,
an inflammatory response, or abnormal lymphocytes that may have been counted as monocytes by
an automated cell counter.

32. **D** In normal erythrocytic maturation, Hgb formation begins in the polychromatic normoblast and is
seen as a pink coloration of the cytoplasm. The red
cell continues to produce Hgb through the reticulocyte stage of development.

33. Which of the following can shift the hemoglobin-oxygen dissociation curve to the right?
- **A.** Increases in 2,3 DPG
- **B.** Acidosis
- **C.** Hypoxia
- **D.** All of the above

Hematology/Evaluate laboratory data to recognize health and disease states/O$_2$ Dissociation curve/3

34. Which of the following Hgb configurations is characteristic of Hgb H?
- **A.** γ_4
- **B.** α_2-γ_2
- **C.** β_4
- **D.** α_2-β_2

Hematology/Apply knowledge of fundamental biological characteristics/Hemoglobin/2

35. Autoagglutination of red cells at room temperature can result in which of the following?
- **A.** Low RBC count
- **B.** High MCV
- **C.** Low hematocrit
- **D.** All of the above

Hematology/Correlate laboratory data with other laboratory data to assess test results/CBC/3

Answers to Questions 33–35

33. **D** Increases in 2,3-DPG, acidosis, hypoxia, and a rise in body temperature all shift the hemoglobin-oxygen dissociation curve to the right. In anemia, although the number of RBCs is reduced, the cells are more efficient at oxygen delivery because there is an increase in red cell 2,3-DPG . This causes the oxyhemoglobin dissociation curve to shift to the right, allowing more oxygen to be released to the tissues

34. **C** The structure of Hgb H is β_4. Hgb H disease is a severe clinical expression of α–thalassemia in which only one α–gene out of four is functioning.

35. **D** Autoagglutination at room temperature may cause a low RBC count and high MCV from an electronic counter. The Hct will be low because it is calculated from the RBC count. Low RBC count and low Hct cause falsely high calculations of MCH and MCHC.

1. **Hypersplenism is characterized by:**
   A. Polycythemia
   B. Pancytosis
   C. Leukopenia
   D. Myelodysplasia

   Hematology/Correlate clinical and laboratory data/WBCs/Hypersplenism/2

2. **Which of the following organs is responsible for the "pitting process" for RBCs?**
   A. Liver
   B. Spleen
   C. Kidney
   D. Lymph nodes

   Hematology/Apply knowledge of fundamental biological characteristics/Physiology/2

3. **Spherocytes differ from normal red cells in all of the following *except:***
   A. Decreased surface to volume
   B. No central pallor
   C. Decreased resistance to hypotonic saline
   D. Increased deformability

   Hematology/Apply knowledge of fundamental biological characteristics/RBC microscopic morphology/2

4. **Which of the following is *not* associated with hereditary spherocytosis?**
   A. Increased osmotic fragility
   B. An MCHC greater than 36%
   C. Intravascular hemolysis
   D. Extravascular hemolysis

   Hematology/Correlate clinical and laboratory data/Hereditary spherocytosis/2

5. **Which of the following disorders has an increase in osmotic fragility?**
   A. Iron deficiency anemia
   B. Hereditary elliptocytosis
   C. Hereditary stomatocytosis
   D. Hereditary spherocytosis

   Hematology/Evaluate laboratory data to recognize health and disease states/Special test/Osmotic fragility/2

6. **The anemia seen in sickle cell disease is usually:**
   A. Microcytic, normochromic
   B. Microcytic, hypochromic
   C. Normocytic, normochromic
   D. Normocytic, hypochromic

   Hematology/Apply knowledge of fundamental biological characteristics/RBC microscopic morphology/ Hemoglobinopathy/1

Answers to Questions 1–6

1. **C** Hypersplenic conditions are generally described by the following four criteria:(1) cytopenias of one or more peripheral cell lines, (2) splenomegaly, (3) bone marrow hyperplasia, (4) resolution of cytopenia by splenectomy.

2. **B** The spleen is the supreme filter of the body, pitting imperfections from the erythrocyte without destroying the integrity of the membrane.

3. **D** Spherocytes lose their deformability owing to the defect in spectrin, a membrane protein, and are therefore prone to splenic sequestration and hemolysis.

4. **C** Classic features of intravascular hemolysis such as hemoglobinemia, hemoglobinuria, or hemosiderinuria do not occur in hereditary spherocytosis. The hemolysis seen in hereditary spherocytosis is an extravascular rather than an intravascular process.

5. **D** Spherocytic cells have decreased tolerance to swelling and, therefore, hemolyze at a higher concentration of sodium salt compared with normal red cells.

6. **C** Sickle cell disease is a chronic hemolytic anemia classified as a normocytic, normochromic anemia.

7. Which is the major Hgb found in the RBCs of patients with sickle cell trait?
   A. Hgb S
   B. Hgb F
   C. Hgb A_2
   D. Hgb A

Hematology/Apply knowledge of fundamental biological characteristics/Anemia/ Hemoglobinopathy/1

8. Select the amino acid substitution that is responsible for sickle cell anemia.
   A. Lysine is substituted for glutamic acid at the sixth position of the α-chain
   B. Valine is substituted for glutamic acid at the sixth position of the β-chain
   C. Valine is substituted for glutamic acid at the sixth position of the α-chain
   D. Glutamine is substituted for glutamic acid at the sixth position of the β-chain

Hematology/Apply knowledge of fundamental biological characteristics/Hemoglobinopathy/1

9. All of the following are usually found in Hgb C disease *except:*
   A. Hgb C crystals
   B. Target cells
   C. Lysine substituted for glutamic acid at the sixth position of the β–chain
   D. Fast mobility of Hgb C at pH 8.6

Hematology/Apply knowledge of fundamental biological characteristics/Anemia/Hemoglobinopathy/1

10. Which of the following hemoglobins migrates to the same position as Hgb A_2 at pH 8.6?
   A. Hgb H
   B. Hgb F
   C. Hgb C
   D. Hgb S

Hematology/Correlate clinical and laboratory data/ Hemoglobin electrophoresis/1

11. Which of the following electrophoretic results is consistent with a diagnosis of sickle cell trait?
   A. Hgb A: 40%   Hgb S: 35%   Hgb F: 5%
   B. Hgb A: 60%   Hgb S: 40%   Hgb A_2: 2%
   C. Hgb A: 0%   Hgb A_2: 5%   Hgb F: 95%
   D. *Hgb A: 80%   Hgb S: 10%   Hgb A_2: 10%*

Hematology/Evaluate laboratory data to recognize health and disease/Special test/Electrophoresis/2

12. In which of the following conditions will autosplenectomy most likely occur?
   A. Thalassemia major
   B. Hgb C disease
   C. Hgb SC disease
   D. Sickle cell disease

Hematology/Apply knowledge of fundamental biological characteristics/Anemia/Hemoglobinopathy/1

13. Which of the following is most true of paroxysmal nocturnal hemoglobinuria (PNH)?
   A. It is an acquired hemolytic anemia
   B. It is inherited as a sex-linked trait
   C. It is inherited as an autosomal dominant trait
   D. It is inherited as an autosomal recessive trait

Hematology/Apply knowledge of fundamental biological characteristics/PNH/1

14. Hemolytic uremic syndrome (HUS) is characterized by all of the following except:
   A. Hemorrhage
   B. Thrombocytopenia
   C. Hemoglobinuria
   D. Reticulocytopenia

Hematology/Correlate clinical and laboratory data/ HUS/2

Answers to Questions 7–14

7. **D** The major hemoglobin in sickle cell trait is Hgb A, which constitutes 50%–70% of the total. Hgb S comprises 20%–40%, and Hgb A_2 and Hgb F are present in normal amounts.

8. **B** The structural mutation for Hgb S is the substitution of valine for glutamic acid at the sixth position of the β-chain. Because glutamic acid is negatively charged, this decreases its rate of migration toward the anode at pH 8.6.

9. **D** Substitution of a positively charged amino acid for a negatively charged amino acid in Hgb C disease results in a slow electrophoretic mobility at pH 8.6.

10. **C** At pH 8.6, several hemoglobins migrate together. These include Hgb A_2, Hgb C, Hgb E, Hgb 0_{arab}, and Hgb C_{Harlem}. These are located nearest the cathode at pH 8.6.

11. **B** Electrophoresis at alkaline pH usually shows 50%–70% Hgb A, 20%–40% Hgb S, and normal levels of Hgb A_2 in a patient with the sickle cell trait.

12. **D** Autosplenectomy occurs in sickle cell anemia as a result of repeated infarcts to the spleen caused by the overwhelming sickling phenomenon.

13. **A** PNH is an acquired hemolytic anemia with an insidious onset, resulting in a chronic hemolytic state. It most often occurs in middle-aged adults.

14. **D** The hemolytic anemia of HUS is associated with reticulocytosis. The anemia seen in HUS is multifactorial, with characteristic schistocytes and polychromasia commensurate with the anemia.

15. An autohemolysis test is positive in all the following areas *except:*
- **A.** Glucose-6-phosphate dehydrogenase (G6PD) deficiency
- **B.** Hereditary spherocytosis (HS)
- **C.** Pyruvate kinase (PK) deficiency
- **D.** Paroxysmal nocturnal hemoglobinuria (PNH)

Hematology/Correlate clinical and laboratory tests/ Special test/2

16. Which antibody is associated with paroxysmal cold hemoglobinuria (PCH)?
- **A.** Anti-I
- **B.** Anti-i
- **C.** Anti-M
- **D.** Anti-P

Hematology/Apply knowledge of fundamental biological characteristics/Anemia/PCH/1

17. All of the following are associated with hemolytic anemia *except:*
- **A.** Methemoglobinemia
- **B.** Hemoglobinuria
- **C.** Hemoglobinemia
- **D.** Increased haptoglobin

Hematology/Correlate clinical and laboratory data/ Anemia/Hemolytic/2

18. Autoimmune hemolytic anemia is best characterized by which of the following?
- **A.** Increased levels of plasma C3
- **B.** Spherocytic red cells
- **C.** Decreased osmotic fragility
- **D.** Decreased unconjugated bilirubin

Hematology/Correlate clinical and laboratory data/ Anemia/Hemolytic/2

19. "Bite cells" are usually seen in patients with:
- **A.** Rh null trait
- **B.** Chronic granulomatous disease
- **C.** G6PD deficiency
- **D.** PK deficiency

Hematology/Correlate clinical and laboratory data/RBC microscopic morphology/1

20. The morphological classification of anemias is based on which of the following?
- **A.** M:E (myeloid:erythroid) ratio
- **B.** Prussian blue stain
- **C.** RBC indices
- **D.** Reticulocyte count

Hematology/Correlate clinical and laboratory disease/ RBC microscopic morphology/1

Answers to Questions 15–20

15. D The autohemolysis test is positive in G6PD and PK deficiencies and in HS but is normal in PNH because lysis in PNH requires sucrose to enhance complement binding. The addition of glucose, sucrose, or adenosine triphosphate (ATP) corrects the autohemolysis of HS. Autohemolysis of PK can be corrected by ATP.

16. D PCH is caused by the anti-P antibody, a cold autoantibody that binds to the patient's RBCs at low temperatures and fixes complement. In the classic Donath-Landsteiner test, hemolysis is demonstrated in a sample placed at 4°C that is then warmed to 37°C.

17. D Haptoglobin is a protein that binds to free Hgb. The increased free Hgb in intravascular hemolysis causes depletion of haptoglobin.

18. B Spherocytes are characteristic of autoimmune hemolytic anemia and result in an increased osmotic fragility. In autoimmune hemolytic anemias (AIHAs), production of autoantibodies against one's own red cells causes hemolysis or phagocytic destruction of RBCs. A positive direct antiglobulin (DAT or Coombs') test identifies in vivo antibody-coated and complement-coated red cells. A positive DAT distinguishes AIHA from other types of hemolytic anemia that produce spherocytes. Those AIHAs that produce complement-binding antibodies cause a depletion of C3. Those not associated with intravascular hemolysis cause an increase in unconjugated bilirubin.

19. C In patients with G6PD deficiency the red cells are unable to reduce nicotinamide adenine dinucleotide phosphate (NADP) to NADPH; consequently, Hgb is denatured and Heinz bodies are formed. "Bite cells" appear in the peripheral circulation as a result of splenic pitting of Heinz bodies.

20. C RBC indices classify the anemia morphologically. Anemias can be classified morphologically by the use of laboratory data, physiologically based upon the mechanism, and clinically based upon an assessment of symptoms.

21. Which of the following is a common finding in aplastic anemia?

A. A monoclonal disorder
B. Tumor infiltration
C. Peripheral blood pancytopenia
D. Defective DNA synthesis

Hematology/Apply knowledge of fundamental biological characteristics/Aplastic anemia/1

22. Congenital dyserythropoietic anemias (CDAs) are characterized by:

A. Bizarre multinucleated erythroblasts
B. Cytogenetic disorders
C. Megaloblastic erythropoiesis
D. An elevated M:E ratio

Hematology/Apply knowledge of fundamental biological characteristics/Anemia/Characteristics/2

23. Microangiopathic hemolytic anemia is characterized by:

A. Target cells and Cabot rings
B. Toxic granulation and Döhle bodies
C. Pappenheimer bodies and basophilic stippling
D. Schistocytes and nucleated RBCs

Hematology/Correlate clinical and laboratory data/RBC microscopic morphology/Anemia/2

24. Which antibiotic(s) is(are) most often implicated in the development of aplastic anemia?

A. Sulfonamides
B. Penicillin
C. Tetracycline
D. Chloramphenicol

Hematology/Correlate clinical and laboratory data/ Aplastic anemia/1

25. Sickle cell disorders are:

A. Hereditary, intracorpuscular RBC defects
B. Hereditary, extracorpuscular RBC defects
C. Acquired, intracorpuscular RBC defects
D. Acquired, extracorpuscular RBC defects

Hematology/Apply knowledge of fundamental biological concepts/2

26. Which of the following conditions may produce spherocytes in a peripheral smear?

A. Pelger-Huët anomaly
B. Pernicious anemia
C. Autoimmune hemolytic anemia
D. Sideroblastic anemia

Hematology/Evaluate laboratory data to recognize health and disease states/Morphology/3

Answers to Questions 21–26

21. **C** Aplastic anemia has many causes, such as chemical, drug, or radiation poisoning; congenital aplasia; and Fanconi's syndrome. All result in depletion of hematopoietic precursors of all cell lines, leading to peripheral blood pancytopenia.

22. **A** There are four classifications of CDAs, each characterized by ineffective erythropoiesis, increased unconjugated bilirubin, and bizarre multinucleated erythroid precursors.

23. **D** Microangiopathic hemolytic anemia is a condition resulting from shear stress to the erythrocytes. Fibrin strands are laid down within the microcirculation, and red cells become fragmented as they contact fibrin through the circulation process.

24. **D** Chloramphenicol is the drug most often implicated in acquired aplastic anemia. About half of the cases occur within 30 days after therapy and about half of the cases are reversible. Penicillin, tetracycline, and sulfonamides have been implicated in a small number of cases.

25. **A** Sickle cell disorders are intracorpuscular red cell defects that are hereditary and result in defective Hgbs being produced. The gene for sickle cell can be inherited either homozygously or heterozygously.

26. **C** Spherocytes are produced in autoimmune hemolytic anemia. Spherocytes may be produced by one of three mechanisms. First, they are a natural morphological phase of normal red cell senescence. Second, they are produced when the cell surface-to-volume ratio is decreased, as seen in hereditary spherocytosis. And third, they may be produced as a result of antibody coating of the red cells. As the antibody-coated red cells travel through the spleen, the antibodies and portions of the red cell membrane are removed by macrophages. The membrane repairs itself; hence the red cell's morphology changes from a biconcave disk to a spherocyte.

27. A patient's peripheral smear reveals numerous NRBCs, marked variation of red cell morphology, and pronounced polychromasia. In addition to a decreased Hgb and decreased Hct values, what other CBC parameters may be anticipated?
- **A.** Reduced platelets
- **B.** Increased MCHC
- **C.** Increased MCV
- **D.** Decreased red-cell distribution width (RDW)

Hematology/Correlate lab data with clinical picture/Complete blood count/2

28. What red cell inclusion may be seen in the peripheral blood smear of a patient postsplenectomy?
- **A.** Toxic granulation
- **B.** Howell-Jolly bodies
- **C.** Malarial parasites
- **D.** Siderotic granules

Hematology/Correlate clinical laboratory data/ Inclusions/1

29. Reticulocytosis usually indicates:
- **A.** Response to inflammation
- **B.** Neoplastic process
- **C.** Aplastic anemia
- **D.** Red cell regeneration

Hematology/Correlate laboratory data for clinical condition/Morphology/3

30. Hereditary pyropoikilocytosis (HP) is a red cell membrane defect characterized by:
- **A.** Increased pencil-shaped cells
- **B.** Increased oval macrocytes

- **C.** Misshapen budding fragmented cells
- **D.** Bite cells

Hematology/Evaluate laboratory data to recognize health and disease states/Red cell membrane/2

Answers to Questions 27–30

27. **C** This patient's abnormal peripheral smear indicates marked red cell regeneration, causing many reticulocytes to be released from the marrow. Since reticulocytes are larger than mature RBCs, the MCV will be slightly elevated.

28. **B** As a result of splenectomy, Howell-Jolly bodies may be seen in great numbers. One of the main functions of the spleen is the pitting function, which allows inclusions to be removed from the red cell without destroying the cell membrane.

29. **D** Reticulocytes are polychromatophilic macrocytes, and the presence of reticulocytes indicates red cell regeneration. The bone marrow's appropriate response to anemia is to deliver red cells prematurely to the peripheral circulation. In this way, reticulocytes and possibly nucleated red cells may be seen in the peripheral smear.

30. **C** HP is a membrane defect characterized by a spectrin abnormality and thermal instability. The MCV is decreased and the red cells appear to be budding and fragmented.

1. The osmotic fragility test result in a patient with thalassemia major would most likely be:
   A. Increased
   B. Decreased
   C. Normal
   D. Decreased after incubation at 37°C

   Hematology/Correlate clinical and laboratory data/Microscopic morphology/Osmotic fragility/1

2. All of the following are characteristic findings in a patient with iron deficiency anemia *except:*
   A. Microcytic, hypochromic red cell morphology
   B. Elevated platelet count along with small platelets
   C. Decreased total iron-binding capacity (TIBC)
   D. Increased RBC protoporphyrin

   Hematology/Correlate clinical and laboratory data/ Anemia/Iron deficiency/2

3. Iron deficiency anemia may be distinguished from anemia of chronic infection by:
   A. Serum iron level
   B. Red cell morphology
   C. Red cell indices
   D. Total iron-binding capacity

   Hematology/Evaluate laboratory data to recognize health and disease states/Anemia/3

4. Which anemia has red cell morphology similar to that seen in iron deficiency anemia?
   A. Sickle cell anemia
   B. Thalassemia syndrome
   C. Pernicious anemia
   D. Hereditary spherocytosis

   Hematology/Correlate laboratory data with other laboratory data to assess test results/Anemia/RBC microscopic morphology/2

5. Iron deficiency anemia is characterized by:
   A. Decreased plasma iron, decreased % saturation, increased total iron-binding capacity (TIBC)
   B. Decreased plasma iron, decreased plasma ferritin, normal RBC porphyrin
   C. Decreased plasma iron, decreased % saturation, decreased TIBC
   D. Decreased plasma iron, increased % saturation, decreased TIBC

   Hematology/Evaluate laboratory data to recognize health and disease states/Anemia/Iron deficiency/2

Answers to Questions 1–5

1. **B** Numerous target cells are present in thalassemia major patients. Because target cells have increased surface volume, the osmotic fragility is decreased.

2. **C** There is an increase in TIBC and in RBC protoporphyrin because of a decreased level of iron in iron deficiency anemia. Morphological characteristics of iron deficiency anemia include a microcytic, hypochromic blood picture. Platelets are usually small and increased in number.

3. **D** In iron deficiency anemia, the serum iron level is decreased and the total iron-binding capacity is increased. In chronic disease the iron is trapped in reticuloendothelial (RE) cells and therefore is unavailable to the red cells. Serum iron and TIBC are both decreased.

4. **B** Iron deficiency anemia and thalassemia are both classified as microcytic, hypochromic anemias. Iron deficiency anemia is caused by defective heme synthesis, whereas thalassemia is caused by decreased globin chain synthesis.

5. **A** Iron deficiency anemia is characterized by decreased plasma iron, increased TIBC, decreased % saturation, and microcytic, hypochromic anemia. Iron deficiency occurs in three phases: iron depletion, iron-deficient erythropoiesis, and iron deficiency anemia.

6. Storage iron is usually best determined by:
  A. Serum transferrin levels
  B. Hgb values
  C. Myoglobin values
  D. Serum ferritin levels

Hematology/Apply knowledge of basic laboratory procedures/Iron/1

7. All of the following are associated with sideroblastic anemia *except:*
  A. Increased serum iron
  B. Ringed sideroblasts
  C. Dimorphic blood picture
  D. Increased RBC protoporphyrin

Hematology/Evaluate laboratory data to recognize health and disease states/Anemia/Sideroblastic/3

8. What is the basic hematological defect seen in patients with thalassemia major?
  A. DNA synthetic defect
  B. Hgb structure
  C. β-Chain synthesis
  D. Hgb phosphorylation

Hematology/Apply knowledge of fundamental biological characteristics/Hemoglobinopathy/1

9. Which of the following is the primary Hgb in patients with thalassemia major?
  A. Hgb D
  B. Hgb A
  C. Hgb C
  D. Hgb F

Hematology/Correlate clinical and laboratory disease/Hemoglobin/Hemoglobinopathy/1

10. A patient has a Hct of 30%, a hemoglobin of 8g/dL, and a RBC count of 4.0×10^{12}/L. What is the morphological classification of this anemia?
  A. Normocytic normochromic
  B. Macrocytic hypochromic
  C. Microcytic hypochromic
  D. Normocytic hyperchromic

Hematology/Evaluate laboratory data to recognize health and disease states/Hemoglobinopathy/Characteristics/3

11. In which of the following conditions is Hgb A_2 elevated?
  A. Hgb H
  B. Hgb SC disease
  C. β-Thalassemia minor
  D. Hgb S trait

Hematology/Correlate laboratory results with disease states/2

12. Which of the following parameters may be similar for the anemia of inflammation and iron deficiency anemia?
  A. Normocytic indices
  B. Decreased serum iron concentration
  C. Ringed sideroblasts
  D. Pappenheimer bodies

Hematology/Correlate laboratory data to recognize health and disease states/2

Answers to Questions 6–12

6. **D** Ferritin enters the serum from all ferritin-producing tissues and therefore is considered to be a good indicator of body storage iron. Because iron stores must be depleted before anemia develops, low serum ferritin levels precede the fall in serum iron associated with iron deficiency anemia.

7. **D** Sideroblastic anemia has a decreased red cell protoporphyrin. The defect in sideroblastic anemia involves ineffective erythropoiesis. The failure to produce RBC protoporphyrin occurs because the nonheme iron is trapped in the mitochondria and is unavailable to be recycled.

8. **C** In thalassemia major there is little or no production of the β-chain, resulting in severely depressed or no synthesis of Hgb A. Severe anemia is seen, along with skeletal abnormalities and marked splenomegaly. The patient is usually supported with transfusion therapy.

9. **D** Patients with thalassemia major are unable to synthesize the β-chain; hence little or no Hgb A is produced. However, γ-chains continue to be synthesized and lead to variable elevations of Hgb F in these patients.

10. **C** The indices will provide a morphological classification of this anemia. The MCV is 75 fL (reference range 80–96 fL), the MCH is 20.0 pg (reference range 27–33 pg), and the MCHC is 26.6% (reference range 33%–36%). Therefore, the anemia is microcytic hypochromic.

11. **C** Hgb A_2 is part of the normal complement of adult Hgb. This Hgb is elevated in β-thalassemia minor because the individual with this condition has only one normal β-gene; consequently, there is a slight elevation of Hgb A_2 and Hgb F.

12. **B** Thirty to fifty percent of the individuals with the anemia of chronic inflammation demonstrate a microcytic hypochromic blood picture with decreased serum iron. Serum iron is decreased because it is unable to escape from the RE cells to be delivered to the pronormoblast in the bone marrow.

MACROCYTIC/ NORMOCHROMIC ANEMIAS

1. Which morphological classification is characteristic of megaloblastic anemia?
   A. Normocytic, normochromic
   B. Microcytic, normochromic
   C. Macrocytic, hypochromic
   D. Macrocytic, normochromic

   Hematology/Correlate clinical and laboratory data/ Microscopic morphology/RBC/2

2. A Schilling test gives the following results: Part I: 2% excretion of radioactive vitamin B_{12} (normal = 5%–35%); Part II: 8% excretion of radioactive vitamin B_{12} after intrinsic factor was given with vitamin B_{12} (normal = 7%–10%). These results indicate:
   A. Tropical sprue
   B. Transcobalamin deficiency
   C. Blind loop syndrome
   D. Pernicious anemia

   Hematology/Evaluate laboratory data to recognize health and disease states/Special test/3

3. All of the following are characteristics of megaloblastic anemia *except*:
   A. Pancytopenia
   B. Elevated reticulocyte count
   C. Hypersegmented neutrophils
   D. Macrocytic erythrocyte indices

   Hematology/Correlate clinical and laboratory data/Anemia/Megaloblastic/2

4. A patient with a vitamin B_{12} anemia is given a high dosage of folate. Which of the following is expected as a result of this treatment?
   A. An improvement in neurological problems
   B. An improvement in hematological abnormalities
   C. No expected improvement
   D. Toxicity of the liver and kidneys

   Hematology/Select course of action/Anemia/Therapy/2

5. Which of the disorders below causes ineffective erythropoiesis?
   A. G6PD deficiency
   B. Liver disease
   C. Hgb C disease
   D. Pernicious anemia

   Hematology/Evaluate laboratory data to recognize health and disease states/RBC physiology/2

Answers to Questions 1–5

1. **D** Megaloblastic macrocytic anemia is normochromic because there is no defect in the Hgb synthesis. These anemias are a group of asynchronized anemias characterized by defective nuclear maturation due to defective deoxyribonucleic acid (DNA) synthesis. This abnormality accounts for the megaloblastic features in the bone marrow and the macrocytosis in the peripheral blood.

2. **D** Pernicious anemia is caused by a lack of intrinsic factor, which prevents vitamin B_{12} absorption. An abnormal excretion in Part I indicates that vitamin B_{12} was not absorbed through the intestine. Normal excretion of labeled B_{12} after administration of intrinsic factor in Part II of the Schilling test indicates pernicious anemia.

3. **B** Megaloblastic anemias are associated with an ineffective erythropoiesis and therefore a decrease in the reticulocyte count.

4. **B** Administration of folic acid to a patient with vitamin B_{12} deficiency will improve the hematological abnormalities; however, the neurological problems will continue. This helps to confirm the correct diagnosis of vitamin B_{12} deficiency.

5. **D** Ineffective erythropoiesis is caused by destruction of erythroid precursor cells prior to their release from the bone marrow. Pernicious anemia results from defective DNA synthesis; it is suggested that the asynchronous development of red cells renders them more liable to intramedullary destruction.

6. A 50-year-old patient is suffering from pernicious anemia. Which of the following laboratory data are most likely for this patient?
   A. RBC = 2.5×10^{12}/L; WBC = 12,500/μL (12.5×10^9/L); PLT = 250,000/μL (250×10^9/L)
   B. RBC = 4.5×10^{12}/L; WBC = 6500/μL (6.5×10^9/L); PLT = 150,000/μL (150×10^9/L)
   C. RBC = 3.0×10^{12}/L; WBC = 5000/μL (5.0×10^9/L); PLT = 750,000/μL (750×10^9/L)
   D. RBC = 2.5×10^{12}/L; WBC = 2500/μL (2.5×10^9/L); PLT = 50,000/μL (50×10^9/L)

   Hematology/Correlate clinical and laboratory data/Microscopic morphology/RBC/2

7. Which of the following may be seen in the peripheral blood smear of a patient with obstructive liver disease?
   A. Schistocytes
   B. Macrocytes
   C. Howell-Jolly bodies
   D. Microcytes

   Hematology/Apply principles of basic laboratory procedures/Microscopic morphology/2

8. The macrocytes typically seen in megaloblastic processes are:
   A. Crescent-shaped
   B. Teardrop-shaped
   C. Ovalocytic
   D. Pencil-shaped

   Hematology/Apply principles of basic laboratory procedures/Microscopic morphology/Differential/1

9. Which of the following are most characteristic of the red cell indices associated with megaloblastic anemias?
   A. MCV 99 fl, MCH 28 pg, MCHC 31%
   B. MCV 62 fL, MCH 27 pg, MCHC 30%
   C. MCV 125 fL, MCH 36 pg, MCHC 34%
   D. MCV 78 fL, MCH 23 pg, MCHC 30%

   Hematology/Correlate clinical and laboratory data/Megaloblastic anemia/2

10. A patient has 80 nucleated red blood cells per 100 leukocytes. In additon to increased polychromasia on the peripheral smear, what other finding may be present on the CBC?
    A. Increased platelets
    B. Increased MCV
    C. Increased Hct
    D. Increased red blood cell count

    Hematolology/Correlate clinical and laboratory data/Megaloblastic anemia/2

Answers to Questions 6–10

6. **D** Patients with pernicious anemia demonstrate a pancytopenia with low WBC, PLT, and RBC counts. Because this is a megaloblastic process and a DNA maturation defect, all cell lines are affected. In the bone marrow, this results in abnormally large precursor cells, maturation asynchrony, hyperplasia of all cell lines, and a low M:E ratio.

7. **B** Patients with obstructive liver disease may have red blood cells that have an increased tendency toward the deposition of lipid on the surface of the red cell. Consequently, the red cells are larger or more macrocytic than normal red cells.

8. **C** Macrocytes in true megaloblastic conditions are oval macrocytes as opposed to the round macrocytes that are usually seen in alcoholism and obstructive liver disease.

9. **C** The red cell indices in a patient with megaloblastic anemia are macrocytic and normochromic. The macrocytosis is prominent, with an MCV ranging from 100 to 130 fL.

10. **B** The patient will have an increased MCV. One of the causes of a macrocytic anemia that is not megaloblastic is an increased reticulocyte count, here noted as increased polychromasia. Reticulocytes are polychromatic macrocytes; therefore, the MCV is slightly increased.

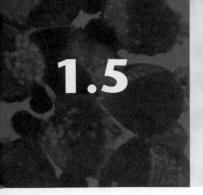

1.5 QUALITATIVE/QUANTITATIVE WHITE BLOOD CELL DISORDERS

1. Which of the following is an unusual complication that may occur in infectious mononucleosis?
   A. Splenic infarctions
   B. Dactylitis
   C. Hemolytic anemia
   D. Giant platelets

   Hematology/Evaluate laboratory data to recognize health and disease states/Infectious mononucleosis/3

2. In a patient with human immunodeficiency virus (HIV) infection, one should expect to see:
   A. Shift to the left in WBCs
   B. Target cells
   C. Reactive lymphocytes
   D. Pelgeroid cells

   Hematology/Evaluate laboratory data to recognize health and disease states/AIDS/Microscopic morphology/1

3. Which inclusions may be seen in leukocytes?
   A. Döhle bodies
   B. Basophilic stippling
   C. Malarial parasites
   D. Howell-Jolly bodies

   Hematology/Apply knowledge of fundamental characteristics/WBC inclusions/1

4. Which of the following is contained in the primary granules of the neutrophil?
   A. Lactoferrin
   B. Myeloperoxidase
   C. Histamine
   D. Alkaline phosphatase

   Hematology/Apply knowledge of fundamental biological characteristics/WBC kinetics/2

5. What is the typical range of relative lymphocyte percentage in the peripheral blood smear of a 1-year-old?
   A. 1%–6%
   B. 27%–33%
   C. 35%–58%
   D. 50%–70%

   Hematology/Evaluate laboratory data to recognize health and disease states/Differential normal values/3

1. **C** Occasionally patients with infectious mononucleosis develop a potent cold agglutinin with anti-I specificity. This cold autoantibody can cause strong hemolysis and a hemolytic anemia.

2. **C** HIV infection brings about several hematological abnormalities seen on peripheral smear examination; most patients demonstrate reactive lymphocytes and have granulocytopenia.

3. **A** Döhle bodies are RNA-rich areas within polymorphonuclear neutrophils (PMNs) that are oval and light blue in color. Although often associated with infectious states, they are seen in a wide range of conditions and toxic reactions, including hemolytic and pernicious anemias, chronic granulocytic leukemia, and therapy with antineoplastic drugs. The other inclusions are associated with erythrocytes.

4. **B** Myeloperoxidase, lysozyme, and acid phosphatase are enzymes that are contained in the primary granules of neutrophils. The contents of secondary and tertiary granules include lactoferrin, collagenase, NADPH oxidase, and alkaline phosphatase.

5. **D** The mean relative lymphocyte percentage for a 1-year-old is 61% compared to the mean lymphocyte percentage of 35% for an adult.

6. Qualitative and quantitative neutrophil changes noted in response to infection include all of the following *except:*
   A. Neutrophilia
   B. Pelgeroid hyposegmentation
   C. Toxic granulation
   D. Vacuolization

Hematology/Apply knowledge of fundamental biological characteristics/WBC microscopic morphology/2

7. Neutropenia is present in patients with which absolute neutrophil counts?
   A. $<1.5 \times 10^9$/L
   B. $<5.0 \times 10^9$/L
   C. $<10.0 \times 10^9$/L
   D. $< 15.0 \times 10^9$/L

Hematology/Evaluate laboratory data to recognize health and disease states/Differential normal values/3

8. The morphological characteristic(s) associated with the Chédiak-Higashi syndrome is/are:
   A. Pale blue cytoplasmic inclusions
   B. Giant lysosomal granules
   C. Small, dark-staining granules and condensed nuclei
   D. Nuclear hyposegmentation

Hematology/Recognize morphological changes associated with disease/WBC inclusion/2

9. The familial condition of Pelger-Huët anomaly is important to recognize because this disorder must be differentiated from:
   A. Infectious mononucleosis
   B. May-Hegglin anomaly
   C. A shift-to-the-left increase in immature granulocytes
   D. G6PD deficiency

Hematology/Recognize morphological changes associated with disease/WBC inclusion/2

10. What is the expected laboratory finding in a patient with a cytomegalovirus (CMV) infection?
   A. Heterophile antibody: positive
   B. Epstein-Barr virus (EBV)–immunoglobulin (IgM): positive
   C. Direct antiglobulin test (DAT): positive
   D. CMV–IgM: positive

Hematology/Evaluate laboratory data to recognize health and disease states/Differential normal values/2

11. Neutrophil phagocytosis and particle ingestion are associated with an increase in oxygen utilization referred to as respiratory burst. What are the two most important products of this biochemical reaction?
   A. Hydrogen peroxide and superoxide anion
   B. Lactoferrin and NADPH oxidase

   C. Cytochrome b and collagenase
   D. Alkaline phosphatase and ascorbic acid

Hematology/Apply knowledge of fundamental biological characteristics/WBC kinetics/3

Answers to Questions 6–11

6. **B** Neutrophil changes associated with infection may include neutrophilia, shift to the left, toxic granulation, Döhle bodies, and vacuolization. Pelgeroid hyposegmentation is noted in neutrophils from individuals with the congenital Pelger-Huët anomaly and as an acquired anomaly induced by drug ingestion or secondary to conditions such as leukemia.

7. **A** Neutropenia is defined as an absolute decrease in the number of circulating neutrophils. This condition is present in patients having neutrophil counts of less than 1.5×10^9/L.

8. **B** Chédiak-Higashi syndrome is a disorder of neutrophil phagocytic dysfunction caused by depressed chemotaxis and delayed degranulation. The degranulation disturbance is attributed to interference from the giant lysosomal granules.

9. **C** Pelger-Huët anomaly is a benign familial condition reported in 1 out of 6000 individuals. Care must be taken to differentiate Pelger-Huët cells from the numerous band neutrophils and metamyelocytes that may be observed during severe infection or a *shift-to-the-left* immaturity in granulocyte stages.

10. **D** If both the heterophile antibody test and the EBV-IgM tests are negative in a patient with reactive lymphocytosis and a suspected viral infection, the serum should be analyzed for IgM antibodies to CMV. CMV belongs to the herpes virus family and is endemic worldwide. CMV infection is the most common cause of heterophile-negative infectious mononucleosis.

11. **A** The biochemical products of the respiratory burst that are involved with neutrophil particle ingestion during phagocytosis are hydrogen peroxide and superoxide anion. The activated neutrophil discharges the enzyme NADPH oxidase into the phagolysosome, where it converts O_2 to superoxide anion (O_2^-), which is then reduced to hydrogen peroxide (H_2O_2).

12. Which of the morphological findings are characteristic of reactive lymphocytes?
   A. High nuclear:cytoplasmic ratio
   B. Prominent nucleoli
   C. Basophilic cytoplasm
   D. All of the above

Hematology/Recognize morphological changes associated with disease/WBC morphology/2

Answer to Question 12

12. **D** Both reactive lymphocytes and blasts may have basophilic cytoplasm, a high N:C ratio, and the presence of prominent nucleoli. Blasts, however, have an extremely fine nuclear chromatin staining pattern as viewed on a Wright-Giemsa–stained smear.

1. **Auer rods may be seen in all of the following** *except*:
   A. Acute myelomonocytic leukemia (M4)
   B. Acute lymphoblastic leukemia
   C. Acute myeloid leukemia without maturation (M1)
   D. Acute promyelocytic leukemia (M3)

   Hematology/Apply knowledge of fundamental biological characteristics/Acute leukemia/1

2. **Which type of anemia is usually present in a patient with acute leukemia?**
   A. Microcytic, hyperchromic
   B. Microcytic, hypochromic
   C. Normocytic, normochromic
   D. Macrocytic, normochromic

   Hematology/Correlate clinical and laboratory data/RBC microscopic morphology/Anemia/2

3. **In leukemia, which term describes a peripheral blood finding of leukocytosis with a shift to the left, accompanied by occasional nucleated red cells?**
   A. Myelophthisis
   B. Dysplasia
   C. Leukoerythroblastosis
   D. Megaloblastosis

   Hematology/Apply knowledge of fundamental biological characteristics/WBC differential/3

4. **The basic pathophysiological mechanisms responsible for producing signs and symptoms in leukemia include all of the following** *except*:
   A. Replacement of normal marrow precursors by leukemic cells causing anemia
   B. Decrease in functional leukocytes causing infection
   C. Hemorrhage secondary to thrombocytopenia
   D. Decreased erythropoietin production

   Hematology/Correlate clinical and laboratory data/Leukemia/2

5. **Which type of acute myeloid leukemia is called the true monocytic leukemia and follows an acute or subacute course characterized by monoblasts, promonocytes, and monocytes?**
   A. Acute myeloid leukemia, minimally differentiated
   B. Acute myeloid leukemia without maturation
   C. Acute myelomonocytic leukemia
   D. Acute monocytic leukemia

   Hematology/Evaluate laboratory data to make identifications/Leukemia/2

Answers to Questions 1–5

1. **B** Auer rods are not seen characteristically in lymphoblasts. They may be seen in myeloblasts, promyelocytes, and monoblasts.

2. **C** Acute leukemia is usually associated with a normocytic normochromic anemia. Anemia in acute leukemia is usually present from the onset and may be severe; however, there is no inherent nutritional deficiency leading to either a microcytic, hypochromic, or megaloblastic process.

3. **C** The presence of immature leukocytes and nucleated red cells is denoted leukoerythroblastosis. Myelophthisis refers to replacement of bone marrow by a disease process such as a neoplasm. The development of abnormal tissue is called dysplasia.

4. **D** A normal physiological response to anemia would be an increase in the kidney's production of erythropoietin. The accumulation of leukemic cells in the bone marrow leads to marrow failure, which is manifested by anemia, thrombocytopenia, and granulocytopenia.

5. **D** Acute monocytic leukemia has an incidence of between 1% and 8% of all acute leukemias. It has a distinctive clinical manifestation of monocytic involvement resulting in skin and gum hyperplasia. The WBC count is markedly elevated, and prognosis is poor.

6. In which age group does acute lymphoblastic leukemia occur with the highest frequency?
  A. 1–15 years
  B. 20–35 years
  C. 45–60 years
  D. 60–75 years

Hematology/Correlate clinical and laboratory data/Leukemia/1

7. Disseminated intravascular coagulation (DIC) is most often associated with which of the following types of acute leukemia?
  A. Acute myeloid leukemia without maturation
  B. Acute promyelocytic leukemia
  C. Acute myelomonocytic leukemia
  D. Acute monocytic leukemia

Hematology/Evaluate laboratory data to recognize health and disease states/Leukemia/DIC/2

8. An M:E ratio of 10:1 is most often seen in:
  A. Thalassemia
  B. Leukemia
  C. Polycythemia vera
  D. Myelofibrosis

Hematology/Evaluate laboratory data to recognize health and disease states/Leukemia/M:E/2

9. Which of the following is a characteristic of Auer rods?
  A. They are composed of azurophilic granules
  B. They stain periodic acid–Schiff (PAS)-positive
  C. They are predominantly seen in chronic myelogeneous leukemia (CML)
  D. The are nonspecific esterase-positive

Hematology/Apply knowledge of fundamental biological characteristics/Leukocytes/Auer rods/1

10. SITUATION: The following laboratory values are seen:

WBCs	6.0×10^9/L	Hgb 6.0 g/dL
RBCs	1.90×10^{12}/L	Hct 18.5%
Platelets	130×10^9/L	Serum vitamin B_{12} and folic acid: normal

WBC Differential	Bone Marrow
6% PMNs	40% myeloblasts
40% lymphocytes	60% promegaloblasts
4% monocytes	40 megaloblastoid NRBCs/100 WBCs
50% blasts	

These results are most characteristic of:
  A. Pernicious anemia
  B. Acute myeloid leukemia without maturation
  C. Acute erythroid leukemia
  D. Acute myelomonocytic leukemia

Hematology/Evaluate laboratory data to make identifications/Leukemia/3

11. A 24-year-old man with Down's syndrome presents with a fever, pallor, lymphadenopathy, and hepatosplenomegaly. His CBC results are as follows:

WBCs	10.8×10^9/L	
RBCs	1.56×10^{12}/L	8% PMNs
Hgb	3.3 g/dL	25% lymphocytes
Hct	11%	67% PAS-positive blasts
Platelets	2.5×10^9/L	

These findings are suggestive of:
  A. Hodgkin's lymphoma
  B. Myeloproliferative disorder
  C. Leukemoid reaction
  D. Acute lymphocytic leukemia

Hematology/Evaluate laboratory data to recognize health and disease states/Leukemia/3

Answers to Questions 6–11

6. **A** Acute lymphoblastic leukemia (ALL) usually affects children from ages 1–15 and is the most common type of acute leukemia in this age group. In addition, ALL constitutes the single most prevalent malignancy in pediatric patients.

7. **B** The azurophilic granules in the leukemic promyelocytes in patients with acute promyelocytic leukemia contain thromboplastic substances. These activate soluble coagulation factors, which when released into the blood cause DIC.

8. **B** A disproportionate increase in the myeloid component of the bone marrow is usually the result of a leukemic state. The normal M:E ratio is approximately 1.5–3.0.

9. **A** Auer rods are a linear projection of primary, azurophilic granules and are present in the cytoplasm of myeloblasts and monoblasts in patients with acute leukemia.

10. **C** Pernicious anemia results in pancytopenia and low vitamin B_{12} concentrations. In acute erythroid leukemia more than 50% of nucleated bone marrow cells are erythroid and more than 30% non-erythroid cells are blasts.

11. **D** Common signs of acute lymphocytic leukemia are hepatosplenomegaly (65%), lymphadenopathy (50%), and fever (60%). Anemia and thrombocytopenia are usually present and the WBC count is variable. The numerous lymphoblasts are generally PAS-positive.

12. **SITUATION:** A peripheral smear shows 75% blasts. These stain positive for both Sudan black B (SBB) and peroxidase (Px). Given these values, which of the following disorders is most likely?
   A. Acute myelocytic leukemia (AML)
   B. CML
   C. Acute undifferentiated leukemia (AUL)
   D. ALL

   Hematology/Evaluate laboratory data to recognize health and disease states/Leukemia/Cytochemical stains/3

13. In myeloid cells, the stain that selectively identifies phospholipid in the membranes of both primary and secondary granules is:
   A. PAS
   B. Myeloperoxidase
   C. Sudan black B stain
   D. Terminal deoxynucleotidyl transferase (TdT)

   Hematology/Apply principles of special procedures/ Leukemia/Cytochemical stains/3

14. Sodium fluoride may be added to the naphthyl ASD acetate (NASDA) esterase reaction. The fluoride is added to inhibit a positive reaction with:
   A. Megakaryocytes
   B. Monocytes
   C. Erythrocytes
   D. Granulocytes

   Hematology/Apply principles of special procedures/ Leukocytes/Cytochemical stains/2

15. Leukemic lymphoblasts reacting with anti-CALLA (common acute lymphoblastic leukemia antigen) are characteristically seen in:
   A. B-cell ALL
   B. T-cell ALL
   C. Null-cell ALL
   D. Common ALL

   Hematology/Evaluate laboratory data to recognize health and disease states/Leukemia/Immunochemical reactions/3

16. Which of the following reactions are often positive in ALL but are negative in AML?
   A. Terminal deoxynucleotidyl transferase and PAS
   B. Chloroacetate esterase and nonspecific esterase
   C. Sudan black B and peroxidase
   D. New methylene blue and acid phosphatase

   Hematology/Apply principles of special procedures/ Leukemia/Special tests/2

17. A patient's peripheral blood smear and bone marrow both show 70% blasts. These cells are negative for Sudan black B stain. Given these data, which of the following is the most likely diagnosis?
   A. Acute myeloid leukemia
   B. Chronic lymphocytic leukemia

   C. Acute promyelocytic leukemia
   D. Acute lymphocytic leukemia

   Hematology/Apply principles of special procedures/ Leukemia/Cytochemical stains/2

Answers to Questions 12–17

12. **A** AML blasts stain positive for Sudan black B and peroxidase. Usually fewer than 10% blasts are found in the peripheral smear of patients with CML, unless there has been a transition to blast crisis. The organelles in the cells of AUL are not mature enough to stain positive for SBB or Px. Blasts in ALL are characteristically negative with these stains.

13. **C** Phospholipids, neutral fats, and sterols are stained by Sudan black B. The PAS reaction stains intracellular glycogen. Myeloperoxidase is an enzyme present in the primary granules of myeloid cells and to a lesser degree in monocytic cells. Terminal deoxynucleotidyl transferase is a DNA polymerase found in thymus-derived and some bone marrow–derived lymphocytes.

14. **B** NASDA stains monocytes (and monoblasts) and granulocytes (and myeloblasts). The addition of fluoride renders the monocytic cells (and blasts) negative, thus allowing for differentiation from the granulocytic cells, which remain positive.

15. **D** The majority of non-T, non-B ALL blast cells display the common ALL antigen (CALLA) marker. Lymphoblasts of common ALL are TdT-positive and CALLA-positive but do not have surface membrane IgM or μ chains and are pre-B lymphoblasts. Common ALL has a lower relapse rate and better prognosis than other immunological subtypes of B-cell ALL.

16. **A** PAS is positive in about 50% of ALL with L1 and L2 morphology but is negative in ALL with L3 morphology (B-cell ALL). Terminal deoxynucleotidyl transferase is positive in all types of ALL except L3. Both terminal deoxynucleotidyl transferase and PAS are negative in AML.

17. **D** Sudan black B stains phospholipids and other neutral fats. It is the most sensitive stain for granulocytic precursors. Lymphoid cells rarely stain positive for it. As 70% lymphoblasts would never be seen in CLL, the correct response is ALL.

18. How does the World Health Organization classification of myeloproliferative disorders differ from the French-American-British (FAB) classification scheme for acute leukemias?

A. It encompases all of the myeloproliferative diseases, including CML

B. It combines the acute lymphocytic and myelogenous leukemias into a single subtype

C. It groups all myelo- and lymphoproliferative diseases into two subtypes

D. It expands the classification of the acute myeloblastic leukemias

Hematology/Leukemias/Apply knowledge of special procedures/Classification/2

19. In addition to morphology, cytochemistry, and immunophenotyping, the WHO classification of myelo- and lymphoproliferative disorders is based upon which characteristic?

A. Proteomics

B. Cytogenetic abnormalities

C. Carbohydrate-associated tumor antigen production

D. Cell signaling and adhesion markers

Hematology/Leukemias/Apply knowledge of special procedures/Classification/1

20. The WHO classification of AML is best characterized by which of the following statements?

A. At least 30% of nucleated bone marrow cells must be blasts

B. Four subtypes with commonly occurring translocations encompass most cases of AML

C. The subtypes include both FAB M0–M7 and all myelodysplastic syndromes

D. The subtypes include all known cytogenetic abnormalities associated with AML

Hematology/Apply knowledge of special procedures/Leukemias/Classification/2

18. **A** The WHO classification system includes four categories for neoplasms of myeloid lineage: myeloproliferative diseases (MPDs), which includes the chronic leukemias, myelodysplastic/myeloproliferative diseases (MDS/MPD), myelodysplastic syndromes (MDSs), and acute myeloid leukemia (AML). It also classifies lymphoproliferative diseases into six categories that include ALLs, non-Hodgkin's and Hodgkin's lymphomas. An 11th category is composed of mast cell disorders. The FAB classification is confined to AML and consists of eight subtypes (M0–M7). The WHO classification divides AML into five subgroups.

19. **B** In addition to morphology, cytochemical stains, and flow cytometry, the WHO classification relies heavily on chromosomal and molecular abnormalities.

20. **B** The WHO classification of AML requires that ≥20% of nucleated bone marrow cells be blasts, while the FAB classification generally requires ≥30%. Therefore, the WHO scheme places refractory anemia with excess blasts in transformation (RAEB-T) into the AML category of diseases. WHO classifies AML into five subgroups: These are acute myeloid leukemias with commonly occurring cytogenetic translocations; acute myeloid leukemia with multilineage dysplasia; acute myeloid leukemia and myelodysplastic syndromes related to therapy; acute leukemia of ambiguous lineage; and acute myeloid leukemia not categorized above.

Of these, the first subgroup accounts for the majority of cases and consists of four subtypes.

1. Acute myeloid leukemia with t(8;21). This results in fusion of the AML gene on chromosome 8 with the ETO gene on chromosome 21 (AML1/ETO), a translocation commonly seen in FAB M2.

2. Acute promyelocytic leukemia t(15;17)(q22;q 11-12). This results in fusion of the PML gene on chromosome 15 with the RARα gene on chromosome 17 (PML/RARα), a translocation commonly associated with M3.

3. Acute myeloid leukemia with eosinophilia inv(16)(p13;q11) or t(16;16)(q13;q11). This causes fusion of the CBF gene and MYH11 gene on chromosome 16 (CBF/MYH11), and is commonly associated with FAB M4Eo.

4. Acute myeloid leukemia with 11q23 abnormalities. This is associated with translocations involving the MLL gene on chromosome 11. It is not associated with any of the FAB subtypes.

LYMPHOPROLIFERATIVE/ MYELOPROLIFERATIVE DISORDERS

1. Repeated phlebotomy in patients with polycythemia vera (PV) may lead to the development of:
   A. Folic acid deficiency
   B. Sideroblastic anemia
   C. Iron deficiency anemia
   D. Hemolytic anemia

   Hematology/Evaluate laboratory data to recognize health and disease states/Anemia/2

2. In essential thrombocythemia, the platelets are:
   A. Increased in number and functionally abnormal
   B. Normal in number and functionally abnormal
   C. Decreased in number and functional
   D. Decreased in number and functionally abnormal

   Hematology/Evaluate laboratory data to recognize health and disease states/CBC/Platelets/2

3. Which of the following cells is considered *pathognomonic* for Hodgkin's disease?
   A. Niemann-Pick cells
   B. Reactive lymphocytes
   C. Flame cells
   D. Reed-Sternberg cells

   Hematology/Evaluate laboratory data to recognize health and disease states/Lymphoma/1

4. In myelofibrosis, the characteristic abnormal red blood cell morphology is that of:
   A. Target cells
   B. Schistocytes
   C. Teardrop cells
   D. Ovalocytes

   Hematology/Correlate clinical and laboratory data/RBC microscopic morphology/1

5. PV is characterized by:
   A. Increased plasma volume
   B. Pancytopenia
   C. Decreased oxygen saturation
   D. Absolute increase in total red cell mass

   Hematology/Evaluate laboratory data to recognize health and disease states/RBC/Leukemia/2

Answers to Questions 1–5

1. **C** Iron deficiency anemia is a predictable complication of therapeutic phlebotomy because approximately 250 mg of iron is removed with each unit of blood.

2. **A** In essential thrombocythemia, the platelet count is extremely elevated. These platelets are abnormal in function, leading to both bleeding and thrombotic diathesis.

3. **D** The morphological common denominator in Hodgkin's lymphoma is the Reed-Sternberg (RS) cell. It is a large, binucleated cell with a dense nucleolus surrounded by clear space. These characteristics give the RS cell an "owl's eye" appearance. Niemann-Pick cells (foam cells) are histiocytes containing phagocytized sphingolipids that stain pale blue and impart a foam-like texture to the cytoplasm. Flame cells are plasma cells with distinctive red cytoplasm. They are sometimes seen in the bone marrow of patients with multiple myeloma.

4. **C** The marked amount of fibrosis, both medullary and extramedullary, accounts for the irreversible red cell morphological change to a teardrop shape. The red cells are "teared" as they attempt to pass through the fibrotic tissue.

5. **D** The diagnosis of PV requires the demonstration of an increase in red cell mass. Pancytosis may also be seen in about two thirds of PV cases. The plasma volume is normal or slightly reduced, and the arterial oxygen saturation is usually normal.

6. Features of secondary polycythemia include all of the following *except*:
   A. Splenomegaly
   B. Decreased oxygen saturation
   C. Increased red cell mass
   D. Increased erythropoietin

Hematology/Evaluate laboratory data to recognize health and disease states/RBC disorder/2

7. The erythrocytosis seen in relative polycythemia occurs because of:
   A. Decreased arterial oxygen saturation
   B. Decreased plasma volume of circulating blood
   C. Increased erythropoietin levels
   D. Increased erythropoiesis in the bone marrow

Hematology/Correlate clinical and laboratory data/RBC disorder/2

8. In PV, what is characteristically seen in the peripheral blood?
   A. Panmyelosis
   B. Pancytosis
   C. Pancytopenia
   D. Panhyperplasia

Hematology/Apply knowledge of fundamental biological characteristics/Polycythemia/1

9. The leukocyte alkaline phosphatase (LAP) stain on a patient gives the following results: 10(0); 48(1+); 38(2+); 3(3+); 1(4+). Calculate the LAP score.
   A. 100
   B. 117
   C. 137
   D. 252

Hematology/Calculate/LAP score/3

10. CML is distinguished from leukemoid reaction by which of the following?
   A. CML: low LAP; leukemoid: high LAP
   B. CML: high LAP; leukemoid: low LAP
   C. CML: high WBC; leukemoid; normal WBC
   D. CML: high WBC; leukemoid: high WBC

Hematology/Evaluate laboratory and clinical data to specify additional tests/Leukemia/2

11. Which of the following occurs in idiopathic myelofibrosis?
   A. Myeloid metaplasia
   B. Leukoerythroblastosis
   C. Fibrosis of the bone marrow
   D. All of the above

Hematology/Evaluate laboratory data to recognize health and disease states/Leukemia/3

12. What influence does the Philadelphia (Ph^1) chromosome have on the prognosis of patients with chronic myelocytic leukemia?
   A. It is not predictive.
   B. The prognosis is better if Ph^1 is present.
   C. The prognosis is worse if Ph^1 is present.
   D. The disease usually transforms into AML when Ph^1 is present.

Hematology/Evaluate laboratory data to recognize health and disease states/Genetic theory and principle/CML/2

Answers to Questions 6–12

6. **A** Splenomegaly is a feature of PV but not characteristic of secondary polycythemia. The red cell mass is increased in both primary polycythemia (PV) and secondary polycythemia. Erythropoietin is increased and oxygen saturation is decreased in secondary polycythemia.

7. **B** Relative polycythemia is caused by a reduction of plasma rather than an increase in red blood cell volume or mass. Red cell mass is increased in both PV and secondary polycythemia, but erythropoietin levels are high only in secondary polycythemia.

8. **B** PV is a myeloproliferative disorder characterized by uncontrolled proliferation of erythroid precursors. However, production of all cell lines is usually increased. Panhyperplasia is a term used to describe the cellularity of the bone marrow in PV.

9. **C** One hundred mature neutrophils are counted and scored. The LAP score is calculated as: (the number of 1+ cells × 1) + (2+ cells × 2) + (3+ cells × 3) + (4+ cells × 4). That is, 48 + 76 + 9 + 4 = 137. The reference range is approximately 20–130.

10. **A** CML causes a low LAP score, whereas an elevated or normal score occurs in a leukemoid reaction. CML cannot be distinguished by WBC count since both CML and a leukemoid reaction have a high count.

11. **D** Anemia, fibrosis, myeloid metaplasia, thrombocytosis, and leukoerythroblastosis occur in idiopathic myelofibrosis.

12. **B** Ninety percent of patients with CML have the Philadelphia chromosome. This appears as a long arm deletion of chromosome 22 but is actually a translocation between the long arms of chromosomes 22 and 9. The prognosis for CML is better if the Philadelphia chromosome is present. Often, a second chromosomal abnormality occurs in CML before blast crisis.

13. Which of the following is/are commonly found in CML?
 A. Many teardrop-shaped cells
 B. Intense LAP staining
 C. A decrease in granulocytes
 D. An increase in basophils

 Hematology/Evaluate laboratory data to recognize health and disease states/CML/3

14. Multiple myeloma and Waldenström's macroglobulinemia have all the following in common *except*:
 A. Monoclonal gammopathy
 B. Hyperviscosity of the blood
 C. Bence-Jones protein in the urine
 D. Osteolytic lesions

 Hematology/Evaluate laboratory data to recognize health and disease states/Myeloma/ Characteristics/2

15. What is the characteristic finding seen in the peripheral smear of a patient with multiple myeloma?
 A. Microcytic hypochromic cells
 B. Intracellular inclusion bodies
 C. Rouleaux
 D. Hypersegmented neutrophils

 Hematology/Apply knowledge of fundamental biological characteristics/Myeloma/RBC microscopic morphology/1

16. In which of the following conditions does LAP show the least activity?
 A. Leukemoid reactions
 B. Idiopathic myelofibrosis
 C. PV
 D. CML

 Hematology/Correlate clinical and laboratory data/LAP score/CML/1

17. A striking feature of the peripheral blood of a patient with CML is a:
 A. Profusion of bizarre blast cells
 B. Normal number of typical granulocytes
 C. Presence of granulocytes at different stages of development
 D. Pancytopenia

 Hematology/Evaluate laboratory data to recognize health and disease states/WBCs/CML/2

18. Which of the following is often associated with CML but *not* with AML?
 A. Infections
 B. WBCs greater than 20.0×10^9/L
 C. Hemorrhage
 D. Splenomegaly

 Hematology/Correlate clinical and laboratory data/CML/Characteristics/2

19. All of the following are associated with the diagnosis of multiple myeloma *except*:
 A. Marrow plasmacytosis
 B. Lytic bone lesions
 C. Serum and/or urine M component (monoclonal protein)
 D. Philadelphia chromosome

 Hematology/Correlate clinical and laboratory data/Myeloma/2

Answers to Questions 13–19

13. **D** CML is marked by an elevated WBC count demonstrating various stages of maturation, hypermetabolism, and a minimal LAP staining. An increase in basophils and eosinophils is a common finding. Pseudo–Pelger-Huët cells and thrombocytosis may be present. The marrow is hypercellular with a high M:E ratio (e.g., 10:1).

14. **D** Osteolytic lesions indicating destruction of the bone as evidenced by radiography is seen in multiple myeloma but not in Waldenström's macroglobulinemia. In addition, Waldenström's gives rise to a lymphocytosis that does not occur in multiple myeloma and differs in the morphology of the malignant cells.

15. **C** Rouleaux is observed in multiple myeloma patients as a result of increased viscosity and decreased albumin/globulin ratio. Multiple myeloma is a plasma cell dyscrasia that is characterized by an overproduction of monoclonal immunoglobulin.

16. **D** Chronic myelogenous leukemia shows the least LAP activity, whereas the LAP score is slightly to markedly increased in each of the other states.

17. **C** The WBC count in CML is often higher than 100×10^9/L, and the peripheral smear shows a granulocyte progression from myeloblast to segmented neutrophil.

18. **D** Splenomegaly is seen in more than 90% of CML patients, but it is not a characteristic finding in AML. Infections, hemorrhage, and elevated WBC counts may be seen in both CML and AML.

19. **D** The Ph[1] chromosome is a diagnostic marker for CML. Osteolytic lesions, monoclonal gammopathy, and bone marrow infiltration by plasma cells constitute the triad of diagnostic markers for multiple myeloma.

20. Multiple myeloma is most difficult to distinguish from:
  A. Chronic lymphocytic leukemia
  B. Acute myelogenous leukemia
  C. Benign monoclonal gammopathy
  D. Benign adenoma

Hematology/Apply knowledge of fundamental biological characteristics/Myeloma/2

21. The pathology of multiple myeloma includes which of the following?
  A. Expanding plasma cell mass
  B. Overproduction of monoclonal immunoglobulins
  C. Production of osteoclast activating factor (OAF) and other cytokines
  D. All of the above

Hematology/Apply knowledge of fundamental biological characteristics/Immunological manifestation of disease/Immunoglobulins/2

22. Waldenström's macroglobulinemia is a malignancy of the:
  A. Lymphoplasmacytoid cells
  B. Adrenal cortex
  C. Myeloblastic cell lines
  D. Erythroid cell precursors

Hematology/Apply knowledge of fundamental biological characteristics/Immunological manifestation of disease/Plasma cell dyscrasia/2

23. Cells that exhibit a positive stain with acid phosphatase and are not inhibited with tartaric acid are characteristically seen in:
  A. Infectious mononucleosis
  B. Infectious lymphocytosis
  C. Hairy cell leukemia
  D. T-cell acute lymphoblastic leukemia

Hematology/Apply principles of special procedures/Leukemia/Cytochemical stains/2

Answers to Questions 20–23

20. **C** Benign monoclonal gammopathies have peripheral blood findings similar to those in myeloma. However, a lower concentration of monoclonal protein is usually seen. There are no osteolytic lesions, and the plasma cells comprise less than 10% of nucleated cells in the bone marrow. About 30% become malignant, and therefore the term monoclonal gammopathy of undetermined significance (MGUS) is the designation used to describe this condition.

21. **D** Mutated plasmablasts in the bone marrow undergo clonal replication and expand the plasma cell mass. Normal bone marrow is gradually replaced by the malignant plasma cells leading to pancytopenia. Most malignant plasma cells actively produce immunoglobulins. In multiple myeloma, the normally controlled and purposeful production of antibodies is replaced by the inappropriate production of even larger amounts of useless immunoglobulin molecules. The normally equal production of light chains and heavy chains may be imbalanced. The result is the release of excess free light chains or free heavy chains. The immunoglobulins produced by a clone of myeloma cells are identical. Any abnormal production of identical antibodies is referred to by the general name of monoclonal gammopathy. Osteoclasts are bone cells active in locally resorbing bone and releasing calcium into the blood. Nearby osteoblasts are equally active in utilizing calcium in the blood to form new bone. Multiple myeloma interrupts this balance by the secretion of at least two substances. These are interleukin-6 (IL-6) and osteoclast-activating factor (OAF). As its name implies, OAF stimulates osteoclasts to increase bone resorption and release of calcium, which leads to lytic lesions of the bone.

22. **A** Waldenström's macroglobulinemia is a malignancy of the lymphoplasmacytoid cells, which manufacture IgM. Although the cells secrete immunoglobulin, they are not fully differentiated into plasma cells and lack the characteristic perinuclear halo, deep basophilia, and eccentric nucleus characteristic of classic plasma cells.

23. **C** A variable number of malignant cells in hairy cell leukemia (HCL) will stain positive with tartrate-resistant acid phosphatase (TRAP+). Although this cytochemical reaction is fairly specific for HCL, TRAP activity has occasionally been reported in B-cell and rarely T-cell leukemia.

1. A 19-year-old man came to the Emergency Room with severe joint pain, fatigue, cough, and fever. Review the following laboratory results:

WBCs	21.0×10^9/L
RBCs	3.23×10^{12}/L
Hgb	9.6 g/dL
PLT	252×10^9/L

Differential: 17 band neutrophils; 75 segmented neutrophils; 5 lymphocytes; 2 monocytes; 1 eosinophil; 26 NRBCs

What is the corrected WBC count?
A. 8.1×10^9/L
B. 16.7×10^9/L
C. 21.0×10^9/L
D. 80.8×10^9/L

Hematology/Calculate/WBCs corrected for NRBCs/2

2. A manual WBC count is performed using the Unopette system. Eighty WBCs are counted in the four large corner squares of a Neubauer hemocytometer. The dilution is 1:100. What is the total WBC count?
A. 4.0×10^9/L
B. 8.0×10^9/L
C. 20.0×10^9/L
D. 200.0×10^9/L

Hematology/Calculate/Cell Count/2

3. A manual RBC count is performed on a pleural fluid using the Unopette system. The RBC count in the large center square of the Neubauer hemocytometer is 125, and the dilution is 1:200. What is the total RBC count?

A. 27.8×10^9/L
B. 62.5×10^9/L
C. 125.0×10^9/L
D. 250.0×10^9/L

Hematology/Calculate/Cell Count/2

Answers to Questions 1–3

1. **B** The formula for correcting the WBC count for the presence of NRBCs is:

   Total WBC × 100 or (21.0 × 100) ÷ 126 = 16.7×10^9/L

   where total WBC = WBCs × 10^9/L, 100 is the number of WBCs counted in the differential, and 126 is the sum of NRBCs plus WBCs counted in the differential.

2. **C** The formula for calculating manual cell counts using a hemocytometer is:

   # cells × 10 (depth factor) × dilution factor divided by the area counted in mm², or

   (80 × 10 × 100) ÷ 4 = 20,000/μL or 20.0 × 10^9/L

3. **D** Regardless of the cell or fluid type, the formula for calculating manual cell counts using a hemocytometer is:

   # cells × 10 (depth factor) × dilution factor divided by the area counted in mm², or

   (125 × 10 × 200) ÷ 1 = 250,000/μL or 250.0 × 10^9/L

4. Review the scatterplot of white blood cells shown. Which section of the scatterplot denotes the number of monocytes?

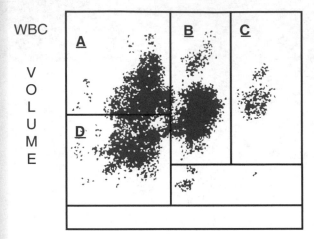

WBC

VOLUME

DF 1

A. A
B. B
C. C
D. D

Hematology/Apply basic principles to interpret results/Automated cell counting/2

5. Review the following automated CBC values.

WBCs	17.5×10^9/L (flagged)	MCV	86.8 fL
RBCs	2.89×10^{12}/L	MCH	28.0 pg
Hgb	8.1 g/dL	MCHC	32.3%
Hct	25.2%	PLT	217×10^9/L

Many sickle cells were observed upon review of the peripheral blood smear. Based on this finding and the above results, what automated parameter of this patient is most likely inaccurate and what follow-up test should be done to accurately assess this parameter?

A. MCV/perform reticulocyte count
B. Hct/perform manual Hct
C. WBC/perform manual WBC count
D. Hgb/perform serum:saline replacement

Hematology/Apply knowledge to identify sources of error/Instrumentation/3

6. Review the following CBC results on a 2-day-old baby girl:

WBCs	15.2×10^9/L	MCV	105 fL
RBCs	5.30×10^{12}/L	MCH	34.0 pg
Hgb	18.5 g/dL	MCHC	33.5%
Hct	57.9%	PLT	213×10^9/L

These results indicate:
A. Macrocytic anemia
B. Microcytic anemia
C. Liver disease
D. Normal values for a 2-day-old infant

Hematology/Apply knowledge of fundamental biological characteristics/Normal values/2

Answers to Questions 4–6

4. **A** White blood cell identification is facilitated by analysis of the impedance, conductance, and light-scattering properties of the WBCs. The scatterplot represents the relationship between volume (x axis) and light scatter (y axis). Monocytes account for the dots in section A, neutrophils are represented in section B, eosinophils in section C, and lymphocytes are denoted in section D.

5. **C** When an automated WBC count is performed using a hematology analyzer, the RBCs are lysed to allow enumeration of the WBCs. Sickle cells are often resistant to lysis within the limited time frame (less than 1 minute), during which the RBCs are exposed to the lysing reagent and the WBCs are subsequently counted. As a result, the nonlysed RBCs are counted along with the WBCs, thus falsely increasing the WBC count. When an automated cell counting analyzer indicates a review flag for the WBC count, and sickle cells are noted on peripheral smear analysis, a manual WBC count must be performed. The manual method allows optimal time for sickle cell lysis and accurate enumeration of the WBCs.

6. **D** During the first week of life an infant has an average Hct of 55 mL/dL. This value drops to a mean of 43 mL/dL by the first month of life. The mean MCV of the first week is 108 fL; after 2 months the average MCV is 96 fL. The mean WBC count during the first week is approximately 18×10^9/L, and this drops to an average of 10.8×10^9/L after the first month. The platelet count of newborns falls within the same normal range as adults.

7. Review the following scatterplot, histograms, and automated values on a 21-year-old college student.

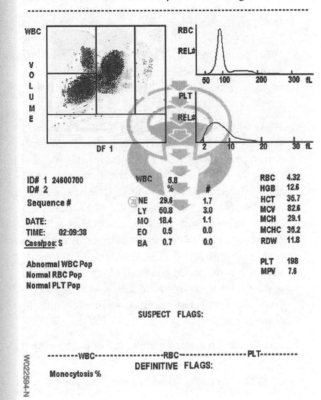

ID# 1 24600700
ID# 2

Sequence #

DATE:
TIME: 02:09:38
Cass/pos: S

Abnormal WBC Pop
Normal RBC Pop
Normal PLT Pop

	%	#
NE	29.6	1.7
LY	50.8	3.0
MO	18.4	1.1
EO	0.5	0.0
BA	0.7	0.0

WBC	5.8

RBC	4.32
HGB	12.6
HCT	35.7
MCV	82.6
MCH	29.1
MCHC	35.2
RDW	11.8
PLT	198
MPV	7.6

SUSPECT FLAGS:

--------WBC------------------RBC-----------------PLT---------
DEFINITIVE FLAGS:
Monocytosis %

W022594-N

WBC Differential: 5 band neutrophils; 27 segmented neutrophils; 60 atypical lymphocytes; 6 monocytes; 1 eosinophil; 1 basophil

What is the presumptive diagnosis?
A. Infectious mononucleosis
B. Monocytosis
C. Chronic lymphocytic leukemia
D. β-Thalassemia

Hematology/Apply knowledge to identify sources of error/Instrumentation/3

Answer to Question 7

7. A Lymphocytosis with numerous atypical lymphocytes is a hallmark finding consistent with the diagnosis of infectious mononucleosis. The automated results demonstrated abnormal WBC subpopulations, specifically lymphocytosis as well as monocytosis. However, on peripheral smear examination 60 atypical lymphocytes and only 6 monocytes were noted. Atypical lymphocytes are often misclassified by automated cell counters as monocytes. Therefore the automated analyzer differential must not be released and the manual differential count must be relied upon for diagnostic interpretation.

8. Review the following scatterplot, histograms, and automated values on a 61-year-old woman.

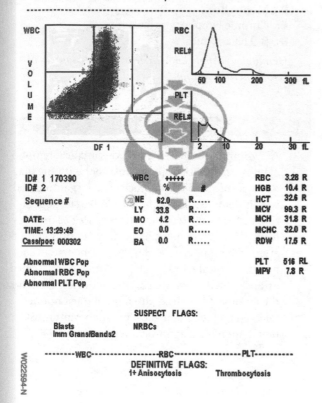

WBC Differential: 14 band neutrophils; 50 segmented neutrophils; 7 lymphocytes; 4 monocytes; 10 metamyelocytes; 8 myelocytes; 1 promyelocyte; 3 eosinophils; 3 basophils; 2 NRBCs/100 WBCs

What is the presumptive diagnosis?
A. Leukemoid reaction
B. Chronic myelocytic leukemia
C. Acute myelocytic leukemia
D. Megaloblastic leukemia

Hematology/Evaluate laboratory data to recognize health and disease states/Instrumentation/3

9. Review the automated results from the previous question. Which parameters can be released without further follow-up verification procedures?
A. WBC and relative percentages of WBC populations
B. RBCs and PLTs
C. Hgb and Hct
D. None of the automated counts can be released without verification procedures.

Hematology/Apply knowledge to identify sources of error/Instrumentation/3

---

8. **B** The ++++ on the printout indicates that the WBC count exceeds the upper linearity of the analyzer ($>99.9 \times 10^9$/L). This markedly elevated WBC count, combined with the spectrum of immature granulocytic cells seen on peripheral smear examination, indicates the diagnosis of chronic myelocytic leukemia.

9. **D** All of the automated results have R or review flags indicated; none can be released without verification procedures. The specimen must be diluted to bring the WBC count within the linearity range of the analyzer. When enumerating the RBC count, the analyzer does not lyse the WBCs and actually counts them in with the RBC count. As such, the RBC count is falsely elevated because of the increased number of WBCs. Therefore, after an accurate WBC count has been obtained, this value can be subtracted from the RBC count to obtain a true RBC count. For example, using the values for this patient:

Step 1: Obtain accurate WBC count by diluting the sample 1:10.

$$\text{WBC} = 41.0 \times 10 \text{ (dilution)} = 410 \times 10^9/\text{L}$$

Step 2: Convert this value to cells per 10^{12} in order to subtract from the RBC count.

$$410 \times 10^9/\text{L} = 0.41 \times 10^{12}/\text{L}$$

Step 3: Subtract the WBC count from the RBC count to get an accurate RBC count.

$$3.28 \text{ (original RBC)} - 0.41 \text{ (true WBC)} =$$
$$2.87 \times 10^{12}/\text{L} = \text{accurate RBC}$$

The Hct may be obtained by microhematocrit centrifugation. The true MCV may be obtained using the standard formula.

$$\text{MCV} = (\text{Hct} \div \text{RBC}) \times 10$$

where RBC = RBC count in millions per microliter.

Additionally, the platelet count must be verified by smear estimate or performed manually.

10. Refer to the following scatterplot, histograms, and automated values on a 45-year-old man. What follow-up verification procedure is indicated before releasing these results?

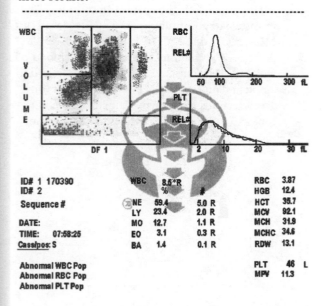

ID# 1 170390
ID# 2
Sequence #

DATE:
TIME: 07:58:25
Cassipos: S

Abnormal WBC Pop
Abnormal RBC Pop
Abnormal PLT Pop

	%	#		
WBC	8.5*R		RBC	3.87
NE	59.4	5.0 R	HGB	12.4
LY	23.4	2.0 R	HCT	35.7
MO	12.7	1.1 R	MCV	92.1
EO	3.1	0.3 R	MCH	31.9
BA	1.4	0.1 R	MCHC	34.6
			RDW	13.1
			PLT	46 L
			MPV	11.3

SUSPECT FLAGS:
NRBCs

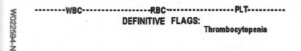

DEFINITIVE FLAGS:
Thrombocytopenia

A. Redraw blood sample using a sodium citrate tube; multiply PLTs × 1.11
B. Dilute the WBCs 1:10; multiply × 10
C. Perform plasma blank Hgb to correct for lipemia
D. Warm specimen at 37°C for 15 minutes; rerun specimen

Hematology/Apply knowledge to identify sources of error/Instrumentation/3

Answer to Question 10

10. A The platelet clumping phenomenon is often induced in vitro by the anticoagulant EDTA. Redrawing a sample from the patient using a sodium citrate tube usually corrects this phenomenon and allows accurate platelet enumeration. The platelet count must be multiplied by 1.11 to adjust for the amount of sodium citrate. Platelet clumps cause a spurious decrease in the platelet count by automated methods. The WBC value has an R (review) flag because the platelet clumps have been falsely counted as WBCs; therefore, a manual WBC count is indicated.

11. Refer to the following scatterplot, histograms, and automated values on a 52-year-old woman. What follow-up verification procedure is indicated before releasing these results?

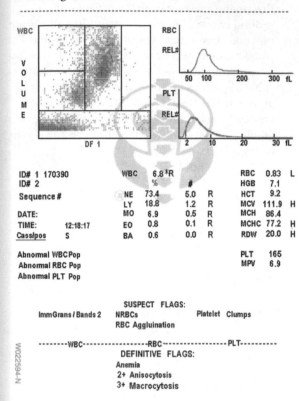

ID# 1 170390	WBC	6.8 ✶R		RBC	0.83	L
ID# 2		%	#	HGB	7.1	
Sequence #	NE	73.4	5.0 R	HCT	9.2	
	LY	18.8	1.2 R	MCV	111.9	H
DATE:	MO	6.9	0.5 R	MCH	86.4	
TIME: 12:18:17	EO	0.8	0.1 R	MCHC	77.2	H
Cass/pos S	BA	0.6	0.0 R	RDW	20.0	H

Abnormal WBC Pop   PLT 165
Abnormal RBC Pop   MPV 6.9
Abnormal PLT Pop

SUSPECT FLAGS:

ImmGrans/Bands 2   NRBCs   Platelet Clumps
                  RBC Aggluination

--------WBC-----------------RBC-----------------PLT---------
DEFINITIVE FLAGS:
Anemia
2+ Anisocytosis
3+ Macrocytosis

A. Redraw specimen using a sodium citrate tube; multiply PLT × 1.11
B. Dilute the WBCs 1:10; multiply × 10
C. Perform plasma blank Hgb to correct for lipemia
D. Warm the specimen at 37°C for 15 minutes; rerun the specimen

Hematology/Apply knowledge to identify sources of error/Instrumentation/3

11. D The presence of a high titer cold agglutinin in a patient with cold autoimmune hemolytic anemia will interfere with automated cell counting. The most remarkable findings are a falsely elevated MCV, MCH, and MCHC as well as a falsely decreased RBC count. The patient's red blood cells will quickly agglutinate in vitro when exposed to ambient temperatures below body temperature. To correct this phenomenon, incubate the EDTA tube at 37°C for 15–30 minutes and then rerun the specimen.

12. Refer to the following scatterplot, histograms, and automated values on a 33-year-old woman. What follow-up verification procedure is indicated before releasing these results?

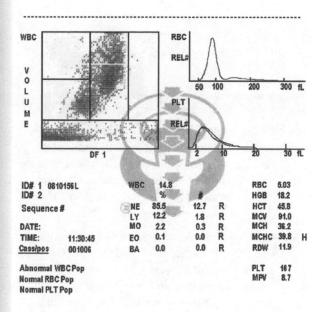

ID# 1 0810156L
ID# 2
Sequence #

DATE:
TIME: 11:30:45
Cass/pos 001006

Abnormal WBC Pop
Normal RBC Pop
Normal PLT Pop

	WBC	14.8				RBC	5.03
		%	#			HGB	18.2
NE	85.5	12.7	R		HCT	45.8
LY	12.2	1.8	R		MCV	91.0
MO	2.2	0.3	R		MCH	36.2
EO	0.1	0.0	R		MCHC	39.8 H
BA	0.0	0.0	R		RDW	11.9

PLT 167
MPV 8.7

SUSPECT FLAGS:

Imm Grans / Bands 2

--------WBC------------------RBC-----------------PLT----------
DEFINITIVE FLAGS:
Leukocytosis
Neutrophilia %

W022594-N

A. Perform a manual hematocrit and redraw the sample using a sodium citrate tube; multiply PLT × 1.11

B. Dilute the WBC 1:10; multiply × 10

C. Perform plasma blank Hgb to correct for lipemia

D. Warm the specimen at 37°C for 15 minutes; rerun the specimen

Hematology/Apply knowledge to identify sources of error/Instrumentation/3

12. C The rule of thumb regarding the Hgb/Hct correlation dictates that Hgb × 3 ≈ Hct (± 3). This rule is violated in this patient; therefore, a follow-up verification procedure is indicated. Additionally, the MCHC is markedly elevated in these results, and an explanation for a falsely increased Hgb should be investigated. Lipemia can be visualized by centrifuging the EDTA tube and observing for a milky white plasma. To correct for the presence of lipemia, a plasma Hgb value (baseline Hgb) should be ascertained using the patient's plasma and subsequently subtracted from the original falsely elevated Hgb value. The following formula can be used to correct for lipemia.

Whole blood Hgb − [(Plasma Hgb)
(1 − Hct/100)] = Corrected Hgb

13. Refer to the following scatterplot, histograms, and automated values on a 48-year-old man. What follow-up verification procedure is indicated before releasing the five-part WBC differential results?

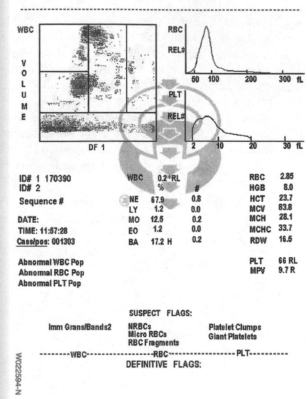

ID# 1 170390
ID# 2
Sequence #
DATE:
TIME: 11:57:28
Cass/pos: 001303

WBC	0.2*RL		RBC	2.85
	%	#	HGB	8.0
NE	67.9	0.8	HCT	23.7
LY	1.2	0.0	MCV	83.8
MO	12.5	0.2	MCH	28.1
EO	1.2	0.0	MCHC	33.7
BA	17.2 H	0.2	RDW	16.5

Abnormal WBC Pop
Abnormal RBC Pop
Abnormal PLT Pop

PLT	66 RL
MPV	9.7 R

SUSPECT FLAGS:

Imm Grans/Bands2	NRBCs	Platelet Clumps
	Micro RBCs	Giant Platelets
	RBC Fragments	

--------WBC-----------------RBC-------------------PLT----------
DEFINITIVE FLAGS:

W022594-N

A. Dilute WBCs 1:10; multiply × 10
B. Redraw the sample using a sodium citrate tube; multiply WBC × 1.11
C. Prepare buffy coat peripheral blood smears and perform a manual differential
D. Warm specimen at 37°C for 15 minutes; rerun specimen

Hematology/Select course of action/Instrumentation/3

14. Review the following CBC results on a 70-year-old man:

WBCs	58.2 × 10⁹/L	MCV	98 fL
RBCs	2.68 × 10¹²/L	MCH	31.7 pg
Hgb	8.5 g/dL	MCHC	32.6%
Hct	26.5 mL/dL%	PLT	132 × 10⁹/L

Differential: 96 lymphocytes; 2 band neutrophils; 2 segmented neutrophils; 25 smudge cells/100 WBCs

What is the most likely diagnosis based on these values?
A. Acute lymphocytic leukemia
B. Chronic lymphocytic leukemia (CLL)
C. Infectious mononucleosis
D. Myelodysplastic syndrome

Hematology/Evaluate laboratory data to recognize health and disease states/Leukemia/2

Answers to Questions 13–14

13. **C** The markedly decreased WBC count (0.2 × 10⁹/L) indicates that a manual differential is necessary and very few leukocytes will be available for differential cell counting. To increase the yield and thereby facilitate counting, differential smears should be prepared using the buffy coat technique.

14. **B** CLL is a disease of the elderly, classically associated with an elevated WBC count and relative and absolute lymphocytosis. CLL is twice as common in men, and smudge cells (WBCs with little or no surrounding cytoplasm) are usually present in the peripheral blood smear. CLL may occur with or without anemia or thrombocytopenia. The patient's age and lack of blasts rule out acute lymphocytic leukemia. Similarly, the patient's age and the lack of atypical lymphocytes make infectious mononucleosis unlikely. Myelodysplastic syndromes may involve the erythroid, granulocytic, or megakaryocytic cell lines but not the lymphoid cells.

15. Refer to the following scatterplot, histograms, and automated values on a 28-year-old woman who had preoperative laboratory testing. A manual WBC differential was requested by her physician. The WBC differential was not significantly different from the automated five-part differential; however, the technologist noted 3+ elliptocytes/ovalocytes while reviewing the RBC morphology. What is the most likely diagnosis for this patient?

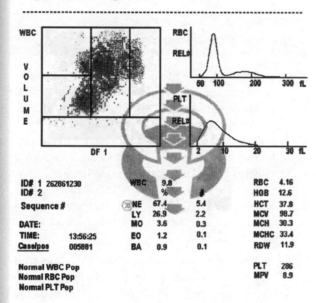

ID# 1 262861230	WBC	9.8		RBC	4.16
ID# 2	%	#		HGB	12.6
Sequence #	NE	67.4	5.4	HCT	37.8
	LY	26.9	2.2	MCV	98.7
DATE:	MO	3.6	0.3	MCH	30.3
TIME: 13:56:25	EO	1.2	0.1	MCHC	33.4
Cass/pos 005881	BA	0.9	0.1	RDW	11.9
				PLT	286
Normal WBC Pop				MPV	8.9
Normal RBC Pop					
Normal PLT Pop					

SUSPECT FLAGS:

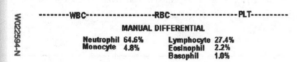

--------WBC-----------------RBC-----------------PLT----------
MANUAL DIFFERENTIAL

Neutrophil	64.6%	Lymphocyte	27.4%
Monocyte	4.8%	Eosinophil	2.2%
		Basophil	1.0%

A. Disseminated intravascular coagulation (DIC)
B. Hereditary elliptocytosis (ovalocytosis)
C. Cirrhosis
D. Hgb C disease

Hematology/Evaluate laboratory data to recognize health and disease states/2

16. A 25-year-old woman saw her physician with symptoms of jaundice, acute cholecystitis, and an enlarged spleen. On investigation, numerous gallstones were discovered. Review the following CBC results:

WBCs	11.1 × 10⁹/L	MCV	100 fL
RBCs	3.33 × 10¹²/L	MCH	34.5 pg
Hgb	11.5 g/dL	MCHC	37.5%
Hct	31.6 mL/dL	PLT	448 × 10⁹/L

WBC Differential: 13 band neutrophils; 65 segmented neutrophils; 15 lymphocytes; 6 monocytes; 1 eosinophil

RBC morphology: 3+ spherocytes, 1+ polychromasia

What follow-up laboratory test would provide valuable information for this patient?
A. Osmotic fragility
B. Hgb electrophoresis
C. G6PD assay
D. Methemoglobin reduction test

Hematology/Evaluate laboratory data to recognize health and disease states/2

15. **B** The finding of ovalocytes as the predominant RBC morphology in peripheral blood is consistent with the diagnosis of hereditary elliptocytosis (HE), or ovalocytosis. This disorder is relatively common and can range in severity from an asymptomatic carrier to homozygous HE with severe hemolysis. The most common clinical subtype is associated with no or minimal hemolysis. Therefore, HE is usually associated with a normal RBC histogram and cell indices and will go unnoticed without microscopic evaluation of the peripheral smear.

16. **A** The osmotic fragility test is indicated as a confirmatory test for the presence of numerous spherocytes, and individuals with hereditary spherocytosis (HS) have an increased osmotic fragility. The MCHC is elevated in more than 50% of patients with spherocytosis, and this parameter can be used as a clue to the presence of HS. Spherocytes have a decreased surface-to-volume ratio, probably resulting from mild cellular dehydration.

17. Refer to the following scatterplot, histograms, and automated values on a 53-year-old man who had preoperative laboratory testing. What is the most likely diagnosis for this patient?

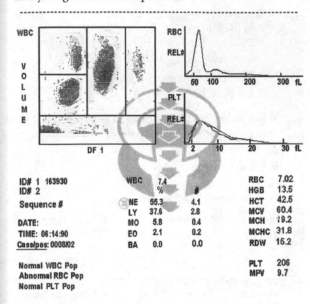

ID# 1 163930
ID# 2
Sequence #

DATE:
TIME: 06:14:90
Cass/pos: 0008/02

Normal WBC Pop
Abnormal RBC Pop
Normal PLT Pop

	WBC	7.4			RBC	7.02
		%	#		HGB	13.5
	NE	55.3	4.1		HCT	42.5
	LY	37.6	2.8		MCV	60.4
	MO	5.8	0.4		MCH	19.2
	EO	2.1	0.2		MCHC	31.8
	BA	0.0	0.0		RDW	16.2
					PLT	206
					MPV	9.7

SUSPECT FLAGS:

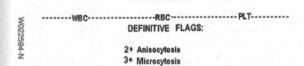

--------WBC-----------------RBC-------------------PLT----------
DEFINITIVE FLAGS:

2+ Anisocytosis
3+ Microcytosis

A. Iron deficiency anemia (IDA)
B. Polycythemia vera (PV)
C. Sideroblastic anemia
D. β-Thalassemia minor

Hematology/Evaluate laboratory data to recognize health and disease states/2

18. Review the following CBC results:

WBCs	11.0×10^9/L	MCV	85.0 fL
RBCs	3.52×10^{12}/L	MCH	28.4 pg
Hgb	10.0 g/dL	MCHC	33.4%
Hct	29.9 mL/dL	PLT	155×10^9/L
12 NRBCs/100 WBC			

RBC Morphology: Moderate polychromasia, 3+ target cells, few schistocytes

Which of the following additional laboratory tests would yield informative diagnostic information for this patient?
A. Osmotic fragility
B. Hgb electrophoresis
C. Sugar water test
D. Bone marrow examination

Hematology/Correlate laboratory data with other laboratory data to assess test results/3

Answers to Questions 17–18

17. D β-Thalassemia minor can easily be detected by noting an abnormally elevated RBC count, an Hct that does not correlate with the elevated RBC count, in conjunction with a decreased MCV. Although thalassemia and IDA are both microcytic, hypochromic processes, thalassemia can be differentiated from IDA because in IDA the RBC count, Hgb, and Hct values are usually decreased along with the MCV. Although the RBC count is increased in PV, the Hct must also be higher than 50% to consider a diagnosis of PV.

18. B The findings of a moderate anemia, numerous target cells seen on a peripheral blood smear, as well as the presence of NRBCs are often associated with hemoglobinopathies. Hemoglobin electrophoresis at alkaline pH is a commonly performed test to correctly diagnose the type of hemoglobinopathy.

BIBLIOGRAPHY

1. Harmening, D.: Clinical Hematology and Fundamentals of Hemostasis, ed 4. F.A. Davis, Philadelphia, 2002.
2. Handin, R.I., Lux, S.E., and Stossel, T.P.: Principles and Practice of Hematology. J.B. Lippincott, Philadelphia, 1995.
3. Jandl, J.H.: Blood Pathophysiology. Blackwell Scientific, Cambridge, England, 1991.
4. Koepke, J.A.: Practical Laboratory Hematology. Churchill Livingstone, New York, 1991.
5. Lotspeich-Steininger, C.A., Stein-Martin, E.A., and Koepke, J.A. (eds.): Clinical Hematology: Principles, Procedures, Correlations. JB Lippincott, Philadelphia, 1992.
6. McKenzie, S.B.: Textbook of Hematology. Lea & Febiger, Philadelphia, 1988.
7. Turgeon, M.L.: Clinical Hematology: Theory and Procedures, ed 2. Little, Brown & Company, Boston, 2005.
8. Williams, W. (ed.): Hematology. McGraw-Hill, New York, 1995.

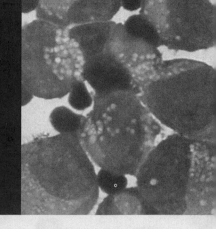

CHAPTER **2**

Hemostasis

2.1   COAGULATION/FIBRINOLYTIC SYSTEMS

2.2   PLATELET/VASCULAR DISORDERS

2.3   COAGULATION SYSTEM DISORDERS

2.4   INHIBITORS, THROMBOTIC DISORDERS, AND ANTICOAGULANT DRUGS

2.5   PROBLEM SOLVING IN HEMOSTASIS

1. The anticoagulant of choice for most routine coagulation studies is:
   A. Sodium oxalate
   B. Sodium citrate
   C. Heparin
   D. Ethlyenediaminetetraacetic acid (EDTA)

   Hemostasis/Select methods/Reagents/Specimen collection and handling/Specimen/1

2. Which ratio of anticoagulant-to-blood is correct for coagulation procedures?
   A. 1:4
   B. 1:5
   C. 1:9
   D. 1:10

   Hemostasis/Select methods/Reagents/Specimen collection and handling/Specimen/1

3. Which results would be expected for the prothrombin time (PT) and activated partial thromboplastin time (APTT) in a patient with polycythemia?
   A. Both prolonged
   B. Both shortened
   C. Normal PT, prolonged APTT
   D. Both normal

   Hemostasis/Correlate clinical and laboratory data/Coagulation tests/2

4. What reagents are used in the PT test?
   A. Thromboplastin and sodium chloride
   B. Thromboplastin and potassium chloride
   C. Thromboplastin and calcium
   D. Actin and calcium chloride

   Hemostasis/Select methods/Reagents/Coagulation tests/1

5. Which test would be abnormal in a patient with Stuart-Prower factor (factor X) deficiency?
   A. PT only
   B. APTT only
   C. PT and APTT
   D. Thrombin time

   Hemostasis/Correlate clinical and laboratory data/Coagulation tests/2

Answers to Questions 1–5

1. **B** The anticoagulant of choice for most coagulation procedures is sodium citrate (3.2%). Because factors V and VIII are more labile in sodium oxalate, heparin neutralizes thrombin, and EDTA inhibits thrombin's action on fibrinogen, these anticoagulants are not used for routine coagulation studies.

2. **C** The optimum ratio of anticoagulant to blood is one part anticoagulant to nine parts of blood. The anticoagulant supplied in this amount is sufficient to bind all the available calcium, thereby preventing clotting.

3. **A** The volume of blood in a polycythemic patient contains so little plasma that excess anticoagulant remains and is available to bind to reagent calcium, thereby resulting in prolongation of the PT and APTT. For more accurate results, the plasma:anticoagulant ratio can be modified by decreasing the amount of anticoagulant in the collection tube using the following formula: $(0.00185)(V)(100-H) = C$, where V = blood volume in mL; H = patient's Hct; and C = volume of anticoagulant. A new sample should be drawn to rerun the PT and APTT.

4. **C** Thromboplastin and calcium (combined into a single reagent) replace the tissue thromboplastin and calcium necessary in vivo to activate factor VII to factor VIIa. This ultimately generates thrombin from prothrombin via the coagulation cascade.

5. **C** Stuart-Prower factor (factor X) is involved in the common pathway of the coagulation cascade; therefore, its deficiency prolongs both the PT and APTT. Activated factor X along with factor V in the presence of calcium and platelet factor III (PF3) converts prothrombin (factor II) to the active enzyme thrombin (factor IIa).

6. Which clotting factor is *not* measured by PT and APTT tests?
   A. Factor VIII
   B. Factor IX
   C. Factor V
   D. Factor XIII

   Hemostasis/Apply principles of basic laboratory procedures/Coagulation tests/1

7. A modification of which procedure can be used to measure fibrinogen?
   A. PT
   B. APTT
   C. Thrombin time
   D. Fibrin degradation products

   Hemostasis/Apply principles of basic laboratory procedures/Coagulation tests/2

8. Which of the following characterizes vitamin K?
   A. It is required for biological activity of fibrinolysis
   B. Its activity is enhanced by heparin therapy
   C. It is required for carboxylation of glutamate residues of some coagulation factors
   D. It is made by the endothelial cells

   Hemostasis/Apply knowledge of fundamental biological characteristics/Vitamin K/2

9. Which statement about the fibrinogen/fibrin degradation product test is correct?
   A. It detects early degradation products
   B. It is decreased in disseminated intravascular coagulation (DIC)
   C. It evaluates the coagulation system
   D. It detects late degradation products

   Hemostasis/Apply principles of basic laboratory procedures/FDPs/2

10. Which of the following platelet aggregating agents demonstrates a monophasic aggregation curve when used in optimal concentration?
    A. Thrombin
    B. Collagen
    C. Adenosine diphosphate (ADP)
    D. Epinephrine

    Hemostasis/Apply knowledge of fundamental biological characteristics/Aggregating agents/1

11. Which coagulation test(s) would be abnormal in a vitamin K–deficient patient?
    A. PT only
    B. PT and APTT
    C. Fibrinogen level
    D. Thrombin time

    Hemostasis/Correlate clinical and laboratory data/Coagulation tests/2

12. Which of the following is correct regarding the international normalized ratio (INR)?
    A. It uses the International Sensitivity Ratio (ISR)
    B. It standardizes PT results
    C. It standardizes APTT results
    D. It is used to monitor heparin therapy

    Hemostasis/Apply knowledge of fundamental biological characteristics/INR/2

Answers to Questions 6–12

6. **D** Factor XIII is not measured by the PT or APTT. Factor XIII (fibrin stabilizing factor) is a transamidase. It creates covalent bonds between fibrin monomers formed during the coagulation process to produce a stable fibrin clot. In the absence of factor XIII, the hydrogen bonded fibrin polymers are soluble in 5M urea or in 1% monochloroacetic acid.

7. **C** Fibrinogen can be quantitatively measured by a modification of the thrombin time by diluting the plasma, since the thrombin clotting time of diluted plasma is inversely proportional to the concentration of fibrinogen (principle of Clauss method).

8. **C** Vitamin K is necessary for activation of vitamin K–dependent clotting factors (II, VII, IX, and X) . This activation is accomplished by carboxylation of glutamic acid residues of the inactive clotting factors. The activity of vitamin K is not enhanced by heparin therapy. Vitamin K is present in a variety of foods and is also the only vitamin made by the organisms living in the intestine.

9. **D** The fibrin degradation product (FDP) test detects the late degradation products (fragments D and E) and not the early ones (fragments X and Y).

10. **B** Collagen is the only commonly used agent that demonstrates a single-wave (monophasic) response preceded by a lag time.

11. **B** Patients with vitamin K deficiency exhibit decreased production of functional prothrombin proteins (factors II, VII, IX, and X). Decreased levels of these factors prolong both the PT and APTT.

12. **B** INR is used to standarize PT results to adjust for the difference in thromboplastin reagents made by different manufacturers and used by various institutions. The INR calculation uses the International sensitivity index (ISI) value and is used to monitor an oral anticoagulant such as warfarin. INR is not used to standarize APTT testing

13. Which of the following is referred to as an endogenous activator of plasminogen?
  A. Streptokinase
  B. Transamidase
  C. Tissue plasminogen activator
  D. Stuart-Prower factor

Hemostasis/Apply knowledge of fundamental biological characteristics/Plasminogen/2

14. Which protein is the primary inhibitor of the fibrinolytic system?
  A. Protein C
  B. Protein S
  C. α_2-Antiplasmin
  D. α_2-Macroglobulin

Hemostasis/Apply knowledge of fundamental biological characteristics/Plasmin/1

15. Which of the following statements is correct regarding the D-dimer test?
  A. Levels are decreased in DIC
  B. Test detects polypeptides A and B
  C. Test detects fragments D and E
  D. Test has a negative predictive value

Hemostasis/Apply principles of basic laboratory procedures/D-dimer/2

16. A protein that plays a role in both coagulation and platelet aggregation is:
  A. Factor I
  B. Factor VIII
  C. Factor IX
  D. Factor XI

Hemostasis/Apply knowledge of fundamental biological characteristics/Clotting factors/2

17. A standard 4.5 mL blue top tube filled with 3.0 mL of blood was submitted to the laboratory for PT and APTT tests. The sample is from a patient undergoing surgery the following morning for a tonsillectomy. Which of the following is the necessary course of action by the technologist?
  A. Run both tests in duplicate and report the average result
  B. Reject the sample and request a new sample
  C. Report the PT result
  D. Report the APTT result

Hemostasis/Select methods/Reagents/Specimen collection and handling/Specimen/2

18. Which statement is correct regarding sample storage for the prothrombin time test?
  A. Stable for 24 hours if the sample is capped
  B. Stable for 24 hours if the sample is refrigerated at 4°C
  C. Stable for 4 hours if the sample is stored at 4°C
  D. Should be run within 8 hours

Hemostasis/Select methods/Reagents/Specimen collection and handling/Specimen/2

Answers to Questions 13–18

13. **C** Tissue plasminogen activator (tPA) is an endogenous (produced in the body) activator of plasminogen. It is released from the endothelial cells by the action of protein C. It converts plasminogen to plasmin. Streptokinase is an exogenous (not made in the body) activator of plasminogen.

14. **C** α_2-Antiplasmin is the main inhibitor of plasmin. It inhibits plasmin by forming a 1:1 stoichiometric complex with any free plasmin in the plasma and, therefore, prevents the binding of plasmin to fibrin and fibrinogen.

15. **D** D-dimer evaluates fibrin degradation. It is a nonspecific screening test that is increased in many conditions in which fibrinolysis is increased, such as DIC and fibrinolytic therapy. The D-dimer test is widely used to rule out thrombosis and thrombotic activities. The negative predictive value of a test is the probability that a person with a negative result is free of the disease the test is meant to detect. Therefore, a negative D-dimer test rules out thrombosis and hence further laboratory investigations are not required.

16. **A** Factor I (fibrinogen) is necessary for platelet aggregation along with the glycoprotein IIb/IIIa complex. Factor I is also a substrate in the common pathway of coagulation. Thrombin acts on fibrinogen to form fibrin clots.

17. **B** A standard blue top tube contains 4.5 mL blood + 0.5 mL sodium citrate. The tube should be 90% full. A tube with 3.0 mL blood should be rejected as quantity not sufficient (QNS). QNS samples alter the necessary blood to an anticoagulant ratio of 9:1. The excess anticoagulant in a QNS sample binds to the reagent calcium, thereby resulting in prolongation of the PT and APTT.

18. **A** According to Clinical Laboratory Standards Institute (CLSI, formerly NCCLS) guidelines, plasma samples for PT testing are stable for 24 hours at room temperature if capped. Refrigerating the sample causes cold activation of factor VII and, therefore, shortened PT results. The APTT samples are stable for 4 hours if stored at 4°C.

19. In primary fibrinolysis, the fibrinolytic activity results in response to:
   A. Increased fibrin formation
   B. Spontaneous activation of fibrinolysis
   C. Increased fibrin monomers
   D. DIC

Hemostasis/Apply knowledge of fundamental biological characteristics/Fibrinolysis/2

20. Plasminogen deficiency is associated with:
   A. Bleeding
   B. Thrombosis
   C. Increased fibrinolysis
   D. Increased coagulation

Hemostasis/Correlate clinical and laboratory data/ Plasminogen/2

19. **B** Primary fibrinolysis is a rare pathological condition in which a spontaneous systemic fibrinolysis occurs. Plasmin is formed in the absence of coagulation activation and clot formation. Primary fibrinolysis is associated with increased production of plasminogen and plasmin, decreased plasmin removal from the circulation, and spontaneous bleeding.

20. **B** Plasminogen deficiency is associated with thrombosis. Plasminogen is an important component of the fibrinolytic system. Plasminogen is activated to plasmin, which is necessary for degradation of fibrin clots to prevent thrombosis. When plasminogen is deficient, plasmin is not formed, causing a defect in the clot lysing processes.

1. **Thrombotic thrombocytopenic purpura (TTP) is characterized by:**
   A. Prolonged PT
   B. Increased platelet aggregation
   C. Thrombocytosis
   D. Prolonged APTT

   Hemostasis/Correlate clinical and laboratory data/ Platelet/2

2. **Thrombocytopenia may be associated with:**
   A. Postsplenectomy
   B. Hypersplenism
   C. Acute blood loss
   D. Increased proliferation of pluripotential stem cells

   Hemostasis/Apply knowledge of fundamental biological characteristics/Platelets/2

3. **Aspirin prevents platelet aggregation by inhibiting the action of which enzyme?**
   A. Phospholipase
   B. Cyclo-oxygenase
   C. Thromboxane A_2 synthetase
   D. Prostacyclin synthetase

   Hemostasis/Apply knowledge of fundamental biological characteristics/Platelets/1

4. **Normal platelet adhesion depends upon:**
   A. Fibrinogen
   B. Glycoprotein Ib
   C. Glycoprotein IIb, IIIa complex
   D. Calcium

   Hemostasis/Apply knowledge of fundamental biological characteristics/Platelets/1

5. **Which of the following test results is normal in a patient with classic von Willebrand's disease ?**
   A. Bleeding time
   B. Activated partial thromboplastin time
   C. Platelet count
   D. Factor VIII:C and von Willebrand's factor (VWF) levels

   Hemostasis/Correlate clinical and laboratory data/Platelet disorders/3

Answers to Questions 1–5

1. **B** Thrombotic thrombocytopenic purpura (TTP) is a quantitative platelet disorder associated with increased intravascular platelet activation and aggregation resulting in thrombocytopenia. The PT and APTT results are normal in TTP.

2. **B** Hypersplenism is associated with thrombocytopenia. In this condition, up to 90% of platelets can be sequestered in the spleen, causing decreases in circulatory platelets. Postsplenectomy, acute blood loss, and increased proliferation of pluripotential stem cells are associated with thrombocytosis.

3. **B** Aspirin prevents platelet aggregation by inhibiting the activity of the enzyme cyclo-oxygenase. This inhibition prevents the formation of thromboxane A_2 (TXA2), which serves as a potent platelet aggregator.

4. **B** Glycoprotein Ib is a platelet receptor for VWF. Glycoprotein Ib and VWF are both necessary for a normal platelet adhesion. Other proteins that play a role in platelet adhesion are glycoproteins V and IX.

5. **C** Von Willebrand's disease is an inherited, qualitative platelet disorder resulting in increased bleeding time, prolonged APTT, and decreased factor VIII:C and VWF levels. The platelet count and morphology are generally normal in von Willebrand's disease.

6. Bernard-Soulier syndrome is associated with:
  A. Decreased bleeding time
  B. Decreased factor VIII assay
  C. Thrombocytopenia and giant platelets
  D. Abnormal platelet aggregation to ADP

  Hemostasis/Correlate clinical and laboratory data/
  Platelet disorders/3

7. When performing platelet aggregation studies, which set of platelet aggregation results would most likely be associated with Bernard-Soulier syndrome?
  A. Normal platelet aggregation to collagen, ADP, and ristocetin
  B. Normal platelet aggregation to collagen, ADP, and epinephrine; decreased aggregation to ristocetin
  C. Normal platelet aggregation to epinephrine and ristocetin; decreased aggregation to collagen and ADP
  D. Normal platelet aggregation to epinephrine, ristocetin, and collagen; decreased aggregation to ADP

  Hemostasis/Correlate clinical and laboratory data/
  Platelet disorders/3

8. Which set of platelet responses would be most likely associated with Glanzmann's thrombasthenia?
  A. Normal platelet aggregation to ADP and ristocetin; decreased aggregation to collagen
  B. Normal platelet aggregation to collagen; decreased aggregation to ADP and ristocetin
  C. Normal platelet aggregation to ristocetin; decreased aggregation to collagen, ADP, and epinephrine
  D. Normal platelet aggregation to ADP; decreased aggregation to collagen and ristocetin

  Hemostasis/Correlate clinical and laboratory data/
  Platelet disorders/3

9. Which of the following is a characteristic of acute idiopathic thrombocytopenic purpura?
  A. Spontaneous remission within a few weeks
  B. Predominantly seen in adults
  C. Nonimmune platelet destruction
  D. Insidious onset

  Hemostasis/Apply knowledge of fundamental biological
  characteristics/Platelet disorders/2

10. TTP differs from DIC in that:
  A. APTT is normal in TTP but prolonged in DIC
  B. Schistocytes are not present in TTP but are present in DIC
  C. Platelet count is decreased in TTP but normal in DIC
  D. PT is prolonged in TTP but decreased in DIC

  Hemostasis/Correlate clinical and laboratory data/
  Platelet disorders/3

11. Several hours after birth, a baby boy develops petechiae and purpura and a hemorrhagic diathesis.

The platelet count is 18×10^9/L. What is the most likely explanation for the low platelet count?
  A. Drug-induced thrombocytopenia
  B. Secondary thrombocytopenia
  C. Isoimmune neonatal thrombocytopenia
  D. Neonatal DIC

  Hemostasis/Correlate clinical and laboratory data/
  Platelet disorders/3

Answers to Questions 6–11

6. **C** Bernard-Soulier syndrome is associated with thrombocytopenia and giant platelets. It is a qualitative platelet disorder caused by the deficiency of glycoprotein Ib. In Bernard-Soulier syndrome, platelet aggregation to ADP is normal and bleeding time is prolonged. Factor VIII assay is not indicated for this diagnosis.

7. **B** Bernard-Soulier syndrome is a disorder of platelet adhesion caused by deficiency of glycoprotein Ib. Platelet aggregation is normal in response to collagen, ADP, and epinephrine but abnormal in response to ristocetin.

8. **C** Glanzmann's thrombasthenia is a disorder of platelet aggregation. Platelet aggregation is normal in response to ristocetin but abnormal in response to collagen, ADP, and epinephrine.

9. **A** Acute idiopathic thrombocytopenic purpura is an immune-mediated disorder found predominantly in children. It is commonly associated with infection (primarily viral). It is characterized by abrupt onset, and spontaneous remission usually occurs within several weeks.

10. **A** In DIC, the PT and APTT are both prolonged, the platelet count is decreased, and schistocytes are seen in the peripheral smear. Thrombotic thrombocytopenic purpura is a platelet disorder in which platelet aggregation increases, resulting in thrombocytopenia. Schistocytes are present in TTP as a result of microangiopathic hemolytic anemia; however, the PT and APTT are both normal.

11. **C** Isoimmune neonatal thrombocytopenia is similar to the hemolytic disease of the fetus and newborn. It results from immunization of the mother by fetal platelet antigens. The maternal antibody produced is most often directed against the platelet A^1 (Pl^{A1}) antigen on the fetal red cells. The maternal antibodies cross the placenta, resulting in thrombocytopenia in the fetus. Isoimmune neonatal thrombocytopenia is reported rarely with other platelet antigens such as Pl^{A2}.

12. Which of the following is associated with post-transfusion purpura (PTP)?
    A. Nonimmune thrombocytopenia/alloantibodies
    B. Immune-mediated thrombocytopenia/alloantibodies
    C. Immune-mediated thrombocytopenia/autoantibodies
    D. Nonimmune-mediated thrombocytopenia/autoantibodies

    Hemostasis/Apply knowledge of fundamental biological characteristics/Platelet disorders/2

13. Hemolytic uremic syndrome (HUS) is associated with:
    A. Fever, thrombocytosis, anemia, and renal failure
    B. Fever, granulocytosis, and thrombocytosis
    C. *Escherichia coli* 0157:H7
    D. Leukocytosis and thrombocytosis

    Hemostasis/Apply knowledge of fundamental biological characteristics/Platelet disorders/2

14. Storage pool deficiencies are defects of:
    A. Platelet adhesion
    B. Platelet aggregation
    C. Platelet granules
    D. Platelet production

    Hemostasis/Apply knowledge of fundamental biological characteristics/Platelet disorders/1

15. Lumi-aggregation measures:
    A. Platelet aggregation only
    B. Platelet aggregation and ATP release
    C. Platelet adhesion
    D. Platelet glycoprotein Ib

    Hemostasis/Select methods/Reagents/Specimen collection and handling/Aggregometry/1

16. Neurological findings may be commonly associated with which of the following disorders?
    A. HUS
    B. TTP
    C. ITP
    D. PTP

    Hemostasis/Apply knowledge of fundamental biological characteristics/Platelet function/1

17. Which of the following is correct regarding acquired thrombotic thrombocytopenic purpura?
    A. Autoimmune disease
    B. Decreased VWF
    C. Decreased platelet aggregation
    D. Decreased platelet adhesion

    Hemostasis/Apply knowledge of fundamental biological characteristics/Platelet disorders/2

18. Hereditary hemorrhagic telangiectasia is a disorder of:
    A. Platelets
    B. Clotting proteins
    C. Fibrinolysis
    D. Connective tissue

    Hemostasis/Apply knowledge of fundamental biological characteristics/Vascular disorders/2

Answers to Questions 12–18

12. **B** Post-transfusion purpura is an alloantibody-mediated thrombocytopenia. Thrombocytopenia occurs about 1 week after transfusion with platelet-contaminated products. PTP is believed to result from an anamnestic immune response. In the majority of cases the alloantibody produced is against platelet antigen A^1 (Pl^{A1}), also referred to as HPA-1a.

13. **C** HUS is caused by *E. coli* 0157:H7. It is associated with ingestion of *E. coli*– contaminated foods and is commonly seen in children. The clinical manifestations in HUS are fever, diarrhea, thrombocytopenia, microangiopathic hemolytic anemia, and renal failure.

14. **C** Storage pool deficiencies are defects of platelet granules. Most commonly, a decrease in platelet dense granules is present with decreased release of ADP, ATP, calcium, and serotonin from platelet-dense granules.

15. **B** Lumi-aggregation measures platelet aggregation and ATP release. It is performed on whole blood diluted with saline. Platelet aggregation is measured by impedance, whereas ATP release is measured by addition of luciferin to a blood sample. There is no ATP release in storage pool deficiencies.

16. **B** TTP is characterized by neurological problems, fever, thrombocytopenia, microangiopathic hemolytic anemia, and renal failure.

17. **A** Acquired TTP is an autoimmune disease associated with autoantibodies produced against VWF cleaving enzyme (ADAMTS-13). This deficiency results in an increase in plasma VWF and consequently increased platelet aggregation and thrombocytopenia.

18. **D** Hereditary hemorrhagic telangiectasia (Osler-Weber-Rendu syndrome) is a connective tissue disorder associated with telangiectases of the mucous membranes and skin. Lesions may develop on the tongue, lips, palate, face, hands, nasal mucosa, and throughout the gastrointestinal tract. This disorder is an autosomal dominant condition that usually manifests itself in adolescence or early adulthood.

19. Which of the following prevents platelet aggregation?
   A. Thromboxane A_2
   B. Thromboxane B_2
   C. Prostacyclin
   D. Antithrombin

   Hemostasis/Apply knowledge of fundamental biological characteristics/Platelets/2

20. Which defect characterizes Gray's syndrome?
   A. Platelet adhesion defect
   B. Dense granule defect
   C. Alpha granule defect
   D. Coagulation defect

   Hemostasis/Apply knowledge of fundamental biological characteristics/Platelet disorders/2

Answers to Questions 19–20

19. **C** Prostacyclin is released from the endothelium and is an inhibitor of platelet aggregation. Thromboxane A_2 promotes platelet aggregation. Thromboxane B_2 is an oxidized form of thromboxane A_2 and is excreted in the urine. Antithrombin is a physiological anticoagulant.

20. **C** Gray's syndrome is a platelet granule defect associated with a decrease in alpha granules resulting in decreased production of alpha granule proteins such as platelet factor 4 and beta thromboglobulin. Alpha granule deficiency results in the appearance of agranular platelets when viewed on a Wright's-stained blood smear.

1. The APTT is sensitive to a deficiency of which clotting factor?

   A. Factor VII
   B. Factor X
   C. PF3
   D. Calcium

   Hemostasis/Evaluate laboratory data to recognize health and disease states/Factor deficiency/2

2. Which test result would be normal in a patient with dysfibrinogenemia?

   A. Thrombin time
   B. APTT
   C. PT
   D. Immunological fibrinogen level

   Hemostasis/Correlate clinical and laboratory data/Factor deficiency/3

3. A patient with a prolonged PT is given intravenous vitamin K. The PT corrects to normal after 24 hours. What clinical condition most likely caused these results?

   A. Necrotic liver disease
   B. Factor X deficiency
   C. Fibrinogen deficiency
   D. Obstructive jaundice

   Hemostasis/Correlate clinical and laboratory data/ Vitamin K deficiency/3

4. A prolonged APTT and PT are corrected when mixed with normal plasma. Which factor is most likely deficient?

   A. V
   B. VIII
   C. IX
   D. XI

   Hemostasis/Evaluate laboratory data to recognize health and disease states/Factor deficiency/2

5. A prolonged APTT is corrected with factor VIII– deficient plasma but not with factor IX–deficient plasma. Which factor is deficient?

   A. V
   B. VIII
   C. IX
   D. X

   Hemostasis/Evaluate laboratory data to recognize health and disease states/Factor deficiency/2

Answers to Questions 1–5

1. **B** The APTT is sensitive to the deficiency of coagulation factors in the intrinsic pathway (factors XII, XI, IX, and VIII) and the common pathway (factors X, V, II, and I).

2. **D** The level of plasma fibrinogen determined immunologically is normal. In a patient with dysfibrinogenemia, fibrinogen is not polymerized properly, causing abnormal fibrinogen-dependent coagulation tests.

3. **D** Obstructive jaundice contributes to coagulation disorders by preventing vitamin K absorption. Vitamin K is fat-soluble and requires bile salts for absorption. Parenteral administration of vitamin K bypasses the bowel; hence the need for bile salts.

4. **A** Factor V, a common pathway factor deficiency, is most likely suspected, since both PT and APTT are prolonged and both are corrected when mixed with normal plasma.

5. **C** Since the prolonged APTT is not corrected with a factor IX–deficient plasma, factor IX is suspected to be deficient in the test plasma.

6. Which of the following is a characteristic of classic hemophilia A?
   A. Prolonged bleeding time
   B. Autosomal recessive inheritance
   C. Mild to severe bleeding episodes
   D. Prolonged PT

Hemostasis/Correlate clinical and laboratory data/ Hemostasis/Hemophilia/2

7. Refer to the following results:

   PT = prolonged

   APTT = prolonged

   Platelet count = decreased

   Bleeding time = increased

Which disorder may be indicated?
   A. Factor VIII deficiency
   B. von Willebrand's disease
   C. DIC
   D. Factor IX deficiency

Hemostasis/Correlate clinical and laboratory data/DIC/3

8. Which of the following is a predisposing condition for the development of DIC?
   A. Adenocarcinoma
   B. Idiopathic thrombocytopenic purpura (ITP)
   C. Post-transfusion purpura (PTP)
   D. Heparin-induced thrombocytopenia (HIT)

Hemostasis/Correlate clinical and laboratory data/ DIC/1

9. Factor XII deficiency is associated with:
   A. Bleeding episodes
   B. Epistaxis
   C. Decreased risk of thrombosis
   D. Increased risk of thrombosis

Hemostasis/Apply knowledge of fundamental biological characteristics/Factor deficiency/2

10. The following results were obtained on a patient: prolonged bleeding time, normal platelet count, normal PT, and prolonged APTT. Which of the following disorders is most consistent with these results?
   A. Hemophilia A
   B. Hemophilia B
   C. von Willebrand's disease
   D. Glanzmann's thrombasthenia

Hemostasis/Correlate clinical and laboratory data/von Willebrand's disease/3

11. The following laboratory results have been obtained from a 40-year-old woman: PT = 20 sec; APTT = 50 sec; thrombin time = 18 sec. What is the most probable diagnosis?
   A. Factor VII deficiency
   B. Factor VIII deficiency

   C. Factor X deficiency
   D. Hypofibrinogenemia

Hemostasis/Correlate clinical and laboratory data/Factor deficiency/3

Answers to Questions 6–11

6. **C** Hemophilia A (factor VIII deficiency) is characterized by mild to severe bleeding episodes, depending upon the concentration of factor VIII:C . Hemophilia A is inherited as a sex-linked disease. Bleeding time and prothrombin time are both normal in hemophilia A.

7. **C** In DIC, there is a diffuse intravascular generation of thrombin and fibrin. As a result, coagulation factors and platelets are consumed, resulting in decreased platelet count and increased PT, APTT, and bleeding time.

8. **A** Adenocarcinoma can liberate procoagulant (thromboplastic) substances that can activate prothrombin intravascularly. ITP is a thrombocytopenia caused by an autoantibody; PTP is a thrombocytopenia caused by an alloantibody directed against antigen-positive transfused platelets; HIT results from an antibody to heparin-PF4 complex causing thrombocytopenia in 1%–5% of patients who are on heparin therapy. In some affected persons thrombosis may also occur.

9. **D** Factor XII–deficient patients commonly have thrombotic episodes. Factor XII is the contact activator of the intrinsic pathway of coagulation. It also plays a major role in the fibrinolytic system by activating plasminogen to form plasmin. Hemorrhagic manifestations are not associated with factor XII deficiency because thrombin generated by the extrinsic pathway can activate factor XI to XIa, and factor VIIa/TF can activate factor IX to IXa.

10. **C** von Willebrand's disease is a disorder of platelet adhesion associated with decreased VWF and factor VIII, causing prolonged bleeding time and APTT. Hemophilia A and B are caused by factors VIII and IX deficiency, respectively, Bleeding time is normal in factor VIII and IX deficiencies and the APTT is prolonged. Glansmann's thrombasthenia is a platelet aggregation defect in which the APTT is normal.

11. **D** Fibrinogen (factor I) is a clotting protein of the common pathway and is evaluated by the thrombin time. In hypofibrinogenemia (fibrinogen concentration <100 mg/dL), the PT, APTT, and TT are prolonged. In factor VII deficiency the APTT is normal; in factor VIII deficiency the PT is normal; and in factor X deficiency the TT is normal.

12. When performing a factor VIII activity assay, a patient's plasma is mixed with:
  A. Normal patient's plasma
  B. Factor VIII deficient plasma
  C. Plasma with a high concentration of factor VIII
  D. Normal control plasma

Hemostasis/Apply principles of basic laboratory procedures/Coagulation tests/2

13. The **most suitable** product for treatment of factor VIII deficiency is:
  A. Fresh frozen plasma
  B. Factor VIII concentrate
  C. Prothrombin complex concentrate
  D. Factor V Leiden

Hemostasis/Correlate clinical and laboratory data/ Treatment/2

14. Which of the following is associated with an increased bleeding time and an abnormal platelet aggregation test?
  A. Factor VIII deficiency
  B. Factor VIII inhibitor
  C. Lupus anticoagulant
  D. Afibrinogenemia

Hemostasis/Correlate clinical and laboratory data/Factor deficiency/2

15. Refer to the following results:

  PT = normal

  APTT = prolonged

  Bleeding time= increased

  Platelet count = normal

  Platelet aggregation to ristocetin = abnormal

Which of the following disorders may be indicated?
  A. Factor VIII deficiency
  B. DIC
  C. von Willebrand's disease
  D. Factor IX deficiency

Hemostasis/Correlate clinical and laboratory data/DIC/2

16. Which results are associated with hemophilia A?
  A. Prolonged APTT, normal PT
  B. Prolonged PT and APTT
  C. Prolonged PT, normal APTT
  D. Normal PT and APTT

Hemostasis/Correlate clinical and laboratory data/ Hemophilia/2

17. Fibrin monomers are increased in which of the following conditions?
  A. Primary fibrinolysis
  B. DIC

  C. Factor VIII deficiency
  D. Fibrinogen deficiency

Hemostasis/Correlate clinical and laboratory data/DIC/2

Answers to Questions 12–17

12. **B** Coagulation factor assays are based upon the ability of the patient's plasma to correct any specific factor-deficient plasma. To measure for factor VIII activity in a patient's plasma, diluted patient plasma is mixed with a factor VIII–deficient plasma . An APTT test is performed on the mixture. Each laboratory should calculate its own normal ranges based on patient population, reagents, and the instrument used. An approximate range of 50%–150% is considered normal.

13. **B** Factor VIII concentrate (human or recombinant) is the treatment of choice for patients with factor VIII deficiency. Fresh frozen plasma contains factor VIII; however, it is no longer used as the primary treatment for factor VIII deficiency. Prothrombin complex concentrate is used to treat patients with factor VIII inhibitor.

14. **D** Fibrinogen is a plasma protein that is essential for platelet aggregation and fibrin formation. In afibrinogenemia both platelet function tests (bleeding time and platelet aggregation) are abnormal.

15. **C** VWF is involved in both platelet adhesion and coagulation via complexing with factor VIII. Therefore, in von Willebrand's disease (deficiency or functional abnormality of VWF) factor VIII is also decreased, causing an abnormal APTT as well as abnormal platelet function tests (bleeding time and platelet aggregation to ristocetin). The platelet count and the PT are not affected in VWF deficiency.

16. **A** Hemophilia A is associated with factor VIII deficiency. Factor VIII is a factor in the intrinsic coagulation pathway that is evaluated by the APTT and not the PT test. The PT test evaluates the extrinsic and common pathways.

17. **B** Increased fibrin monomers result from coagulation activation. DIC is an acquired condition associated with spontaneous activation of coagulation and fibrinolysis. In primary fibrinolysis, the fibrinolytic system is activated and fibrin monomers are normal.

18. Which of the following is associated with multiple factor deficiencies?

A. An inherited disorder of coagulation
B. Severe liver disease
C. Dysfibrinogenemia
D. Lupus anticoagulant

Hemostasis/Correlate clinical and laboratory data/Factor deficiency/2

19. Normal PT and APTT results in a patient with a poor wound healing may be associated with:

A. Factor VII deficiency
B. Factor VIII deficiency
C. Factor XII deficiency
D. Factor XIII deficiency

Hemostasis/Correlate clinical and laboratory data/Factor deficiency/2

20. Fletcher factor (prekallikrein) deficiency may be associated with:

A. Bleeding
B. Thrombosis
C. Thrombocytopenia
D. Thrombocytosis

Hemostasis/Correlate clinical and laboratory data/Factor deficiency/2

21. One of the complications associated with a severe hemophilia A is:

A. Hemarthrosis
B. Mucous membrane bleeding
C. Mild bleeding during surgery
D. Immune-mediated thrombocytopenia

Hemostasis/Apply knowledge of fundamental biological characteristics/Hemophilia/1

22. The most common subtype of classic von Willebrand's disease is:

A. Type 1
B. Type 2A
C. Type 2B
D. Type 3

Hemostasis/Apply knowledge of fundamental biological characteristics/von Willebrand's disease/2

Answers to Questions 18–22

18. **B** Most of the clotting factors are made in the liver. Therefore, severe liver disease results in multiple factor deficiencies. An inherited disorder of coagulation is commonly associated wth a single factor deficiency. Lupus anticoagualant is directed against the phospholipid-dependent coagulation factors. Dysfibrinogenemia results from an abnormal fibrinogen molecule.

19. **D** Factor XIII deficiency can lead to impaired wound healing and may cause severe bleeding problems. Factor XIII is a fibrin stabilizing factor that changes the fibrinogen bonds in fibrin polymers to stable covalent bonds. Factor XIII is not involved in the process of fibrin formation and, therefore, the PT and APTT are both normal.

20. **B** Fletcher factor (prekallikrein) is a contact factor. Activated prekallikrein is named kallikrein and is involved in activation of factors XII to XIIa. Like factor XII deficiency, Fletcher factor deficiency may be associated with thrombosis.

21. **A** In severe hemophilia A, factor VIII activity is less than 1%, resulting in a severe bleeding diathesis such as hemarthrosis (bleeding into the joints).

22. **A** VWF is a multimeric plasma glycoprotein that results in different subtypes of von Willebrand's disease with varied severity. The most common subtype is subtype 1, and 70%–80% of these cases are associated with mild bleeding. Subtype 3 involves the total absence of the von Willebrand's molecule and is associated with severe bleeding. Subtypes 2A and 2B result in deficiency of intermediate and/or high molecular weight portions of the von Willebrand molecule and are associated with 10%–12% and 3%–6% of cases of von Willebrand's disease, respectively.

1. **Which characteristic describes antithrombin (AT)?**
   A. It is synthesized in megakaryocytes
   B. It is activated by protein C
   C. It is a cofactor of heparin
   D. It is a pathological inhibitor of coagulation

   Hemostasis/Apply knowledge of fundamental biological characteristics/AT/1

2. **Which laboratory test is affected by heparin therapy?**
   A. Thrombin time
   B. Fibrinogen assay
   C. Bleeding time
   D. Reptilase time

   Hematology/Apply knowledge of fundamental biological characteristics/Hemostasis/Heparin/2

3. **An abnormal APTT caused by a pathological circulating anticoagulant is:**
   A. Corrected with factor VIII–deficient plasma
   B. Corrected with factor IX–deficient plasma
   C. Corrected with normal plasma
   D. Not corrected with normal plasma

   Hemostasis/Correlate clinical and laboratory data/Special test/2

4. **The lupus anticoagulant is directed against:**
   A. Factor VIII
   B. Factor IX
   C. Factor X
   D. Phospholipid

   Hemostasis/Apply knowledge of fundamental biological characteristics/Lupus anticoagulant/2

5. **Which statement about Coumadin (warfarin) is accurate?**
   A. It is a vitamin B antagonist.
   B. It is not recommended for pregnant and lactating women
   C. It needs antithrombin as a cofactor
   D. APTT test is used to monitor its dosage

   Hemostasis/Apply knowledge of fundamental biological characteristics/Warfarin/2

Answers to Questions 1–5

1. **C** Antithrombin is heparin cofactor and it is the most important naturally occurring physiological inhibitor of blood coagulation. It represents about 75% of antithrombotic activity and is an α_2 globulin made by the liver.

2. **A** Heparin is an antithrombin drug and therefore increases the thrombin time test. Reptilase is a thrombin-like snake venom protease that converts fibrinogen to fibrin. Reptilase time is not affected by heparin. Heparin therapy has no effect on either fibrinogen assay or bleeding time.

3. **D** In the presence of a pathological circulating anticoagulant, a mixing test using a normal plasma does not correct the abnormal APTT. These anticoagulants are pathological substances and are endogenously produced. They are either directed against a specific clotting factor or against a group of factors. A prolonged APTT due to a factor deficiency is corrected when mixed with a normal plasma. Factors VIII and IX deficient plasmas are used for assaying factor VIII and IX activities, repectively.

4. **D** The lupus anticoagulant reacts with phospholipids rather than clotting proteins and therefore interferes with phospholipid-dependent coagulation assays.

5. **B** Coumadin (warfarin) crosses the placenta and is present in human milk; it is not recommended for pregnant and lactating women. Warfarin is a vitamin K antagonist drug that retards synthesis of the active form of vitamin K–dependent factors (II, VII, IX, and X). Antithrombin is heparin (not warfarin) cofactor. The International Normalized Ratio (INR) is used to monitor the dosage.

6. Which statement regarding protein C is correct?
   A. It is a vitamin K–independent zymogen
   B. It is activated by fibrinogen
   C. It activates cofactors V and VIII
   D. Its activity is enhanced by protein S

Hemostasis/Apply knowledge of fundamental biological characteristics/Protein C/1

7. Which of the following is an appropriate screening test for the diagnosis of lupus anticoagulant?
   A. Thrombin time test
   B. Diluted Russell's viper venom test (DRVVT)
   C. D-dimer test
   D. FDP test

Hemostasis/Correlate clinical and laboratory data/Lupus anticoagulant/2

8. Which of the following is most commonly associated with activated protein C resistance (APCR)?
   A. Bleeding
   B. Thrombosis
   C. Epistaxis
   D. Menorrhagia

Hemostasis/Correlate clinical and laboratory data/APCR/2

9. A 50-year-old white man has been on heparin for the past 7 days. Which combination of the tests is expected to be abnormal?
   A. PT and APTT only
   B. APTT, TT only
   C. APTT, TT, fibrinogen assay
   D. PT, APTT, TT

Hemostasis/Correlate clinical and laboratory data/Heparin therapy/3

10. Mrs. Smith has the following laboratory results and no bleeding history:

> APTT: prolonged
>
> APTT: results on a 1:1 mixture of the patient plasma with normal plasma are:
>
> > Preincubation: prolonged APTT
> >
> > 2 hours' incubation: prolonged APTT

These results are consistent with:
   A. Factor VIII deficiency
   B. Factor VIII inhibitor
   C. Lupus anticoagulant
   D. Protein C deficiency

Hemostasis/Correlate clinical and laboratory data/LA/3

Answers to Questions 6–10

6. **D** Protein S functions as a cofactor of protein C and as such enhances its activity. Activated protein C inactivates factors Va and VIIIa.

7. **B** Russell's viper venom (RVV) reagent contains factors X and V, activating enzymes that are strongly phospholipid-dependent. The reagent contains RVV, calcium ions, and phospholipid. In the presence of phospholipid autoantibodies such as lupus anticoagulant, the reagent's phospholipid is partially neutralized. causing prolongation of the clotting time. Thrombin time evaluates fibrinogen; FDP and D-dimer tests evaluate fibrinogen and fibrin degradation products.

8. **B** Activated protein C resistance is the single most common cause of inherited thrombosis. In 90% of individuals, the cause is gene mutation of factor V (Leiden factor V). Affected individuals are predisposed to thrombosis, mainly after age 40. Heterozygous individuals may not manifest thrombosis unless other clinical conditions coexist.

9. **D** Heparin is a therapeutic anticoagulant with an antithrombin activity. Heparin also inhibits factors XIIa, XIa, Xa, and IXa. In patients receiving heparin therapy, the PT, APTT, and TT are all prolonged. Quantitative fibrinogen assay, however, is not affected by heparin therapy.

10. **C** Mixing studies differentiate factor deficiencies from factor inhibitors. Lupus anticoagulant is associated with thrombosis and it is directed against phospholipid-dependent coagulation tests such as APTT. In patients with lupus anticoagulant, the APTT on the mixture of patient's plasma with normal plasma remains prolonged immediately after mixing and following 2 hours of incubation. Factor VIII deficiency and factor VIII inhibitor are associated with bleeding. Factor VIII inhibitor is time- and temperature-dependent. The prolonged APTT may be corrected immediately after mixing and becomes abnormally prolonged following incubation. In factor VIII deficiency the prolonged APTT would be corrected after mixing the patient's plasma with normal plasma.

11. Thrombin-thrombomodulin complex is necessary for activation of:
  A. Protein C
  B. Antithrombin
  C. Protein S
  D. Factors V and VIII

Hemostasis/Apply knowledge of fundamental biological characteristics/Thrombomodulin/2

12. What test is used to monitor heparin therapy?
  A. INR
  B. APTT
  C. TT
  D. PT

Hemostasis/Correlate clinical and laboratory data/ Heparin therapy/3

13. What test is commonly used to monitor warfarin therapy?
  A. INR
  B. APTT
  C. TT
  D. Ecarin time

Hemostasis/Correlate clinical and laboratory data/ Warfarin therapy/3

14. What clotting factors (cofactors) are inhibited by protein S?
  A. V and X
  B. Va and VIIIa
  C. VIII and IX
  D. VIII and X

Hemostasis/Correlate clinical and laboratory data/ Clotting factors/3

15. Which drug promotes fibrinolysis?
  A. Warfarin
  B. Heparin
  C. Urokinase
  D. Aspirin

Hemostasis/Correlate clinical and laboratory data/Therapy/3

16. Diagnosis of lupus anticoagulant is confirmed by which of the following criteria?
  A. Decreased APTT
  B. Correction of the APPT by mixing studies
  C. Neutralization of the antibody by high concentration of platelets
  D. Confirmation that abnormal coagulation tests are time- and temperature-dependent

Hemostasis/Correlate clinical and laboratory data/LA/3

Answers to Questions 11–16

11. **A** Protein C is activated by thrombin-thrombomodulin complex. Thrombomodulin (TM) is a transmembrane protein that accelerates protein C activation 1000-fold by forming a complex with thrombin. When thrombin binds to TM, it loses its clotting function, including activation of factors V and VIII. Activated protein C deactivates factors Va and VIIIa. Protein S is a cofactor necessary for the activation of protein C.

12. **B** Heparin dosage may be monitored by the APTT test. Heparin dose is adjusted to an APTT of 1.5–2.5 times the upper reference limit of the laboratory. This level of APTT is equivalent to plasma heparin levels of 0.3 to 0.7 U/mL. The PT would be prolonged in heparin therapy, but the test is not as sensitive as the APTT. Heparin inhibits thrombin and therefore causes a prolonged TT. The TT test, however, is not used to monitor heparin therapy.

13. **A** Warfarin is a vitamin K antagonist drug. It inhibits vitamin K–dependent factors (II, VII, IX, and X) and other vitamin K–dependent proteins such as proteins C and S. Warfarin therapy is monitored by the INR. An INR of 2.0–3.0 is used as the target when monitoring warfarin therapy for prophylaxis and treatment of DVT. A higher dose of warfarin (giving an INR of 2.5–3.5) is required for patients with mechanical heart valves.

14. **B** Factors Va and VIIIa are deactivated by protein S and activated protein C.

15. **C** Urokinase is a thrombolytic drug commonly used to treat acute arterial thrombosis. Urokinase can also be used for the treatment of venous thromboembolism, myocardial infarction, and clotted catheters. Warfarin and heparin are anticoagulant drugs, whereas aspirin prevents platelet aggregation by inhibiting cyclo-oxygenase.

16. **C** The International Society of Hemostasis and Thrombosis has recommended four criteria for the diagnosis of lupus anticoagulant: (1) a prolongation of one or more of the phospholipid-dependent clotting tests such as APTT or DRVVT; (2) the presence of an inhibitor confirmed by mixing studies (not corrected); (3) evidence that the inhibitor is directed against phospholipids by neutralizing the antibodies with a high concentration of platelets (platelet neutralization test); (4) lack of any other causes for thrombosis. Lupus inhibitor is not commonly time- and temperature-dependent.

17. Which of the following abnormalities is consistent with the presence of lupus anticoagulant?
  A. Decreased APTT/bleeding complications
  B. Prolonged APTT/thrombosis
  C. Prolonged APTT/thrombocytosis
  D. Thrombocytosis/thrombosis

Hemostasis/Correlate clinical and laboratory data/ LA/3

18. Which of the following is a characteristic of low molecular weight heparin (LMWH)?
  A. Generally requires monitoring
  B. Specifically acts on factor Va
  C. Has a longer half-life than unfractionated heparin
  D. Can be used as a fibrinolytic agent

Hemostasis/Apply knowledge of fundamental biological characteristics/LMWH/1

19. Which of the following tests is most likely to be abnormal in patients taking aspirin?
  A. Platelet morphology
  B. Platelet count
  C. Bleeding time
  D. Prothrombin time

Hemostasis/Correlate clinical and laboratory data/ Aspirin therapy/2

20. Which of the following is associated with antithrombin deficiency?
  A. Thrombocytosis
  B. Thrombosis
  C. Thrombocytopenia
  D. Bleeding

Hemostasis/Correlate clinical and laboratory data/ Inhibitors/2

21. Which of the following may be associated with thrombotic events?
  A. Decreased protein C
  B. Increased fibrinolysis
  C. Afibrinogenemia
  D. ITP

Hemostasis/Correlate clinical and laboratory data/ Protein C/2

22. Aspirin resistance may be associated with:
  A. Bleeding
  B. Factor VIII deficiency
  C. Thrombosis
  D. Thrombocytosis

Hemostasis/Correlate clinical and laboratory data/ Aspirin resistance/2

23. A prolonged thrombin time and a normal reptilase time are indicative of:
  A. Afibrinogenemia
  B. Hypofibrinogenemia

  C. Aspirin therapy
  D. Heparin therapy

Hemostasis/Correlate clinical and laboratory data/Heparin therapy/2

Answers to Questions 17–23

17. B Lupus anticoagulant interferes with phospholipids in the APTT reagent, resulting in prolongation of APTT. However, in vivo, lupus anticoagulant decreases fibrinolytic activity, causing an increased risk of thrombosis. It does not result in a bleeding tendency unless there is a coexisting thrombocytopenia or other coagulation abnormality.

18. C Low molecular weight heparin (LMWH) is a small glycosaminoglycan that is derived from unfractionated heparin (UFH). The LMWH has a low affinity for plasma proteins and endothelial cells and therefore has a longer half-life. The half-life of the drug does not depend on the dosage. LMWH has an inhibitory effect on factors Xa and IIa. It does not require routine monitoring except in patients with renal disease or in pediatric patients.

19. C Aspirin is an antiplatelet drug. It prevents platelet aggregation, causing prolonged bleeding time. Aspirin has no effect on platelet count, platelet morphology, or clotting factors.

20. B Antithrombin is a physiological anticoagulant. It inhibits factors IIa, Xa, IXa, XIa, and XIIa. Deficiency of antithrombin is associated with thrombosis. Thrombotic events may be primary (in the absence of trigging factor) or may be associated with another risk factor such as pregnancy or surgery.

21. A Protein C is a physiological inhibitor of coagulation. It is activated by thrombin-thrombomodulin complex. Activated protein C inhibits cofactors Va and VIIIa. The deficiency of protein C is associated with thrombosis. Increased fibrinolysis, afibrinogenemia, and ITP are associated with bleeding.

22. C Up to 22% of patients taking aspirin become resistant to aspirin's antiplatelet effect. Patients who are aspirin-resistant have a higher rate of thrombosis (heart attacks and strokes).

23. D Heparin is an antithrombin drug causing prolonged TT in patients who are on heparin therapy. Reptilase is a thrombin-like snake venom protease that is able to clot fibrinogen. Reptilase time is not affected by heparin or LMWH. Reptilase time is prolonged in afibrinogenemia and hypofibrinogenemia. Aspirin therapy has no effect on TT or reptilase time.

24. Screening tests for thrombophilia should be performed:
A. On all pregnant women because of the thrombotic risk
B. On patients with a negative family history
C. On patients with thrombotic events occurring at a young age
D. On patients who are receiving anticoagulant therapy

25. Prothrombin G20210A is characterized by which of the following causes and conditions?
A. Single mutation of prothrombin molecule/bleeding
B. Single mutation of prothrombin molecule/thrombosis
C. Decreased levels of prothrombin in plasma/thrombosis
D. Increased levels of prothrombin in plasma/bleeding

Hemostasis/Correlate clinical and laboratory data/Prothrombin/3

26. Factor V Leiden promotes thrombosis by preventing:
A. Deactivation of factor Va
B. Activation of factor V
C. Activation of protein C
D. Activation of protein S

Hemostasis/Correlate clinical and laboratory data/Factor V Leiden/3

27. The incidence of antiphospholipid antibodies in the general population is:
A. <1%
B. 2%
C. 10%
D. 20%

Hemostasis/Apply knowledge of fundamental biological characteristics/LA/1

28. Which of the following laboratory tests is helpful in the diagnosis of aspirin resistance?
A. APTT
B. PT
C. Platelet count and morphology
D. Platelet aggregation

Hemostasis/Correlate clinical and laboratory data/Aspirin resistance/3

29. Which of the following complications may occur as a result of decreased tissue factor pathway inhibitor (TFPI)?
A. Increased hemorrhagic episodes
B. Increased thrombotic risk
C. Impaired platelet plug formation
D. Immune thrombocytopenia

Hemostasis/Apply knowledge of fundamental biological characteristics/Thrombosis/2

30. Factor VIII inhibitors occur in _____of patients with factor VIII deficiency?
A. 40%–50%
B. 30%–40%
C. 25%–30%
D. 10%–20%

Hemostasis/Apply knowledge of fundamental biological characteristics/Inhibitors/1

Answers to Questions 24–30

24. **C** Laboratory tests for evaluation of thrombophilia are justified in young patients with thrombotic events, in patients with a positive family history after a single thrombotic event, in those with recurrent spontaneous thrombosis, and in pregnancies associated with thrombosis.

25. **B** Prothrombin G20210A is defined as a single point mutation of the prothrombin gene, resulting in increased concentration of plasma prothrombin and thereby a risk factor for thrombosis. Prothrombin G20210A is the second most common cause of inherited hypercoagulability (behind factor V Leiden). It has the highest incidence in whites from southern Europe. The thrombotic episodes generally occur before age 40.

26. **A** Factor V Leiden is a single point mutation in the factor V gene that inhibits factor Va inactivation by protein C. Activated protein C enhances deactivation of factors Va and VIIIa.

27. **B** The incidence of antiphospholipid antibodies in the general population is about 2%.

28. **D** Currently, the platelet aggregation test is considered the gold standard for evaluation of aspirin resistance. In aspirin resistance, platelet aggregation is not inhibited by aspirin ingestion. Aspirin resistance has no effect on platelet count and morphology.

29. **B** Tissue factor pathway inhibitor (TFPI) is released from the vasculature and is the most important inhibitor of the extrinsic pathway. TFPI inhibits factors Xa and VIIa-TF complex. Therefore, the deficiency of TFPI is associated with thrombosis.

30. **D** Factor VIII inhibitors (antibodies) occur in 10%–20% of patients with factor VIII deficiency receiving factor VIII replacement.

31. Which therapy and resulting mode of action are appropriate for the treatment of a patient with a high titer of factor VIII inhibitors?
    A. Factor VIII concentrate to neutralize the antibodies
    B. Recombinant factorVIIa (rVIIa) to activate the common pathway
    C. Factor X concentrate to activate the common pathway
    D. Fresh frozen plasma to replace factor VIII

    Hemostasis/Apply knowledge of fundamental biological characteristics/Inhibitors/2

32. The Bethesda assay is used for which determination?
    A. Lupus anticoagulant titer
    B. Factor VIII inhibitor titer
    C. Factor V Leiden titer
    D. Protein S deficiency

    Hemostasis/Select methods/Reagents/Special tests/2

33. Hyperhomocysteinemia may be a risk factor for:
    A. Bleeding
    B. Thrombocytopenia
    C. Thrombosis
    D. Thrombocytopenia

    Hemostasis/Correlate clinical and laboratory data/Thrombosis/2

34. Which drug may be associated with deep venous thrombosis (DVT)?
    A. Aspirin
    B. tPA
    C. Oral contraceptives
    D. Plavix

    Hemostasis/Apply knowledge of fundamental biological characteristics/Thrombophilia/2

35. Hirudin may be used for the treatment of which of the following conditions?
    A. DVT
    B. Hemorrhage
    C. TTP
    D. Thrombocytosis

    Hemostasis/Apply knowledge of fundamental biological characteristics/Therapy/2

36. Heparin-induced thrombocytopenia results from:
    A. Antibodies to heparin
    B. Antibodies to platelets
    C. Antibodies to PF4
    D. Antibodies to heparin+PF4 complex

    Hemostasis/Apply knowledge of fundamental biological characteristics/Heparin treatment/2

Answers to Questions 31–36

31. **B** Recombinant factor VII (rVIIa) is effective for the treatment of a high titer factor VIII inhibitor. Factor VIIa can directly activate factors X to Xa in the absence of factors VIII and IX. Recombinant factor VIIa does not stimulate anamnestic responses in patients with factor VIII inhibitor. Factor VIII concentrate is used for a low titer VIII inhibitor. Factor X concentrate and FFP are not the treatments of choice for factor VIII inhibitor.

32. **B** The Bethesda assay is a quantitative assay for factor VIII inhibitor. In this assay normal plasma is incubated with different dilutions of the patient's plasma or a normal control. The inhibitor inactivates factor VIII present in normal plasma following incubation for 2 hours at 37°C. The residual activities in the sample are determined, and the inhibitor titer is calculated.

33. **C** Elevated plasma homocysteine is a risk factor for the development of venous thrombosis. Homocystinemia may be inherited or acquired. Acquired homocystinemia is caused by the dietary deficiencies of vitamins B_6, B_{12}, and folic acid.

34. **C** Oral contraceptive drugs are acquired risk factors for thrombosis. Aspirin and Plavix are antiplatelet drugs and tPA is a fibrinolytic drug used for the treatment of thrombosis.

35. **A** Hirudin is an inhibitor of thrombin and is used as an alternative to heparin for the treatment of thrombotic disorders such as DVT and thromboembolism in patients who have developed heparin-induced thrombocytopenia.

36. **D** Heparin-induced thrombocytopenia and thrombosis are immune processes caused by the production of antibodies to heparin-PF4 complex. This immune complex binds to platelet Fc receptors causing platelet activation and formation of platelet microparticles that in turn induce hypercoagulability and thrombocytopenia.

37. Which laboratory test is used to screen for activated protein C resistance?
   A. Mixing studies with normal plasma
   B. Mixing studies with factor-deficient plasma
   C. Modified APTT with and without activated protein C
   D. Modified PT with and without activated protein C

Hemostasis/Select methods/Reagents/Special tests/2

38. Ecarin clotting time may be used to monitor:
   A. Heparin therapy
   B. Warfarin therapy
   C. Fibrinolytic therapy
   D. Hirudin therapy

Hemostasis/Select methods/Reagents/Special tests/2

39. Which of the following may interfere with the activated protein C resistance (APCR) screening test?
   A. Lupus anticoagulant
   B. Protein C deficiency
   C. Antithrombin deficiency
   D. Protein S deficiency

Hemostasis/Correlate clinical and laboratory/Special tests/2

40. Thrombophilia may be associated with which of the following disorders?
   A. Afibrinogenemia
   B. Hypofibrinogenemia
   C. Factor VIII inhibitor
   D. Hyperfibrinogenemia

Hemostasis/Apply knowledge of fundamental biological characteristics/Fibrinogen/2

Answers to Questions 37–40

37. **C** Activated protein C resistance can be evaluated by a two-part APTT test. The APTT is measured on patient's plasma with and without the addition of activated protein C (APC). The result is expressed as the ratio of the APTT with APC to the APTT without APC. The normal ratio is 2 to 5. Patients with APCR have a lower ratio than the reference range. A positive screening test should be followed by a confirmatory test such as polymerase chain reaction (PCR) for factor V Leiden.

38. **D** Ecarin clotting time, a snake venom-based clotting assay, may be used to monitor hirudin therapy. The APTT is insensitive to hirudin levels above 0.6 mg/L, and this insensitivity may result in a drug overdose despite a monitoring protocol. Heparin therapy is monitored by the APTT; warfarin therapy is monitored by the INR. Fibrinolytic therapy may be monitored by D-dimer and fibrinogen assays.

39. **A** The lupus anticoagulant interferes with the APCR screening assay based on the APTT ratio with and without APC addition. Persons with the lupus anticoagulant have a prolonged APTT that renders the test invalid for APCR screening.

40. **D** Hyperfibrinogenemia is a risk factor for thrombophilia. Fibrinogen is an acute phase reactant and may be increased in inflammation, stress, obesity, smoking, and medications such as oral contraceptives. Hypofibrinogenemia, afibrinogenemia, and factor VIII inhibitors are associated with bleeding.

1. Patient History

A 3-year-old male was admitted to a hospital with scattered petechiae and epistaxis. The patient had normal growth and had no other medical problems except for chicken pox three weeks earlier. His family history was unremarkable.

Laboratory Results		
	Patient	**Reference Range**
PT:	11 sec	10–13 sec
APTT:	32 sec	28–37 sec
Platelet Count:	18,000/μL	150–450 $\times$ 10^3/μL
Bleeding time:	21 min	2–8 min

These clinical manifestations and laboratory results are consistent with which condition?

A. TTP

B. DIC

C. ITP

D. HUS

Hemostasis/Evaluate laboratory data to recognize health and disease states/Platelet disorders/3

Answer to Question 1

1. **C** These clinical manifestations and laboratory results are consistent with ITP. ITP is an autoimmune thrombocytopenia. In children, acute ITP thrombocytopenia occurs following a viral infection, as is the case in this 3-year-old patient. Clinical manifestations are associated with petechiae, purpura, and mucous membrane bleedings such as epistaxis and gingival bleeding. Abnormal laboratory tests include a very low platelet count and a prolonged bleeding time. Other causes of thrombocytopenia should be ruled out in patients with ITP

2. Patient History

A 12-year-old white male has the following symptoms: visible bruising on arms and legs, bruising after sports activities, and excessive postoperative hemorrhage following tonsillectomy 3 months ago. His family history revealed that his mother suffers from heavy menstrual bleeding, and his maternal grandfather had recurrent nosebleeds and bruising.

Laboratory Results

	Patient	Reference Range
Platelet Count:	350,000/µL	200–450×10^3/µL
Bleeding time:	15 min	3–8 min
PT:	11.0 sec	10–12 sec
APTT:	70 sec	28–37 sec
TT:	13 sec	10–15 sec

Platelet Aggregation

Normal aggregation with collagen, epinephrine, ADP
Abnormal aggregation with ristocetin

Confirmatory Tests	Patient	Reference Range
VWF:Rco	25%	45%–140%
VIII:C	20%	50%–150%
WWF:antigen	10%	45%–185%

These clinical manifestations and laboratory results are consistent with which diagnosis?
A. Factor VIII deficiency
B. von Willebrand's disease
C. Glanzmann's thrombasthenia
D. Bernard-Soulier syndrome

Hemostasis/Evaluate laboratory data to recognize health and disease states/Platelet disorders/3

3. The following results are obtained from a patient who developed severe bleeding:

Prolonged PT and APTT

Platelet count = 100×10^9/L

Fibrinogen = 40 mg/dL

Which of the following blood products should be recommended for transfusion?
A. Factor VIII concentrate
B. Platelets
C. Fresh frozen plasma
D. Cryoprecipitate

4. A 30-year-old woman develops signs and symptoms of thrombosis in her left lower leg following 5 days of heparin therapy. The patient had open-heart surgery 3 days previously and has been on heparin ever since. Which of the following would be the most helpful in making the diagnosis?

A. Fibrinogen assay
B. Prothrombin time
C. Platelet counts
D. Increased heparin dose

Hemostasis/Correlate clinical and laboratory data/Heparin therapy/3

Answers to Questions 2–4

2. **B** These clinical manifestations and laboratory results are consistent with von Willebrand's disease. von Willebrand's disease is an inherited bleeding disorder caused by abnormal platelet adhesion. Platelet adhesion depends on VWF and glycoprotein Ib. In von Willebrand's disease, VWF is deficient or dysfunctional. VWF promotes secondary hemostasis by acting as a carrier for factor VIII. Deficienct or dysfunctional VWF results in decreased factor VIII and therefore abnormal secondary hemostasis. The clinical manifestations associated with von Willebrand's disease are easy bruising, epistaxis, and bleeding after surgery. Abnormal laboratory test results are increased bleeding time and abnormal platelet aggregation to ristocetin, which is corrected on addition of normal plasma containing VWF. Activated partial thromboplastin time (APTT) is prolonged as a result of the deficiency of factor VIII. Factor VIII activity (VIII:C), VWF ristocetin cofactor activity (VWF:Rco), and VWF:antigenic activity (VWF:antigen) are all abnormal. The platelet count and prothrombin time are normal in von Willebrand's disease.

3. **D** Cryoprecipitate contains fibrinogen, factor VIII, and VWF. Fresh frozen plasma has all of the clotting factors; however, it is not the best choice if cryoprecipitate is available.

4. **C** The platelet count should be checked every other day in patients receiving heparin therapy. Heparin-induced thrombocytopenia (HIT) should be suspected in patients who are not responding to heparin therapy and/or are developing thrombocytopenia (50% below the baseline value) and thrombotic complications while on heparin therapy. Increase in heparin dose should be avoided in patients with the clinical symptoms of thrombosis while they are receiving heparin. Fibrinogen assay and PT are not the appropriate assays for monitoring heparin therapy, nor are they used to test for HIT.

5. The following laboratory results were obtained on a 25-year-old woman with menorrhagia after delivery of her second son. The patient has no previous bleeding history.

Normal platelet count; normal bleeding time; normal PT; prolonged APTT

Mixing of the patient's plasma with normal plasma corrected the prolonged APTT on immediate testing. However, mixing followed by a 2-hr incubation at 37°C caused a prolonged APTT. What is the most probable cause of these laboratory results?
A. Lupus anticoagulant
B. Factor VIII deficiency
C. Factor IX deficiency
D. Factor VIII inhibitor

Hemostasis/Correlate clinical and laboratory data/Inhibitors/3

6. A 62-year-old female presents with jaundice and the following laboratory data:

Peripheral blood smear: macrocytosis, target cells

Platelet count: 355 × 10⁹/L

PT: 25 sec (reference range =10–14)

APTT: 65 sec (reference range = 28–36)

Transaminases: elevated (AST:ALT>1)

Total and direct bilirubin: elevated

These clinical presentations and laboratory results are consistent with:

A. Inherited factor VII deficiency
B. DIC
C. Cirrhosis of the liver
D. von Willebrand's disease

Hemostasis/Correlate clinical and laboratory data/Coagulation disorders/3

7. When performing a mixing study, the patient's APTT is corrected to 12% of normal. What is the most appropriate interpretation of these findings?
A. The APTT is considered corrected
B. The APTT is considered uncorrected
C. The mixing study needs to be repeated
D. A circulating anticoagulant can be ruled out

Hemostasis/Correlate clinical and laboratory data/Mixing studies/3

5. **D** Factor VIII inhibitor is found in 10%–20% of hemophilia patients receiving replacement therapy. It may also develop in patients with immunological problems, women after childbirth, and patients with lymphoproliferative and plasma cell disorders, or it may develop in response to medications. Factor VIII inhibitor is an IgG immunoglobulin with an inhibitory effect that is time- and temperature-dependent. The presence of factor VIII inhibitor causes an elevated APTT in the face of a normal prothrombin time. Mixing studies in factors VIII and IX deficiencies will correct the prolonged APTT both at the immediate mixing stage and after incubation for 2 hours. The APTT would not be corrected by mixing studies if lupus anticoagulant was present. In addition, lupus anticoagulant is not associated with bleeding unless it coexists with thrombocytopenia.

6. **C** The clinical presentation and laboratory results in this patient are indicative of cirrhosis of the liver. Most of the clotting factors are made in the liver. A decrease in multiple clotting factors is associated with a prolonged PT and APTT. Macrocytosis and target cells are present in liver disease. The liver changes the unconjugated bilirubin to conjugated bilirubin. Conjugated bilirubin is excreted into the intestines, where the bilirubin is then converted to urobilinogen and excreted into the stool. In cirrhosis of the liver both necrosis and obstruction caused by scarring produce an increase in unconjugated and conjugated bilirubin, respectively. In addition, the liver enzymes are elevated.

7. **C** In mixing studies, correction occurs if a prolonged APTT result drops to within 10% of the result of normal human plasma. Only 50% factor activity is required for a normal PT or APTT. Clotting results >15% are not considered corrected, and results between 10–15% should be repeated. A circulating anticoagulant typically results in failure to correct the APTT with normal plasma.

8. A standard blue top tube filled appropriately (with 4.5 mL blood) was submitted to the laboratory for preoperative PT and APTT testing. The results of both tests were elevated. The patient's PT and APTT from the previous day were within normal limits, and he is not on heparin therapy. Which is the most appropriate first step to investigate the abnormal results?
- **A.** Report the result as obtained
- **B.** Perform a mixing study
- **C.** Check the sample for a clot
- **D.** Report the APTT only

Hemostasis/Apply knowledge to identify sources of errors/Proper samples/3

9. A plasma sample submitted to the lab for PT testing has been stored for 25 hours at 4°C. The PT result is shortened. What is the most probable cause?
- **A.** Factor VII deficiency
- **B.** Activation of factor VII due to exposure to cold temperature
- **C.** Lupus inhibitor
- **D.** Factor X inhibitor

Hemostasis/Apply knowledge to identify sources of errors/Sample storage/3

10. The APTT results are not elevated in a patient receiving heparin. Which of the following factors may be associated with the lack of response to heparin therapy in this patient?
- **A.** Protein C deficiency
- **B.** Antithrombin deficiency
- **C.** Protein S deficiency
- **D.** Factor VIII deficiency

Hemostasis/Correlate clinical and laboratory data/Inhibitors/3

11. A 50-year-old patient was admitted to the emergency room complaining of pain in her right leg. Her leg was red, swollen, and warm to the touch. Deep venous thrombosis was suspected, and the patient was started on heparin therapy. Which of the following is (are) the proper protocol to evaluate patients receiving heparin therapy?
- **A.** A baseline APTT and platelet count; APTT testing every 6 hours until the target is reached.
- **B.** Repeat APTT after 5 days postheparin therapy to adjust the therapeutic dose.
- **C.** Monitor the platelet count daily and every other day after heparin therapy is completed
- **D.** Monitor PT daily to adjust the therapeutic dose

Hemostasis/Correlate clinical and laboratory data/heparin therapy/2

Answers to Questions 8–11

8. **C** A clot can form because of inadequate mixing of the sample after venipuncture, if the blood fills the evacuated tube at a slow rate, or with traumatic venipuncture. In vitro, blood clots result in consumption of the clotting factors and therefore prolongation of PT, APTT, and other clot-based assays. If the clotting factors have been activated but the clot formation is incomplete, it may result in shortening of the PT and APTT. Checking the sample for a clot is the most reasonable step in this case.

9. **B** Samples for evaluation of PT are stable for 24 hours if kept at room temperature. Prolonged exposure to cold will activate factor VII, resulting in decreased PT results.

10. **B** Antithrombin deficiency in patients receiving heparin therapy may lead to heparin resistance and therefore lack of prolongation of APTT results. Antithrombin is heparin cofactor and as such increases heparin activities by 1000-fold. The deficiency of AT is associated with a poor response to heparin therapy.

11. **A** The baseline platelet count and APTT should be performed on all patients prior to administration of heparin. The response to heparin therapy varies among different patients for the following reasons: heparin half-life is decreased in extended thrombosis, and the anticoagulant activities of heparin change based upon nonspecific binding of heparin to plasma proteins. Therefore, heparin therapy should be closely monitored. Heparin dosage can be monitored by an APTT or activated clotting time (ACT) test but not by the PT. In addition, the platelet count should be monitored regularly during heparin therapy, since a decrease of the platelet count to 50% below the baseline value is significant and may be associated with HIT.

12. Patient History:

A 46-year-old female was admitted to the emergency room with complaints of headache, dizziness, lethargy, nausea, vomiting, and weakness. The patient had a gastrectomy procedure 4 months earlier to remove adenocarcinoma of the stomach. She was placed on mitomycin therapy. Diagnostic procedures indicated recurrence of the carcinoma.

Admission CBC results:

	Patient	Reference Range
WBC	17.1×10^9/L	$4.8–10.8 \times 10^9$/L
RBC	2.29×10^{12}/L	$3.80–5.50 \times 10^{12}$/L
Hgb	8.1 g/dL	12.0–15.2 g/dL
Hct	23%	37%–46%
MCV	95.7 fL	79–101 fL
MCH	35.4 pg	27–33 pg
MCHC	35.0 g/dL	31–34 g/dL
RDW	18.5	11.5–14.5
PLT	48.0×10^9/L	$140–450 \times 10^9$/L
MPV	11.2	7.4–9.4

Differential Counts (%)

Segmented neutrophils	79	30%–70%
Band neutrophils	3	0%–10%
Lymphocytes	11	20%–50%
Monocytes	6	2%–12%
Basophils	1	0%–2%
NRBCs (/100 WBCs)	3	0
Manual platelet count:	18×10^9/L	$140–450 \times 10^9$/L
Marked anisocytosis		none
Marked RBC fragmentation		none
PT, APTT, and TT:	Normal	

Additional Laboratory Data:

Urinalysis	Patient	Reference Range
pH	5.0	5-7
Protein	300 mg/dL	0-15 mg/dL
RBC	60–100/μL	0-5/μL
Casts	10/hpf granular and hyaline	Not detectable
Creatinine	3.1 mg/dL	0.7-1.3 mg/dL
BUN	39 mg/dL	8-22 mg/dL
Haptoglobin	5.0 mg/dL	50–150 mg/dL

These clinical manifestations and laboratory results are consistent with:
A. ITP
B. von Willebrand's disease
C. TTP
D. DIC

Hemostasis/Correlate clinical and laboratory data/ Platelet Disorders/3

Answer to Question 12

12. **C** The clinical manifestations and laboratory results in this patient are consistent with TTP. The clinical manifestations of TTP include microangiopathic hemolytic anemia (MAHA), thrombocytopenia, fever, renal failure, and neurological symptoms. The neurological symptoms in this patient are manifested by headache, dizziness, nausea, and vomiting. Weakness and lethargy are signs and symptoms of anemia. Low hemoglobin and hematocrit with normal MCV and MCHC indicate a normocytic/normochromic anemia. The presence of schistocytes on the peripheral blood with low platelet counts and low haptoglobin are consistent with microangiopathic hemolytic anemia. The high blood urea nitrogen and creatinine levels are characteristic of renal failure. The platelet count, performed on admission, was done on a hematology analyzer and was falsely elevated because of the presence of microcytes or fragmented red cells. The manual platelet count was much lower and correlates with the platelet estimate on the peripheral smear. The coagulation tests are normal in TTP. In von Willebrand's disease, the platelet count is normal and the APTT is usually abnormal. ITP is characterized by thrombocytopenia but HA is not. Although DIC is associated with a low platelet count and HA, it is characterizted by abnormal coagulation studies. The acute onset of symptoms may be related to mitomycin used for the treatment of gastric carcinoma in this patient.

13. Patient History

A 1-year-old infant was admitted to the hospital with recurrent epistaxis for the past 5 days. The past medical history revealed easy bruising and a severe nosebleed at 3 months of age, necessitating transfusion therapy. The mother had had a severe nosebleed 8 years ago. The father was reported to bleed easily after lacerations. The patient was transfused with 2 units of packed red cells upon admission.

Admission Laboratory Results

	Patient	Reference Range
Hgb:	4.5 g/dL	13-15 g/dL
Platelet count:	249 × 10⁹/L	150-450 × 10⁹/L
Bleeding time:	15 min	3-8 min
PT:	11.2 sec	11–13 sec
APTT:	34 sec	28–37 sec

Additional Laboratory Tests

Factor VIII assay	70%	50%–150%
Platelet aggregation:	Abnormal to ADP, epinephrine, and thrombin; normal to ristocetin	

These clinical manifestations and laboratory results are consistent with which condition?
A. von Willebrand's disease
B. Bernard-Soulier syndrome
C. Glanzmann's thrombasthenia
D. Factor VIII deficiency

Hemostasis/Correlate clinical and laboratory data/ Platelet disorders /3

14. Patient History:

A 30-year-old female was referred to the hospital for evaluation for multiple spontaneous abortions and current complaint of pain and swelling in her right leg. Her family history is unremarkable.

Laboratory Tests:	Patient	Reference Range
PT:	14.5 sec	11–13 sec
APTT:	63.0 sec	28–37 sec
Thrombin time:	12.0 sec	10–15 sec
Mixing Study APTT: Preincubation and after 2-hour incubation at 37°C	57.0 sec	
Platelet Neutralization Procedure:		
Patient plasma + freeze-thawed platelets	APTT: 35.0 sec	
Patient plasma + saline	APTT: 59.0 sec	
Anticardiolipin antibodies done by ELISA:	Negative	

These clinical manifestations and laboratory results are consistent with:

A. Factor VIII inhibitor
B. Factor VIII deficiency
C. Anticardiolipin antibodies
D. Lupus anticoagulant

Hemostasis/Correlate clinical and laboratory data/ Platelet disorders /3

Answers to Questions 13–14

13. **C** These clinical manifestations and laboratory results are consistent with Glansmann's thrombasthenia. Epistaxis and easy bruising are characteristics of platelet disorders. The positive family history is indicative of an inherited bleeding disorder. Laboratory tests reveal low hemoglobin levels due to epistaxis. The normal platelet count rules out any quantitative platelet disorder. The platelet count is typically low in Bernard-Soulier syndrome. The bleeding time test evaluates in vivo platelet function and number. Normal PT and APTT combined with a normal factor VIII assay rule out coagulation disorders. The laboratory test that confirms an inherited platelet disorder is platelet aggregation studies. Platelet aggregation is normal to ristocetin and abnormal to ADP, epinephrine, and thrombin. These results are consistent with Glansmann's thrombasthenia. Platelet aggregation is abnormal to ristocetin in von Willebrand disease and Bernard-Soulier syndrome.

14. **D** These clinical manifestations and laboratory results are consistent with lupus anticoagulant. Pain and swelling in ther right leg may be indicative of thrombosis. As many as 48% of women with repeated spontaneous abortions have lupus anticoagulant or/and antibody to phospholipid such as anticardiolipin antibodies. The unremarkable family history in this patient rules out an inherited thrombotic disorder. A normal TT rules out fibrinogen disorders. A prolonged PT and APTT in the absence of bleeding history eliminate the diagnosis of factor deficiency, including factor VIII deficiency. The APTT performed on a mixture of patient plasma and normal plasma did not correct. This result is indicative of an inhibitor. However, since the patient is not bleeding, factor VIII inhibitor is not indicated. A negative anticardiolipin antibody result rules out anticardiolipin antibodies' being responsible for the patient's clinical symptoms. The laboratory tests that confirm the presence of a lupus anticoagulant are a prolonged APTT that is not corrected when mixed with normal plasma and that is neutralized by preincubation with platelets (an excess of platelet phospholipid neutralizes the antibody, resulting in a normal APTT).

15. A 60-year-old patient was admitted to a hospital for a liver biopsy. The biopsy was scheduled for 11:00 a.m. The coagulation results performed at the time of admission revealed a prolonged PT with an INR of 4.5. What is the most appropriate course of action?
  - **A.** Proceed with biopsy, since a prolonged PT is expected in liver disease.
  - **B.** Postpone the procedure for a couple of days
  - **C.** Cancel the procedure and start the patient on vitamin K therapy
  - **D.** Put patient on vitamin K and proceed with the procedure immediately.

Hemostasis/Correlate clinical and laboratory data/INR/3

16. A fresh blood sample was sent to the laboratory at 8:00 a.m. for a PT test. At 4:00 p.m., the doctor requested an APTT test to be done on the same sample. What should the technologist do?
  - **A.** Rerun APTT on the 8:00 a.m. sample and report the result
  - **B.** Request a new sample for APTT
  - **C.** Run APTT in duplicates and report the average
  - **D.** Mix the patient plasma with normal plasma and run the APTT

Hemostasis/Select methods/Reagents/Specimen collection and handling/Specimen/3

17. An APTT test is performed on a patient and the result is 50 sec (reference range 27–37 sec). The instrument flags the result owing to failure of the delta check. The patient had an APTT of 35 sec the previous day. The technologist calls the nursing unit to check whether the patient is on heparin therapy. The patient is not receiving heparin. What is the next appropriate step?
  - **A.** Check the family history for an inherited factor VIII deficiency
  - **B.** Check to see if the patient has received any other anticoagulant medications
  - **C.** Perform mixing studies
  - **D.** Perform a factor VIII assay

Hemostasis/Evaluate laboratory data to recognize health and disease states/Anticoagulant drugs/3

Answers to Questions 15–17

15. **C** Liver biopsy in a patient with a prolonged PT and a high INR could be life-threatening. In this patient, the prolonged PT is likely caused by liver disease. Vitamin K is stored in the liver and is essential for activation of factors II, VII, IX, and X. Vitamin K needs bile (secreted by the liver) for its absorption. In liver disease characterized by obstruction, bile is not secreted into the GI tract and therefore vitamin K is poorly absorbed. The most logical course of action is to recommend the following: start the patient on vitamin K therapy, repeat the PT test 4 days after starting vitamin K administration, and cancel the biopsy until the patient's PT returns to normal.

16. **B** According to Clinical Laboratory Standards Institute (CLSI) guidelines, samples for APTT should be centrifuged and tested within 2 hours after collection. However, the sample is stable for 4 hours if stored at 4°C. APTT evaluates the clotting factors in the intrinsic and common coagulation pathways, including factor VIII (intrinsic) and factor V (common). Factors VIII and V are cofactors necessary for fibrin formation. However, they are both labile. Storage beyond 4 hours causes falsely elevated APTT results. The technologist should request a new sample for the APTT.

17. **B** Traditional anticoagulant drugs such as heparin and warfarin are well known. There are new anticoagulant drugs available for the treatment and prevention of thrombosis. Some of these new drugs have antithrombin effects and therefore increase PT, APTT, and TT results. Examples of these drugs are hirudin, which inhibits thrombin, and danaparoid, which inhibits factor Xa.

18. A patient was put on heparin therapy postoperatively
for prevention of thrombosis. The patient had the following laboratory results on admission: Platelet count
= 350 ×10⁹/L; PT = 12 sec (reference: 10–13 sec);
APTT = 35 sec (reference: 28–37). After 6 days of
heparin therapy, the patient complained of pain and
swelling in her left leg. Her platelet count dropped to
85 × 10⁹/L and her APTT result was 36 sec. The physician suspected heparin-induced thrombocytopenia
(HIT) and ordered a platelet aggregation test to be
performed immediatly. The heparin-induced platelet
aggregation test result was negative. Heparin therapy
was continued. Several days later, the patient developed a massive clot in her left leg that necessitated
amputation.

Which of the following should have been recognized
or initiated?
- **A.** The patient should have been placed on LMWH
- **B.** The heparin dose should have been increased
- **C.** The negative platelet aggregation does not rule out
  HIT
- **D.** The patient should have been placed on warfarin
  therapy

Hemostasis/Correlate clinical and laboratory data/HIT/3

19. A 50-year-old female was admitted to a hospital for a
hip replacement surgery. The preoperative tests were
performed and the results showed a Hgb of 13.5 g/dL;
Hct = 42%; PT = 12 sec; APTT = 36 sec. The patient
was bleeding during surgery and the postoperative
test results revealed a Hgb = 5.0 g/dL; Hct = 16%; PT
= 8 sec; and APTT = 25 sec.

What steps should be taken before releasing these
results?
- **A.** No follow-up steps are needed; report the results as
  obtained
- **B.** Report Hgb and Hct results, adjust the
  anticoagulant volume, and redraw a new sample
  for PT and APTT
- **C.** Call the nurse and ask if the patient is receiving
  heparin
- **D.** Since the patient is severely anemic, multiply the
  PT and APTT results by two and report the results

18. C Heparin therapy should be stopped immediately
when clinical symptoms indicate HIT. The blood
sample should be tested at least 4 hours after
heparin therapy is discontinued. Early sampling for
HIT testing may give a false-negative result due to
the neutralization of antibody by heparin. LMWH
should not be used in patients who develop HIT,
since LMWH drugs can also cause HIT. Warfarin
therapy can be started in patients who respond to
heparin therapy as soon as the APTT is increased to
1.5 times the baseline APTT. Heparin therapy must
overlap warfarin therapy until the INR reaches a
stable theraputic range (2.0–3.0). Warfarin therapy
could not be used in this patient because she did
not respond to heparin therapy. The first step in the
treatment of HIT is discontinuation of heparin,
including intravenous catheter flushes, heparin-
coated indwelling catheters, unfractionated heparin,
and LMWH.

19. B The anticoagulant-to-blood ratio should be
adjusted for PT and APTT tests in patients with a
severe anemia. The standard anticoagulant volume
(0.5 mL) is not sufficient for the large quantity of
plasma in these patients, causing unreliable PT and
APTT results. The low Hgb and Hct in this patient
were due to severe bleeding during surgery. To get
accurate PT and APTT results, the amount of anticoagulant is adjusted according to the following
formula: $(0.00185)(V)(100-H) = C$, where V =
blood volume in mL; H = patient's Hct; and C =
volume of anticoagulant. A new sample should be
drawn to rerun the PT and APTT. There are other
causes for decreased PT and APTT, such as increased fibrinogen and increased factor VIII; however, the preanalytical variables affecting unreliable
results should be ruled out first. Heparin therapy
would increase PT and APTT.

20. Patient and Family History

A 45- year-old woman visited her doctor complaining of easy bruising and menorrhagia occuring for the past few weeks. The patient had no history of excessive bleeding during childbirth several years earlier nor during a tonsillectomy in childhood. Her family history was unremarkable.

Laboratory Tests:	Patient	Reference Range
PT	45 sec	11–13 sec
APTT	125 sec	28–37 sec
Thrombin Time	14.0 sec	10–15 sec

Mixing studies (patient plasma + normal plasma): PT = 40 sec; APTT = 90 sec

Patelet count and morphology = normal

Liver function tests = normal

These clinical manifestations and laboratory results are consistant with:

A. Factor VIII inhibitor

B. Factor V inhibitor

C. Factor VIII deficiency

D. Lupus anticoagulant

Hemostasis/Correlate clinical and laboratory data/Heparin therapy/3

Answer to Question 20

20. B The lack of a positive family history in this patient indicates the presence of an acquired coagulopathy. Since both PT and APTT tests are abnormal, the clotting factor involved is most probably in the common pathway. The lack of correction by mixing studies suggests the presence of an inhibitor. Factor V antibodies are the most common antibodies among the clotting factors of the common pathway (I, II, V, and X). Factor V antibodies are reported to be associated with surgery, some antibiotics such as streptomycin, patients who are exposed to blood products, or the bovine form of "fibrin glue." Patients with antibodies to factor V may require long-term therapy with immunosuppressive drugs. Acute bleeding episodes may be treated by platelet transfusions. The PT test is normal in patients with factor VIII deficiency and factor VIII inhibitor. Lupus anticoagulant is not present with bleeding unless associated with coexisting thrombocytopenia.

BIBLIOGRAPHY

1. Bick, R.L.: Disorders of Thrombosis and Hemostasis. ed 3. Lippincott Williams and Wilkins, Philadelphia, 2002.
2. Coleman, R.W., Hirsh, J., Marder, V. J., et al.: Hemostasis and Thrombosis, Basic Principles and Clinical Practice. ed 5. Lippincott Williams and Wilkins, Philadelphia, 2006.
3. Greer, J.P., Foester, J., Lukens, J, et al.: Wintrobe's Clinical Hematology. ed 11, Vol 2. Lippincott Williams and Wilkins, Philadelphia, 2004.
4. Nathan, D.G., Orkin, S. H., Ginsburg, D., et al.: Hematology of Infancy and Childhood. ed 6, Vol 2. W.B.Saunders, Philadelphia, 2003.
5. Lichtman, M.A., Beutler, E., Kaushansky, K., et al: Williams Hematology. ed 7. McGraw-Hill, New York 2006.

CHAPTER **3**

Immunology

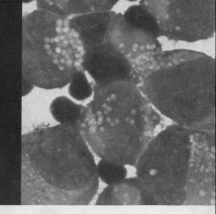

3.1   BASIC PRINCIPLES OF IMMUNOLOGY

3.2   IMMUNOLOGICAL PROCEDURES

3.3   INFECTIOUS DISEASES

3.4   AUTOIMMUNE DISEASES

3.5   HYPERSENSITIVITY

3.6   IMMUNOGLOBULINS, COMPLEMENT, AND CELLULAR TESTING

3.7   TUMOR TESTING AND TRANSPLANTATION

3.8   IMMUNOLOGY PROBLEM SOLVING

1. From the following, identify a specific component of the adaptive immune system that is formed in response to antigenic stimulation:
   A. Lysozyme
   B. Complement
   C. Commensal organisms
   D. Immunoglobulin

   Immunology/Apply knowledge of fundamental biological characteristics/Immune system/Complement/1

2. Which two organs are considered the primary lymphoid organs in which immunocompetent cells originate and mature?
   A. Thyroid and Peyer's patches
   B. Thymus and bone marrow
   C. Spleen and mucosal-associated lymphoid tissue (MALT)
   D. Lymph nodes and thoracic duct

   Immunology/Apply knowledge of fundamental biological characteristics/Immune system/Organs/1

3. What type of B cells are formed after antigen stimulation?
   A. Plasma cells and memory B cells
   B. Mature B cells
   C. Antigen-dependent B cells
   D. Receptor-activated B cells

   Immunology/Apply knowledge of fundamental biological characteristics/Immune system/Cells/1

4. T cells travel from the bone marrow to the thymus for maturation. What is the correct order of the maturation sequence for T cells in the thymus?
   A. Bone marrow to the cortex; after thymic education, released back to peripheral circulation
   B. Maturation and selection occur in the cortex; migration to the medulla; release of mature T cells to secondary lymphoid organs
   C. Storage in either the cortex or medulla; release of T cells into the peripheral circulation
   D. Activation and selection occur in the medulla; mature T cells are stored in the cortex until activated by antigen

   Immunology/Apply knowledge of fundamental biological characteristics/Immune system/Cells/1

Answers to Questions 1–4

1. **D** Immunoglobulin is a specific part of the adaptive immune system and is formed only in response to a specific antigenic stimulation. Complement, lysozyme, and commensal organisms all act non-specifically as a part of the adaptive immune system. These three components do not require any type of specific antigenic stimulation.

2. **B** The bone marrow and thymus are considered primary lymphoid organs because immunocompetent cells either originate or mature in them. Some immunocompetent cells mature or reside in the bone marrow (the source of all hematopoietic cells) until transported to the thymus, spleen, or Peyer's patches, where they process antigen or manufacture antibody. T lymphocytes, after originating in the bone marrow, travel to the thymus to mature and differentiate.

3. **A** Mature B cells exhibit surface immunoglobulin that may cross-link a foreign antigen, thus forming the activated B cell and leading to capping and internalization of antigen. The activated B cell gives rise to plasma cells that produce and secrete immunoglobulins and memory cells that reside in lymphoid organs.

4. **B** Immature T cells travel from the bone marrow to the thymus to mature into functional T cells. Once in the thymus, T cells undergo a selection and maturation sequence that begins in the cortex and moves to the medulla of the thymus. Thymic factors such as thymosin and thymopoietin and cells within the thymus such as macrophages and dendritic cells assist in this sequence. After completion of the maturation cycle, T cells are released to secondary lymphoid organs to await antigen recognition and activation.

5. Which cluster of differentiation (CD) marker appears during the first stage of T-cell development and remains present as an identifying marker for T cells?
   A. CD1
   B. CD2
   C. CD3
   D. CD4 or CD8

Immunology/Apply principles of basic laboratory procedures/T cells/Markers/1

6. Which markers are found on mature, peripheral helper T cells?
   A. CD1, CD2, CD4
   B. CD2, CD3, CD8
   C. CD1, CD3, CD4
   D. CD2, CD3, CD4

Immunology/Apply knowledge of fundamental biological characteristics/T cells/Markers/1

7. Which T cell expresses the CD8 marker and acts specifically to kill tumors or virally infected cells?
   A. Helper T
   B. T suppressor
   C. T cytotoxic
   D. T inducer/suppressor

Immunology/Apply knowledge of fundamental biological characteristics/T cells/Cytokines/1

8. How are cytotoxic T cells (T_C cells) and natural killer (NK) cells similar?
   A. Require antibody to be present
   B. Effective against virally infected cells
   C. Recognize antigen in association with HLA class II markers
   D. Do not bind to infected cells

Immunology/Apply knowledge of fundamental biological characteristics/Lymphocytes/Function/1

9. What is the name of the process by which phagocytic cells are attracted to a substance such as a bacterial peptide?
   A. Diapedesis
   B. Degranulation
   C. Chemotaxis
   D. Phagotaxis

Immunology/Apply knowledge of fundamental biological characteristics/Immune system/Cells/1

10. All of the following are immunological functions of complement *except*:
   A. Induction of an antiviral state
   B. Opsonization
   C. Chemotaxis
   D. Anaphylatoxin formation

Immunology/Apply knowledge of fundamental biological characteristics/Complement/Function/1

Answers to Questions 5–10

5. B The CD2 marker appears during the first stage of T-cell development and can be used to differentiate T cells from other lymphocytes. This T-lymphocyte receptor binds sheep red blood cells (RBCs). This peculiar characteristic was the basis for the classic E rosette test once used to enumerate T cells in peripheral blood. CD2 is not specific for T cells, however, and is also found on large granular lymphocytes (LGL or natural killer [NK]cells).

6. D Mature, peripheral helper T cells have the CD2 (E rosette), CD3 (mature T cell), and CD4 (helper) markers.

7. C T cytotoxic cells recognize antigen in association with major histocompatibility complex (MHC) class I complexes and act against target cells that express foreign antigens. These include viral antigens and the human leukocyte antigens (HLA) that are the target of graft rejection.

8. B Both T_C and NK cells are effective against virally infected cells, and neither requires antibody to be present to bind to infected cells. NK cells do not exhibit MHC class restriction, whereas activation of T_C cells requires the presence of MHC class I molecules in association with the viral antigen.

9. C Chemotaxis is the process by which phagocytic cells are attracted toward an area where they detect a disturbance in the normal functions of body tissues. Products from bacteria and viruses, complement components, coagulation proteins, and cytokines from other immune cells may all act as chemotactic factors.

10. A Complement components are serum proteins that function in opsonization, chemotaxis, and anaphylatoxin formation but do not induce an antiviral state in target cells. This function is performed by interferons.

11. Which complement component is found in both the classic and alternative pathways?
  A. C1
  B. C4
  C. Factor D
  D. C3

Immunology/Apply knowledge of fundamental biological characteristics/Complement/Components/1

12. Which immunoglobulin(s) help(s) initiate the classic complement pathway?
  A. IgA and IgD
  B. IgM only
  C. IgG and IgM
  D. IgG only

Immunology/Apply knowledge of fundamental biological characteristics/Complement/Activation/1

13. How is complement activity destroyed in vitro?
  A. Heating serum at 56°C for 30 min
  B. Keeping serum at room temperature of 22°C for 1 hour
  C. Heating serum at 37°C for 45 min
  D. Freezing serum at 0°C for 24 hours

Immunology/Apply knowledge of fundamental biological characteristics/Complement/Activation/1

14. What is the purpose of C3a, C4a, and C5a, the split-products of the complement cascade?
  A. To bind with specific membrane receptors of lymphocytes and cause release of cytotoxic substances
  B. To cause increased vascular permeability, contraction of smooth muscle, and release of histamine from basophils
  C. To bind with membrane receptors of macrophages to facilitate phagocytosis and the removal of debris and foreign substances
  D. To regulate and degrade membrane cofactor protein after activation by C3 convertase

Immunology/Apply knowledge of fundamental biological characteristics/Complement/Anaphylatoxins/1

15. Which region of the immunoglobulin molecule can bind antigen?
  A. Fab
  B. Fc
  C. C_L
  D. C_H

Immunology/Apply knowledge of fundamental biological characteristics/Immunoglobulin/Structure/1

16. Which region determines whether an immunoglobulin molecule can fix complement?
  A. V_H
  B. C_H
  C. V_L
  D. C_L

Immunology/Apply knowledge of fundamental biological characteristics/Immunoglobulin/Structure/1

Answers to Questions 11–16

11. **D** C3 is found in both the classic and alternative (alternate) pathways of the complement system. In the classic pathway, C3b forms a complex on the cell with C4b2a that enzymatically cleaves C5. In the alternative pathway, C3b binds to an activator on the cell surface. It forms a complex with factor B called C3bBb which, like C4b2a3b, can split C5.

12. **C** Both IgG and IgM are the immunoglobulins that help to initiate the activation of the classic complement pathway. IgM is a more potent complement activator, however.

13. **A** Complement activity in serum in vitro is destroyed by heating the serum at 56°C for 30 min. In test procedures where complement may interfere with the test system, it may be necessary to destroy complement activity in the test sample by heat inactivation.

14. **B** C3a, C4a, and C5a are split-products of the complement cascade that participate in various biological functions such as vasodilation and smooth muscle contraction. These small peptides act as anaphylatoxins, e.g., effector molecules that participate in the inflammatory response to assist in the destruction and clearance of foreign antigens.

15. **A** The Fab (fragment antigen binding) is the region of the immunoglobulin molecule that can bind antigen. Two Fab fragments are formed from hydrolysis of the immunoglobulin molecule by papain. Each consists of a light chain and the V_H and C_{H1} regions of the heavy chain. The variable regions of the light and heavy chains interact, forming a specific antigen-combining site.

16. **B** The composition and structure of the constant region of the heavy chain determine whether that immunoglobulin will fix complement. The Fc fragment (fragment crystallizable) is formed by partial immunoglobulin digestion with papain and includes the C_{H2} and C_{H3} domains of both heavy chains. The complement component C1q molecule will bind to the C_{H2} region of an IgG or IgM molecule.

17. Which immunoglobulin class(es) has/have a J chain?
  A. IgM
  B. IgE and IgD
  C. IgM and sIgA
  D. IgG3 and IgA

Immunology/Apply knowledge of fundamental biological characteristics/Immunoglobulin/Structure/1

18. Which immunoglobulin appears first in the primary immune response?
  A. IgG
  B. IgM
  C. IgA
  D. IgE

Immunology/Apply knowledge of fundamental biological characteristics/Immunoglobulin/Function/1

19. Which immunoglobulin appears in highest titer in the secondary response?
  A. IgG
  B. IgM
  C. IgA
  D. IgE

Immunology/Apply knowledge of fundamental biological characteristics/Immunoglobulin/Function/1

20. Which immunoglobulin(s) can cross the placenta?
  A. IgG
  B. IgM
  C. IgA
  D. IgE

Immunology/Apply knowledge of fundamental biological characteristics/Immunoglobulin/Function/1

21. Which immunoglobulin cross-links mast cells to release histamine?
  A. IgG
  B. IgM
  C. IgA
  D. IgE

Immunology/Apply knowledge of fundamental biological characteristics/Immunoglobulin/Function/1

22. All of the following are functions of immunoglobulins *except*:
  A. Neutralizing toxic substances
  B. Facilitating phagocytosis through opsonization
  C. Interacting with T_C cells to lyse viruses
  D. Combining with complement to destroy cellular antigens

Immunology/Apply knowledge of fundamental biological characteristics/Immunoglobulin/Function/1

23. Which of the following antigens is classified as an MHC class II antigen?
  A. HLA-A
  B. HLA-B
  C. HLA-C
  D. HLA-DR

Immunology/Apply knowledge of fundamental biological characteristics/MHC/HLA antigens/1

Answers to Questions 17–23

17. **C** Both IgM and secretory IgA have a J chain joining individual molecules together; the J chain in IgM joins five molecules and the J chain in sIgA joins two molecules.

18. **B** The first antibody to appear in the primary immune response to an antigen is IgM. The titer of antiviral IgM (e.g., IgM antibody to cytomegalovirus [anti-CMV]) is more specific for acute or active viral infection than IgG and may be measured to help differentiate active from prior infection.

19. **A** A high titer of IgG characterizes the secondary immune response. Consequently, IgG antibodies make up about 80% of the total immunoglobulin concentration in normal serum.

20. **A** IgG is the only immunoglobulin class that can cross the placenta. All subclasses of IgG can cross the placenta, but IgG2 crosses more slowly. This process requires recognition of the Fc region of the IgG by placental cells. These cells take up the IgG from the maternal blood and secrete it into the fetal blood, providing humoral immunity to the neonate for the first few months after delivery.

21. **D** IgE is the immunoglobulin that cross-links with basophils and mast cells. IgE causes the release of such immune response modifiers as histamine and mediates an allergic immune response.

22. **C** Cytotoxic T cells lyse virally infected cells directly, without requirement for specific antibody. The T_C cell is activated by viral antigen that is associated with MHC class I molecules on the surface of the infected cell. The activated T_C cell secretes several toxins, such as tumor necrosis factor, which destroy the infected cell and virions.

23. **D** The MHC region is located on the short arm of chromosome 6 and codes for antigens expressed on the surface of leukocytes and tissues. The MHC region genes control immune recognition; their products include the antigens that determine transplantation rejection. HLA-DR antigens are expressed on B cells. HLA-DR2, DR3, DR4, and DR5 antigens show linkage with a wide range of autoimmune diseases.

24. Which MHC class of antigens is necessary for antigen recognition by CD4-positive T cells?
  A. Class I
  B. Class II
  C. Class III
  D. No MHC molecule is necessary for antigen recognition.

Immunology/Apply knowledge of fundamental biological characteristics/MHC/Function/1

25. Which of the following are products of HLA class III genes?
  A. T-cell immune receptors
  B. HLA-D antigens on immune cells
  C. Complement proteins C2, C4, and Factor B
  D. Immunoglobulin V_L regions

Immunology/Apply knowledge of fundamental biological characteristics/MHC/Function/1

26. What molecule on the surface of most T cells recognizes antigen?
  A. IgT, a four-chain molecule that includes the tau heavy chain
  B. MHC protein, a two-chain molecule encoded by the HLA region
  C. CD3, consisting of six different chains
  D. TcR, consisting of two chains, alpha and beta

Immunology/Apply knowledge of fundamental biological characteristics/TcR/Function/1

27. The T-cell antigen receptor is similar to immunoglobulin molecules in that it:
  A. Remains bound to the cell surface and is never secreted
  B. Contains V and C regions on each of its chains
  C. Binds complement
  D. Can cross the placenta and provide protection to a fetus

Immunology/Apply knowledge of fundamental biological characteristics/TcR/Function/2

28. Toll-like receptors are found on which cells?
  A. T cells
  B. Dendritic cells
  C. B cells
  D. Large granular lymphocytes

Immunology/Apply knowledge of fundamental biological characteristics/Innate immune system/Toll-like Receptors/1

29. Macrophages produce which of the following proteins during antigen processing?
  A. IL-1 and IL-6
  B. γ-Interferon
  C. IL-4, IL-5, and IL-10
  D. Complement components C1 and C3

Immunology/Apply knowledge of fundamental biological characteristics/Innate immune system/Toll cytokines/2

Answers to Questions 24–29

24. **B** Helper T lymphocytes (CD4-positive T cells) recognize antigens only in the context of a class II molecule. Because class II antigens are expressed on macrophages, monocytes, and B cells, the helper T-cell response is mediated by interaction with processed antigen on the surface of these cells.

25. **C** Complement components C2 and C4 of the classic pathway and Factor B of the alternative pathway are class III molecules. HLA-A, HLA-B, and HLA-C antigens are classified as class I antigens, and HLA-D, HLA-DR, HLA-DQ, and HLA-DP antigens as class II antigens.

26. **D** T cells have a membrane bound receptor (T-cell receptor or TcR) that is antigen specific. This two-chain molecule consists of a single α-chain, similar to an immunoglobulin light chain, and a single β-chain, similar to an immunoglobulin heavy chain. Some T cells may express a γ/δ receptor instead of the α-β molecule. There is no τ heavy chain. MHC and CD3 molecules are present on T cells, but they are not the molecules that give antigen specificity to the cell.

27. **B** The antigen binding regions of both the α- and β-chains of the T-cell receptor are encoded by V genes that undergo rearrangement similar to that observed in immunoglobulin genes. The α-chain gene consists of V and J segments, similar to an immunoglobulin light chain. The β-chain consists of V, D, and J segments, similar to an immunoglobulin heavy chain. The α- and β-chains each have a single C region gene encoding the constant region of the molecule. While answer A is true for T cell receptors, it is not true for immunoglobulins that can be cell-bound or secreted. Answers C and D are true for certain immunoglobulin heavy chain isotypes but are not true for the T cell receptor.

28. **B** Toll-like receptors (TLR) are the primary antigen recognition protein of the innate immune system. They are found on antigen-presenting cells such as dendritic cells and macrophages. Eleven TLRs have been described. TLRs recognize certain structural motifs common to infecting organisms. TLR 4, for example, recognizes bacterial lipopolysaccharide (LPS). The name comes from their similarity to the Toll protein in *Drosophila*.

29. **A** Interleukin-1 (IL-1) and IL-6 are proinflammatory macrophage-produced cytokines. In addition to their inflammatory properties, they activate T-helper cells during antigen presentation. γ-Interferon, IL-4, 5, and 10 are all produced by T cells. Complement components are produced by a variety of cells but are not part of the macrophage antigen presentation process.

30. A superantigen, such as toxic shock syndrome toxin-1 (TSST-1), bypasses the normal antigen processing stage by binding to and cross-linking:

A. A portion of an immunoglobulin molecule and complement component C1

B. Toll-like receptors and an MHC class 1 molecule

C. A portion of an immunoglobulin and a portion of a T-cell receptor

D. A portion of a T-cell receptor and an MHC class II molecule

Immunology/Apply knowledge of fundamental biological characteristics/Antigen Processing/Superantigens/2

Answer to Question 30

30.   D A superantigen binds to the V β portion of the T-cell receptor and an MHC class II molecule. This binding can activate T cells without the involvement of an antigen-presenting cell. In some individuals, a single V β protein that recognizes TSST-1 is expressed on up to 10%–20% of T cells. The simultaneous activation of this amount of T cells causes a heavy cytokine release, resulting in the vascular collapse and pathology of toxic shock syndrome.

1. The interaction between an individual antigen and antibody molecule depends upon several types of bonds such as ionic bonds, hydrogen bonds, hydrophobic bonds, and van der Waals forces. How is the strength of this attraction characterized?
   A. Avidity
   B. Affinity
   C. Reactivity
   D. Valency

Immunology/Apply principles of basic laboratory procedures/1

2. A laboratory is evaluating an enzyme-linked immunosorbent assay (ELISA) for detecting an antibody to cyclic citrullinated peptide (CCP), which is a marker for rheumatoid arthritis. The laboratory includes serum from healthy volunteers and patients with other connective tissue diseases in the evaluation. These specimens determine which factor of the assay:
   A. Sensitivity
   B. Precision
   C. Bias
   D. Specificity

Immunology/Apply principles of basic laboratory procedures/RA/2

3. The detection of precipitation reactions depends on the presence of maximal proportions of antigen and antibody. A patient's sample contains a large amount of antibody, but the reaction in a test system containing antigen is negative. What has happened?
   A. Performance error
   B. Low specificity
   C. A shift in the zone of equivalence
   D. Prozone phenomenon

Immunology/Apply principles of basic laboratory procedures/3

4. Which part of the radial immunodiffusion (RID) test system contains the antisera?
   A. Center well
   B. Outer wells
   C. Gel
   D. Antisera may be added to any well.

Immunology/Apply principles of basic laboratory procedures/RID/Principle/1

Answers to Questions 1–4

1. **B.** Affinity refers to the strength of a single antibody-antigen interaction. Avidity is the strength of interactions between many different antibodies in a serum against a particular antigen (i.e., the sum of many affinities).

2. **D.** Specificity is defined as a negative result in the absence of the disease. The non–rheumatoid arthritis specimens would be expected to test negative if the assay has high specificity. Precision is the ability of the assay to repeatedly yield the same results on a single specimen. Both bias and sensitivity calculations would include specimens from rheumatoid arthritis specimens. Although those specimens would be included in the evaluation, they are not listed in the question.

3. **D** Although performance error and low specificity should be considered, if a test system fails to yield the expected reaction, excessive antibody preventing a precipitation reaction is usually the cause. Prozone occurs when antibody molecules saturate the antigen sites, preventing cross-linking of the antigen-antibody complexes by other antibody molecules. Because the antigen and antibody do not react at equivalence, a visible product is not formed, leading to a false-negative result.

4. **C** In an RID test system, for example, one measuring hemopexin concentration, the gel would contain the antihemopexin. A standardized volume of serum containing the antigen is added to each well. Antigen diffuses from the well into the gel and forms a precipitin ring by reaction with antibody. At equivalence, the area of the ring is proportional to antigen concentration.

5. What is the interpretation when an Ouchterlony plate shows crossed lines between wells 1 and 2 (antigen is placed in the center well and antisera in wells 1 and 2)?
   A. No reaction between wells 1 and 2
   B. Partial identity between wells 1 and 2
   C. Nonidentity between wells 1 and 2
   D. Identity between wells 1 and 2

   Immunology/Apply principles of basic laboratory procedures/Ouchterlony techniques/Interpretation/2

6. Why is radioimmunoassay (RIA) or enzyme immunoassay (EIA) the method of choice for detection of certain analytes, such as hormones, normally found in low concentrations?
   A. Because of low cross-reactivity
   B. Because of high specificity
   C. Because of high sensitivity
   D. Because test systems may be designed as both competitive and noncompetitive assays

   Immunology/Apply principles of basic laboratory procedures/RIA/1

7. What comprises the indicator system in an ELISA for detecting antibody?
   A. Enzyme-conjugated antibody + chromogenic substrate
   B. Antigen-conjugate + chromogenic substrate
   C. Enzyme + antigen
   D. Substrate + antigen

   Immunology/Apply principles of basic laboratory procedures/ELISA/1

8. What outcome results from improper washing of a tube or well after adding the enzyme-antibody conjugate in an ELISA system?
   A. Result will be falsely decreased
   B. Result will be falsely increased
   C. Result will be unaffected
   D. Result is impossible to determine

   Immunology/Apply knowledge to identify sources of error/ELISA/3

9. What would happen if the color reaction phase is prolonged in one tube or well of an ELISA test?
   A. Result will be falsely decreased
   B. Result will be falsely increased
   C. Result will be unaffected
   D. Impossible to determine

   Immunology/Apply knowledge to identify sources of error/ELISA/3

10. The absorbance of a sample measured by ELISA is greater than the highest standard. What corrective action should be taken?
    A. Extrapolate an estimated value from the highest reading
    B. Repeat the test using a standard of higher concentration
    C. Repeat the assay using one-half the volume of the sample
    D. Dilute the test sample

    Immunology/Evaluate laboratory data to take corrective action according to predetermined criteria/ELISA/3

Answers to Questions 5–10

5. **C** Crossed lines indicate nonidentity between wells 1 and 2. The antibody from well 1 recognizes a different antigenic determinant than the antibody from well 2.

6. **C** RIA is extremely sensitive, but because of strict regulations for handling radioactive materials and safety concerns, it is used only when an alternative method is unavailable. The sensitivity of EIA methods producing fluorescent and chemiluminescent products can be equivalent to that of RIA. These detection systems have greatly diminished the number of analytes that must be measured by RIA.

7. **A** The ELISA test measures antibody using immobilized reagent antigen. The antigen is fixed to the walls of a tube or bottom of a microtiter well. Serum is added (and incubated) and the antibody binds, if present. After washing, the antigen-antibody complexes are detected by adding an enzyme labeled anti-immunoglobulin. Unbound enzyme label is removed by washing, and the bound enzyme label is detected by adding chromogenic substrate. The enzyme catalyzes the conversion of substrate to colored product.

8. **B** If unbound enzyme-conjugated anti-immunoglobulin is not washed away, it will catalyze conversion of substrate to colored product, yielding a falsely elevated result.

9. **B** If the color reaction is not stopped within the time limits specified by the procedure, the enzyme will continue to act on the substrate, producing a falsely elevated test result.

10. **D** Usually when a test sample reads at a value above the highest standard in an ELISA test, it is diluted and measured again. In those instances where no additional clinical value can be obtained by dilution, the result may be reported as greater than the highest standard (citing the upper reportable limit of the assay).

11. A patient was suspected of having a lymphoprolifera-tive disorder. After several laboratory tests were com-pleted, the patient was found to have an IgMκ paraprotein. In what sequence should the laboratory tests leading to this diagnosis have been performed?
    A. Serum and urine protein electrophoresis followed by immunofixation electrophoresis (IFE) on the positives
    B. Immunoelectrophoresis (IEP) of serum followed by IFE of serum if positive
    C. IEP of serum followed by protein electrophoresis of serum if positive
    D. Either serum protein electrophoresis or IEP could have led to the final conclusion. Only a single test should have been performed

Immunology/Evaluate laboratory data to reach conclu-sions/IFE/3

12. An IFE performed on a serum sample showed a nar-row dark band in the lanes containing anti-γ and anti-λ. How should this result be interpreted?
    A. Abnormally decreased IgG concentration
    B. Abnormal test result demonstrating monoclonal IgGλ
    C. Normal test result
    D. Impossible to determine without densitometric quantitation

Immunology/Evaluate laboratory data to make identifi-cations/IFE/2

13. Which type of nephelometry is used to measure immune complex formation almost immediately after reagent has been added?
    A. Rate
    B. Endpoint
    C. Continuous
    D. One-dimensional

Immunology/Apply principles of basic laboratory proce-dures/Nephelometry/1

14. An immunofluorescence microscopy assay (IFA) was performed, and a significant antibody titer was reported. Positive and negative controls performed as expected. However, the clinical evaluation of the patient was not consistent with a positive finding. What is the most likely explanation of this situation?
    A. The clinical condition of the patient changed since the sample was tested
    B. The pattern of fluorescence was misinterpreted
    C. The control results were misinterpreted
    D. The wrong cell line was used for the test

Immunology/Apply principles of basic laboratory proce-dures/IFA/3

Answers to Questions 11–14

11. **A** Serum and urine protein electrophoresis should be performed initially to detect the presence of an abnormal immunoglobulin which demonstrates restricted electrophoretic mobility. A patient pro-ducing only monoclonal light chains may not show any abnormal serum finding because the light chains may be excreted in the urine. A positive find-ing for either serum or urine should be followed by IFE on the positive specimen. This is required to confirm the presence of monoclonal immunoglob-ulin, to identify the heavy and light chain type, and to determine whether free monoclonal light chains are being produced.

12. **B** A *narrow* dark band formed in both the lane containing anti-γ and anti-λ indicates the presence of a monoclonal IgG λ immunoglobulin. A diffuse dark band would indicate a polyclonal increase in IgG that often accompanies chronic inflammatory disorders such as systemic lupus erythematosus (SLE).

13. **A** Rate nephelometry is used to measure formation of small immune complexes as they are formed under conditions of antibody excess. The rate of increase in photodetector output is measured within seconds or minutes and increases with increasing antigen concentration. Antigen concen-tration is determined by comparing the rate for the sample to that for standards using an algorithm that compensates for nonlinearity. In endpoint neph-elometry, reactions are read after equivalence. Immune complexes are of maximal size but may have a tendency to settle out of solution, thereby decreasing the amount of scatter.

14. **B** In an IFA, for example, an antinuclear antibody (ANA) test, the fluorescence pattern must be corre-lated correctly with the specificity of the antibodies. Both pathological and nonpathological antibodies can occur, and antibodies may be detected at a sig-nificant titer in a patient whose disease is inactive. Failure to correctly identify subcellular structures may result in misinterpretation of the antibody specificity, or a false-positive caused by nonspecific fluorescence.

15. What corrective action should be taken when an indeterminate pattern occurs in an indirect IFA?
  A. Repeat the test using a larger volume of sample
  B. Call the physician
  C. Have another person read the slide
  D. Dilute the sample and retest

Immunology/Evaluate laboratory data to take corrective action according to predetermined criteria/IFA/3

16. Which statement best describes passive agglutination reactions used for serodiagnosis?
  A. Such agglutination reactions are more rapid because they are a single-step process
  B. Reactions require the addition of a second antibody
  C. Passive agglutination reactions require biphasic incubation
  D. Carrier particles for antigen such as latex particles are used

Immunology/Apply principles of basic laboratory procedures/Agglutination/1

17. What has happened in a titer, if tube Nos. 5–7 show a stronger reaction than tube Nos.1–4?
  A. Prozone reaction
  B. Postzone reaction
  C. Equivalence reaction
  D. Poor technique

Immunology/Evaluate data to determine possible inconsistent results/Serological titration/3

18. What is the titer in tube No. 8 if tube No. 1 is undiluted and dilutions are doubled?
  A. 64
  B. 128
  C. 256
  D. 512

Immunology/Calculate/Serological titration/2

19. The directions for a slide agglutination test instruct that after mixing the patient's serum and latex particles, the slide must be rotated for 2 minutes. What would happen if the slide were rotated for 10 minutes?
  A. Possible false-positive result
  B. Possible false-negative result
  C. No effect
  D. Depends on the amount of antibody present in the sample

Immunology/Apply principles of basic laboratory procedures/Agglutination/3

20. Which outcome indicates a negative result in a complement fixation test?
  A. Hemagglutination
  B. Absence of hemagglutination
  C. Hemolysis
  D. Absence of hemolysis

Immunology/Apply principles of basic laboratory procedures/Complement fixation/1

Answers to Questions 15–20

15. **D** An unexpected pattern may indicate the presence of more than one antibody. Diluting the sample may help to clearly show the antibody specificities, if they are found in different titers. If the pattern is still atypical, a new sample should be collected and the test repeated.

16. **D** Most agglutination tests used in serology employ passive or indirect agglutination where carrier particles are coated with the antigen. The carrier molecule is of sufficient size so that the reaction of the antigen with antibody results in formation of a complex that is more easily visible.

17. **A** In tubes Nos.1–4, insufficient antigen is present to give a visible reaction because excess antibody has saturated all available antigen sites. After dilution of antibody, tubes Nos.1–4 have the equivalent concentrations of antigen and antibody to allow formation of visible complexes.

18. **B** The antibody titer is reciprocal of the highest dilution of serum giving a positive reaction. For doubling dilutions, each tube has 1/2 the amount of serum as the previous tube. Because the first tube was undiluted (neat), the dilution in tube No. 8 is $(1/2)^7$ and the titer equals 2^7 or 128.

19. **A** Failure to follow directions, as in this case where the reaction was allowed to proceed beyond the recommended time, may result in a false-positive reading. Drying on the slide may lead to a possible erroneous positive reading.

20. **C** In complement fixation, hemolysis indicates a negative test result. The absence of hemolysis indicates that complement was fixed in an antigen-antibody reaction and, therefore, that the specific complement binding antibody was present in the patient's serum. Consequently it was not available to react in the indicator system.

21. What effect does selecting the wrong gate have on the results when cells are counted by flow cytometry?
   A. No effect
   B. Failure to count the desired cell population
   C. Falsely elevated results
   D. Impossible to determine

Immunology/Apply principles of basic laboratory procedures/Flow cytometry//3

22. Which statement best describes immunophenotyping?
   A. Lineage determination by detecting antigens on the surface of the gated cells using fluorescent antibodies
   B. Identification of cell maturity using antibodies to detect antigens within the nucleus
   C. Identification and sorting of cells by front and side-scatter of light from a laser
   D. Analysis of cells collected by flow cytometry using traditional agglutination reactions

Immunology/Apply principles of basic laboratory procedures/Flow cytometry/1

23. A flow cytometry scattergram of a bone marrow sample shows a dense population of cells located in-between normal lymphoid and normal myeloid cells. What is the most likely explanation?
   A. The sample was improperly collected
   B. An abnormal cell population is present
   C. The laser optics are out of alignment
   D. The cells are most likely not leukocytes

Immunology/Apply principles of basic laboratory procedures/Flow cytometry/3

Answers to Questions 21–23

21. B Gating is the step performed to select the proper cells to be counted. Failure to properly perform this procedure will result in problems in isolating and counting the desired cells. It is impossible to determine if the final result would be falsely elevated or falsely lowered by problems with gating.

22. A Immunophenotyping refers to classification of cells (lineage and maturity assignment) using a panel of fluorescent-labeled antibodies directed against specific surface antigens on the cells. Antibodies are referred to by their CD (cluster of differentiation) number. Monoclonal antibodies having a common CD number do not necessarily bind to the same epitope but recognize the same antigen on the cell surface. Reactivity of the selected cells with a panel of antibodies differentiates lymphoid from myeloid cells and identifies the stage of cell maturation.

23. B Lymphoid cells and myeloid cells display in predictable regions of the scatterplot because of their characteristic size and density. Lymphoid cells cause less forward and side scatter from the laser than do myeloid cells. A dense zone of cells in between those regions is caused by the presence of a large number of abnormal cells, usually blasts. The lineage of the cells can be determined by immunophenotyping with a panel of fluorescent-labeled antibodies.

1. Which serum antibody response usually characterizes the primary (early) stage of syphilis?
   A. Antibodies against syphilis are undetectable
   B. Detected 1–3 weeks after appearance of the primary chancre
   C. Detected in 50% of cases before the primary chancre disappears
   D. Detected within 2 weeks after infection

Immunology/Correlate laboratory data with physiological processes/Syphilis/Testing/1

2. What substance is detected by the rapid plasma reagin (RPR) and Venereal Disease Research Laboratory (VDRL) tests for syphilis?
   A. Cardiolipin
   B. Reagin
   C. Specific antibody
   D. *Treponema pallidum*

Immunology/Apply knowledge of fundamental biological characteristics/Syphilis/Testing/1

3. What type of antigen is used in the RPR card test?
   A. Live treponemal organisms
   B. Killed suspension of treponemal organisms
   C. Cardiolipin
   D. Tanned sheep cells

Immunology/Apply principles of basic laboratory procedures/Syphilis/Testing/1

4. Which of the following is the most sensitive test to detect congenital syphilis?
   A. VDRL
   B. RPR
   C. Microhemagglutinin test for *T. pallidum* (MHA-TP)
   D. Polymerase chain reaction (PCR)

Immunology/Apply principles of basic laboratory procedures/Syphilis/Testing/1

5. A biological false-positive reaction is *LEAST* likely with which test for syphilis?
   A. VDRL
   B. Fluorescent *T. pallidum* antibody absorption test (FTA-ABS)
   C. RPR
   D. All are equally likely to detect a false-positive result.

Immunology/Apply principles of basic laboratory procedures/Syphilis/Testing/1

Answers to Questions 1–5

1. **B** During the primary stage of syphilis, about 90% of patients develop antibodies between 1 and 3 weeks after the appearance of the primary chancre.

2. **B** Reagin is the name for a nontreponemal antibody that appears in the serum of syphilis-infected persons. Reagin reacts with cardiolipin, a lipid-rich extract of beef heart and other animal tissues.

3. **C** Cardiolipin is extracted from animal tissues, such as beef hearts, and attached to carbon particles. In the presence of reagin, the particles will agglutinate.

4. **D** The PCR will amplify a very small amount of DNA from *T.. pallidum* and allow for detection of the organism in the infant. Antibody tests such as VDRL and RPR may detect maternal antibody only, not indicating if the infant has been infected.

5. **B** The FTA-ABS test is more specific for *T. pallidum* than nontreponemal tests such as the VDRL and RPR and would be least likely to detect a biological false-positive result. The FTA-ABS test uses heat-inactivated serum that has been absorbed with the Reiter strain of *T. pallidum* to remove nonspecific antibodies. Nontreponemal tests have a biological false-positive rate of 1%–10%, depending upon the patient population tested. False-positive findings are caused commonly by infectious mononucleosis (IM), SLE, viral hepatitis, and human immunodeficiency virus (HIV) infection.

6. A 12-year-old girl has symptoms of fatigue and a localized lymphadenopathy. Laboratory tests reveal a peripheral blood lymphocytosis, a positive RPR, and a positive spot test for IM. What test should be performed next?
   A. HIV test by ELISA
   B. VDRL
   C. Epstein-Barr virus (EBV) specific antigen test
   D. MHA-TP

   Immunology/Correlate laboratory data with physiological processes/Syphilis/Testing/3

7. Which test is most likely to be positive in the tertiary stage of syphilis?
   A. FTA-ABS
   B. RPR
   C. VDRL
   D. Reagin screen test (RST)

   Immunology/Correlate laboratory data with physiological processes/Syphilis/Testing/3

8. What is the most likely interpretation of the following syphilis serological results?

   RPR: reactive; VDRL: reactive; MHA-TP: nonreactive
   A. Neurosyphilis
   B. Secondary syphilis
   C. Syphilis that has been successfully treated
   D. Biological false-positive

   Immunology/Correlate laboratory data with physiological processes/Syphilis/Testing/2

9. Which specimen is the sample of choice to evaluate latent or tertiary syphilis?
   A. Serum sample
   B. Chancre fluid
   C. CSF
   D. Joint fluid

   Immunology/Correlate laboratory data with physiological processes/Syphilis/Testing/1

10. Interpret the following quantitative RPR test results.

    RPR titer: weakly reactive 1:8; reactive 1:8–1:64
    A. Excess antibody, prozone effect
    B. Excess antigen, postzone effect
    C. Equivalence of antigen and antibody
    D. Impossible to interpret; testing error

    Immunology/Correlate laboratory data with physiological processes/Syphilis/Testing/2

Answers to Questions 6–10

6. **D** The patient's symptoms are nonspecific and could be attributed to many potential causes. However, the patient's age, lymphocytosis, and serological results point to infectious mononucleosis (IM). The rapid spot test for antibodies seen in IM is highly specific. The EBV-specific antigen test is more sensitive but is unnecessary when the spot test is positive. HIV infection is uncommon at this age and is often associated with generalized lymphadenopathy and a normal or reduced total lymphocyte count. IM antibodies are commonly implicated as a cause of biological false-positive nontreponemal tests for syphilis. Therefore, a treponemal test for syphilis should be performed to document this phenomenon in this case.

7. **A** The FTA-ABS or one of the treponemal tests is more likely to be positive than a nontreponemal test in the tertiary stage of syphilis. In some cases, systemic lesions have subsided by the tertiary stage and the nontreponemal tests become seronegative. Although the FTA-ABS is the most sensitive test for tertiary syphilis, it will be positive in both treated and untreated cases.

8. **D** A positive reaction with nontreponemal antigen and a negative reaction with a treponemal antigen is most likely caused by a biological false-positive nontreponemal test.

9. **C** Latent syphilis usually begins after the second year of untreated infection. In some cases the serological tests become negative. However, if neurosyphilis is present, cerebrospinal fluid serology will be positive and the CSF will display increased protein and pleocytosis characteristic of central nervous system infection.

10. **A** This patient may be in the secondary stage of syphilis and is producing large amounts of antibody to *T. pallidum* sufficient to cause antibody excess in the test. The test became strongly reactive only after the antibody was diluted.

11. Tests to identify infection with HIV fall into which three general classification types of tests?
   A. Tissue culture, antigen, and antibody tests
   B. Tests for antigens, antibodies, and nucleic acid
   C. DNA probe, DNA amplification, and Western blot tests
   D. ELISA, Western blot, and Southern blot tests

Immunology/Apply principles of basic laboratory procedures/HIV/Testing/1

12. Which tests are considered screening tests for HIV?
   A. ELISA and rapid antibody tests
   B. Immunofluorescence, Western blot, radioimmuno-precipitation assay
   C. Culture, antigen capture assay, DNA amplification
   D. Reverse transcriptase and messenger RNA (mRNA) assay

Immunology/Apply principles of basic laboratory procedures/HIV/Testing/1

13. Which tests are considered confirmatory tests for HIV?
   A. ELISA and rapid antibody tests
   B. Immunofluorescence assay (IFA), Western blot test, and polymerase chain reaction
   C. Culture, antigen capture assay, polymerase chain reaction
   D. Reverse transcriptase and mRNA assay

Immunology/Apply principles of basic laboratory procedures/HIV/Testing/1

14. Which is most likely a positive Western blot result for infection with HIV?
   A. Band at p24
   B. Band at gp60
   C. Bands at p24 and p31
   D. Bands at p24 and gp120

Immunology/Evaluate laboratory data to recognize health and disease states/HIV/Western blot/2

15. A woman who has had five pregnancies subsequently tests positive for HIV by Western blot. What is the most likely reason for this result?
   A. Possible cross-reaction with herpes or EBV antibodies
   B. Interference from medication
   C. Cross-reaction with HLA antigens in the antigen preparation
   D. Possible technical error

Immunology/Evaluate laboratory data to recognize health and disease states/HIV/Western blot/3

16. Interpret the following results for HIV infection.

ELISA: positive; repeat ELISA: negative; Western blot: no bands
   A. Positive for HIV
   B. Negative for HIV

   C. Indeterminate
   D. Further testing needed

Immunology/Evaluate laboratory data to recognize health and disease states/HIV/Testing/2

Answers to Questions 11–16

11. **B** Two common methods for detecting antibodies to HIV are the ELISA and Western blot tests. Two common methods for detecting HIV antigens are ELISA and immunofluorescence. Two common methods for detecting HIV genes are the Southern blot test and DNA amplification using the polymerase chain reaction to detect viral nucleic acid in infected lymphocytes.

12. **A** ELISA and rapid antibody tests (usually agglutination tests) are screening tests for HIV. The latter use polystyrene beads coated with HIV antigens to give visible agglutination following incubation with serum containing anti-HIV.

13. **B** IFAs, Western blot, and PCR tests are generally used as confirmatory tests for HIV. PCR, however, is more often used for early detection of HIV infection, for documenting infant HIV infection, and for following antiviral therapy.

14. **D** To be considered positive by Western blot testing, bands must be found for at least two of the following three HIV proteins: gp41, p24, and gp120 or 160. The p24 band denotes antibody to a *gag* protein. The gp160 is the precursor protein from which gp120 and gp41 are made; these are *env* proteins.

15. **C** Multiparous women often have HLA antibodies. The Western blot antigens are derived from HIV grown in human cell lines having HLA antigens. A cross-reaction with HLA antigen(s) in the Western blot could have occurred.

16. **B** These results are not indicative of an HIV infection and may be due to a testing error in the first ELISA assay. Known false-positive ELISA reactions occur in autoimmune diseases, syphilis, alcoholism, and lymphoproliferative diseases. A sample is considered positive for HIV if it is repeatedly positive by ELISA or other screening method and positive by a confirmatory method.

17. Interpret the following results for HIV infection. ELISA: positive; Western blot: indeterminate; radioimmunoprecipitation assay (RIPA): negative
  A. Positive for human immunodeficiency virus, HIV-1
  B. Positive for human immunodeficiency virus, HIV-2
  C. Cross-reaction; biological false-positive result
  D. Impossible to determine

Immunology/Evaluate laboratory data to recognize health and disease states/HIV/Testing/2

18. What is the most likely explanation when antibody tests for HIV are negative but a polymerase chain reaction test performed 1 week later is positive?
  A. Probably not HIV infection
  B. Patient is in the "window phase" before antibody production
  C. Tests were performed incorrectly
  D. Clinical signs may be misinterpreted

Immunology/Correlate laboratory data with physiological processes/HIV/Testing/3

19. What criteria constitute the classification system for HIV infection?
  A. CD4-positive T-cell count and clinical symptoms
  B. Clinical symptoms, condition, duration, and number of positive bands on Western blot
  C. Presence or absence of lymphadenopathy
  D. Positive bands on Western blot and CD8-positive T-cell count

Immunology/Apply knowledge of fundamental biological characteristics/HIV/Helper T/1

20. What is the main difficulty associated with the development of an HIV vaccine?
  A. The virus has been difficult to culture; antigen extraction and concentration are extremely laborious
  B. Human trials cannot be performed
  C. Different strains of the virus are genetically diverse
  D. Anti-idiotype antibodies cannot be developed

Immunology/Apply principles of basic immunology/HIV/Vaccines/2

21. Which T-helper to T-suppressor ratio ($T_h:T_s$) is most likely in a patient with acquired immunodeficiency syndrome (AIDS)?
  A. 2:1
  B. 3:1
  C. 2:3
  D. 1:2

Immunology/Correlate laboratory data with physiological processes/HIV/Testing/2

22. What is a disadvantage of using a culture technique for diagnosis of HIV infection?
  A. Time consuming
  B. Large amounts of sample required
  C. Difficult to grow
  D. Difficult to measure growth

Immunology/Apply principles of basic laboratory procedures/HIV/Culture/1

Answers to Questions 17–22

17. C Because the Western blot test did not show a definite positive pattern, the RIPA assay was conducted to rule out cross-reactivity. The RIPA, highly specific for HIV, was negative. Therefore, the antibody detected in the other two assays is considered to be a biological false-positive reaction.

18. B In early seroconversion, patients may not be making enough antibodies to be detected by antibody tests. The period between infection with HIV and the appearance of detectable antibodies is called the *window phase*. Although this period has been reduced to a few weeks by sensitive enzyme immunoassays, patients at high risk or displaying clinical conditions associated with HIV disease should be tested again after waiting several more weeks.

19. A The classification system for HIV infection is based upon a combination of CD4-positive T-cell count (helper T cells) and various categories of clinical symptoms. Classification is important in determining treatment options and the progression of the disease.

20. C Vaccine development has been difficult primarily because of the genetic diversity among different strains of the virus, and new strains are constantly emerging. HIV-1 can be divided into two groups designated M (for main) and O (for outlier). The M group is further divided into 10 subtypes, designated A–J, based upon differences in the nucleotide sequence of the *gag* gene. A vaccine has yet to be developed that is effective for all of the subgroups of HIV-1.

21. D An inverted $T_h:T_s$ (less than 1.0) is a common finding in an AIDS patient. The Centers for Disease Control and Prevention requires a CD4-positive (helper T) cell count of less than 200/μL or 14% in the absence of an AIDS-defining illness (e.g., *Pneumocystis carinii* pneumonia) in the case surveillance definition of AIDS.

22. A The major disadvantage of culture techniques is that growth is very slow and then requires performance of a nucleic acid or antigen assay (e.g., immunofluorescence) to identify the virus.

23. Which method is used to test for HIV infection in infants who are born to HIV-positive mothers?
   A. ELISA
   B. Western blot test
   C. Polymerase chain reaction
   D. Viral culture

Immunology/Apply principles of special procedures/HIV/1

24. What is the most likely cause when a Western blot or ELISA is positive for all controls and samples?
   A. Improper pipetting
   B. Improper washing
   C. Improper addition of sample
   D. Improper reading

Immunology/Evaluate laboratory data to recognize problems/HIV/Testing/3

25. What constitutes a diagnosis of viral hepatitis?
   A. Abnormal test results for liver enzymes
   B. Clinical signs and symptoms
   C. Positive results for hepatitis markers
   D. All of the above

Immunology/Evaluate laboratory data to recognize health and disease states/Hepatitis/Testing/2

26. Which of the following statements regarding infection with hepatitis D virus is true?
   A. Occurs in patients with HIV infection
   B. Does not progress to chronic hepatitis
   C. Occurs in patients with hepatitis B
   D. Is not spread through blood or sexual contact

Immunology/Apply knowledge of fundamental biological characteristics/Hepatitis/1

27. All of the following hepatitis viruses are spread through blood or blood products *except*:
   A. Hepatitis A
   B. Hepatitis B
   C. Hepatitis C
   D. Hepatitis D

Immunology/Apply knowledge of fundamental biological characteristics/Hepatitis/1

28. Which hepatitis B marker is the best indicator of early acute infection?
   A. HBsAg
   B. HBeAg
   C. Anti-HBc
   D. Anti-HBs

Immunology/Correlate laboratory data with physiological processes/Hepatitis/Testing/2

Answers to Questions 23–28

23. **C** ELISA and Western blot primarily reflect the presence of maternal antibody. The PCR uses small amounts of blood and does not rely on the antibody response. PCR amplifies small amounts of viral nucleic acid and can detect less than 200 copies of viral RNA per milliliter of plasma. These qualities make PCR ideal for the testing of infants. PCR methods for HIV RNA include the Roche Amplicor reverse-transcriptase assay, the branched DNA (bDNA) signal amplification method, and the nucleic acid sequence-based amplification (NASBA) method.

24. **B** Improper washing may not remove unbound enzyme conjugated anti-human globulin, and every sample may appear positive.

25. **D** To diagnose a case of hepatitis, the physician must consider clinical signs as well as laboratory tests that measure liver enzymes and hepatitis markers.

26. **C** Hepatitis D virus is an RNA virus that requires the surface antigen or envelope of the hepatitis B virus for entry into the hepatocyte. Consequently, hepatitis D virus can infect only patients who are coinfected with hepatitis B.

27. **A** Hepatitis A is spread through the fecal-oral route and is the cause of infectious hepatitis. Hepatitis A virus has a shorter incubation period (2–7 weeks) than hepatitis B virus (1–6 months). Epidemics of hepatitis A virus can occur, especially when food and water become contaminated with raw sewage. Hepatitis E virus is also spread via the oral-fecal route and, like hepatitis A virus, has a short incubation period.

28. **A** Hepatitis B surface antigen (HBsAg) is the first marker to appear in hepatitis B virus infection. It is usually detected within 4 weeks of exposure (prior to the rise in transaminases) and persists for about 3 months after serum enzyme levels return to normal.

29. Which is the first antibody detected in serum after infection with hepatitis B virus (HBV)?
- **A.** Anti-HBs
- **B.** Anti-HBc
- **C.** Anti-HBe
- **D.** All are detectable at the same time

Immunology/Correlate laboratory data with physiological processes/Hepatitis/Testing/2

30. Which antibody persists in low-level carriers of hepatitis B virus?
- **A.** IgM anti-HBc
- **B.** IgG anti-HBc
- **C.** IgM anti-HBe
- **D.** IgG anti-HBs

Immunology/Correlate laboratory data with physiological processes/Hepatitis/Testing/2

31. What is the most likely explanation when a patient has clinical signs of viral hepatitis but tests negative for hepatitis A IgM, hepatitis B surface antigen, and hepatitis C Ab?
- **A.** Tests were performed improperly
- **B.** The patient does not have hepatitis
- **C.** The patient may be in the "core window"
- **D.** Clinical evaluation was performed improperly

Immunology/Correlate laboratory data with physiological processes/Hepatitis/Testing/3

32. Which hepatitis B markers should be performed on blood products?
- **A.** HBsAg and anti-HBc
- **B.** Anti-HBs and anti-HBc
- **C.** HBeAg and HBcAg
- **D.** Anti-HBs and HBeAg

Immunology/Apply principles of laboratory operations/Hepatitis/Testing/1

33. Which hepatitis antibody confers immunity against reinfection with hepatitis B virus?
- **A.** Anti-HBc IgM
- **B.** Anti-HBc IgG
- **C.** Anti-HBe
- **D.** Anti-HBs

Immunology/Correlate laboratory data with physiological processes/Hepatitis/Testing/1

34. Which test, other than serological markers, is most consistently elevated in viral hepatitis?
- **A.** Antinuclear antibodies
- **B.** Alanine aminotransferase (ALT)
- **C.** Absolute lymphocyte count
- **D.** Lactate dehydrogenase

Immunology/Correlate laboratory data with physiological processes/Hepatitis/Testing/1

Answers to Questions 29–34

29. **B** Antibody to the hepatitis B core antigen (anti-HBc) is the first detectable hepatitis B antibody. It persists in the serum for 1–2 years postinfection and is found in the serum of asymptomatic carriers of HBV. Because levels of total anti-HBc are high after recovery, IgM anti-HBc is a more useful marker for acute infection. Both anti-HBc and anti-HBs can persist for life, but only anti-HBs is considered protective.

30. **B** IgG antibodies to the hepatitis B core antigen (anti-HBc) can be detected in carriers who are HBsAg- and anti-HBs-negative. These persons are presumed infective even though the level of HBsAg is too low to detect. No specific B core IgG test is available, however. This patient would be positive in the anti-B core total antibody assay and negative in the anti-HB core IgM test.

31. **C** The patient may be in the "core window," the period of hepatitis B infection when both the surface antigen and surface antibody are undetectable. The IgM anti-hepatitis B core and the anti-hepatitis B core total antibody assays would be the only detectable markers in the serum of a patient in the core window phase of hepatitis B infection.

32. **A** Blood products are tested for HBsAg, an early indicator of infection, and anti-HBc, a marker that may persist for life. Following recovery from HBV infection, some patients demonstrate negative serology for HBsAg and anti-HBs but are positive for anti-HBc. Such patients are considered infective.

33. **D** Anti-HBs appears later in infection than anti-HBc and is used as a marker for immunity following infection or vaccination rather than for diagnosis of current infection.

34. **B** ALT is a liver enzyme and may be increased in hepatic disease. Highest levels occur in acute viral hepatitis, reaching 20–50 times the upper limit of normal.

35. If only anti-HBs is positive, which of the following can be ruled out?
- **A.** Hepatitis B virus vaccination
- **B.** Distant past infection with hepatitis B virus
- **C.** Hepatitis B immune globulin (HBIG) injection
- **D.** Chronic hepatitis B virus infection

Immunology/Correlate laboratory data with physiological processes/Hepatitis/Testing/2

36. Interpret the following results for EBV infection: IgG and IgM antibodies to viral capsid antigen (VCA) are positive.
- **A.** Infection in the past
- **B.** Infection with a mutual enhancer virus such as HIV
- **C.** Current infection
- **D.** Impossible to interpret; need more information

Immunology/Correlate laboratory data with physiological processes/EBV/Testing/2

37. Which statement concerning non-Forssman antibody is true?
- **A.** It is not absorbed by guinea pig antigen
- **B.** It is absorbed by guinea pig antigen
- **C.** It does not agglutinate horse RBCs
- **D.** It does not agglutinate sheep RBCs

Immunology/Apply principles of basic laboratory procedures/IM/Testing/1

38. Given a heterophile antibody titer of 224, which of the results below indicate IM?

	Absorption with guinea pig kidney	Absorption with beef cells
A.	Two-tube titer reduction	Five-tube titer reduction
B.	No titer reduction	No titer reduction
C.	Five-tube titer reduction	Five-tube titer reduction
D.	Five-tube titer reduction	No titer reduction

Immunology/Evaluate laboratory data to recognize health and disease states/IM/Testing/2

39. Given a heterophile antibody titer of 224, which of the results below indicate serum sickness?

	Absorption with guinea pig kidney	Absorption with beef cells
A.	Two-tube titer reduction	Five-tube titer reduction
B.	No titer reduction	No titer reduction
C.	Five-tube titer reduction	Five-tube titer reduction
D.	Five-tube titer reduction	No titer reduction

Immunology/Evaluate laboratory data to recognize health and disease states/Serum sickness/Testing/2

40. Given a heterophile antibody titer of 224, which of the results below indicate an error in testing?

	Absorption with guinea pig kidney	Absorption with beef cells
A.	Two-tube titer reduction	Five-tube titer reduction
B.	No titer reduction	No titer reduction
C.	Five-tube titer reduction	Five-tube titer reduction
D.	Five-tube titer reduction	No titer reduction

Immunology/Evaluate laboratory data to determine possible inconsistent results/IM/Testing/2

Answers to Questions 35–40

35. D Persons with chronic HBV infection show a positive test result for anti-HBc (IgG or total) and HBsAg but not anti-HBs. Patients with active chronic hepatitis have not become immune to the virus.

36. C Antibodies to both IgG and IgM VCA are found in a current infection with EBV. The IgG antibody may persist for life, but the IgM anti-VCA disappears within 4 months after the infection resolves.

37. A Non-Forssman antibody is not absorbed by guinea pig antigen. This is one of the principles of the Davidsohn differential test for antibodies to IM. These antibodies are non-Forssman; they are absorbed by sheep, horse, or beef RBCs but not by guinea pig kidney. Therefore, a heterophile titer remaining higher after absorption with guinea pig kidney than with beef RBCs indicates IM.

38. A Antibodies to infectious mononucleosis (non-Forssman antibodies) are not neutralized or absorbed by guinea pig antigen (but are absorbed by beef cell antigen). A positive test is indicated by at least a four-tube reduction in the heterophile titer after absorption with beef cells and no more than a three-tube reduction in titer after absorption with guinea pig kidney.

39. C In serum sickness, antibodies are neutralized by both guinea pig kidney and beef cell antigens, and at least a three-tube (eightfold) reduction in titer should occur after absorption with both.

40. B An individual with a 56 or higher titer in the presumptive test (significant heterophile antibodies) has either Forssman antibodies, non-Forssman antibodies, or both. A testing error has occurred if no reduction in the titer of antibody against sheep RBCs is observed after absorption because absorption should remove one or both types of sheep RBC agglutinins.

41. Blood products are tested for which virus before being transfused to newborns?
A. EBV
B. Human T-lymphotropic virus II (HTLV-II)
C. Cytomegalovirus (CMV)
D. Hepatitis D virus

Immunology/Apply principles of laboratory operations/CMV/Testing/1

42. What is the endpoint for the antistreptolysin O (ASO) latex agglutination assay?
A. Highest serum dilution that shows no agglutination
B. Highest serum dilution that shows agglutination
C. Lowest serum dilution that shows agglutination
D. Lowest serum dilution that shows no agglutination

Immunology/Apply principles of basic laboratory procedures/ASO/Interpretation/1

43. Interpret the following antistreptolysin O (ASO) results.

Tube Nos. 1–4 (Todd unit 125): no hemolysis; Tube No. 5 (Todd unit 166): hemolysis
A. Positive Todd unit 125
B. Positive Todd unit 166
C. Negative
D. Impossible to interpret

Immunology/Evaluate laboratory data to make identifications/ASO/Interpretation/2

44. Which control shows the correct result for a valid ASO test?
A. SLO control, no hemolysis
B. Red cell control, no hemolysis
C. Positive control, hemolysis in all tubes
D. Hemolysis in both SLO and red cell control

Immunology/Apply principles of basic laboratory procedures/ASO/Controls/1

45. A streptozyme test was performed, but the result was negative, even though the patient showed clinical signs of a streptococcal throat infection. What should be done next?
A. Either ASO or anti-deoxyribonuclease B (anti-DNase B) testing
B. Another streptozyme test using diluted serum
C. Antihyaluronidase testing
D. Wait for 3–5 days and repeat the streptozyme test

Immunology/Evaluate laboratory data to recognize health and disease states/ASO/Testing/3

46. Rapid assays for influenza that utilize specimens obtained from nasopharyngeal swabs detect:
A. IgM anti-influenza
B. IgA anti-influenza

C. IgA-influenza Ag immune complexes
D. Influenza antigen

Immunology/Evaluate laboratory data to recognize health and disease states/2

41. C CMV can be life-threatening if transmitted to a newborn through a blood product. HTLV-II is a rare virus, which like HIV, is a T-cell tropic RNA retrovirus. The virus has been associated with hairy cell leukemia, but this is not a consistent finding.

42. B The latex test for ASO includes latex particles coated with streptolysin O. Serial dilutions are prepared and the highest dilution showing agglutination is the endpoint.

43. A An ASO titer is expressed in Todd units as the last tube that neutralizes (*no* visible hemolysis) the streptolysin O (SLO). Most laboratories consider an ASO titer significant if it is 166 Todd units or higher. However, people with a recent history of streptococcal infection may demonstrate an ASO titer of 166 or higher; demonstration of a rise in titer from acute to convalescent serum is required to confirm a current streptococcal infection. ASO is commonly measured using a rapid latex agglutination assay. These tests show agglutination when the ASO concentration is 200 IU/mL or higher.

44. B The red cell control contains no SLO and should show no hemolysis. The SLO control contains no serum and should show complete hemolysis. An ASO titer cannot be determined unless both the RBC and SLO controls demonstrate the expected results.

45. A A streptozyme test is used for screening and contains several of the antigens associated with streptococcal products. Because some patients produce an antibody response to a limited number of streptococcal products, no single test is sufficiently sensitive to rule out infection. Clinical sensitivity is increased by performing additional tests when initial results are negative. The streptozyme test generally shows more false-positives and false-negatives than ASO and anti-DNase. A positive test for anti-hyaluronidase occurs in a smaller number of patients with recent streptococcal infections than ASO and anti-DNase.

46. D The rapid influenza assays are antigen detection methods. They are designed to detect early infection, before antibody is produced.

47. How can interfering cold agglutinins be removed from a test sample?
- **A.** Centrifuge the serum and remove the top layer
- **B.** Incubate the clot at 1°–4°C for several hours, then remove serum
- **C.** Incubate the serum at 56°C in a water bath for 30 minutes
- **D.** Use an anticoagulated sample

Immunology/Apply principles of special procedures/Cold agglutinins/Testing/2

48. All tubes (dilutions) except the negative control are positive for cold agglutinins. This indicates:
- **A.** Contaminated red cells
- **B.** A rare antibody against red cell antigens
- **C.** The sample was stored at 4°C prior to separating serum and cells
- **D.** Further serial dilution is necessary

Immunology/Select course of action/Cold agglutinins/Testing/3

49. All positive cold agglutinin tubes remain positive after 37°C incubation except the positive control. What is the most likely explanation for this situation?
- **A.** High titer cold agglutinins
- **B.** Contamination of the test system
- **C.** Antibody other than cold agglutinins
- **D.** Faulty water bath

Immunology/Evaluate laboratory data to determine possible inconsistent results/Cold agglutinins/Testing/3

50. Which increase in antibody titer (dilution) best indicates an acute infection?
- **A.** From 1:2 to 1:8
- **B.** From 1:4 to 1:16
- **C.** From 1:16 to 1:256
- **D.** From 1:64 to 1:128

Immunology/Correlate laboratory data with physiological processes/Antibody titers/1

51. Which of the following positive antibody tests may be an indication of recent vaccination or early primary infection for rubella in a patient with no clinical symptoms?
- **A.** Only IgG antibodies positive
- **B.** Only IgM antibodies positive
- **C.** Both IgG and IgM antibodies positive
- **D.** Fourfold rise in titer for IgG antibodies

Immunology/Apply principles of basic laboratory procedures/Rubella/Testing/2

52. Why is laboratory diagnosis difficult in cases of Lyme disease?
- **A.** Clinical response may not be apparent upon initial infection; IgM antibody may not be detected until 3–6 weeks after the infection

- **B.** Laboratory tests may be designed to detect whole *Borrelia burgdorferi,* not flagellar antigen found early in infection
- **C.** Most laboratory tests are technically demanding and lack specificity
- **D.** Antibodies formed initially to *B. burgdorferi* may cross-react in antigen tests for autoimmune diseases

Immunology/Correlate clinical signs with laboratory procedures/Lyme disease/Testing/2

Answers to Questions 47–52

47. **B** Cold agglutinins will attach to autologous red cells if incubated at 1°–4°C. The absorbed serum will be free of cold agglutinins.

48. **D** Cold agglutinins may be measured in patients who have cold agglutinin disease, a cold autoimmune hemolytic anemia. In such cases, titers can be as high as 10^6. If all tubes (dilutions) for cold agglutinins are positive, except the negative control, then a high titer of cold agglutinins is present in the sample. Further serial dilutions should be performed.

49. **C** Cold agglutinins do not remain reactive above 30°C, and agglutination must disperse following incubation at 37°C. The most likely explanation when agglutination remains after 37°C incubation is that a warm alloantibody or autoantibody is present.

50. **C** A fourfold or greater increase in antibody titer is usually indicative of an acute infection. In most serological tests a single high titer is insufficient evidence of acute infection unless specific IgM antibodies are measured because age, individual variation, immunological status, and history of previous exposure (or vaccination) cause a wide variation in normal serum antibody titers.

51. **B** If only IgM antibodies are positive, this result indicates a recent vaccination or an early primary infection.

52. **A** Lyme disease is caused by *B. burgdorferi,* a spirochete, and typical clinical symptoms such as rash or erythema chronicum migrans may be lacking in some infected individuals. Additionally, IgM antibody is not detectable by laboratory tests until 3–6 weeks after a tick bite, and IgG antibody develops later.

53. Serological tests for which disease may give a false-positive result if the patient has Lyme disease?
    A. AIDS
    B. Syphilis
    C. Cold agglutinins
    D. Hepatitis C

Immunology/Evaluate laboratory data to determine possible inconsistent results/Lyme disease/Testing/3

54. In monitoring an HIV-infected patient, which parameter may be expected to be the most sensitive indicator of the effectiveness of antiretroviral treatment?
    A. HIV antibody titer
    B. CD4:CD8 ratio
    C. HIV viral load
    D. Absolute total T-cell count

Immunology/Correlate clinical and laboratory data/ HIV/2

55. A renal transplant recipient is found to have a rising creatinine level and reduced urine output. The physician orders a "Urine PCR" assay. When you call to find out what organism the physician wants to identify, you are told:
    A. Hepatitis C virus
    B. *Legionella pneumophila*
    C. EBV
    D. BK virus

Immunology/Apply knowledge of fundamental biological characteristics/Transplant/Virus/2

56. A newborn is to be tested for a vertically transmitted HIV infection. Which of the following tests is most useful?
    A. HIV PCR
    B. CD4 count
    C. Rapid HIV antibody test
    D. HIV IgM antibody test

Immunology/Select test/Neonatal HIV/2

57. Which of the following methods used for HIV identification is considered a signal amplification technique?
    A. Branched chain DNA analysis
    B. DNA PCR
    C. Reverse transcriptase PCR
    D. Nucleic acid sequence based assay (NASBA)

Immunology/Apply knowledge of special procedures/ Molecular/HIV/1

58. Which of the following fungal organisms is often diagnosed by a serum antigen detection test as opposed to a serum antibody detection assay?
    A. *Histoplasma*
    B. *Cryptococcus*
    C. *Candida*
    D. *Aspergillus*

Immunology/Apply knowledge of special procedures/ Fungal testing/2

Answers to Questions 53–58

53. **B** Lyme disease is caused by a spirochete and may give positive results with some specific treponemal antibody tests for syphilis.

54. **C** The HIV viral load will rise or fall in response to treatment more quickly than any of the other listed parameters. The absolute CD4 count is also an indicator of treatment effectiveness and is used in resource poor areas that might not have facilities for molecular testing available. Note that the absolute CD4 count is not one of the choices, however.

55. **D** BK virus is a polyoma virus that can cause renal and urinary tract infections. The virus is an opportunistic pathogen and has become a well-recognized cause of poor renal function in kidney transplant recipients. Antibody testing is not practical or useful for this infection. The principal diagnostic assays are urinary cytology, and specific BK virus PCR testing in urine and serum. Although *Legionella pneumophila* can be diagnosed through a urinary antigen assay, that organism is not a primary cause of renal insufficiency in transplant patients.

56. **A** Neonatal HIV diagnosis is performed by screening for the presence of the virus. The current antibody tests are either IgG-specific or an IgG/IgM combination assay. Thus an infant whose mother is HIV-positive will also be positive in the HIV antibody assay. Although the CD4 count may be a useful assay to determine disease activity, there are many causes of reduced CD4 numbers and this assay should not be used to diagnose HIV infection.

57. **A** Branched chain DNA is a signal amplification technique, i.e., if you start with one copy of the gene you finish with one copy. The detection reagent is amplified, increasing the sensitivity of the assay to levels on par with target amplification techniques such as PCR and NASBA.

58. **B** The *Cryptococcus* antibody response is not a reliable indicator of a current infection; thus, an antigen assay is normally used to monitor the disease. The antigen assay may be used in serum or spinal fluid and will decline in response to treatment much faster than a traditional antibody test. A urinary antigen test is available for histoplasmosis, although antibody assays are also used for diagnosing *Histoplasma* infections.

59. Your cytology laboratory refers a Papanicolaou smear specimen to you for an assay designed to detect the presence of a virus associated with cervical cancer. You perform:
A. An ELISA assay for anti HSV-2 antibodies
B. A molecular assay for HSV-2
C. An ELISA assay for HPV antibodies
D. A molecular assay for HPV

Immunology/Select course of action/Virus testing/Methods/3

60. An immunosuppressed patient has an unexplained anemia. The physician suspects a parvovirus B19 infection. A parvovirus IgM test is negative. The next course of action is to tell the physician:
A. The patient does not have parvovirus
B. A convalescent specimen is recommended in 4 weeks to determine if a fourfold rise in titer has occurred
C. A parvovirus PCR is recommended
D. That a recent transfusion for the patient's anemia may have resulted in a false negative assay and the patient should be retested in 4 weeks

Immunology/Select course of action/Virus testing/Parvovirus/3

59. **D** Cervical cell atypia and cervical cancer are associated with specific high risk serotypes of human papilloma virus (HPV) infections. Although HPV antibody assays are available, they are not serotype-specific, nor do they relate to disease activity. Thus molecular probe assays are the tests of choice to detect high-risk HPV infection. Although HSVC-2 is associated with genital herpesvirus, that virus has not been shown to cause cervical cancer.

60. **C** A negative IgM assay rarely rules out an infection. While a convalescent specimen may be useful in many cases, in an immunosuppressed patient the convalescent specimen may remain negative in the presence of an infection. Thus a parvovirus PCR is the preferred choice in this case. A false-negative result could conceivably be caused by multiple whole blood or plasma transfusions, but retesting for antibody a month later would not be beneficial to the patient.

AUTOIMMUNE DISEASES

1. What is a general definition for autoimmunity?
   A. Increase of tolerance to self-antigens
   B. Loss of tolerance to self-antigens
   C. Increase in clonal deletion of mutant cells
   D. Manifestation of immunosuppression

Immunology/Apply knowledge of fundamental biological characteristics/Autoimmunity/Definition/1

2. An antinuclear antibody test is performed on a specimen from a 55-year-old woman who has unexplained joint pain. The IFA result is a titer of 40 and a homogeneous pattern. The appropriate follow-up for this patient is:
   A. Anti-DNA assay
   B. ENA testing
   C. Retest ANA in 3–6 months
   D. CH50 complement assay

Immunology/Correlate laboratory data with physiological processes/IF/2

3. Which disease is likely to show a rim (peripheral) pattern in an immunofluorescence (IF) microscopy test for ANA?
   A. Mixed connective tissue disease (MCTD)
   B. Rheumatoid arthritis
   C. Systemic lupus erythematosus
   D. Scleroderma

Immunology/Correlate laboratory data with physiological processes/IF/2

4. A patient's specimen is strongly positive in an ANA ELISA. Which of the following would *not* be an appropriate follow up to this result?
   A. Immunofluorescence test on HEp-2 cells
   B. Specific ENA ELISA tests
   C. Specific anti-DNA ELISA
   D. Rheumatoid factor assay

Immunology/Select test/ANA/IF/2

5. What type of antibodies are represented by the solid or homogeneous pattern in the immunofluorescence test for antinuclear antibodies?
   A. Antihistone antibodies
   B. Anticentromere antibodies
   C. Anti-ENA (anti-Sm and anti-RNP) antibodies
   D. Anti-RNA antibodies

Immunology/Correlate laboratory data with physiological processes/IF/1

Answers to Questions 1–5

1. B Autoimmunity is a loss of tolerance to self-antigens and the subsequent formation of autoantibodies.

2. C Approximately 25% of women in this age range may have low titer positive ANA assays with no demonstrable connective tissue disease. A patient with anti-DNA positive SLE would be expected to have a much higher titer (>160) in an IFA assay. A similar titer would be expected for an ENA positive specimen, although the pattern would be speckled. Complement testing would not be indicated with this low titer in a 55-year-old female.

3. C The rim or peripheral pattern seen in indirect immunofluorescence techniques is most commonly found in cases of active SLE. The responsible autoantibody is highly correlated to anti–double-stranded DNA (anti-dsDNA).

4. D The ANA ELISA is a screening assay. A positive result may be followed up by more specific antibody ELISA tests or an ANA immunofluorescence test to determine pattern and titer. The ANA ELISA does not screen for rheumatoid factor.

5. A Antihistone antibodies (and also anti-DNA antibodies) cause the solid or homogeneous pattern, which is commonly found in patients with SLE, RA, mixed connective tissue disease, and Sjögren's syndrome. Antibodies to the centromere of chromosomes is a marker for the CREST (calcinosis, Raynaud's phenomenon, esophageal dysfunction, sclerodactyly, and telangiectasia) form of systemic sclerosis.

6. What disease is indicated by a high titer of anti-Sm (anti-Smith) antibody?
   A. Mixed connective tissue disease (MCTD)
   B. RA
   C. SLE
   D. Scleroderma

   Immunology/Correlate laboratory data with physiological processes/IF/2

7. Which disease is *LEAST* likely when a nucleolar pattern occurs in an immunofluorescence test for antinuclear antibodies?
   A. MCTD
   B. Sjögren's syndrome
   C. SLE
   D. Scleroderma

   Immunology/Correlate laboratory data with physiological processes/IF/2

8. What antibodies are represented by the nucleolar pattern in the immunofluorescence test for antinuclear antibodies?
   A. Antihistone antibodies
   B. Anti-dsDNA antibodies
   C. Anti-ENA (anti-Sm and anti-RNP) antibodies
   D. Anti-RNA antibodies

   Immunology/Correlate laboratory data with physiological processes/IF/1

9. Which test would best distinguish between SLE and MCTD?
   A. Ouchterlony or ELISA test for anti-SM and anti-RNP
   B. Immunofluorescence testing using *Crithidia* as substrate
   C. Slide agglutination testing
   D. Laboratory tests cannot distinguish between these disorders

   Immunology/Evaluate laboratory data to recognize and report the need for additional testing/Autoimmune/ Testing/3

10. An ANA test on HEp-2 cells shows nucleolar staining in interphase cells and dense chromatin staining in mitotic cells. The most likely cause of this staining pattern is:
    A. Antifibrillarin antibody
    B. Antiribosomal p antibody
    C. A serum with nucleolar and homogeneous patterns
    D. Technical artifact

    Immunology/Correlate laboratory data with physiological processes/IF/1

11. Which immunofluorescence pattern indicates the need for ENA testing by Ouchterlony immunodiffusion or ELISA assays?

    A. Homogeneous or solid
    B. Peripheral or rim
    C. Speckled
    D. Nucleolar

    Immunology/Evaluate laboratory data to recognize and report the need for additional testing/Autoimmune/ Testing/3

Answers to Questions 6–11

6. **C** High titer anti-Sm is indicative of SLE. Anti-Sm is one of two antibodies against saline extractable nuclear antigens, the other being anti-RNP. These antibodies cause a speckled pattern of immunofluorescence.

7. **A** All of the diseases except MCTD may cause a nucleolar pattern of immunofluorescence. Nucleolar fluorescence is caused by anti-RNA antibodies and is seen in about 50% of patients with scleroderma.

8. **D** Anti-RNA antibodies are represented by the nucleolar pattern. This pattern may be seen in most systemic autoimmune diseases and is especially common in patients with scleroderma. Anti-RNA and anti-Sm are not usually found in patients with mixed connective tissue disease. This is a syndrome involving aspects of SLE, RA, scleroderma, and polymyositis. The immunofluorescence pattern most often seen in MCTD is the speckled pattern caused by anti-RNP.

9. **A** The Ouchterlony (double) immunodiffusion assay may be used to identify and differentiate anti-Sm from anti-RNP. ELISA assays, using purified or recombinant antigens, are also available for this testing. Anti-Sm with or without anti-RNP is found in approximately one third of SLE patients. Anti-RNP in the absence of anti-Sm is found in over 95% of MCTD patients.

10. **A** Antifibrillarin antibody has this appearance. Ribosomal p antibody has nucleolar staining and a background homogeneous and cytoplasmic stain. A combination nucleolar/homogeneous specimen will also show homogeneous staining in the interphase cells. This pattern is not seen in typical technical artifacts.

11. **C** A speckled pattern is often due to the presence of antibodies against the extractable nuclear antigens, such as Sm, RNP, SSA and SSB. Homogenous and rim patterns suggest antibodies to double-stranded DNA. The homogeneous pattern may also be seen with antibodies to deoxyribonuclear protein, which is not an ENA. Nucleolar patterns often indicate antibodies to RNA or fibrillarin.

12. Which of the following is used in rapid slide tests for detection of rheumatoid factors?
   A. Whole IgM molecules
   B. Fc portion of the IgG molecule
   C. Fab portion of the IgG molecule
   D. Fc portion of the IgM molecule

   Immunology/Apply knowledge of fundamental biological characteristics/RA/Testing/1

13. Which of the following methods is *LEAST* likely to give a definitive result for the diagnosis of RA?
   A. Nephelometric measurement of anti-IgG
   B. Agglutination testing for rheumatoid factor
   C. ELISA of anti-IgG
   D. Immunofluorescence testing for antinuclear antibodies

   Immunology/Select routine laboratory procedures/ Autoimmune/RA/Testing/1

14. Which disease might be indicated by antibodies to smooth muscle?
   A. Atrophic gastritis
   B. Active chronic hepatitis
   C. Myasthenia gravis
   D. Sjögren's syndrome

   Immunology/Apply knowledge of fundamental biological characteristics/Autoimmune/Testing/1

15. Antibodies to thyroid peroxidase can be detected by using agglutination assays. Which of the following diseases may show positive results with this type of assay?
   A. Graves' disease and Hashimoto's thyroiditis
   B. Myasthenia gravis
   C. Granulomatous thyroid disease
   D. Addison's disease

   Immunology/Select routine laboratory procedures/ Autoimmune/Testing/1

16. What is the main use of laboratory tests to detect antibodies to islet cells and insulin in cases of insulin-dependent diabetes mellitus (IDDM)?
   A. To regulate levels of injected insulin
   B. To diagnose IDDM
   C. To rule out the presence of other autoimmune diseases
   D. To screen susceptible individuals prior to destruction of β cells

   Immunology/Select routine laboratory procedures/ Autoimmune/IDDM/Testing/1

Answers to Questions 12–16

12. **B** Rheumatoid factors react with the Fc portion of the IgG molecule and are usually IgM. This is the basis of rapid agglutination tests for RA. Particles of latex or cells are coated with IgG. Addition of serum containing rheumatoid factor results in visible agglutination.

13. **D** Patients with RA often show a homogeneous pattern of fluorescence in tests for antinuclear antibodies. However, this pattern is seen in a wide range of systemic autoimmune diseases and in many normal persons at a titer below 10. The other three methods may be used to identify anti-IgG, which is required to establish a diagnosis of RA.

14. **B** Antibodies to smooth muscle are found in the serum of up to 70% of patients with active chronic hepatitis and up to 50% of patients with primary biliary cirrhosis.

15. **A** Antibodies to thyroid peroxidase may be detected in both Graves' disease (hyperthyroidism) and Hashimoto's thyroiditis (hypothyroidism). If a positive result is found to thyroid peroxidase, thyroxine levels can be measured to distinguish between the two diseases.

16. **D** Fasting hyperglycemia is the primary finding used to diagnose IDDM. For individuals with an inherited susceptibility to the development of IDDM, laboratory tests for the detection of antibodies to islet cells and insulin may help to initiate early treatment before complete destruction of β cells.

1. Which of the following is a description of a type I hypersensitivity reaction?
   A. Ragweed antigen cross-links with IgE on the surface of mast cells causing release of preformed mediators and resulting in symptoms of an allergic reaction
   B. Anti-Fy^a from a pregnant woman crosses the placenta and attaches to the Fy^a antigen-positive red cells of the fetus, destroying the red cells
   C. Immune complex deposition occurs on the glomerular basement membrane of the kidney, leading to renal failure
   D. Exposure to poison ivy causes sensitized T cells to release lymphokines that cause a localized inflammatory reaction

   Immunology/Apply knowledge of fundamental biological characteristics/Hypersensitivity/2

2. Why is skin testing the most widely used method to test for a type I hypersensitivity reaction?
   A. It causes less trauma and is more cost-effective than other methods
   B. It has greater sensitivity than in vitro measurements
   C. It is more likely to be positive for IgE-specific allergens than other methods
   D. It may be used to predict the development of further allergen sensitivity

   Immunology/Apply principles of basic laboratory procedures/Hypersensitivity/Testing/1

3. Which in vitro test measures IgE levels against a specific allergen?
   A. Histamine release assay
   B. Radioimmunosorbent test (RIST)
   C. Fluorescent allergosorbent test (FAST)
   D. Precipitin radioimmunosorbent test (PRIST)

   Immunology/Apply principles of basic laboratory procedures/Hypersensitivity/IgE testing/1

Answers to Questions 1–3

1. **A** Type I immediate hypersensitivity (anaphylactic) responses are characterized by IgE molecules binding to mast cells via the Fc receptor. Cross-linking of surface IgE caused by binding of allergens causes the mast cell to degranulate, releasing histamine and other chemical mediators of allergy. Answer B describes a type II reaction; C describes a type III reaction; and D describes a type IV reaction.

2. **B** Skin testing is considered much more sensitive than in vitro tests that measure either total or antigen-specific IgE.

3. **C** The FAST is a fluorescent assay that measures specific IgE; the RIST and PRIST tests are radioimmunoassays that measure total IgE. The FAST procedure has replaced the RAST, or radioallergosorbent assay. The histamine release assay measures the amount of histamine. Allergen-specific IgE assays are available based upon solid-phase enzyme immunoassay. The allergen is covalently bound to a cellulose solid phase and reacts with specific IgE in the serum. After washing, enzyme (β-galactosidase)-labeled monoclonal anti-IgE is added. The unbound antibody-conjugate is washed away and fluorogenic substrate (4-methylumbelliferyl-β-D-galactose) is added. Fluorescence is directly proportional to specific IgE.

4. A patient who is blood group O is accidentally transfused with group A blood. What antibody is involved in this type II reaction?

A. IgM

B. IgE

C. IgG and IgE

D. IgG

Immunology/Apply principles of basic laboratory procedures/Hypersensitivity/Testing/1

5. Which test would measure the coating of red cells by antibody as occurs in hemolytic transfusion reactions?

A. Indirect antiglobulin test (IAT)

B. Direct antiglobulin test (DAT)

C. ELISA

D. Hemagglutination

Immunology/Apply principles of basic laboratory procedures/Hemolytic reaction/1

6. Which test detects antibodies that have attached to tissues, resulting in a type II cytotoxic reaction?

A. Migration inhibition factor assay (MIF)

B. Direct immunofluorescence (IF)

C. Immunofixation electrophoresis (IFE)

D. Hemagglutination

Immunology/Apply principles of basic laboratory procedures/Hemolytic reaction/1

7. Which of the following conditions will most likely result in a false-negative DAT test?

A. Insufficient washing of RBCs

B. Use of heavy chain specific polyclonal anti-human Ig

C. Use of excessive centrifugal force

D. Use of a sample obtained by finger puncture

Immunology/Apply knowledge to identify sources of error/Hemolytic reaction/3

8. Which of the following tests is used to detect circulating immune complexes in the serum of some patients with systemic autoimmune diseases such as rheumatoid arthritis?

A. Direct immunofluorescence

B. Enzyme immunoassay

C. Assay of cryoglobulins

D. Indirect antiglobulin test

Immunology/Apply knowledge of fundamental biological characteristics/Hypersensitivity/1

9. All of the following tests may be abnormal in a type III immune complex reaction *except*:

A. C1q-binding assay by ELISA

B. Raji cell assay

C. CH$_{50}$ level

D. Mitogen response

Immunology/Apply principles of special laboratory procedures/Hypersensitivity/Testing/1

Answers to Questions 4–9

4. **A** IgG and IgM are the antibodies involved in a type II cytotoxic reaction. Naturally occurring anti-A in the form of IgM is present in the blood of a group O individual and would cause an immediate transfusion reaction. Cell destruction occurs when antibodies bind to cells causing destruction via complement activation, thereby triggering intravascular hemolysis.

5. **B** The DAT test measures antibody that has already coated RBCs in vivo. Direct antiglobulin and direct immunofluorescence tests use anti-immunoglobulin to detect antibody sensitized cells.

6. **B** The direct IF test detects the presence of antibody that may cause a type II cytotoxic reaction. For example, renal biopsies from patients with Goodpasture's syndrome exhibit a smooth pattern of fluorescence along the basement membrane after reaction with fluorescein isothiocyanate (FITC) conjugated anti-immunoglobulin. The reaction detects antibodies against the basement membrane of the glomeruli.

7. **A** Insufficient washing can cause incomplete removal of excess or unbound immunoglobulins and other proteins, which may neutralize the antiglobulin reagent.

8. **C** Most autoimmune diseases involve the formation of antigen-antibody complexes that deposit in the tissues, causing local inflammation and necrosis induced by complement activation, phagocytosis, WBC infiltration, and lysosomal damage. Some patients make monoclonal or polyclonal antibodies with rheumatoid factor activity that bind to serum immunoglobulins, forming aggregates that are insoluble at 4°C. These circulating immune complexes are detected by allowing a blood sample to clot at 37°C, transferring the serum to a sedimentation rate tube, and then incubating the serum at 4°C for 3 days.

9. **D** Mitogen stimulation is used to measure T-cell, B-cell, and null-cell responsiveness, which is important in patients displaying anergy and other signs of immunodeficiency. The C1q assay and the Raji cell assays detect circulating immune complexes that are present during a type III reaction. The CH$_{50}$ level is usually decreased owing to complement activation by the immune complexes. Raji cells are derived from a malignant B-cell line that demonstrates C3 receptors but no surface membrane immunoglobulin. Immune complexes that have fixed complement will bind to Raji cells and can be identified using radiolabeled or enzyme labeled anti-immunoglobulin. More recently, a C3 binding ELISA assay has replaced the Raji cell procedure.

10. What immune elements are involved in a positive skin test for tuberculosis?
  A. IgE antibodies
  B. T cells and macrophages
  C. NK cells and IgG antibody
  D. B cells and IgM antibody

Immunology/Apply knowledge of fundamental biological characteristics/Hypersensitivity/1

11. A patient receives a transfusion of packed red cells and fresh frozen plasma and develops an anaphylactic, nonhemolytic reaction. She reports receiving a transfusion 20 years earlier. She had no reaction to the previous transfusion, but she did feel "poorly" a few weeks later. Which of the following transfused substances most likely elicited the reaction?
  A. IgA
  B. Group A antigen
  C. Rho (D) antigen
  D. An antigen belonging to the Duffy system

Immunology/Apply knowledge of fundamental biological characteristics/Immune Deficiency/Hypersensitivity/3

12. A patient deficient in the C3 complement component would be expected to mount a normal:
  A. Type I and IV hypersensitivity response
  B. Type II and IV hypersensitivity response
  C. Type I and III hypersensitivity response
  D. Type II and III hypersensitivity response

Immunology/Apply knowledge of fundamental biological characteristics/Immune Deficiency/Hypersensitivity/2

Answers to Questions 10–12

10. **B** T cells and macrophages are the immune elements primarily responsible for the clinical manifestations of a positive tuberculosis test. Reactions usually take 72 hours to reach peak development and are characteristic of localized type IV cell-mediated hypersensitivity. The skin reaction is characterized by a lesion containing a mononuclear cell infiltrate.

11. **A** The fact that this is a nonhemolytic reaction suggests that a non–red cell antigen may be involved. Selective IgA deficiency occurs in approximately 1 in 700 individuals and is often asymptomatic. Individuals deficient in IgA may make an antibody against the α heavy chain if they are exposed to IgA via a transfusion. This antibody may lead to a serum sickness reaction if the IgA is still present after antibody formation. This could explain the "poor feeling" the patient had after the initial transfusion. A subsequent transfusion may lead to an Arthus reaction if IgG anti-IgA is present or an anaphylactic reaction if IgE anti-IgA is present.

12. **A** Complement is involved in types II and III hypersensitivity; thus an individual deficient in C3 will be deficient in those responses. The complement deficiency should have no effect on IgE (type I) or cell mediated (type IV) hypersensitivities.

1. **Which of the following symptoms in a young child may indicate an immunodeficiency syndrome?**
   - **A.** Anaphylactic reactions
   - **B.** Severe rashes and myalgia
   - **C.** Recurrent bacterial, fungal, and viral infections
   - **D.** Weight loss, rapid heartbeat, breathlessness

   Immunology/Apply knowledge of fundamental biological characteristics/T cell/Testing/1

2. **What screening test should be performed first in a young patient suspected of having an immune dysfunction disorder?**
   - **A.** Complete blood count (CBC) and white cell differential
   - **B.** Chemotaxis assay
   - **C.** Complement levels
   - **D.** Bone marrow biopsy

   Immunology/Apply knowledge of fundamental biological characteristics/Testing/2

3. **Which test should be performed when a patient has a reaction to transfused plasma products?**
   - **A.** Immunoglobulin levels
   - **B.** T-cell count
   - **C.** Hemoglobin levels
   - **D.** Red cell enzymes

   Immunology/Evaluate laboratory and clinical data to specify additional tests/Testing/3

4. **What is the "M" component in monoclonal gammopathies?**
   - **A.** IgM produced in excess
   - **B.** μ Heavy chain produced in excess
   - **C.** Malignant proliferation of B cells
   - **D.** Monoclonal antibody or cell line

   Immunology/Apply knowledge of fundamental biological characteristics/Immunoglobulin/Testing/1

5. **A child suspected of having an inherited humoral immunodeficiency disease is given diphtheria/tetanus vaccine. Two weeks after the immunization, his level of antibody to the specific antigens is measured. Which result is expected for this patient?**
   - **A.** Increased levels of specific antibody
   - **B.** No change in the level of specific antibody
   - **C.** An increase in IgG-specific antibody but not IgM-specific antibody
   - **D.** Increased levels of nonspecific antibody

   Immunology/Evaluate laboratory data/Immunoglobulins/Testing/2

Answers to Questions 1–5

1. **C** An immunodeficiency syndrome should be considered in a young child who has a history of recurrent bacterial, fungal, and viral infections manifested after the disappearance of maternal IgG. Immunodeficiency disorders may involve deficiencies in production and/or function of lymphocytes and phagocytic cells or a deficiency in production of a complement factor. Choice of laboratory tests is based upon the patient's clinical presentation, age, and history.

2. **A** The first screening tests performed in the initial evaluation of a young patient who is suspected of having an immune dysfunction are the CBC and differential. White blood cells that are decreased in number or abnormal in appearance may indicate further testing.

3. **A** A reaction to plasma products may be found in an IgA-deficient person who has formed anti-IgA antibodies. Immunoglobulin levels would aid in this determination. Selective IgA deficiency is the most common immunodeficiency disease and is characterized by serum IgA levels below 5 mg/dL. IgA is usually absent from secretions, but the B-cell count is usually normal.

4. **D** The "M" component refers to any monoclonal protein or cell line produced in a monoclonal gammopathy such as multiple myeloma.

5. **B** In an immunodeficient patient, the expected levels of specific antibody to the antigens in the vaccine would be decreased or not present. This response provides evidence of deficient antibody production.

6. Which disease may be expected to show an IgM spike on an electrophoretic pattern?
   A. Hypogammaglobulinemia
   B. Multicystic kidney disease
   C. Waldenström's macroglobulinemia
   D. Wiskott-Aldrich syndrome

   Immunology/Evaluate laboratory data to make identifications/Immunoglobulins/Testing/2

7. In testing for DiGeorge's syndrome, what type of laboratory analysis would be most helpful in determining the number of mature T cells?
   A. Complete blood count
   B. Nitroblue tetrazolium (NBT) test
   C. T-cell enzyme assays
   D. Flow cytometry

   Immunology/Evaluate laboratory data to make identifications/T cells/Testing/2

8. Interpret the following description of an immunofixation electrophoresis assay of urine. Dense wide bands in both the κ and λ lanes. No bands present in the heavy chain lanes.
   A. Normal
   B. Light chain disease
   C. Increased polyclonal Fab fragments
   D. Multiple myeloma

   Immunology/Evaluate laboratory data to make identifications/Immunoglobulins/Testing/2

9. Free monoclonal light chains are often present in the serum of multiple myeloma patients, and may be useful for disease monitoring. Which of the following assays would be recommended to detect the presence of serum free light chains?
   A. Serum protein electrophoresis
   B. Urine immunofixation
   C. Nephelometry
   D. ELISA

   Immunology/Evaluate laboratory and clinical data to specify additional tests/Testing/2

10. What is measured in the CH_{50} assay?
    A. RBC quantity needed to agglutinate 50% of antibody
    B. Complement needed to lyse 50% of RBCs
    C. Complement needed to lyse 50% of antibody-sensitized RBCs
    D. Antibody and complement needed to sensitize 50% of RBCs

    Immunology/Apply principles of basic laboratory procedures/Complement/Testing/1

---

6. **C** Waldenström's macroglobulinemia is a malignancy of plasmacytoid lymphocytes involving both the bone marrow and lymph nodes. The malignant cells secrete monoclonal IgM and are in transition from B cells to plasma cells. In contrast to multiple myeloma, osteolytic bone lesions are not found.

7. **D** DiGeorge's syndrome is caused by a developmental failure or hypoplasia of the thymus, and results in a deficiency of T lymphocytes and cell-mediated immune function. The T-cell count is low, but the level of immunoglobulins is usually normal. Flow cytometry is most helpful in determining numbers and subpopulations of T cells.

8. **C** Heavy wide bands seen with both anti-κ and anti-λ antisera indicate excessive light chain excretion. Light chain disease would show a heavy restricted band for one of the light chain reactions but not both. The finding of excess λ and κ chains indicates a polyclonal gammopathy with increased immunoglobulin turnover and excretion of the light chains as Fab fragments.

9. **C** Serum free light chains are a sensitive indicator of a monoclonal gammopathy. They are often not present in sufficient quantity to show a band on a protein electrophoresis gel. Detecting light chains in the urine is not an indicator of what the serum levels may be. Serum immunoglobulin heavy and light chains are most commonly measured by rate or endpoint nephelometry. ELISA assays are most often used to measure specific antibody levels, not to quantitate immunoglobulin heavy or light chain isotypes.

10. **C** The CH_{50} is the amount of complement needed to lyse 50% of standardized hemolysin-sensitized sheep RBCs. It is expressed as the reciprocal of the serum dilution resulting in 50% hemolysis. Low levels are associated with deficiency of some complement components and active systemic autoimmune diseases in which complement is being consumed.

11. What type of disorders would show a decrease in C3, C4, and CH_{50}?
    A. Autoimmune disorders such as SLE and RA
    B. Immunodeficiency disorders such as common variable immunodeficiency
    C. Tumors
    D. Bacterial, viral, fungal, or parasitic infections

    Immunology/Evaluate laboratory data to make identifications/Complement/Testing/2

12. All of the following tests measure phagocyte function *except*:
    A. Leukocyte adhesion molecule analysis
    B. Hydrogen peroxide production
    C. NBT test
    D. IL-2 (interleukin-2) assay

    Immunology/Apply principles of basic laboratory procedures/Phagocyte/Testing/1

Answers to Questions 11–12

11. **A** The pattern of decreased C3, C4, and CH_{50} indicates classic pathway activation. This results in consumption of complement and is associated with SLE, serum sickness, subacute bacterial endocarditis, and other immune complex diseases. The inflammatory response seen in malignancy and acute infections gives rise to an increase in complement components. Immunodeficiency caused by an inherited deficiency in complement constitutes only about 1% of immunodeficiency diseases. Such disorders reduce the CH_{50} but involve a deficient serum level of only one complement factor.

12. **D** Hydrogen peroxide and NBT tests are used to diagnose chronic granulomatous disease, an inherited disorder in which phagocytic cells fail to kill microorganisms owing to a defect in peroxide production (respiratory burst). Leukocyte adhesion deficiency is associated with a defect in the production of integrin molecules on the surface of WBCs and their granules. IL-2 is a cytokine produced by activated T_h and B cells. It causes B-cell proliferation and increased production of antibody, interferon, and other cytokines. IL-2 can be measured by EIA and is used to detect transplant rejection, which is associated with an increase in the serum and urine levels.

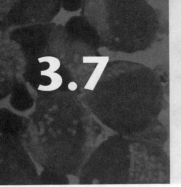

3.7 TUMOR TESTING AND TRANSPLANTATION

1. A patient had surgery for colorectal cancer, after which he received chemotherapy for 6 months. The test for carcinoembryonic antigen (CEA) was normal at this time. One year later, the bimonthly CEA was elevated (above 10 ng/mL). An examination and biopsy revealed the recurrence of a small tumor. What was the value of the results provided by the CEA test in this clinical situation?
   A. Diagnostic information
   B. Information for further treatment
   C. Information on the immunological response of the patient
   D. No useful clinical information in this case

   Immunology/Apply principles of basic laboratory procedures/Tumor/Testing/1

2. A carbohydrate antigen 125 assay (CA-125) was performed on a woman with ovarian cancer. After treatment the levels fell significantly. An examination performed later revealed the recurrence of the tumor, but the CA 125 levels remained low. How can this finding be explained?
   A. Test error
   B. CA-125 was the wrong laboratory test; α-fetoprotein (AFP) is a better test to monitor ovarian cancer
   C. CA-125 may not be sensitive enough when used alone to monitor tumor development
   D. CA-125 is not specific enough to detect only one type of tumor

   Immunology/Apply principles of basic laboratory procedures/Tumor/Testing/3

3. What is the correct procedure upon receipt of a test request for human chorionic gonadotropin (hCG) on the serum from a 60-year-old man?
   A. Return the request; hCG is not performed on men
   B. Perform a qualitative hCG test to see if hCG is present

   C. Perform the test; hCG may be increased in testicular tumors
   D. Perform the test but use different standards and controls

   Immunology/Correlate laboratory data with physiological processes/Tumor/HCG/3

Answers to Questions 1–3

1. **B** CEA is a glycoprotein that is elevated in about 60% of patients with colorectal cancer and one-third or more patients with pulmonary, gastric, and pancreatic cancers. CEA may be positive in smokers, patients with cirrhosis, Crohn's disease, and other nonmalignant conditions. Because sensitivity for malignant disease is low, CEA is not recommended for use as a diagnostic test. However, an elevated CEA after treatment is evidence of tumor recurrence and the need for second-look surgery.

2. **C** CA-125 is a tumor associated carbohydrate antigen that is elevated in 70%–80% of patients with ovarian cancer and about 20% of patients with pancreatic cancer. While an increase in CA-125 may indicate recurrent or progressive disease, failure to do so does not necessarily indicate the absence of tumor growth.

3. **C** hCG is normally tested for in pregnancy; it is increased in approximately 60% of patients with testicular tumors and a lower percentage of those with ovarian, GI, breast, and pulmonary tumors. Malignant cells secreting hCG may produce only the β-subunit; therefore, qualitative and quantitative tests that detect only intact hormone may not be appropriate.

4. Would an hCG test using a monoclonal antibody against the β-subunit of hCG likely be affected by an increased level of follicle-stimulating hormone (FSH)?
  A. Yes, the β-subunit of FSH is identical to that of hCG
  B. No, the test would be specific for the β-subunit of hCG
  C. Yes, a cross-reaction would occur because of structural similarities
  D. No, the structure of FSH and hCG are not at all similar

Immunology/Evaluate laboratory data to check for sources of error/hCG/Testing/3

5. Which of the following substances, sometimes used as a tumor marker, is increased two- or threefold in a normal pregnancy?
  A. Alkaline phosphatase (ALP)
  B. Calcitonin
  C. Adrenocortocotropic hormone (ACTH)
  D. Neuron-specific enolase

Immunology/Tumor markers/Testing/1

6. What is an advantage of performing a prostate specific antigen (PSA) test for prostate cancer?
  A. PSA is stable in serum and not affected by a digital-rectal examination
  B. PSA is increased only in prostatic malignancy
  C. A normal serum level rules out malignant prostatic disease
  D. The percentage of free PSA is elevated in persons with malignant disease

Immunology/Correlate laboratory data with physiological processes/Tumor/PSA/1

7. Which method is the most sensitive for quantitation of AFP?
  A. Double immunodiffusion
  B. Electrophoresis
  C. Enzyme immunoassay
  D. Particle agglutination

Immunology/Select appropriate method/AFP/1

Answers to Questions 4–7

4. **B** Luteinizing hormone, FSH, and hCG share a common α-subunit but have different β subunits. A test for hCG using a monoclonal antibody would be specific for hCG provided that the antibody was directed against an antigenic determinant on the carboxy terminal end of the β subunit.

5. **A** Isoenzymes of ALP are sometimes used as tumor markers but have a low specificity because they are also increased in nonmalignant diseases. These include the placental-like (heat-stable) ALP isoenzymes, which are found (infrequently) in some malignancies such as cancer of the lung; bone-derived ALP, which is a marker for metastatic bone cancer; and the fast-migrating liver isoenzyme, which is a marker for metastatic liver cancer. ACTH is secreted as an ectopic hormone in some patients with cancer of the lung. Calcitonin is a hormone produced by the medulla of the thyroid and is increased in the serum of patients with medullary thyroid carcinoma. Neuron-specific enolase is an enzyme that is used as a tumor marker primarily for neuroblastoma.

6. **A** PSA is a glycoprotein with protease activity that is specific for the prostate gland. High levels may be caused by prostate malignancy, benign prostatic hypertrophy, or prostatitis, but PSA is not increased by physical examination of the prostate. PSA has a sensitivity of 80% and a specificity of about 75% for prostate cancer. The sensitivity is sufficiently high to warrant its use as a screening test, but sensitivity for stage A cancer is below 60%. Most of the serum PSA is bound to protease inhibitors such as α_1-antitrypsin and α_1-antichymotrypsin. Patients with borderline PSA levels (4–10 ng/mL) and a low percentage of free PSA are more likely to have cancer of the prostate than patients with a normal percentage of free PSA.

7. **C** AFP is a glycoprotein that is produced in about 80%–90% of patients with hepatoma and in a lower percentage of patients with other tumors, including retinoblastoma, breast, uterine, and pancreatic cancer. The upper reference limit for serum is only 10 ng/mL, which requires a sensitive method of assay such as EIA. The high analytical sensitivity of immunoassays permits detection of reduced AFP levels in maternal serum associated with Down's syndrome, as well as elevated levels associated with spina bifida.

8. How is HLA typing used in the investigation of genetic diseases?
  A. For prediction of the severity of the disease
  B. For genetic linkage studies
  C. For direct diagnosis of disease
  D. Is not useful in this situation

Immunology/Correlate clinical and laboratory data/HLA typing/1

9. Select the best donor for a man, blood type AB, in need of a kidney transplant.
  A. His brother, type AB, HLA matched for class II antigens
  B. His mother, type B, HLA matched for class I antigens
  C. His cousin, type O, HLA matched for major class II antigens
  D. Cadaver donor, type O, HLA matched for some class I and II antigens

Immunology/Correlate data with other laboratory data to assess test results/Transplantation/Testing/3

10. Interpret the following microcytotoxicity result: A9 and B12 cells damaged; A1 and Aw19 cells intact.
  A. Positive for A1 and Aw19; negative for A9 and B12
  B. Negative for A1 and Aw19; positive for A9 and B12
  C. Error in test system; retest
  D. Impossible to determine

Immunology/Evaluate laboratory data to make identifications/Transplantation/Testing/2

11. Which method, classically used for HLA-D typing, is often used to determine the compatibility between a living organ donor and recipient?
  A. Flow cytometry
  B. Mixed lymphocyte culture (MLC)
  C. Primed lymphocyte test (PLT)
  D. Restriction fragment length polymorphism (RFLP)

Immunology/Apply principles of special procedures/Transplantation/HLA typing/1

12. **SITUATION:** Cells type negative for all HLA antigens. What is the most likely cause?
  A. Too much supravital dye was added
  B. Rabbit complement is inactivated
  C. All leukocytes are dead
  D. Antisera is too concentrated

Immunology/Evaluate laboratory data to check for sources of error/HLA typing/3

13. What method may be used for tissue typing instead of serological HLA typing?
  A. PCR
  B. Southern blotting
  C. RFLP
  D. All of the above

Immunology/Apply principles of special procedures/Transplantation/HLA typing/1

8. **B** HLA typing is useful in predicting some genetic diseases and for genetic counseling because certain HLA types show strong linkage to some diseases. HLA typing is not specifically used to diagnose a disease or assess its severity. In linkage studies a disease gene can be predicted because it is located next to the locus of a normal gene with which it segregates. For example, the relative risk of developing ankylosing spondylitis is 87% in persons who are positive for HLA-B27. Analysis of family pedigrees for the linkage marker and disease can be used to determine the probability that a family member will inherit the disease gene.

9. **A** A twin or sibling donor of the same blood type and HLA matched for class II antigens is the best donor in this situation. Class II antigens (HLA-D, HLA-DR, DQ, and DP) determine the ability of the transplant recipient to recognize the graft. The HLA genes are located close together on chromosome 6, and crossover between HLA genes is rare. Siblings with closely matched class II antigens most likely inherited the same class I genes. The probability of siblings inheriting the same HLA haplotypes from both parents is 1:4.

10. **B** The microcytotoxicity test is based upon the reaction of specific antisera and HLA antigens on test cells. Cells damaged by the binding of antibody and complement are detected with a supravital dye such as eosin.

11. **B** Flow cytometry can be used in transplantation to type serologically defined HLA antigens. The one-way mixed lymphocyte reaction is used to identify HLA-D antigens on the donor's lymphocytes and is used for cross-matching living donors with transplant recipients. The assay is time-consuming and would not be used as part of a work-up for a cadaver donor transplant. HLA-D incompatibility is associated with the recognition phase of allograft rejection. The primed lymphocyte test is used to identify HLA-DP antigens.

12. **B** Inactive rabbit complement may not become fixed to antibodies that have bound test leukocytes; therefore, no lysis of cells will occur. When the supravital dye is added, all cells will appear negative (exclude the dye) for all HLAs.

13. **D** PCR, Southern blotting, and testing for RFLPs may all be used to identify HLA genes. Many laboratories use PCR technology for the routine determination of HLA type.

1. Which of the following serial dilutions contains an incorrect factor?
   - A. 1:4, 1:8, 1:16
   - B. 1:1, 1:2, 1:4
   - C. 1:5, 1:15, 1:45
   - D. 1:2, 1:6, 1:12

   Immunology/Apply knowledge to recognize sources of error/Serological titration/3

2. A patient was tested for syphilis by the RPR method and was reactive. An FTA-ABS test was performed and the result was negative. Subsequent testing showed the patient to have a high titer of anticardiolipin antibodies (ACAs) by the ELISA method. Which routine laboratory test is most likely to be abnormal for this patient?
   - A. Activated partial thromboplastin time (APTT)
   - B. Antismooth muscle antibodies
   - C. Aspartate aminotransferase (AST)
   - D. C3 assay by immunonephelometry

   Immunology/Apply knowledge to recognize sources of error/Anticardiolipin/3

3. Inflammation involves a variety of biochemical and cellular mediators. Which of the following may be increased within 72 hours after an initial infection?
   - A. Neutrophils, macrophages, antibody, complement, α_1-antitrypsin
   - B. Macrophages, T cells, antibody, haptoglobin, fibrinogen
   - C. Neutrophils, macrophages, complement, fibrinogen, C-reactive protein
   - D. Macrophages, T cells, B cells, ceruloplasmin, complement

   Immunology/Apply principles of basic immunologic response/Inflammation/2

1. **D** All the dilutions are multiplied by the same factor in a progression except the last one. 1:2 to 1:6 is × 3, whereas 1:6 to 1:12 is × 2. Threefold dilutions of a 1:2 dilution would result in a 1:6 followed by a 1:18.

2. **A** Approximately 50%–70% of patients with ACA also have the lupus anticoagulant (LAC) in their serum. The LAC is an immunoglobulin that interferes with in vitro coagulation tests: prothrombin time (PT), APTT, and dilute Russell's viper venom time (dRVVT). These tests require phospholipid for the activation of factor X. About 30% of patients with antibodies to cardiolipin or phospholipids have a biological false-positive RPR result. Antismooth muscle is most commonly associated with chronic active hepatitis, and increased AST with necrotic liver diseases. Although ACA and LAC may be associated with SLE, the majority of patients with these antibodies do not have lupus and would have a normal C3 level.

3. **C** The correct list, in which *all* mediators are involved in an inflammatory response within 72 hours after initial infection, is neutrophils, macrophages, complement, fibrinogen, and C-reactive protein. Phagocytic cells, acute phase reactants, and fibrinolytic factors enter the site of inflammation. Antibody and lymphocytes do not enter until later.

4. An 18-month-old boy has recurrent sinopulmonary infections and septicemia. Bruton's X-linked immunodeficiency syndrome is suspected. Which test result would be markedly decreased?
A. Serum IgG, IgA, and IgM
B. Total T-cell count
C. Both B- and T-cell counts
D. Lymphocyte proliferation with phytohemagglutinin stimulation

Immunology/Correlate laboratory data with physiological processes/Immunodeficiency/Testing/2

5. A patient received five units of fresh frozen plasma (FFP) and developed a severe anaphylactic reaction. He has a history of respiratory and gastrointestinal infections. Post-transfusion studies showed all five units to be ABO-compatible. What immunological test would help to determine the cause of this transfusion reaction?
A. Complement levels, particularly C3 and C4
B. Flow cytometry for T-cell counts
C. Measurement of immunoglobulins
D. NBT test for phagocytic function

Immunology/Determine laboratory tests/ Immunodeficiency/Testing/3

6. An IEP and IFE both revealed excessive amounts of polyclonal IgM and low concentrations of IgG and IgA. What is the most likely explanation of these findings and the best course of action?
A. Proper amounts of antisera were not added; repeat both tests
B. Test specimen was not added properly; repeat both procedures
C. Patient has common variable immunodeficiency; perform B-cell count
D. Patient has immunodeficiency with hyper-M; perform immunoglobulin levels

Immunology/Correlate laboratory data with physiological processes/Immunodeficiency/Testing/3

7. **SITUATION:** A 54-year-old man was admitted to the hospital after having a seizure. Many laboratory tests were performed, including an RPR, but none of the results were positive. The physician suspects a case of late (tertiary) syphilis. Which test should be performed next?
A. Repeat RPR, then perform VDRL
B. Treponemal test such as MHA-TP on serum

C. VDRL on CSF
D. No laboratory test is positive for late (tertiary) syphilis

Immunology/Correlate laboratory data with physiological processes/Syphilis/Testing/3

Answers to Questions 4–7

4. **A** A patient with Bruton's X-linked agammaglobulinemia presents with clinical symptoms related to recurrent infections, demonstrated in the laboratory by decreased or absent immunoglobulins. Peripheral blood B cells are absent or markedly reduced, but T cells are normal in number and function. Because phytohemagglutinin is a T-cell mitogen, the lymphocyte proliferation test using PHA would be normal for this patient.

5. **C** The patient had an anaphylactic reaction to a plasma product. This, combined with the history of respiratory and gastrointestinal infections, suggests a selective IgA deficiency. Measurement of immunoglobulins would be helpful in this case. A low serum IgA and normal IgG substantiate the diagnosis of selective IgA deficiency. Such patients frequently produce anti-IgA, which is often responsible for a severe transfusion reaction when ABO-compatible plasma is administered.

6. **D** The same finding on two different procedures decreases the possibility of a technical error. This finding is consistent with an immunodeficiency of IgG and IgA and an abundance of IgM. Patients with common variable immunodeficiency have low serum IgG, IgA, and IgM but a normal number of B cells that exhibit a maturation defect.

7. **B** Serum antibody tests such as RPR and VDRL are often negative in cases of late syphilis. However, treponemal tests remain positive in over 95% of cases. The VDRL test on CSF is the most specific test for diagnosis of neurosyphilis. It should be used as the confirmatory test when the serum treponemal test is positive. However, the CSF VDRL is limited in sensitivity and would not be positive if the serum MHA-TP or FTA-ABS was negative.

8. A patient came to his physician complaining of a rash, severe headaches, stiff neck, and sleep problems. Laboratory tests of significance were an elevated sedimentation rate (ESR) and slightly increased liver enzymes. Further questioning of the patient revealed that he had returned from a hunting trip in upstate New York 4 weeks ago. His physician ordered a serological test for Lyme disease, and the assay was negative. What is the most likely explanation of these results?
A. The antibody response is not sufficient to be detected at this stage
B. The clinical symptoms and laboratory results are not characteristic of Lyme disease
C. The patient likely has an early infection with hepatitis B virus
D. Laboratory error has caused a false-negative result

Immunology/Correlate laboratory data with physiological processes/Lyme testing/Testing/3

9. A 19-year-old girl came to her physician complaining of a sore throat and fatigue. Upon physical examination, lymphadenopathy was noted. Reactive lymphocytes were noted on the differential, but a rapid test for IM antibodies was negative. Liver enzymes were only slightly elevated. What test(s) should be ordered next?
A. Hepatitis testing
B. EBV serological panel
C. HIV confirmatory testing
D. Bone marrow biopsy

Immunology/Correlate laboratory data with physiological processes/EBV/Testing/3

10. A patient received two units of RBCs following surgery. Two weeks after the surgery, the patient was seen by his physician and exhibited mild jaundice and slightly elevated liver enzymes. Hepatitis testing, however, was negative. What should be done next?
A. Nothing until more severe or definitive clinical signs develop
B. Repeat hepatitis testing immediately
C. Repeat hepatitis testing in a few weeks
D. Check blood bank donor records and contact donor(s) of transfused units

Immunology/Correlate laboratory data with physiological processes/Hepatitis/Testing/3

11. A hospital employee has just received the third dose of hepatitis vaccine. She wants to donate blood next week. Which of the following results are expected from the hepatitis screen, and will she be allowed to donate blood?
A. HBsAg, positive; anti-HBc, negative. She may donate
B. HBsAg, negative; anti-HBc, positive. She may not donate

C. HBsAg, positive; anti-HBc, positive. She may not donate
D. HBsAg, negative; anti-HBc, negative. She may donate

Immunology/Correlate laboratory data with physiological processes/Hepatitis/Testing/3

12. A pregnant woman came to her physician with a maculopapular rash on her face and neck. Her temperature was 37.7°C (100°F). Rubella tests for both IgG and IgM antibody were positive. What positive test(s) would reveal a diagnosis of congenital rubella syndrome in her baby after birth?
A. Positive rubella tests for both IgG and IgM antibody
B. Positive rubella test for IgM
C. Positive rubella test for IgG
D. No positive test is revealed in congenital rubella syndrome

Immunology/Correlate laboratory data with physiological processes/Rubella/Testing/3

Answers to Questions 8–12

8. A The antibody response to *B. burgdorferi* may not develop until several weeks after initial infection. The antibody test should be followed by a test such as PCR to detect the DNA of the organism. Regardless of the test outcome, if the physician suspects Lyme disease, treatment should begin immediately.

9. B An EBV serological panel would give a more accurate assessment than a rapid slide IM test. The time of appearance of the various antibodies to the viral antigens differ according to the clinical course of the infection.

10. C The level of HBsAg may not have reached detectable levels, and antibodies to HBc and HCV would not have yet developed. Waiting 1 or 2 weeks and repeating the tests may reveal evidence of hepatitis virus infection.

11. D She may donate if she is symptom-free. The response to hepatitis B vaccine would include a positive result for anti-HBs, a test not normally a part of routine donor testing. She will be negative for HBsAg and anti-HBc.

12. B A finding of IgG is not definitive for congenital rubella syndrome because IgG crosses the placenta from the mother; however, demonstration of IgM, even in a single neonatal sample, is diagnostic.

13. **SITUATION:** A patient with RA has acute pneumonia but a negative throat culture. The physician suspects an infection with *Mycoplasma pneumoniae* and requests an IgM-specific antibody test. The test is performed directly on serial dilutions of serum less than 4 hours old. The result is positive, giving a titer of 1:32. However, the test is repeated 3 weeks later, and the titer remains at 1:32. What best explains these results?

   A. IgM-specific antibodies do not increase fourfold between acute and convalescent serum
   B. The results are not significant because the initial titer was not accompanied by a positive test for cold agglutinins
   C. Rheumatoid factor caused a false-positive test result
   D. Insufficient time had elapsed between measurement of acute and convalescent samples

   Immunology/Apply knowledge to recognize sources of error/IgM testing/3

14. A patient has a prostate specific antigen level of 60 ng/mL the day before surgery to remove a localized prostate tumor. One week following surgery the serum PSA was determined to be 8 ng/mL by the same method. What is the most likely cause of these results?

   A. Incomplete removal of the malignancy
   B. Cross-reactivity of the antibody with another tumor antigen
   C. Testing too soon after surgery
   D. Hook effect with the PSA assay

   Immunology/Apply knowledge to recognize inconsistent results/Tumor markers/3

15. A patient with symptoms associated with SLE and scleroderma was evaluated by immunofluorescence microscopy for ANAs using the HEp-2 cell line as substrate. The cell line displayed a mixed pattern of fluorescence that could not be separated by serial dilutions of the serum. Which procedure would be most helpful in determining the antibody profile of this patient?

   A. Use of a different tissue substrate
   B. Absorption of the serum using the appropriate tissue extract
   C. Ouchterlony technique
   D. ELISA tests for nuclear antigens

   Immunology/Apply knowledge to identify laboratory tests/ANA/Testing/3

Answers to Questions 13–15

13. **C** The IgM-specific antibody test for *M. pneumoniae* detects antibodies to mycoplasmal membrane antigens and, unlike cold agglutinins, is specific for *M. pneumoniae*. A positive result (titer of 1:32 or higher) occurs during the acute phase in about 87% of *M. pneumoniae* infections and does not need to be confirmed by assay of convalescent serum. However, patients with RA may show a false-positive reaction because rheumatoid factor in their serum can react with the conjugated anti-IgM used in the test. For this reason, serum from patients known or suspected to have rheumatoid factor (RF) must be pretreated. The serum is heated to 56°C to aggregate the RF, and the aggregated immunoglobulin is removed by a chromatography minicolumn.

14. **C** When monitoring the level of a tumor marker for treatment efficacy or recurrence, the half-life of the protein must be considered when determining the testing interval. PSA has a half-life of almost 4 days and would not reach normal levels after surgery for approximately 3–4 weeks. The hook effect is the result of very high antigen levels giving a lower than expected result in a double antibody sandwich assay.

15. **D** Many patients with multiorgan autoimmune disease display symptoms that overlap two or more diseases and have complex mixtures of serum autoantibodies. The HEp-2 substrate is the most sensitive cell line for immunofluorescent microscopy because it contains cells in various mitotic stages, which exposes the serum to more antigens. Use of a nonhuman substrate such as *Crithidia* may help to identify dsDNA antibodies but would not aid in differentiating all of the antibodies in a complex mixture. Ouchterlony immunodiffusion helps to identify specific ANAs but has limited sensitivity. The best method is ELISA because it is more sensitive than immunofluorescence microscopy and can quantitate antibodies to specific antigens. ELISA is often used to measure antibodies to extractable nuclear antigens, which may be partially or completely lost during fixation of cells used for immunofluorescent microscopy. These antibodies cause a speckled pattern and are seen in a wide range of autoimmune diseases. Identification of the ENA specificities is helpful in differentiating these diseases.

16. A patient with joint swelling and pain tested negative for serum RF by both latex agglutination and ELISA methods. What other test would help establish a diagnosis of RA in this patient?

A. Analysis of synovial fluid
B. ANA testing
C. Flow cytometry
D. Complement levels

Immunology/Correlate laboratory data with physiological processes/RA/Testing/3

17. What is the main advantage of the recovery and reinfusion of autologous stem cells?

A. It slows the rate of rejection of transplanted cells
B. It prevents graft-versus-host disease
C. No HLA testing is required
D. Engraftment occurs in a more efficient sequence

Immunology/Apply knowledge of fundamental biological characteristics/Transplantation/2

18. A transplant patient began to show signs of rejection 8 days after receipt of the transplanted organ, and the organ was removed. What immune elements might be found in the rejected organ?

A. Antibody and complement
B. Primarily antibody
C. Macrophages
D. T cells

Immunology/Correlate laboratory data and basic immune response/Transplantation/Rejection/3

19. A patient with ovarian cancer who has been treated with chemotherapy is being monitored for recurrence using serum CA-125, CA-50, and CA 15–3. Six months after treatment the CA 15–3 is elevated, but the CA-125 and CA-50 remain low. What is the most likely explanation of these findings?

A. Ovarian malignancy has recurred
B. CA 15–3 is specific for breast cancer and indicates metastatic breast cancer
C. Testing error occurred in the measurement of CA 15–3 caused by poor analytical specificity
D. The CA 15–3 elevation is spurious and probably benign

Immunology/Correlate laboratory data with physiological processes/Tumor markers/Testing/3

Answers to Questions 16–19

16. **A** Analysis of synovial fluid would help to distinguish RA from other causes of arthritis such as gout and septic arthritis. The absence of rheumatoid factors from serum does not rule out a diagnosis of RA, and more than half of patients who are diagnosed with RA present initially with a negative serum result. The serum RF test will eventually be positive in 80%–90% of patients who meet the clinical criteria for RA. Conversely, a positive test for RF (and ANA) is nonspecific and is not by itself sufficient evidence of RA. Because RF may be present in the fluid from an affected joint before it appears in serum, the evaluation of joint fluid should include this test.

17. **B** The main advantage to the patient for the reinfusion of autologous stem cells is that the procedure prevents graft-versus-host disease, especially in the immunocompromised patient. Although HLA testing is not required, this is not the primary advantage for patient care.

18. **D** Acute rejection occurs within 3 weeks of transplantation. The immune elements most likely to be involved in an acute rejection are T cells in a type IV, delayed hypersensitivity (cell-mediated) reaction. Preformed antibody, and possibly complement, is usually involved in hyperacute (immediate) rejection and chronic rejection.

19. **A** Although CA-125 is the most commonly used tumor marker for ovarian cancer, not all ovarian tumors produce CA-125. Greatest sensitivity in monitoring for recurrence is achieved when several markers known to be increased in the malignant tissue type are measured simultaneously and when the markers are elevated (by malignancy) prior to treatment. In addition to limited sensitivity, no single tumor maker is entirely specific. Carbohydrate and other oncofetal antigens are produced by several malignant and benign conditions. Although testing errors may occur in any situation, measurements of carbohydrate antigens use purified monoclonal antibodies with very low cross-reactivities.

20. An initial and repeat ELISA test for antibodies to HIV-1 are both positive. A Western blot shows a single band at gp160. The patient shows no clinical signs of HIV infection, and the patient's helper T-cell count is normal. Based upon these results, which conclusion is correct?
A. Patient is diagnosed as HIV-1-positive
B. Patient is diagnosed as HIV-2-positive
C. Results are inconclusive
D. Patient is diagnosed as HIV-1-negative

Immunology/Apply knowledge to recognize inconsistent results/HIV/3

21. A woman who has been pregnant for 12 weeks is tested for toxoplasmosis. Her IgM ELISA titer is 2.6 (reference range <1.6), and her IgG ELISA value is 66 (reference range <8). The physician asks you if these results indicated an infection during the past 12 weeks. Which of the following tests would you recommend to determine if the woman was infected during her pregnancy?
A. Toxo PCR on amniotic fluid
B. Toxo IgM on amniotic fluid
C. Toxo IgG avidity
D. Amniotic fluid culture

Immunology/Correlate laboratory data with physiological processes/Time course of immune response/ Toxoplasmosis/Testing/3

22. On January 4, a serum protein electrophoresis on a specimen obtained at your hospital in North Dakota from a 58-year-old shows a band at the β-γ junction. The specimen was also positive for rheumatoid factor. You recommend that an immunofixation test be performed to determine if the band represents a monoclonal immunoglobulin. Another specimen is obtained 2 weeks later by the physician in his office 30 miles away, and the whole blood is submitted to you for the IFE. The courier placed the whole blood specimen in an ice chest for transport. In this specimen, no β-γ band is seen in the serum protein lane, and the IgM lane is very faint. The rheumatoid factor on this specimen was negative. The physician wants to know what's wrong with your laboratory. You tell the physician:
A. Nothing's wrong with our laboratory. The patient had an infection 2 weeks ago that has cleared up
B. Something's wrong with our laboratory. We likely mislabeled one of the specimens. Please resubmit a new specimen and we will test it at no charge

C. You will run the second specimen using a 2-mercaptoethanol treatment that will eliminate IgM aggregates and allow for more sensitive monoclonal IgM detection
D. Redraw another specimen from the patient and that this time separate the serum from the clot in his office before sending the specimen in by courier

Immunology/Correlate laboratory data with physiological processes/Specimen integrity/3

Answers to Questions 20–22

20. **C** The Western blot test is used as a confirmatory test for HIV, but it is not as sensitive as enzyme immunoassay tests using polyvalent HIV antigens derived from cloned HIV genes. The Western blot test is considered positive only if antibodies to two of three viral antigens—p24, gp41, and gp160/120—are detected. The presence of a single band is indeterminate. Over the course of the next 3 months, two or more antibodies will be detected if the patient is HIV-positive; however, antibodies to a single viral protein may be caused by a cross-reaction, and this patient may fail to seroconvert. This result should be reported as indeterminate, and the patient should be retested in 3 months. Alternatively, a more sensitive confirmatory test such as PCR or immunofluorescence may be performed.

21. **C** Although IgM is positive, in toxoplasmosis, specific IgM may remain detectable for a year or more following infection. IgG avidity, or the strength of binding of a serum to the antigen of interest, is a useful method to determine if an infection is recent or in the distant past. IgG avidity will increase with time following an infection. Amniotic fluid testing is not useful for determining when the mother might have been infected.

22. **D** The most likely cause of the discrepant results is the presence of a type II cryoglobulin. This is a monoclonal rheumatoid factor. The protein likely precipitated during the courier ride and was thus in the clot when the laboratory separated the serum.

23. A dialysis patient is positive for both hepatitis B surface antigen and hepatitis B surface antibody. The physician suspects a laboratory error. Do you agree?
- **A.** Yes. No patient should be positive for both HBsAg and HBsAb
- **B.** No. Incomplete dialysis of a patient in the core window phase of hepatitis B infection will yield this result
- **C.** No. It is likely the patient has recently received a hepatitis B booster vaccination and could have these results
- **D.** Perhaps. A new specimen should be submitted to clear up the confusion

Immunology/Correlate laboratory data with physiological processes/Hepatitis/Testing/3

24. You are evaluating an ELISA assay as a replacement for your immunofluorescent antinuclear antibody test. You test 50 specimens in duplicate on each assay. The ELISA assay uses a HEp-2 extract as its antigen source. The correlation between the ELISA and the IFA tests is only 60% (30 of 50 specimens agree). Which of the following is the next best course of action?
- **A.** Test another 50 specimens
- **B.** Perform a competency check on the technologists who performed the tests
- **C.** Order a new lot of both kits and then retest on the new lots.
- **D.** Refer the discrepant specimens for testing by another method.

Immunology/Management Principles/Method Comparison/3

Answers to questions 23–24

23. **C** Hepatitis B surface antigen will remain detectable at low levels following a vaccination for up to 1–2 weeks. Thus, patients who have received a second injection of hepatitis B vaccine may have anti-hepatitis B surface antigen and detectable antigen for a brief period of time. This has been reported more frequently in dialysis and pediatric populations.

24. **D** In this situation you have already tested the specimens in duplicate. Testing an additional 50 specimens will not change the fact that you have 20 discrepant specimens. The best course of action is to determine what antibodies are actually present in these specimens. Then, you can determine whether the ELISA or IFA is a better procedure for detecting the most clinically relevant antibodies. You could perform clinical chart reviews as an alternative, but obtaining that data would be difficult and much of it may be subjective.

BIBLIOGRAPHY

1. Detrick, B., and Hamilton, R. G.: Manual of Molecular and Clinical Laboratory Immunology, ed 7. Washington, DC, ASM Press, 2006.
2. Folds, J., and Normansell, D.: Pocket Guide to Clinical Immunology. Washington, DC, ASM Press, 1999.
3. Kindt, T. J., Osborne, B. A., and Goldsby, R. A.: Kuby Immunology, ed 6. New York, WH Freeman, 2006.
4. Mahon, C., and Tice, D.: Clinical Laboratory Immunology. Upper Saddle River, NJ, Pearson, Prentice-Hall, 2006.
5. Nakamura, R., Burek, L., Cook, L., et al.: Clinical Diagnostic Immunology: Protocols in Quality Assurance and Standardization. Blackwell Publishing, Malden, MA, 1998.
6. Playfair, H.: Immunology at a Glance. Blackwell Publishing, Malden, MA, 2005.
7. Rosen, F. and Geha R.: Case Studies in Immunology. A Clinical Companion, ed 4. Garland Science, New York, 2004.
8. Stites, D.P., Terr, A.I., Parslow, T.G.: Medical Immunology. East Norwalk, CT, Appleton & Lange, 1997.

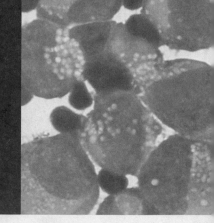

CHAPTER **4**

Immunohematology

4.1   GENETICS AND IMMUNOLOGY OF BLOOD GROUPS

4.2   ABO BLOOD GROUP SYSTEM

4.3   Rh BLOOD GROUP SYSTEM

4.4   TESTING FOR ANTIBODIES

4.5   COMPATIBILITY TESTING

4.6   TRANSFUSION REACTIONS

4.7   COMPONENTS

4.8   DONORS

4.9   HEMOLYTIC DISEASE OF THE NEWBORN

4.10   SEROLOGICAL TESTING OF BLOOD PRODUCTS

4.11   IMMUNOHEMATOLOGY PROBLEM SOLVING

GENETICS AND IMMUNOLOGY OF BLOOD GROUPS

4.1

1. **What type of testing does the blood bank technologist perform when determining the blood group of a patient?**
   A. Genotyping
   B. Phenotyping
   C. Both genotyping and phenotyping
   D. Polymerase chain reaction

   Blood Bank/Apply knowledge of laboratory operations/Genetics/1

2. **If anti-K reacts 3+ with a donor cell with a genotype *KK* and 2+ with a *Kk* cell, the antibody is demonstrating:**
   A. Dosage
   B. Linkage disequilibrium
   C. Homozygosity
   D. Heterozygosity

   Blood Bank/Apply knowledge of fundamental biological characteristics/Genetics/Kell/3

3. **Carla expresses the blood group antigens Fyᵃ, Fyᵇ, and Xgᵃ. James shows expression of none of these antigens. What factor(s) may account for the absence of these antigens in James?**
   A. Gender
   B. Race
   C. Gender and race
   D. Medication or pathological condition

   Blood bank/Apply knowledge of fundamental biological characteristics/Genetics/2

4. **Which of the following statements is true?**
   A. An individual with the *BO* genotype is homozygous for B
   B. An individual with the *BB* genotype is homozygous for B
   C. An individual with the *OO* genotype is heterozygous for O
   D. An individual with the *AB* genotype is homozygous for A and B

   Blood Bank/Apply knowledge of fundamental biological characteristics/Genetics/ABO/1

5. **Which genotype is heterozygous for C?**
   A. DCe/dce
   B. DCE/DCE
   C. Dce/dce
   D. dCE/dCe

   Blood Bank/Apply knowledge of fundamental biological characteristics/Genetics/Rh/2

Answers to Questions 1–5

1. **B** Phenotyping, or the physical expression of a genotype, is the type of testing routinely performed in the blood bank. An individual, for example, may have the AO genotype but phenotypes as group A.

2. **A** Dosage is defined as an antibody reacting stronger with homozygous cells, e.g., KK, than with heterozygous cells, e.g., Kk. In addition to Kell, dosage effect is seen commonly with antigens MN, Ss, FyᵃFyᵇ, JkᵃJkᵇ, and the antigens of the Rh system.

3. **C** The frequency of Duffy antigens Fyᵃ and Fyᵇ varies with race. The Fy(a-b-) phenotype occurs in almost 70% of African Americans and is very rare in whites. The Xgᵃ antigen is X-linked and, therefore, expressed more frequently in women (who may inherit the antigen from either parent) than in men.

4. **B** An individual having the *BB* genotype has inherited the *B* gene from both parents and, therefore, is homozygous for *B*.

5. **A** The genotype *DCe/dce* contains one *C* and one *c* gene and is heterozygous for *C* (and *c*).

115

6. Which genotype(s) will give rise to the Bombay phenotype?
   A. *HH* only
   B. *HH* and *Hh*
   C. *Hh* and *hh*
   D. *hh* only

   Blood Bank/Apply knowledge of fundamental biological characteristics/ABO/Bombay/1

7. Meiosis in cell division is limited to the ova and sperm producing four gametes containing what complement of DNA?
   A. 1N
   B. 2N
   C. 3N
   D. 4N

   Blood bank/Apply knowledge of fundamental biological characteristics/Genetics/1

8. A cell that is not actively dividing is said to be in:
   A. Interphase
   B. Prophase
   C. Anaphase
   D. Telophase

   Blood bank/Apply knowledge of fundamental biological characteristics/Genetics/1

9. Which of the following describes the expression of most blood group antigens?
   A. Dominant
   B. Recessive
   C. Codominant
   D. Corecessive

   Blood bank/Apply knowledge of fundamental biological characteristics/Genetics/1

10. What blood type is not possible for an offspring of *AO* and *BO* mating?
    A. AB
    B. A or B
    C. O
    D. All are possible

    Blood bank/Apply knowledge of fundamental biological characteristics/Genetics/ABO/2

11. The alleged father of a child in a disputed case of paternity is blood group AB. The mother is group O and the child is group O. What type of exclusion is this?
    A. Direct/primary/first order
    B. Probability
    C. Random
    D. Indirect/secondary/second order

    Blood bank/Evaluate laboratory data to verify test results/Genotype/Paternity Testing/2

12. If the frequency of gene Y is 0.4 and the frequency of gene Z is 0.5, one would expect that they should occur together 0.2 (20%) of the time. In actuality, they are found together 32% of the time. This is an example of:
    A. Crossing over
    B. Linkage disequilibrium
    C. Polymorphism
    D. Chimerism

    Blood bank/Apply principles of genetics/3

Answers to Questions 6–12

6. **D** The Bombay phenotype will be expressed only when no H substance is present. The O_h type is expressed by the genotype *hh*. Bombays produce naturally occurring anti-H, and their serum agglutinates group O red cells in addition to red cells from groups A, B, and AB persons.

7. **A** Meiosis involves two nuclear divisions in succession resulting in four gameteocytes with each containing half the number of chromosomes found in somatic cells or 1N.

8. **A** Interphase is the stage in between cell divisions. The cell is engaged in metabolic activity. Chromosomes are not clearly discerned; however, nucleoli may be visible.

9. **C** The inheritance of most blood group genes is codominant, meaning that no gene or allele is dominant over another. For example, a person who is group AB expresses both the A and B antigen on his or her red cells.

10. **D** A mating between AO and BO persons can result in an offspring with a blood type of A, B, AB, or O.

11. **D** A indirect/secondary/second order exclusion occurs when a genetic marker is absent in the child but should have been transmitted by the alleged father. In this case, either A or B should be present in the child.

12. **B** Linkage disquilibrium is a phenomenon in which alleles situated in close proximity on a chromosome associate with one another more than would be expected from individual allelic frequencies.

13. In the Hardy-Weinberg formula, p^2 represents:
   A. The heterozygous population of one allele
   B. The homozygous population of one allele
   C. The recessive allele
   D. The dominant allele

Blood bank/Apply knowledge of fundamental biological characteristics/Genetics/1

14. In this type of inheritance the father carries the trait on his X chromosome. He has no sons with the trait because he passed his Y chromosome to his sons; however, all his daughters will express the trait.
   A. Autosomal dominant
   B. Autosomal recessive
   C. X-linked dominant
   D. X-linked recessive

Blood bank/Apply knowledge of fundamental biological characteristics/Genetics/1

15. Why do IgM antibodies, such as those formed against the ABO antigens, have the ability to directly agglutinate red blood cells (RBCs) and cause visible agglutination?
   A. IgM antibodies are larger molecules and have the ability to bind more antigen
   B. IgM antibodies tend to clump together more readily to bind more antigen
   C. IgM antibodies are found in greater concentrations than IgG molecules
   D. IgM antibodies are not limited by subclass specficity

Blood bank/Apply knowledge of fundamental biological characteristics/Antibodies/1

16. Which of the following enhancement mediums decreases the zeta potential allowing antibody and antigen to come closer together?
   A. LISS
   B. Polyethylene glycol
   C. Polybrene
   D. ZZAP

Blood bank/Apply knowledge of fundamental biological characteristics/Antigens/1

17. This type of antibody response is analogous to an anamnestic antibody reaction.
   A. Primary
   B. Secondary
   C. Tertiary
   D. Anaphylactic

Blood bank/Apply knowledge of fundamental biological characteristics/Antibody/1

18. Which antibodies to a component of complement are contained in the rabbit polyspecific antihuman globulin reagent for detection of in vivo sensitization?
   A. Anti-IgG and anti-C3a
   B. Anti-IgG and anti-C3d
   C. Anti-IgG and anti-IgM
   D. All of the above

Blood bank/Apply knowledge of fundamental biological characteristics/AHG/2

Answers to Questions 13–18

13. **B** In the Hardy-Weinberg formula $p^2 + 2pq + q^2$, p^2 and q^2 represent homozygous expressions and $2pq$ represents heterozygous expression. This formula is used in population genetics to determine the frequency of different alleles.

14. **C** In X-linked dominant inheritance there is absence of male to male transmission since a male passes his Y chromosome to all of his sons and his single X chromosome to all his daughters. All daughters who inherit the affected gene will express the trait. An example of this type of inheritance is the Xg^a blood group.

15. **A** An IgM molecule has the potential to bind up to 10 antigens, as compared to a molecule of IgG, which can bind only two.

16. **A** LISS contains a reduced concentration of NaCl (0.2%) and results in a reduction in charged ions within the ionic cloud, decreasing the zeta potential and facilitating antigen and antibody interaction.

17. **B** An anamnestic response is a secondary immune response in which memory lymphocytes respond rapidly to foreign antigen in producing specific antibody. The antibodies are IgG and are produced at lower doses of antigen than in the primary response.

18. **B** In the DAT (direct antiglobulin test) rabbit polyspecific antisera contains both an anti-human IgG component and an antibody against the C3d component of complement.

1. **Which of the following distinguishes between the blood groups A_1 and A_2?**
   A. A_2 antigen will not react with anti-A; A_1 will react strongly (4+)
   B. An A_2 person may form anti-A_1; an A_1 person will not form anti-A_1
   C. An A_1 person may form anti-A_2; an A_2 person will not form anti-A_1
   D. A_2 antigen will not react with anti-A from a non-immunized donor; A_1 will react with any anti-A

   Blood bank/Apply knowledge of fundamental biological characteristics/ABO blood group/2

2. **A patient's serum is incompatible with O cells. The patient's RBCs give a negative reaction to anti-H lectin. What is the most likely cause of these results?**
   A. The patient may be a subgroup of A
   B. The patient may have an immunodeficiency
   C. The patient may be a Bombay individual
   D. The patient may have developed alloantibodies

   Blood bank/Apply principles of special procedures/ABO blood group/3

3. **What antibodies are formed by a Bombay individual?**
   A. Anti-A and anti-B
   B. Anti-H
   C. Anti-A,B
   D. Anti-A, anti-B, anti-H

   Blood bank/Apply knowledge of fundamental biological characteristics/ABO blood group/Bombay/1

4. **Acquired B antigens have been found in:**
   A. Bombay individuals
   B. Group O persons
   C. All blood groups
   D. Group A persons

   Blood bank/Apply knowledge of fundamental characteristics/ABO/1

Answers to Questions 1–4

1. **B** The group A_1 comprises both A_1 and A antigens. Anti-A will react with both A_1 and A_2 positive RBCs. A person who is group A_2 may form anti-A_1, but an A_1 person will not form anti-A (which would cause autoagglutination).

2. **C** Bombay cells are the only group incompatible with O cells, and the red cells of a Bombay individual show a negative reaction to anti-H because they contain no H antigen.

3. **D** A Bombay individual does not express A, B, or H antigens; therefore, anti-A, anti-B, and anti-H are formed. Because a Bombay individual may form these antibodies, the only compatible blood must be from a Bombay donor.

4. **D** The acquired B phenomenon is seen only in group A persons. The phenomenon arises when microbial deacetylating enzymes modify the A antigen by altering the A-determining sugar (N-acetylgalactosamine) so that it resembles the B-determining sugar, which is D-galactose. Anti-B acidified to a pH of 6.0 does not agglutinate acquired B cells.

5. **Which typing results characterize a secretor who is group O?**
   A. Anti-A + saliva + A cells = positive; anti-B + saliva + B cells = negative; anti-H + saliva + O cells = negative
   B. Anti-A + sailva + A cells = positive; anti-B + saliva + B cells = positive; anti-H + saliva + O cells = positive
   C. Anti-A + saliva + A cells = positive; anti-B + saliva + B cells = positive; anti-H + saliva + O cells = negative
   D. Anti-A + saliva + A cells = negative; anti-B + saliva + B cells = negative; anti-H + saliva + O cells = negative

   Blood bank/Evaluate laboratory data to make identifications/Saliva neutralization/2

6. **Which of the following results is characteristic of an ABO nonsecretor?**
   A. All negative indicator cells for anti-A, anti-B, and anti-H
   B. All positive indicator cells for anti-A, anti-B, and anti-H
   C. Positive indicator cells for anti-A and anti-B; negative for anti-H
   D. Positive indicator cells for anti-H; negative for anti-A and anti-B

   Blood bank/Evaluate laboratory data to make identifications/Saliva neutralization/2

7. **A patient's red blood cells forward type as group O, but the serum agglutinates B cells (4+) only. Your next step would be:**
   A. Extend reverse typing for 15 min
   B. Perform an antibody screen, including a room temperature incubation
   C. Incubate washed red cells with anti-A_1 and anti-A,B for 30 min at room temperature
   D. Test patient's cells with *Dolichos biflorus*

   Blood bank/Apply principles of special procedures/RBC/ABO Discrepancy/3

8. **Which typing results are most likely to occur when a patient has an "acquired B" antigen?**
   A. Anti-A, 4+   Anti-B, 3+ A_1 cells, neg   B cells, neg
   B. Anti-A, 3+   Anti-B, neg A_1 cells, neg   B cells, neg
   C. Anti-A, 4+   Anti-B, 1+ A_1 cells, neg   B cells, 4+
   D. Anti-A, 4+   Anti-B, 4+ A_1 cells, 2+   B cells, neg

   Blood bank/Evaluate laboratory data to recognize problems/ABO discrepancy/2

9. **Which blood group has the least amount of H antigen?**
   A. A_1B
   B. A_2
   C. B
   D. A_1

   Blood bank/Apply knowledge of fundamental biological principles/ABO/1

Answers to Questions 5–9

5. **C** The result is consistent for a secretor group O, in which soluble H antigens from saliva have neutralized anti-H typing reagent. No H antibody is left to react with reagent O cells. No A or B antigens are present in a group O individual, so no A or B antigen is available in the saliva to bind with the anti-A or anti-B antiserum. When A and B cells are added, a positive result is obtained.

6. **B** If no soluble antigens are found in secretions, then antibodies in the reagents are free to bind to the corresponding antigens on red cells. This results in agglutination when anti-A, anti-B, and anti-H are mixed with saliva and the respective antigen-positive RBCs.

7. **C** The strong 4+ reaction in reverse grouping suggests that the discrepancy is in forward grouping. Incubating washed red cells at room temperature with anti-A and anti-A, B will enhance reactions.

8. **C** In forward typing a 1+ reaction with anti-B is suspicious because of the weak reaction and the normal reverse grouping that appears to be group A. This may be indicative of an acquired antigen. In case of acquired B antigen, the reverse grouping is the same as for a group A person. Choice A is indicative of group AB; B is indicative of a group A who may be immunocompromised; D may be caused by a mistyping, an A_2B with anti-A_1, or an alloantibody against antigens on reverse typing cells.

9. **A** The A_1B blood group has the least amount of H antigen. This is due to both A and B epitopes being present on the red cells causing the H epitope's availability to be reduced. Consequently, A_1B red cells demonstrate weak reactions with anti-H lectin.

10. What should be done if all forward and reverse ABO results as well as the autocontrol are positive?
  A. Wash the cells with warm saline; autoadsorb the serum at 4°C
  B. Retype the sample using a different lot number of reagents
  C. Use polyclonal typing reagents
  D. Report the sample as group AB

Blood bank/Evaluate laboratory and clinical data to specify additional tests/RBC/ABO discrepancy/3

11. What should be done if all forward and reverse ABO results are negative?
  A. Perform additional testing such as typing with anti-A$_1$ lectin and anti-A,B
  B. Incubate at 22°C or 4°C to enhance weak expression
  C. Repeat the tests with new reagents
  D. Run an antibody identification panel

Blood bank/Evaluate laboratory and clinical data to specify additional tests/RBC/ABO discrepancy/3

12. N-acetyl-D-galactosamine is the immunodominant carbohydrate that reacts with:
  A. *Arachis hypogaea*
  B. *Salvia sclarea*
  C. *Dolichos biflorus*
  D. *Ulex europaeus*

Blood bank/Apply knowledge of fundamental biological principles/ABO/2

13. A transplant patient was retyped when she was transferred from another hospital. What is the most likely cause of the following results?

| Patient cells: | Anti-A, neg | Anti-B, 4+ |
| Patient serum: | A$_1$ cells, neg | B cells, neg |

  A. Viral infection
  B. Alloantibodies
  C. Immunodeficiency
  D. Autoimmune hemolytic anemia

Blood bank/Evaluate laboratory data to recognize health and disease states/ABO discrepancy/3

14. What reaction would be the same for an A$_1$ and an A$_2$ individual?
  A. Positive reaction with anti-A$_1$ lectin
  B. Positive reaction with A$_1$ cells
  C. Equal reaction with anti-H
  D. Positive reaction with anti-A,B

Blood bank/Evaluate laboratory data to make identifications/ABO discrepancy/2

15. A female patient at 28 weeks' gestation yields the following results:

| Patient cells: | Anti-A, 3+ | Anti-B, 4+ | |
| Patient serum: | A$_1$ cells, neg | B cells, 1+ | O cells, 1+ |

Which of the following could be causing the ABO discrepancy?
  A. Hypogammaglobulinemia
  B. Alloantibody in patient serum
  C. Acquired B
  D. Weak subgroup

Blood bank/Evaluate laboratory data to make identifications/ABO discrepancy/3

Answers to Questions 10–15

10. **A** These results point to a cold autoantibody. Washing the cells with warm saline may elute the autoantibody, allowing a valid forward type to be performed. The serum should be adsorbed using washed cells until the autocontrol is negative. Then the adsorbed serum should be used for the reverse grouping.

11. **B** All negative results may be due to weakened antigens or antibodies. Room temperature or lower incubation temperature may enhance expression of weakened antigens or antibodies.

12. **C** The immunodominant sugar N-acetyl-galactosamine is specific for the A antigen and therefore would react with the A$_1$ lectin *Dolichos biflorus*. The lectin produced from *Arachis hypogaea* contains anti-T activity; *Salvia sclarea* contains anti-Tn, and *Ulex europaeus* contains anti-H.

13. **C** A transplant patient is probably taking immunosuppressive medication to increase graft survival. This can contribute to the loss of normal blood group antibodies as well as other types of antibodies.

14. **D** Anti-A,B should react positively with group A or B and any subgroup of A or B (with the exception of A$_m$). An A$_1$ (not A$_2$) would react with anti-A$_1$ lectin; only an A$_2$ individual with anti-A$_1$ would give a positive reaction with A$_1$ cells; an A$_2$ would react more strongly with anti-H than an A$_1$.

15. **B** The patient is most likely an AB person who has formed a cold reacting alloantibody reacting with B cells and O cells. An identification panel should be performed. An acquired B person or someone with hypogammaglobulinemia should not make an antibody that would agglutinate O cells.

16. Which condition would most likely be responsible for the following typing results?

Patient cells: Anti-A, neg   Anti-B, neg
Patient serum: A₁ cells, neg   B cells, 4+

A. Immunodeficiency
B. Masking of antigens by the presence of massive amounts of antibody
C. Weak or excessive antigen(s)
D. Impossible to determine

Blood bank/Apply principles of basic laboratory procedures/ABO discrepancy/3

17. Which of the following results is discrepant?

Anti-A, neg   Anti-B, 4+
A1 cells, neg   B cells, neg

A. Negative B cells
B. Positive reaction with anti-B
C. Negative A₁ cells
D. No problem with this typing

Blood bank/Evaluate laboratory data to recognize problems/ABO discrepancy/3

18. The following results were found on a 32-year-old female:

Anti-A, mf   Anti-B,neg
A₁ cells, 3+   B cells, 4+

These results are consistent with which ABO subgroup?

A. Aₓ
B. A₃
C. A_el
D. A_y

Blood bank/Evaluate laboratory data to recognize problems/ABO discrepancy/3

19. Which of the following procedures would be most helpful to confirm a weak ABO subgroup?
A. Adsorption-elution
B. Neutralization
C. Elution-diffusion
D. Immunodiffusion-precipitation

Blood bank/Apply principles of special procedures/RBC/ABO discrepancy/3

20. A patient's red cells do not react with anti-A or anti-B but do react weakly with anti-A,B from group O persons. His or her serum agglutinates both A₁ and B cells but not O cells. This patient's blood group is most likely:

A. O
B. Aₘ
C. Aₓ
D. A₃

Blood bank/Evaluate laboratory data to recognize problems/ABO discrepancy/2

Answers to Questions 16–20

16. **C** Excessive A substance, such as may be found in some types of tumors, may be neutralizing the anti-A. Weak A subgroups may fail to react with anti-A and require additional testing techniques (e.g., room temperature incubation) before their expression is apparent.

17. **C** The reverse typing should agree with the forward typing in this result. The 4+ reaction with anti-B indicates group B. A positive reaction is expected with A₁ cells in the reverse group.

18. **B** The A₃ subgroup is characterized by a mixed-field reaction with anti-A and/or anti-A,B, and anti-A₁ may be present in the patient serum. Aₓ red cells usually do not react with anti-A but can react with anti-A,B and can form anti-A₁. A_el red cells do not react with anti-A or anti-A,B but can form anti-A₁. A_y red cells, like A_el red cells, do not react with anti-A or anti-A,B but will not form anti-A₁. All phenotypes mentioned react with anti-H.

19. **A** Adsorption and elution procedures can help confirm A or B specificity when weak reactions are found in corresponding subgroups. This involves incubation of test red cells with corresponding anti-A or anti-B. The antisera adsorb to the red cell antigen if present. This is followed by an elution procedure that is tested against A, B, and O cells to confirm specificity.

20. **C** Aₓ red cells typically will not agglutinate anti-A but will agglutinate anti-A,B and can form anti-A₁. Group O is not the correct choice because of the anti-A,B reaction. Aₘ red cells can react weakly with anti-A and anti-A,B, but do not form anti-A₁. A₃ red cells characteristically yield mixed-field reactions with anti-A.

1. A complete Rh typing for antigens C, c, D, E, and e revealed negative results for C, D, and E. How is the individual designated?
   A. Rh-positive
   B. Rh-negative
   C. positive for c and e
   D. Impossible to determine

   Blood bank/Apply knowledge of fundamental biological characteristics/Rh typing/1

2. How is an individual classified with genotype Dce/dce?
   A. Rh-positive
   B. Rh-negative
   C. Rh$_{null}$
   D. Total Rh

   Blood bank/Apply knowledge of fundamental biological characteristics/Rh typing/2

3. If a patient has a positive direct antiglobulin test, should you perform a weak D test on the cells?
   A. No, the cells are already coated with antibody
   B. No, the cells are Rh$_{null}$
   C. Yes, the immunoglobulin will not interfere with the test
   D. Yes, Rh reagents are enhanced in protein media

   Blood bank/Apply knowledge of fundamental biological characteristics/Rh typing/3

4. Which donor unit is selected for a recipient with anti-c?
   A. r'r
   B. R_0R_1
   C. R_2r'
   D. r'r^y

   Blood bank/Apply knowledge of fundamental biological characteristics/Rh typing/3

5. Which genotype usually shows the strongest reaction with anti-D?
   A. DCE/DCE
   B. Dce/dCe

   C. D—/D—
   D. -CE/-ce

   Blood bank/Apply knowledge of fundamental biological characteristics/Rh typing/1

Answers to Questions 1–5

1. **B** Rh-positive refers to the presence of D antigen; Rh-negative refers to the absence of the D antigen. These designations are for D antigen only and do not involve other Rh antigens.

2. **A** This individual has the D antigen and is classified as Rh-positive. Any genotype containing the D antigen will be considered Rh-positive.

3. **A** If a person has a positive DAT the red cells are coated with immunoglobulin (anti-IgG, anti-C3d, or both). If a test for weak D were performed, the test would yield positive results independent of the presence or absence of the D antigen on red cells.

4. **D** The designation r' is dCe and r^y is dCE, neither of which contains the c antigen. The other three Rh types contain the c antigen and could not be used in transfusion for a person with anti-c.

5. **C** The phenotype that results from D—/D— is classified as enhanced D because it shows a stronger reaction than expected with anti-D. Such cells have a greater amount of D antigen than normal. This is thought to result from a larger quantity of precursors being available to the D genes because there is no competition from other Rh genes.

6. Why is testing for Rh antigens and antibodies different from ABO testing?
   A. ABO reactions are primarily due to IgM antibodies and usually occur at room temperature; Rh antibodies are IgG, and agglutination usually requires a 37°C incubation and enhancement media
   B. ABO antigens are attached to receptors on the outside of the red cell and do not require any special enhancement for testing; Rh antigens are loosely attached to the red cell membrane and require enhancement for detection
   C. Both ABO and Rh antigens and antibodies have similar structures, but Rh antibodies are configured so that special techniques are needed to facilitate binding to Rh antigens
   D. There is no difference in ABO and Rh testing; both may be conducted at room temperature with no special enhancement needed for reaction

Blood bank/Apply knowledge of fundamental biological characteristics/Rh system/1

7. Testing reveals a weak D that reacts 1+ after indirect antiglobulin testing (IAT). How is this result classified?
   A. Rh-positive
   B. Rh-negative, D^u positive
   C. Rh-negative
   D. Rh-positive, D^u positive

Blood bank/Apply knowledge of standard operating procedures/Components/Rh label/2

8. What is one possible genotype for a patient who develops anti-C antibody?
   A. R^1r
   B. R^1R^1
   C. $r'r$
   D. rr

Blood bank/Apply knowledge of fundamental biological characteristics/Rh typing/2

9. A patient developed a combination of Rh antibodies: anti-C, anti-E, and anti-D. Can compatible blood be found for this patient?
   A. It is almost impossible to find blood lacking the C, E, and D antigens
   B. rr blood could be used without causing a problem
   C. R_0R_0 may be used because it lacks all three of these antigens
   D. Although rare, r^yr blood may be obtained from close relatives of the patient

Blood bank/Apply knowledge of fundamental biological characteristics/Rh antibodies/1

10. A patient tests positive for weak D but also appears to have anti-D in his serum. What may be the problem?
   A. Mixup of samples or testing error
   B. Most weak D individuals make anti-D
   C. The problem could be due to a disease state
   D. A D mosaic may make antibodies to missing antigen parts

Blood bank/Apply knowledge to identify sources of error/Rh antibodies/2

11. Which offspring is not possible from a mother who is R^1R^2 and a father who is R^1r?
   A. DcE/DcE
   B. DCe/DCe
   C. DcE/DCe
   D. DCe/dce

Blood bank/Evaluate laboratory data to verify test results/Rh system/paternity testing/2

Answers to Questions 6–11

6. **A** Detection of ABO and Rh antigens and antibodies requires different reaction conditions. ABO antibodies are naturally occurring IgM molecules and react best at room temperature. Rh antibodies are generally immune IgG molecules that result from transfusion or pregnancy. Detection usually requires 37°C incubation and/or enhancement techniques.

7. **A** Blood tested for weak D that shows a 1+ reaction after IAT is classified as Rh-positive. The weak D designation is not noted in the reporting of the result.

8. **D** Only rr (dce/dce) does not contain C antigen. A person will form alloantibodies only to the antigens he or she lacks.

9. **B** The genotype rr (dce/dce) lacks D, C, and E antigens and would be suitable for an individual who has developed antibodies to all three antigens. This is the most common Rh-negative genotype and is found in nearly 14% of white blood donors.

10. **D** The D antigen is made up of different parts designated as a mosaic. If an individual lacks parts of the antigen, he or she may make antibodies to the missing parts if exposed to the whole D antigen.

11. **A** DcE/DcE (R^2R^2) is not possible because R^2 can be inherited only from the mother and is not present in the father.

12. Which genotype would most likely show dosage effect for both C and e antigens?
   A. dce/dce
   B. dCE/dCE
   C. DCE/DCE
   D. DCe/DcE

Blood bank/Evaluate laboratory data to verify test results/Rh system/Rh testing/2

13. What antibodies could an R_1R_1 make if exposed to R_2R_2 blood?
   A. Anti-e and anti-C
   B. Anti-E and anti-c
   C. Anti-E and anti-C
   D. Anti-e and anti-c

Blood bank/Apply knowledge of fundamental biological characteristics/Rh antibodies/2

14. Interpret this phenotype: —-/—-
   A. No problem, Rh-negative
   B. D mosaic
   C. Rh_{null}
   D. Total Rh

Blood bank/Evaluate laboratory data to make identifications/Rh system/Rh antigens/2

15. What techniques are necessary for weak D testing?
   A. Saline + 22°C incubation
   B. Albumin or LISS + 37°C incubation
   C. Saline + 37°C incubation
   D. 37°C incubation + IAT

Blood bank/Apply knowledge of basic laboratory procedure/Rh system/weak D/2

16. A patient types as AB and appears to be Rh-positive on slide typing. What additional test should be performed for tube typing?
   A. Rh-negative control
   B. Direct antiglobulin test (DAT)
   C. Low-protein Rh antisera
   D. No additional testing is needed

Blood bank/Evaluate laboratory data to verify test results/Rh system/2

17. According to the Wiener nomenclature and/or genetic theory of Rh inheritance:
   A. There are three closely linked loci, each with a primary set of allelic genes
   B. The alleles are named R^1, R^2, R^0, r, r′, r″, R^z, and r^y
   C. There are multiple alleles at a single complex locus that determine each Rh antigen
   D. The antigens are named D, C, E, c, and e

Blood bank/Apply knowledge of fundamental biological principles/Rh system/2

18. The Wiener nomenclature for the E antigen is:
   A. hr′
   B. hr″
   C. rh″
   D. Rh_0

Blood bank/Apply knowledge of fundamental biological principles/Rh typing/1

Answers to Questions 12–18

12. **D** In the genotypes DCe/DcE, both C and e (and C and E) are heterozygous, which may result in dosage effect. The agglutination reaction between these antigens and the respective antisera will be weaker than for cells from a homozygote.

13. **B** The R_1R_1 (DCe/DCe) individual does not have the E or c antigen and could make anti-E and anti-c antibodies when exposed to R_2R_2 cells (DcE/DcE).

14. **C** A person who is Rh_{null} shows no Rh antigens on his or her RBCs. Loss of Rh antigens is very unlikely to happen because Rh antigens are integral parts of the RBC membrane. The Rh_{null} phenotype can result from either genetic suppression of the Rh genes or inheritance of amorphic genes at the Rh locus.

15. **D** Weak D testing requires both 37°C incubation and the IAT procedure. Anti-D is an IgG antibody, and attachment of the D antigen is optimized at warmer temperatures. Antihuman globulin in the IAT phase facilitates lattice formation by binding to the antigen-antibody complexes.

16. **A** An Rh-negative control (patient cells in saline or 6% albumin) should be run if a sample appears to be AB-positive. The ABO test serves as the Rh control for other ABO types.

17. **C** Wiener proposed a single locus theory for Rh with multiple alleles determining surface molecules that embody numerous antigens. The Rh gene produces an antigen that contains at least three factors. R_0, R_1, R_2, R^Z, r, r′, r″, r^y are shorthand symbols for the Wiener genes Rh^0, Rh^1, Rh^2, Rh^Z, rh, rh′, rh″, rh^y. $\overline{\overline{rr}}$ is the symbol for the Rh_{null} genotype.

18. **C** rh″ is the Wiener designation for the E antigen. hr′ would be c, hr″ would be e, and Rh_0 is D.

19. Given the following results, what course of action should be followed in order to determine the patient's Rh type?

Anti-A	Anti-B	A₁ cells	B cells	Autocontrol	Anti-D	DAT
4+	Neg	Neg	4+	1+	4+	Neg

A. Rh typing is probably correct; no further action is needed
B. Wash the patient's cells and retype
C. Wash the patient's cells in warm saline and repeat the Rh typing
D. Obtain a new sample and repeat all tests

Blood bank/Evaluate sources of error/Rh system/3

20. What is the purpose of adding antibody-coated red cells to all negative anti-human globulin (AHG) tubes?
A. To ensure proper tube reading
B. To ensure proper cell washing and addition of AHG reagent
C. To check for hemolysis or reaction of complement
D. To check for attachment of additional antibody

Blood bank/Apply principles of basic laboratory procedures/AHG testing/1

Answers to Questions 19–20

19. **C** There appears to be no problem with ABO typing, and no antibody is coating the patient's red cells (negative DAT). The patient's serum may contain a cold-reacting antibody directed only against the patient's own RBCs. Check the patient's records for a previous diagnosis and repeat the Rh typing after washing the cells with warm saline to remove the cold autoantibody.

20. **B** The addition of red cells coated with antibody (Coombs' Check Cells) ensures proper cell washing and the addition of AHG reagent. If the cells agglutinate, then the test was performed properly and the results are valid.

1. A patient has the Lewis phenotype Le(a-b-). An antibody panel reveals the presence of anti-Le^a. Another patient with the phenotype Le(a-b+) has a positive antibody screen: however, a panel reveals no conclusive antibody. Should anti-Le^a be considered as a possibility for the patient with the Le(a-b+) phenotype?
   A. Anti-Le^a should be considered as a possible antibody for this patient
   B. Anti-Le^a may be a possible antibody, but further studies are needed
   C. Anti-Le^a is not a likely antibody because even Le^b individuals secrete some Le^a
   D. Anti-Le^a may be found in saliva but is not detectable in serum

   Blood bank/Apply knowledge of fundamental biological characteristics/Blood groups/2

2. A technologist is having great difficulty resolving an antibody mixture. One of the antibodies is anti-Le^a. This antibody is not clinically significant in this situation, but it needs to be removed to reveal the possible presence of an underlying antibody of clinical significance. What can be done?
   A. Perform an enzyme panel
   B. Neutralize the serum with saliva
   C. Neutralize the serum with hydatid cyst fluid
   D. Use DTT (dithiothreitol) to treat the panel cells

   Blood bank/Apply knowledge of fundamental biological characteristics/Blood groups/3

3. What type of blood should be given an individual who has an anti-Le^b that reacts 1+ at the IAT phase?
   A. Blood that is negative for the Le^b antigen
   B. Blood that is negative for both the Le^a and the Le^b antigens
   C. Blood that is positive for the Le^b antigen
   D. Lewis antibodies are not clinically significant, so any type of blood may be given

   Blood bank/Apply knowledge of fundamental biological characteristics/Blood group antibodies/3

4. Which of the following statements is true concerning the *MN* genotype?
   A. Antigens are destroyed using bleach-treated cells
   B. Dosage effect may be seen for both M and N antigens
   C. Both M and N antigens are impossible to detect because of cross-interference
   D. MN is a rare phenotype seldom found in routine antigen typing

   Blood bank/Apply knowledge of fundamental biological characteristics/Blood groups/2

Answers to Questions 1–4

1. **C** Anti-Le^a is produced primarily by persons with the Le(a-b-) phenotype because Le(a-b+) persons still have some Le^a antigen present in saliva. Although Le^a is not present on their red cells, Le(a-b+) persons do not form anti-Le^a.

2. **B** Saliva from an individual with the Le gene contains the Le^a antigen. This combines with anti-Le^a, neutralizing the antibody. Panel cells treated with DTT (0.2M) lose reactivity with anti-K and other antibodies, but not anti-Le^a. Hydatid cyst fluid neutralizes anti-P_1.

3. **A** Lewis antibodies are generally not considered clinically significant unless they react at 37°C or at the IAT phase; for example, 1+ at IAT. The antibody must be honored in this scenario.

4. **B** Dosage effect is the term used to describe the phenomenon of an antibody that reacts more strongly with homozygous cells than with heterozygous cells. Dosage effect is a characteristic of the genotype *MN* because the M and N antigens are heterozygous on the same cell. This causes a weaker reaction than seen with RBCs of either the *MM* or *NN* genotype, which carry a greater amount of the corresponding antigen.

5. Anti-M is sometimes found with reactivity detected at the immediate spin (IS) phase that persists in strength to the IAT phase. What is the main testing problem with a strong anti-M?
   - **A.** Anti-M may not allow detection of a clinically significant antibody
   - **B.** Compatible blood may not be found for the patient with a strongly reacting anti-M
   - **C.** The anti-M cannot be removed from the serum
   - **D.** The anti-M may react with the patient's own cells, causing a positive autocontrol

   Blood bank/Apply knowledge of fundamental biological characteristics/Blood groups/2

6. A patient is suspected of having paroxysmal cold hemoglobinuria (PCH). Which pattern of reactivity is characteristic of the Donath-Landsteiner antibody, which causes this condition?
   - **A.** The antibody attaches to RBCs at 4°C and causes hemolysis at 37°C
   - **B.** The antibody attaches to RBCs at 37°C and causes agglutination at the IAT phase
   - **C.** The antibody attaches to RBCs at 22°C and causes hemolysis at 37°C
   - **D.** The antibody attaches to RBCs and causes agglutination at the IAT phase

   Blood bank/Apply knowledge of fundamental biological characteristics/Blood group antibodies/1

7. How can interfering anti-P_1 antibody be removed from a mixture of antibodies?
   - **A.** Neutralization with saliva
   - **B.** Agglutination with human milk
   - **C.** Combination with urine
   - **D.** Neutralization with hydatid cyst fluid

   Blood bank/Apply principles of special procedures/Blood group antibodies/1

8. This antibody is frequently seen in warm autoimmune hemolytic anemia.
   - **A.** Anti-Jk^a
   - **B.** Anti-e
   - **C.** Anti-K
   - **D.** Anti-Fy^b

   Blood bank/Apply knowledge of fundamental biological characteristics/Blood group antibodies/1

9. An antibody shows strong reactions in all test phases. All screen and panel cells are positive. The serum is then tested with a cord cell and the reaction is negative. What antibody is suspected?
   - **A.** Anti-i
   - **B.** Anti-I
   - **C.** Anti-H
   - **D.** Anti-p

   Blood bank/Apply principles of special procedures/ Antibody ID/2

10. Which group of antibodies are commonly found as cold agglutinins?
    - **A.** Anti-K, Anti-k, Anti-Js^b
    - **B.** Anti-D, Anti-e, Anti-C
    - **C.** Anti-M, Anti-N
    - **D.** Anti-Fy^a, Anti-Fy^b

    Blood bank/Apply knowledge of fundamental biological characteristics/Blood group antibodies/1

11. Which of the following antibodies characteristically gives a refractile mixed-field appearance?
    - **A.** Anti-K
    - **B.** Anti-Di^a
    - **C.** Anti-Sd^a
    - **D.** Anti-s

    Blood bank/Apply knowledge of fundamental biological characteristics/Blood group antibodies/1

Answers to Questions 5–11

5. **A** While anti-M may not be clinically significant, a strongly reacting anti-M that persists through to the IAT phase may interfere with detection of a clinically significant antibody that reacts only at IAT.

6. **A** The Donath-Landsteiner antibody has anti-P specificity with biphasic activity. The antibody attaches to RBCs at 4°C and then causes the red cells to hemolyze when warmed to 37°C.

7. **D** Hydatid cyst fluid contains P_1 substance, which can neutralize anti-P_1 antibody.

8. **B** Anti-e is frequently implicated in cases of warm autoimmune hemolytic anemia. The corresponding antigen is characterized as high frequency in the Rh system and can mask the presence of other alloantibodies.

9. **B** Adult cells contain mostly I antigen, and anti-I would react with all adult cells found on screen or panel cells. Cord cells, however, contain mostly i antigen and would test negative or only weakly positive with anti-I.

10. **C** Antibodies to the M and N antigens are IgM antibodies commonly found as cold agglutinins.

11. **C** Anti-Sd^a characteristically gives a refractile mixed-field agglutination reaction in the IAT. The refractile characteristic is more evident under the microscope.

12. **What is true concerning the acquisition of K-negative donor units?**
    A. Blood must be provided by rare donor files
    B. Close relatives must be screened as potential donors
    C. Ninety percent of donor units will be K-negative
    D. It depends upon the racial composition of the blood donors

    Blood bank/Calculate/Hemotherapy/1

13. **The k (Cellano) antigen is a high-frequency antigen and is found on most red cells. How often would one expect to find the corresponding antibody?**
    A. Often, because it is a high-frequency antibody
    B. Rarely, because most individuals have the antigen and therefore would not develop the antibody
    C. It depends upon the population because certain racial and ethnic groups show a higher frequency of anti-k
    D. Impossible to determine without consulting regional blood group antigen charts

    Blood bank/Calculate/Hemotherapy/1

14. **Which procedure would help to distinguish between an anti-e and anti-Fyᵃ in an antibody mixture?**
    A. Lower pH of test serum
    B. Run an enzyme panel
    C. Use a thiol reagent
    D. Run a regular panel

    Blood bank/Apply principles of special procedures/ Antibody ID/2

15. **Which characteristics are true of all three of the following antibodies: anti-Fyᵃ, anti-Jkᵃ, anti-K?**
    A. Detected at the IAT phase; may cause hemolytic disease of the newborn (HDN) and transfusion reactions
    B. Not detected with enzyme-treated cells; may cause delayed transfusion reactions
    C. Requires the IAT technique for detection; usually not responsible for causing HDN
    D. Enhanced reactivity with enzyme-treated cells; may cause severe hemolytic transfusion reactions

    Blood bank/Apply principles of special procedures/ Antibody ID/2

16. **A patient is admitted to the hospital. Medical records indicate that the patient has a history of anti-Jkᵇ. When you performed the type and screen, it was negative. You should:**
    A. Crossmatch using Jkᵇ negative units
    B. Crossmatch random units, since the antibody is not demonstrable
    C. Request a new sample because you think they drew the sample from the incorrect patient
    D. All of the above are incorrect

    Blood bank/Apply principles of basic laboratory procedures/Antibody ID/3

17. **A technologist performs an antibody study and finds 1+ and weak positive reactions for several of the panel cells. The reactions do not fit a pattern. Several selected panels and a patient phenotype do not reveal any additional information. The serum is diluted and retested, but the same reactions persist. What type of antibody may be causing these results?**
    A. Antibody to a high frequency antigen
    B. Antibody to a low frequency antigen
    C. High titer low avidity (HTLA)
    D. HLA

    Blood bank/Evaluate laboratory data to make identifications/Antibody ID/3

Answers to Questions 12–17

12. **C** The K antigen is found in approximately 9%–10% of the population. Ninety percent of donor units, therefore, should be negative for the K antigen.

13. **B** The k antigen is found with a frequency of 99.8%; therefore, the k-negative person is rare. Because k-negative individuals are very rare, the occurrence of anti-k is also rare.

14. **B** Enzyme-treated cells will not react with Duffy antibodies. Rh antibodies react more strongly with enzyme-treated panel cells. An enzyme panel, therefore, would enhance reactivity of anti-e and destroy reactivity to anti-Fyᵃ.

15. **A** Anti-Fyᵃ, anti-Jkᵃ, and anti-K are usually detected at IAT and all may cause HDN and transfusion reactions that may be hemolytic. Reactivity with anti-Fya is lost with enzyme-treated red cells, but reactivity with anti-Jkᵃ is enhanced with enzyme-treated red cells. Reactivity with anti-K is unaffected by enzyme-treated red cells.

16. **A** The Kidd antibodies are notorious for disappearing from serum, yielding a negative result for the antibody screen. If a patient has a history of a Kidd antibody, blood must be crossmatched using antigen-negative units. If the patient is transfused with the corresponding antigen, an anamnestic reaction may occur with a subsequent hemolytic transfusion reaction.

17. **C** HTLA antibodies may persist in reaction strength, even when diluted. These antibodies are directed against high-frequency antigens (such as Chᵃ). They are not clinically significant but, when present, are responsible for a high incidence of incompatible crossmatches.

18. An antibody is detected in a pregnant woman and is suspected of being the cause of fetal distress. The antibody reacts at the IAT phase but does not react with DTT-treated cells. This antibody causes in vitro hemolysis. What is the most likely antibody specificity?
   A. Anti-Le^a
   B. Anti-Lu^a
   C. Anti-Lu^b
   D. Anti-Xg^a

Blood bank/Evaluate laboratory data to make identifications/Antibody ID/3

19. What sample is best for detecting complement-dependent antibodies?
   A. Plasma stored at 4°C for no longer than 24 hours
   B. Serum stored at 4°C for no longer than 48 hours
   C. Either serum or plasma stored at 20–24°C no longer than 6 hours
   D. Serum heated at 56°C for 30 min

Blood bank/Apply principles of basic laboratory procedures/Antibody ID/2

20. Which antibody would not be detected by group O screen cells?
   A. Anti-N
   B. Anti-A$_1$
   C. Anti-Di^a
   D. Anti-k

Blood bank/Apply principles of special procedures/Antibody ID/2

21. Refer to Panel 1 below. Which antibody is most likely implicated?
   A. Anti-Fy^b
   B. Anti-Jk^b
   C. Anti-e
   D. Anti-c and anti-K

Blood bank/Apply principles of special procedures/Antibody ID/2

Answers to Questions 18–21

18. **C** Of the antibodies above only Lu^b is detected in the IAT phase, causes in vitro hemolysis, may cause HDN. and does not react with DTT-treated cells.

19. **B** Serum stored at 4°C for no longer than 48 hours preserves complement activity. Plasma is inappropriate because most anticoagulants chelate Ca^{2+} needed for activation of complement. Heating the serum to 56°C destroys complement.

20. **B** ABO antibodies are not detected by group O screen cells, as O cells contain no A or B antigen.

21. **B** The pattern clearly fits that of anti-Jk^b, an antibody that usually reacts best at IAT. The weaker reactions are due to dosage effect found on cells that are heterozygous for Jk^b antigen.

Panel 1

cell	D	C	E	c	e	K	k	Kpa	Kpb	Jsa	Jsb	Fya	Fyb	Jka	Jkb	Xga	Lea	Leb	S	s	M	N	P1	Lua	Lub	37	IAT
1	+	+	O	O	+	O	+	O	+	O	+	O	+	O	+	+	+	O	O	+	O	+	O	O	+	O	2+
2	+	+	O	O	+	+	+	O	+	O	+	+	+	+	+	+	O	+	+	+	O	+	+	O	+	O	1+
3	+	O	+	+	O	O	+	O	+	O	+	+	O	+	+	O	O	+	+	+	+	+	O	+	O	O	1+
4	O	+	O	+	+	O	+	O	+	O	+	+	+	+	+	O	+	O	+	+	+	O	O	+	O	O	1+
5	O	O	+	+	+	+	+	O	+	O	+	+	+	O	O	O	+	O	+	+	+	+	O	+	O	O	O
6	O	O	O	O	+	O	+	O	+	O	+	+	+	+	+	O	+	O	+	+	O	+	O	O	+	O	1+
7	O	O	O	+	+	+	+	O	+	O	+	O	O	+	O	+	O	+	+	O	+	O	+	O	+	O	O
8	O	O	O	+	+	O	+	O	+	O	+	O	+	O	+	+	O	O	+	+	O	+	O	O	+	O	2+
9	+	+	O	O	+	O	+	O	+	O	+	+	+	+	+	+	O	O	+	+	+	+	O	+	O	O	1+
10	+	O	O	+	+	O	+	O	+	O	+	O	O	+	+	+	O	O	O	O	+	O	+	O	+	O	1+

22. Refer to Panel 2 below. Which antibody specificity is most likely present?
  A. Anti-S and anti-E
  B. Anti-E and anti-K
  C. Anti-Le^a and anti-Fy^b
  D. Anti-C and anti-K

Blood bank/Apply principles of special procedures/ Antibody ID/3

23. On Panel 2, which of the following antibodies could not be ruled out?
  A. Anti-Jk^b
  B. Anti-C
  C. Anti-M
  D. Anti-Fy^b

Blood Bank/Apply principles of special procedures/ Antibody ID/2

Answers to Questions 22–23

22. **D** The pattern fits anti-C at 37°C, which becomes stronger at the IAT phase. The additional antibody is anti-K, which appears only at the IAT phase.

23. **B** To rule out an antibody there should be a homozygous cell with the corresponding antigen that fails to react with the serum. Of the choices, anti-C was not ruled out on Panel 2. To rule this antibody out, a cell that is homozygous for C and negative for K (the other probable antibody) would be run against patient serum. A positive reaction supports the presence of anti-C, whereas a negative reaction would rule out anti-C.

Panel 2

cell	D	C	E	c	e	K	k	Kpa	Kpb	Jsa	Jsb	Fya	Fyb	Jka	Jkb	Xga	Lea	Leb	S	s	M	N	P1	Lua	Lub	37	IAT
1	+	+	O	O	+	O	+	O	+	O	+	O	+	O	+	+	+	O	O	+	O	+	O	O	+	1+	2+
2	+	+	O	O	+	+	+	O	+	O	+	+	+	+	+	+	O	+	+	+	O	+	+	O	+	1+	2+
3	+	O	+	+	O	O	+	O	+	O	+	+	O	+	+	O	O	+	+	+	+	+	+	O	+	O	O
4	O	+	O	+	+	O	+	O	+	O	+	+	+	+	+	+	O	+	O	+	+	+	O	O	+	1+	2+
5	O	O	+	+	+	+	+	O	+	O	+	+	+	O	O	O	+	O	+	+	+	+	+	O	+	O	2+
6	O	O	O	O	+	O	+	O	+	O	+	+	+	+	+	+	+	O	+	+	+	O	+	O	+	O	O
7	O	O	O	+	+	+	+	O	+	O	+	O	O	+	O	+	O	+	+	O	+	O	+	O	+	O	2+
8	O	O	O	+	+	O	+	O	+	O	+	O	+	O	+	+	O	O	+	+	+	O	+	O	+	O	O
9	+	+	O	O	+	O	+	O	+	O	+	+	+	+	+	+	+	O	O	+	+	+	+	O	+	1+	1+
10	+	O	O	+	+	O	+	O	+	O	+	O	O	O	+	+	+	O	O	O	O	+	O	+	O	O	O

1. **SITUATION:** An emergency trauma patient requires transfusion. Six units of blood are ordered *stat*. There is no time to draw a patient sample. O-negative blood is released. When will compatibility testing be performed?
   A. Compatibility testing must be performed before blood is issued
   B. Compatibility testing will be performed when a patient sample is available
   C. Compatibility testing may be performed immediately using donor serum
   D. Compatibility testing is not necessary when blood is released in emergency situations

   Blood bank/Apply knowledge of laboratory operations/ Crossmatch/1

2. How would autoantibodies affect compatibility testing?
   A. No effect
   B. The DAT would be positive
   C. ABO, Rh, antibody screen, and crossmatch may show abnormal results
   D. Results would depend on the specificity of autoantibody

   Blood bank/Evaluate laboratory data to make identifications/Antibody ID/3

3. An antibody screen is reactive at the IAT phase of testing with all three screen cells, and the autocontrol is negative. What is a possible explanation for these results?
   A. A cold alloantibody
   B. High frequency alloantibody or a mixture of alloantibodies
   C. A warm autoantibody
   D. A cold and warm alloantibody

   Blood bank/evaluate laboratory data to make identifications/Antibody identifications/3

4. In which case would a minor crossmatch be required?
   A. Transfusion of fresh frozen plasma
   B. Investigation of a transfusion reaction
   C. When the donor is found to have an alloantibody
   D. No situations require minor crossmatching

   Blood bank/Apply knowledge of standard operating procedures/Crossmatch/2

5. Can crossmatching be performed on October 14 using a patient sample drawn on October 12?
   A. Yes, a new sample would not be needed
   B. Yes, but only if the previous sample has no alloantibodies
   C. No, a new sample is needed because the 2-day limit has expired
   D. No, a new sample is needed for each testing

   Blood bank/Apply knowledge of standard operating procedures/Crossmatch/2

Answers to Questions 1–5

1. **B** When patient serum is available, it will be crossmatched with donor cells. Patient serum might contain antibodies against antigens on donor cells that may destroy donor cells. If an incompatibility is discovered, the problem is reported immediately to the patient's physician.

2. **C** Autoantibodies may cause positive reactions with screen cells, panel cells, donor cells, and patient cells. The DAT will be positive; however, the recipient cells are not used in compatibility testing.

3. **B** High-frequency alloantibodies or a mixture of alloantibodies may cause all three screen cells to be positive. A negative autocontrol would rule out autoantibodies.

4. **D** A minor crossmatch consists of recipient red cells and donor serum or plasma. The antibody screen in donor testing has replaced the minor crossmatch in detecting antibodies in donor serum that would be incompatible with recipient cells.

5. **A** Compatibility testing may be performed on a patient sample within 3 days of the scheduled transfusion.

6. A type and screen were performed on a 32-year old woman, and the patient was typed as AB-negative. There are no AB-negative units in the blood bank. What should be done?
   A. Order AB-negative units from a blood supplier
   B. Check inventory of A-, B-, and O-negative units
   C. Ask the patient to make a preoperative autologous donation
   D. Nothing, the blood will probably not be used

   Blood bank/Apply principles of basic laboratory procedures/Crossmatch/2

7. What ABO type(s) may donate to any other ABO type?
   A. A-negative, B-negative, AB-negative, or O-negative
   B. O-negative
   C. AB-negative
   D. AB-negative, A-negative, B-negative

   Blood bank/Apply knowledge of fundamental biological characteristics/Crossmatch/2

8. What type(s) of red cells is (are) acceptable to transfuse to an O-negative patient?
   A. A-negative, B-negative, AB-negative, or O-negative
   B. O-negative
   C. AB-negative
   D. AB-negative, A-negative, B-negative

   Blood bank/Apply knowledge of fundamental biological characteristics/Crossmatch/2

9. A technologist removed four units of blood from the blood bank refrigerator and placed them on the counter. A clerk was waiting to take the units for transfusion. As she checked the paperwork, she noticed that one of the units was leaking onto the counter. What should she do?
   A. Issue the unit if red cells appear normal
   B. Reseal the unit
   C. Discard the unit
   D. Call the medical director and ask for an opinion

   Blood bank/Apply knowledge of standard operating procedures/Crossmatch/1

10. A donor was found to contain anti-K using pilot tubes from the collection procedure. How would this affect the compatibility testing?
    A. The AHG major crossmatch would be positive if the recipient expressed K antigen
    B. The IS (immediate spin) major crossmatch would be positive if recipient was negative for K antigen
    C. The antibody screen done on the recipient would be positive for anti-K
    D. Compatibility testing would not be affected

    Blood bank/Apply principles of basic laboratory procedures/Crossmatch/2

11. Which of the following statements about requirements for an electronic cross-match is *NOT* correct?

    A. The computer system contains logic to prevent assignment and release of ABO incompatible blood
    B. There are concordant results of at least two determinations of the recipient's ABO type on record, one of which is from the current sample
    C. Critical elements of the system have been validated on-site
    D. One determination of the recipient's ABO type is required

    Blood bank/Apply principles of basic laboratory procedures/Crossmatch/1

12. A patient showed positive results with screen cells and four donor units at the IAT phase of testing. The patient autocontrol was negative. What is the most likely antibody?
    A. Anti-H
    B. Anti-S
    C. Anti-Kp^a
    D. Anti-k

    Blood bank/Evaluate laboratory data to make identifications/Incompatible crossmatch/3

Answers to Questions 6–12

6. **B** An AB person is the universal recipient and may receive any blood type; because only a type and screen were ordered and blood may not be used, check inventory for A-negative, B-negative, and O-negative units.

7. **B** An O-negative individual has no A or B antigen and may donate red cells to any other ABO type.

8. **B** An O-negative individual has both anti-A and anti-B and may receive only O-negative red cells.

9. **C** Leaking may indicate a broken seal or a puncture, which indicates possible contamination of the unit, even if the red cells appear normal. The unit should be discarded.

10. **D** Compatibility testing would not be affected if the donor has anti-K in his/her serum. This is because the major crossmatch uses recipient serum and not donor serum. Other tests such as ABO, Rh, and antibody screen on the recipient also would not be affected.

11. **D** ABO determinations must be concordant on at least 2 occasions, including the current sample.

12. **D** Anti-k (Cellano) is a high-frequency alloantibody that would react with screen cells and most donor units. The negative autocontrol rules out autoantibodies. Anti-H and anti-S are cold antibodies and anti-Kp^a is a low-frequency alloantibody.

13. Screening cells and major crossmatch are positive on immediate spin (IS) only, and the autocontrol is negative. Identify the problem.
    A. Cold alloantibody
    B. Cold autoantibody
    C. Abnormal protein
    D. Antibody mixture

    Blood bank/Evaluate laboratory data to make identifications/Incompatible crossmatch/3

14. Six units are crossmatched. Five units are compatible, one unit is incompatible, and the recipient's antibody screen is negative. Identify the problem.
    A. Patient may have an alloantibody to a high-frequency antigen
    B. Patient may have an abnormal protein
    C. Donor unit may have a positive DAT
    D. Donor may have a high-frequency antigen

    Blood bank/Evaluate laboratory data to make identifications/Incompatible crossmatch/3

15. What should be done with a donor unit with a positive DAT?
    A. Discard the unit
    B. Antigen type the unit for high-frequency antigens
    C. Wash the donor cells and use the washed cells for testing
    D. Perform a panel on the incompatible unit

    Blood bank/Apply principles of special procedures/Incompatible crossmatch/3

16. Screening cells, major crossmatch, and patient autocontrol are positive in all phases. Identify the problem.
    A. Specific cold alloantibody
    B. Specific cold autoantibody
    C. Abnormal protein or nonspecific autoantibody
    D. Cold and warm alloantibody mixture

    Blood bank/Evaluate laboratory data to make identifications/Incompatible crossmatch/3

17. A panel study has revealed the presence of patient alloantibodies. What is the first step in a major crossmatch?
    A. Perform a DAT on patient cells and donor units
    B. Antigen type patient cells and any donor cells to be crossmatched
    C. Adsorb any antibodies from the patient serum
    D. Obtain a different enhancement medium for testing

    Blood bank/Apply principles of special procedures/Incompatible crossmatch/1

18. What is the disposition of a donor red blood cell unit that contains an antibody?

    A. The unit must be discarded
    B. Only the plasma may be used to make components
    C. The antibody must be adsorbed from the unit
    D. The red cell unit may be labeled to indicate it contains antibody and released into inventory

    Blood bank/Apply knowledge of laboratory operations/Hemotherapy/Blood components/1

19. Given a situation where screening cells, major crossmatch, autocontrol, and DAT (anti-IgG) are all positive, what procedure should be performed next?
    A. Adsorption using rabbit stroma
    B. Antigen typing of the patient's cells
    C. Elution followed by a cell panel on the eluate
    D. Selected cell panel

    Blood bank/Apply principles of special procedures/Incompatible crossmatch/3

Answers to Questions 13–19

13. **A** A cold alloantibody would show a reaction with screening cells and donor units only at IS phase. The negative autocontrol rules out autoantibodies and abnormal protein.

14. **C** The incompatible donor unit may have an antibody coating the red cells, or the patient may have an alloantibody to a low-frequency antigen. An alloantibody to a high-frequency antigen would agglutinate all units and screening cells.

15. **A** The incompatible unit may have red cells coated with antibody or complement. If red cells are sensitized, then some problem exists with the donor. Discard the unit.

16. **C** An abnormal protein or nonspecific autoantibody would cause antibody screen, crossmatch, and patient autocontrol to be positive. Alloantibodies would not cause a positive patient autocontrol.

17. **B** Antigen typing or phenotyping of the patient's cells confirms the antibody identification; antigen typing of donor cells helps ensure the crossmatch of compatible donor units.

18. **D** The RBC unit may be used in the general blood inventory if it is properly labeled and only cellular elements are used.

19. **C** A positive DAT using anti-IgG indicates that antibodies are coating the patient cells. An eluate would be helpful to remove the antibody, followed by a cell panel in order to identify it.

20. A major crossmatch and screening cells are 2+ at IS, 1+ at 37°C, and negative at the IAT phase. Identify the most likely problem.
   A. Combination of antibodies
   B. Cold alloantibody
   C. Rouleaux
   D. Test error

Blood bank/Evaluate laboratory data to make identifications/Incompatible crossmatch/3

21. What corrective action should be taken when rouleaux causes positive test results?
   A. Perform a saline replacement procedure
   B. Perform an autoadsorption
   C. Run a panel
   D. Perform an elution

Blood bank/Apply principles of special procedures/Testing problem/3

22. All of the following are reasons for performing an adsorption, *except*:
   A. Separation of mixtures of antibodies
   B. Removal of interfering antibodies
   C. Confirmation of weak antigens on red cells
   D. Identification of antibodies causing a positive DAT

Blood bank/Apply principles of special procedures/Antibody identifications/2

23. How long must a recipient sample be kept in the blood bank following compatibility testing?
   A. 3 days
   B. 5 days
   C. 7 days
   D. 10 days

Blood bank/Apply principles of basic laboratory procedures/Compatibility/1

24. What is the crossmatching protocol for platelets and/or plasma?
   A. Perform a reverse grouping on donor plasma
   B. No testing required
   C. Perform a reverse grouping on recipient plasma
   D. Platelets must be HLA-compatible

Blood bank/Apply principles of basic laboratory procedures/Compatibility/2

25. What are the pretransfusion requirements for an autologous transfusion?
   A. ABO and Rh typing
   B. Type and screen
   C. Major crossmatch
   D. All of the above

Blood bank/Apply principles of basic laboratory procedures/Compatibility/1

26. A patient types as AB positive. Two units of blood have been ordered by the physician. Currently, the inventory shows 0 AB units, 10 A positive units, 1 A negative unit, 5 B positive units, and 20 O positive units. Which should be set up for the major crossmatch?
   A. A positive units
   B. O positive units
   C. B positive units
   D. Call blood supplier for type-specific blood

Blood bank/Apply principles of basic laboratory procedures/Compatibility/2

Answers to Questions 20–26

20. **B** The reaction pattern fits that of a cold antibody reacting at IS phase and of sufficient titer to persist at 37°C incubation. The reactions disappear in the IAT phase.

21. **A** Rouleaux may be dispersed or lessened by using the saline replacement technique. This involves recentrifuging the tube, withdrawing serum, and replacing it with 2 drops of saline. The tube is respun and examined for agglutination. If there is no agglutination, then the initial reaction was due to excess protein in serum and not to the presence of a specific alloantibody directed against an antigen on the red cells.

22. **D** Antibodies causing a positive DAT would be coating red cells and would require an elution, not an adsorption, to identify them.

23. **C** According to American Association of Blood Banks Standards, the recipient sample must be kept for 7 days following compatibility testing.

24. **B** For transfusion of platelets or fresh frozen plasma (FFP), there is no required protocol for crossmatching. However, ABO-compatible FFP units should be used.

25. **A** Pretransfusion testing for autologous transfusion includes ABO group and Rh type.

26. **A** The type chosen should be A positive red cell units. Although all choices would be compatible, the first choice should be A positive because this unit will contain residual plasma anti-B. Anti-B is less immunogenic than anti-A, which would be present, although in small amounts, in B positive and O positive units.

27. Which of the following constitutes an abbreviated crossmatch?
  A. ABO, Rh, and antibody screen
  B. ABO, Rh, antibody screen, IS crossmatch
  C. Type and screen
  D. ABO, Rh, IS crossmatch

Blood bank/Apply principles of basic laboratory procedures/Crossmatch/2

28. When may an IS crossmatch be performed?
  A. When a patient is being massively transfused
  B. When there is no history of antibodies and the current antibody screen is negative
  C. When a single unit of red cells is ordered

  D. When a patient has not been transfused in the past 3 months

Blood bank/Apply principles of basic laboratory procedures/Crossmatch/1

Answers to Questions 27–28

27. **B** The abbreviated crossmatch usually consists of a type and screen and an immediate spin crossmatch.

28. **B** The IS crossmatch may be performed when the patient has no history of antibodies and the current antibody screen is negative.

1. A patient had a transfusion reaction. The technologist began the laboratory investigation of the transfusion reaction by assembling pre- and post-transfusion specimens and all paperwork and computer printouts. He checked the patient's records and talked to the nurse in charge of the patient. What should he do first?
   A. Perform a DAT on the posttransfusion sample
   B. Check for a clerical error
   C. Repeat ABO and Rh typing of patient and donor unit
   D. Perform antibody screen on the post-transfusion sample

Blood bank/Apply knowledge of standard operating procedures/Transfusion reaction/2

2. What is the pathophysiological cause surrounding anaphylactic and anaphylactoid reactions?
   A. Antibody in patient serum reacting with donor red blood cells is detected 3 to 7 days after transfusion
   B. Donor plasma has reagins (IgE or IgA) that combine with allergens in patient plasma
   C. A patient deficient in IgE develops IgE antibodies via sensitization from transfusion or pregnancy
   D. A patient deficient in IgA develops IgA antibodies via sensitization from transfusion or pregnancy

Blood bank/Apply knowledge of fundamental biological principles/Transfusion reaction/1

3. A patient has a hemolytic reaction to blood transfused 8 days ago. What is the most likely cause?
   A. Immediate, nonimmunological; probably caused by volume overload
   B. Delayed immunological; probably due to an antibody such as anti-Jk^a
   C. Delayed nonimmunological; probably a result of iron overload
   D. Immediate, immunological; probably due to clerical error, ABO incompatibility

Blood bank/Apply knowledge of fundamental biological characteristics/Transfusion reaction/2

4. What may be found in the serum of a person who is exhibiting signs of TRALI (transfusion-related acute lung injury)?
   A. Red blood cell alloantibody
   B. IgA antibody
   C. Antileukocyte antibody
   D. Allergen

Blood bank/Apply knowledge of fundamental biological characteristics/Transfusion reaction/1

Answers to Questions 1–4

1. **B** Over 90% of transfusion reactions are the result of some type of clerical error. The most time-saving approach would be to check all paperwork before any laboratory testing is performed.

2. **D** Anaphylactic or anaphylactoid reactions are the most severe forms of allergic transfusion reaction and are associated with a deficient or absent IgA in the patient, allowing them the capability to form anti-IgA. These patients must be transfused with washed cellular products.

3. **B** A transfusion reaction that occurs several days after a transfusion of blood products is probably a delayed immunological reaction due to an antibody formed against donor antigens. This is a classic example of a reaction caused by an antibody such as anti-Jk^a.

4. **C** TRALI is associated with antibodies to human leukocyte antigens or neutrophil antigens that react with patient granulocytes causing acute respiratory insufficiency.

5. This type of transfusion reaction occurs in about 1% of all transfusions and results in a 1°C temperature rise or higher. It is associated with blood component transfusion and not related to patient medical condition.
   A. Immediate hemolytic
   B. Delayed hemolytic
   C. Febrile nonhemolytic reaction
   D. Transfusion-related acute lung injury

   Blood bank/Apply knowledge of fundamental biological characteristics/Transfusion reaction/1

6. What would be the result of group A blood given to a group O patient?
   A. Nonimmune transfusion reaction
   B. Immediate hemolytic transfusion reaction
   C. Delayed hemolytic transfusion reaction
   D. Febrile nonhemolytic transfusion reaction

   Blood bank/Apply knowledge of fundamental biological characteristics/Transfusion reaction/2

7. Patient XG received two units of group A positive red cells 2 days ago. Two days later he developed a fever and appeared jaundiced. His blood type was A positive. A transfusion reaction workup was ordered. There were no clerical errors detected. A post-transfusion specimen was collected and a DAT performed. A DAT was positive with monospecific anti-IgG. The plasma was also hemolyzed. An antibody screen and panel studies revealed the presence of anti-Jk^b (post-specimen). The antibody screen on the pretransfusion specimen was negative. Which of the following explains the positive DAT?
   A. The donor cells had a positive DAT
   B. The donor cells were polyagglutinable
   C. The donor cells were likely positive for the Jk^b antigen

   D. The recipient cells were likely positive for the Jk^b antigen

   Blood bank/Apply knowledge of fundamental biological characteristics/Transfusion reaction/3

8. All of the following are part of the preliminary evaluation of a transfusion reaction, *except*:
   A. Check pre- and post-transfusion samples for color of serum
   B. Perform ABO and Rh recheck
   C. DAT on the post-transfusion sample
   D. Panel on pre- and post-transfusion sample

   Blood bank/Apply knowledge of standard operating procedures/Transfusion reaction/1

Answers to Questions 5–8

5. **C** A febrile nonhemolytic transfusion reaction (FNHTR) is defined as a rise in temperature of more than 1°C. The patient has formed antibodies to HLA that react with donor cells.

6. **B** Group A blood given to a group O patient would cause an immediate hemolytic transfusion reaction because a group O patient has anti-A (and anti-B) antibodies and would destroy A cells.

7. **C** This is an example of an anamnestic reaction in which the patient was most likely exposed to the Jk^b antigen at some point in his life, and upon his re-exposure to antigen the antibody titer rose to detectable levels, resulting in a positive DAT and post-transfusion antibody screen.

8. **D** The preliminary evaluation of a transfusion reaction includes checking the color of serum or plasma, performing ABO and Rh checks, and a DAT on the post-transfusion sample. A panel would not be part of the preliminary workup.

4.7

COMPONENTS

1. A male cancer patient with a hemoglobin of 6 g/dL was admitted to the hospital with acute abdominal pain. Small bowel resection was indicated, but the attending physician wanted to raise the patient's hemoglobin to 12 g/dL before surgery. How many units of RBCs would most likely be required to accomplish this?
   A. Two
   B. Three
   C. Six
   D. Eight

   Blood bank/Apply knowledge of fundamental biological characteristics/Blood components/RBCs/2

2. A shipment of packed RBCs, platelets, and leukocyte-reduced RBCs arrived in the same container, at 1°–6°C. What should be done?
   A. Place all units in the 1°–6°C blood bank refrigerator
   B. Reject the shipment
   C. Prepare the RBC units for freezing
   D. Accept red cell products; return or discard the platelets

   Blood bank/Select course of action/Blood components/RBCs/3

3. Four units of packed RBCs were brought to the nurses' station at 10:20 a.m. Two units were transfused immediately, and one unit was transfused at 10:40 a.m. The remaining unit was returned to the blood bank at 11:00 a.m. The units were not refrigerated after leaving the blood bank. What problem(s) is (are) present in this situation?
   A. The only problem is with the returned unit; the 30-min limit has expired and the unit cannot be used
   B. The unit should not have been transfused at 10:40 a.m because the time limit had expired; this unit and the remaining unit should have been returned to the blood bank
   C. The returned unit may be held for this patient for 48 hours but cannot be used for another patient

   D. No problems; all actions were performed within the allowable time limits

   Blood bank/Select course of action/Blood components/ RBCs/3

4. A unit of whole blood is collected at 10:00 am and stored at 20°–24°C. What is the last hour platelet concentrates may be made from this unit?
   A. 4:00 p.m.
   B. 6:00 p.m.
   C. 7:00 p.m.
   D. 8:00 p.m.

   Blood bank/Apply knowledge of standard operating procedures/Blood components/3

Answers to Questions 1–4

1. **C** One unit of RBCs will raise the Hgb level by approximately 1 to 1.5 g/dL, and the Hct by 3%–4%. Results vary depending upon the age of the blood and the blood volume and hydration status of the patient. Six units will raise the hemoglobin to at least 12 g/dL.

2. **D** The transport and storage temperature for RBC products is 1°–6°C. Platelets should be shipped at 20°–24°C in an insulated container to protect them from extreme heat or cold.

3. **A** There is a 30-minute time limit for a unit of RBCs that is not kept under proper storage conditions (1°–6°C).

4. **B** Platelets prepared from whole blood must be processed within 8 hours of collection.

5. Which of the following is acceptable according to the AABB Standards?

A. Rejuvenated RBCs may be made within 3 days of outdate and transfused or frozen within 24 hours of rejuvenation

B. Frozen RBCs must be prepared within 30 min of collection and may be used within 10 years

C. Irradiated RBCs must be treated within 8 hours of collection and transfused within 6 hours

D. Leukocyte-reduced RBCs must be prepared within 6 hours of collection and transfused within 6 hours of preparation

Blood bank/Apply knowledge of laboratory operations/Blood components/RBCs/2

6. Which of the following is true regarding apheresis platelets?

A. The minimum platelet count must be 3.0×10^{11}, pH must be ≥ 6.0

B. The minimum platelet count must be 3.0×10^{10}, pH must be ≤ 6.2

C. The minimum platelet count must be 3.0×10^{11}, pH must be ≥ 6.2

D. The minimum platelet count must be 5.5×10^{10}, pH must be ≤ 6.0

Blood bank/Apply knowledge of laboratory operations/ Blood components/Platelets/1

7. What is the component of choice for a patient with chronic granulomatous disease (CGD)?

A. FFP

B. Granulocytes

C. Cryoprecipitate

D. RBCs

Blood bank/Apply knowledge of laboratory operations/ Blood components/3

8. All of the following statements are true, *except*:

A. Centrifugation is an acceptable method for preparing leukocyte-reduced RBCs

B. Graft-versus-host disease may be prevented by visual inspection of units before transfusion

C. Circulatory overload may be prevented by the administration of packed RBCs

D. Leukodepletion filters may prevent febrile transfusion reactions

Blood bank/Apply principles of special procedures/Blood components/Preparation of Components/1

9. All of the following statements regarding fresh frozen plasma (FFP) are true, *except*:

A. FFP must be prepared within 24 hours of collection

B. After thawing, FFP must be transfused within 24 hours

C. Storage temperature for FFP with a 1-year shelf life is $\leq 18°C$

D. When thawed, FFP must be stored between $1°-6°C$

Blood bank/Apply knowledge of standard operating procedures/Blood components/RBCs/1

10. What may be done to RBCs before transfusion to a patient with cold agglutinin disease in order to reduce the possibility of a transfusion reaction?

A. Irradiate to prevent graft-versus-host-disease

B. Wash with 0.9% saline

C. Warm to 37°C with a blood warmer

D. Transport so that temperature is maintained at $20°-24°C$

Blood bank/Apply knowledge of standard operating procedures/Hemotherapy/RBCs/2

Answers to Questions 5–10

5. **A** Rejuvenated RBCs may be prepared within 3 days of the outdate of the unit and washed and transfused or frozen within 24 hours. A unit of RBCs may be frozen within 6 days of collection. An RBC unit can be irradiated anytime prior to the expiration date; once irradiated the unit must be transfused within 28 days or the original outdate, whichever comes first. Leukocyte-reduced RBCs should be prepared within 6 hours of collection but must be given within 24 hours if prepared using an open system. Leukocyte-reduced RBCs prepared using a closed system may be kept until the original outdate.

6. **C** Single donor platelets prepared by apheresis must contain a minimum of 3.0×10^{11} platelets, and the pH must be 6.2 or greater throughout the shelf-life of the product.

7. **B** Patients with CGD cannot fight bacterial infections because of dysfunctional phagocytic enzymes; granulocyte concentrates are the product of choice for these patients.

8. **B** Although visual inspection is important in evaluating possible bacterial contamination of units, graft-versus-host disease is prevented by irradiation. Irradiation prevents blast transformation of lymphocytes.

9. **A** FFP must be prepared within 8 hours after collection if the anticoagulant is citrate phosphate dextrose (CPD), citrate phosphate double dextrose (CP2D), or citrate phosphate dextrose adenine (CPDA-1), or within 6 hours if the anticoagulant is acid citrate dextrose.

10. **C** A patient having cold agglutinins might have a reaction to a cold blood product. The product should be warmed to 37°C before transfusion.

11. A unit of packed RBCs is split using the open system. One of the half units is used. What may be done with the second half unit?
    A. Must be issued within 24 hours
    B. Must be issued within 48 hours
    C. Must be discarded
    D. Retains the original expiration date

    Blood bank/Apply knowledge of laboratory operations/Blood components/RBCs/2

12. What should be done if a noticeable clot is found in an RBC unit?
    A. Issue the unit; the blood will be filtered
    B. Issue the unit; note the presence of a clot on the release form
    C. Filter the unit in the blood bank before issue
    D. Do not issue the unit

    Blood bank/Select course of action/Hemotherapy/RBCs/2

13. Cryoprecipitate may be used to treat all of the following, *except*:
    A. von Willebrand's disease
    B. Hypofibrinogenemia
    C. Idiopathic thrombocytopenic purpura (ITP)
    D. Factor XIII deficiency

    Blood bank/Select best course of action/Hemotherapy/Cryo/3

14. A transplant patient may receive only type A or AB platelets. There are only type O apheresis platelets available. What device (s) may be used to deplete the incompatible plasma and replace with sterile saline?
    A. Cytospin/irradiator
    B. Water bath/centrifuge
    C. Centrifuge/sterile connecting device
    D. Cell washer/densitometer

    Blood bank/Apply knowledge of standard operating procedures/Blood components/Platelets/2

15. What component(s) is/are indicated for patients who have anti-IgA antibodies?
    A. Whole blood
    B. Packed RBCs
    C. Washed or deglycerolized RBCs
    D. Granulocyte concentrates

    Blood bank/Select course of action/Hemotherapy/RBCs/2

16. FFP can be transfused without regard for:
    A. ABO type
    B. Rh type
    C. Antibody in product
    D. All of the above

    Blood bank/Apply knowledge of standard operating procedures/Blood components/FFP/1

17. What component may not be prepared if whole blood is spun at 1°–6°C?

    A. Packed red cells
    B. Platelets
    C. Leukocyte-reduced red blood cells
    D. FFP

    Blood bank/Apply knowledge of standard operating procedures/Blood components/Processing/1

18. How should units of platelet concentrate be stored?
    A. At room temperature, 20°–24°C, lying horizontally
    B. No other components may be stored with platelets
    C. Platelet units must be stored upright in separate holders
    D. Platelet units require constant agitation at 20°–24°C

    Blood bank/Apply knowledge of standard operating procedures/Blood components/Processing/1

Answers to Questions 11–18

11. **A** The other half unit must be issued within 24 hours if an open system is used to split the unit.

12. **D** A unit having a noticeable clot should not be issued for transfusion to a patient. The clot may be an indication of contamination or bacterial growth.

13. **C** Cryoprecipitate may be used to treat von Willebrand's disease, hypofibrinogenemia, and factor XIII deficiency but is not indicated in ITP. winRho or IVIG is the product of choice for ITP.

14. **C** In the event of an ABO-mismatched stem cell transplant special attention must be paid to the choice of transfused blood products. Type A or AB platelets may be given to a transplant patient who is group O but is given stem cells from a group A donor. Once the stem cells engraft, platelets/plasma must be compatible with the type A cells. If only type O apheresis platelets are available, the product can be spun down using a centrifuge and the plasma can be removed; then a sterile connecting device can be used to aseptically transfer sterile isotonic saline to the platelet product replacing the incompatible plasma.

15. **C** Patients with anti-IgA antibodies should not receive components containing plasma. Plasma contains IgA, and an anaphylactic reaction may ensue. Washed or deglycerolyzed red cells can be issued.

16. **B** FFP can be transfused without regard for Rh type, as FFP is not a cellular product.

17. **B** Whole blood must be spun at 20°–24°C in order to prepare platelets.

18. **D** Platelets require constant agitation to allow proper gas exchange and are stored at 20°–24°C.

19. Transfusion of an irradiated product is indicated in all of the following conditions, *except*:
   A. Exchange transfusion
   B. Bone marrow transplant
   C. Severe combined immunodeficiency syndrome (SCIDS)
   D. Warm autoimmune hemolytic anemia

Blood bank/Select course of action/Hemotherapy/Irradiation/2

20. What percentage of red cells must be retained in leukocyte-reduced red cells?
   A. 85%
   B. 80%
   C. 100%
   D. 75%

Blood bank/Apply knowledge of standard operating procedures/Blood components/1

21. Which of the following is true regarding granulocyte concentrates?
   A. Product must contain a maximum of 1.0×10^{10} granulocytes
   B. The pH must be ≥ 6.0
   C. Product must be crossmatched
   D. Product must be irradiated

Blood bank/Apply knowledge of standard operating procedures/blood components/2

22. What course of action should be taken if a medical technologist inadvertently irradiates a unit of red cells twice?
   A. Issue the unit
   B. Discard the unit
   C. Change the expiration date, then issue the unit
   D. Note on the irradiation sticker that the unit was irradiated twice and issue

Blood bank/Apply knowledge of standard operating procedures/Irradiation/2

23. What component(s) may be shipped together with FFP?
   A. Frozen RBCs and cryoprecipitate
   B. Platelets
   C. Packed RBCs and granulocytes
   D. Double red cell

Blood bank/Apply knowledge of standard operating procedures/Blood components/FFP/1

24. What procedure should be followed in order to prevent contamination of FFP during thawing?
   A. Place the unit directly into a clean water bath
   B. Seal the unit in an outer, separate bag prior to placing in the water bath
   C. Thaw at 1°–6°C
   D. When half-thawed, transfer the FFP to another bag

Blood bank/Apply knowledge of standard operating procedures/Blood components/FFP/1

25. What laboratory testing is required for allogeneic stem cell donors?
   A. ABO, Rh, and antibody screen
   B. ABO, Rh, HLA, infectious disease markers
   C. HLA and infectious disease markers
   D. Only HIV testing

Blood bank/Apply knowledge of standard operating procedures/Blood components/Stem cells/1

26. Which component has the longest expiration date?
   A. Cryoprecipitate
   B. FFP
   C. Frozen RBCs
   D. Platelet concentrate

Blood bank/Apply knowledge of standard operating procedures/Blood components/Expiration date/1

Answers to Questions 19–26

19. **D** WAIHA would not require irradiation unless the patient had an underlying immunosuppressive disorder.

20. **A** A red cell unit that has been leukocyte-reduced must retain 85% of the original red cell mass.

21. **C** Granulocyte concentrates contain a large amount of red cells and must be crossmatched with the recipient's serum before the product can be transfused.

22. **B** If a technologist mistakenly irradiated a unit of red cells more than once, that unit must be discarded because of subsequent potassium accumulation. This does not apply to platelets.

23. **A** FFP requires dry ice for shipment. Frozen RBCs and cryoprecipitate also require dry ice and can be shipped with FFP. Platelets are transported at 20° to 24°C as well as granulocytes, and red cells are shipped at 1 to 10°C.

24. **B** To prevent contamination of FFP during thawing in a water bath, seal the bag of FFP in a separate bag prior to placing it in the water bath.

25. **B** Required testing for an allogeneic stem cell donor includes ABO, Rh, HLA testing, and viral disease markers.

26. **C** Frozen RBCs may be kept for up to 10 years. FFP and cryoprecipitate stored at -18°C or lower expire in 1 year. If FFP is kept at -65°C or lower, the expiration time is 7 years. Platelet concentrates expire in 5 days; however, single donor apheresis platelets expire in 7 days if both aerobic and anaerobic cultures are performed and the laboratory participates in the outcome assessment study on platelets called passport.

27. All of the following are advantages of using single donor rather than random donor platelets, *except*:
A. Less preparation time
B. Less antigen exposure for patients
C. May be HLA-matched
D. No pooling is required

Blood bank/Apply principles of special procedures/Blood components/Platelets/1

28. What is the expiration time of cryoprecipitate once pooled using an open system?
A. 4 hours
B. 6 hours
C. 8 hours
D. 24 hours

Blood bank/Apply knowledge of standard operating procedures/Blood components/Expiration date/1

29. What is the number of white blood cells permitted in a leukoreduced red cell unit?
A. $<5.0 \times 10^{10}$
B. $<5.0 \times 10^{6}$
C. $<8.3 \times 10^{5}$
D. $<8.3 \times 10^{6}$

Blood bank/Apply knowledge of standard operating procedures/Blood components/1

30. **SITUATION:** A cancer patient recently developed a severe infection. The patient's Hgb is 8 g/dL owing to chemotherapy with a drug known to cause bone marrow depression and immunodeficiency. Which blood products are indicated for this patient?

A. Liquid plasma and cryoprecipitate
B. Crossmatched platelets and washed RBCs
C. Factor IX concentrate and FFP
D. Irradiated RBCs, platelets, and granulocytes

Blood bank/Correlate clinical and laboratory data/Blood and components/3

Answers to Questions 27–30

27. **A** Single donor platelets require more preparation time than random donor platelets because they are prepared by apheresis that may require 1–3 hours depending on the methodology used. Pooling random donor platelets in equivalent amounts (usually 5–6 units) may require only a few minutes.

28. **A** When individual cryo units are pooled in an open system, the expiration time is 4 hours; if cryo is pooled using a sterile connecting device, the expiration time is 6 hours.

29. **B** Red cells that have been leukoreduced must have fewer than 5×10^{6} white cells per unit.

30. **D** This cancer patient may be immunocompromised from the medication but needs to receive RBCs for anemia; therefore, irradiated RBCs are indicated. Platelets may be needed to control bleeding, and granulocytes may be indicated for short-term control of severe infection.

1. **Which of the following individuals is acceptable as a blood donor?**
   A. A 29-year-old man who received the hepatitis B vaccine last week
   B. A 21-year-old woman who has had her nose pierced last week
   C. A 30-year-old man who lived in Zambia for 3 years and returned last month
   D. A 54-year-old man who tested positive for hepatitis C (HCV) last year but has no active symptoms of the disease

   Blood bank/Apply knowledge of standard operating procedures/Donor requirements/2

2. **SITUATION:** A 17-year-old girl comes to the blood center to donate blood. She weighs 90 pounds and has a Hgb of 13 g/dL. She tells the interviewer that she helped to care for her older brother for a week last month, who is diagnosed with Crohn's disease. Is she an acceptable donor for the maximum amount of blood allowed?
   A. Yes
   B. No, she is too young
   C. No, her weight is too low
   D. No, her Hgb is too low

   Blood bank/Apply knowledge of standard operating procedures/Donor requirements/1

3. **Which immunization has the longest deferral period?**
   A. HBIG (Hepatitis B immune globulin)
   B. Rubella vaccine
   C. Influenza vaccine
   D. Yellow fever vaccine

   Blood bank/Apply knowledge of standard operating procedures/Donor requirements/1

4. **The following whole blood donors regularly give blood. Which donor may donate on September 10?**
   A. A 40-year-old woman who last donated on July 23
   B. A 28-year-old man who had plateletpheresis on August 24
   C. A 52-year-old man who made an autologous donation 2 days ago
   D. A 23-year-old woman who donated blood for her aunt on August 14

   Blood bank/Apply knowledge of standard operating procedures/Donor requirements/2

Answers to Questions 1–4

1. **A** If the donor is symptom-free, there is no deferral period for the hepatitis B vaccine. Persons who have had body piercing are given a 12-month deferral. Persons who lived in an area endemic for malaria or who received antimalarial drugs are deferred for 3 years. A positive test for the HCV is cause for permanent deferral.

2. **C** Her age and hemoglobin meet donor criteria (17 years or older, 12.5 g/dL or higher). Her weight does not disqualify her from donation, but she is not permitted to donate the maximum volume, 525 mL, including pilot tubes. She would be permitted to donate 10.5 mL per kg (4.77 mL per lb) or 429.5 mL of whole blood inclusive of pilot tubes. The bag should be set to collect 400 mL of blood.

3. **A** Deferral for HBIG injection is 12 months. Deferral for rubella vaccine is 4 weeks. The deferral period for the influenza vaccine and yellow fever vaccine is 2 weeks.

4. **B** A plateletpheresis donor must wait at least 48 hours between donations. The waiting period following an autologous donation is at least 3 days. An 8-week interval must pass between all other types of donations.

5. Which of the following precludes acceptance of a plateletpheresis donor?
  A. Platelet count of 75×10^9/L in a donor who is a frequent platelet donor
  B. Plasma loss of 800 mL from plasmapheresis 1 week ago
  C. Plateletpheresis performed 4 days ago
  D. Aspirin ingested 7 days ago

Blood bank/Apply knowledge of standard operating procedures/Donor requirements/1

6. Which of the following donors could be accepted for whole blood donation?
  A. A former drug addict who has been drug-free for the past 3 years
  B. A triathelete with a pulse of 45 beats per min
  C. A man who is in remission from lymphoma
  D. A woman treated for gonorrhea 8 months ago

Blood bank/Apply knowledge of standard operating procedures/Donor requirements/1

7. Which physical examination result is cause for rejecting a whole blood donor?
  A. Weight of 105 lb
  B. Pulse of 75 beats per min
  C. Temperature of 99.3 °F
  D. Diastolic pressure of 110 mm Hg

Blood bank/Apply knowledge of standard operating procedures/Donor requirements/1

8. Which situation is *not* a cause for indefinite deferral of a donor?
  A. History of contact with prostitutes
  B. Donation of a unit of blood that transmitted hepatitis B virus (HBV) to a recipient
  C. Receipt of human growth hormone 30 years ago
  D. Accidental needle stick 1 year ago; negative for infectious diseases

Blood bank/Apply knowledge of standard operating procedures/Donor requirements/1

9. The tubing on a donor blood collection set begins to leak halfway through a donation. What course of action should be taken?
  A. Repair the leak by placing tape over the tubing
  B. Continue the donation but be careful to use a sterile container to collect the leaking blood
  C. Discontinue the donation
  D. Remove the damaged set and begin collection of another unit from another venous site

Blood bank/Select course of action/Donor processing/ Unacceptable donor set/3

10. Orders are to collect 250 mL of whole blood from an autologous donor. How much anticoagulant would have to be removed from the collection bag in order to collect 250 mL of whole blood?

  A. 15 mL
  B. 20 mL
  C. 28 mL
  D. 33 mL

Blood bank/Apply knowledge of standard operating procedures/Donor collection/3

Answers to Questions 5–10

5. **A** To be eligible for plateletpheresis the platelet count should be $\geq 150 \times 10^9$ for a frequent platelet donor. Plasma loss exceeding 1000 mL would be cause for rejection, 800 mL would not. A donor may donate 24 times in a year but not as frequently as once every 2 days in a 7-day period. A donor cannot ingest aspirin within 36 hours of platelet donation.

6. **B** Athletes may have a pulse below 50 beats per min and may still be acceptable as blood donors. Drug addiction is cause for permanent deferral, as is a major illness like cancer. The deferral period following treatment for syphilis or gonorrhea is 12 months.

7. **D** Diastolic pressure must not be higher than 100 mm Hg. Donors weighing less than 110 pounds may donate 10.5 mL per kg body weight or about 15% of their blood volume. Oral temperature must not be higher than 99.5 °F. Blood pressure limits for donation are 180 mm Hg for systolic and 100 mm Hg for diastolic pressure. The limit for hemoglobin is 12.5 g/dL and for Hct is 38%.

8. **D** An accidental needle stick would not be a cause for indefinite deferral of a donor. The deferral period is 1 year.

9. **C** If the set is leaking, then the sterility of the system has been compromised. The collection set and blood collected must be discarded.

10. **C** When <300 mL are collected in the bag, sufficient anticoagulant must be removed to maintain the proper blood to anticoagulant ratio (10:1.4). To determine the amount of anticoagulant to remove, divide the amount collected (300 mL) by 450 mL, then multiply by 63 mL, which is the standard volume of anticoagulant in a 450-mL bag. This volume is subtracted from 63 mL to give the volume that must be removed. Alternatively, one can divide the amount collected by 100, then multiply by 14. This gives the amount of anticoagulant needed. The amount to remove is calculated by subtracting from 63. In this case $250/100 \times 14 = 35$ mL needed. $63 - 35 = 28$ mL to be removed.

11. A woman begins to breathe rapidly while donating blood. Choose the correct course of action.
   A. Continue the donation; rapid breathing is not a reason to discontinue a donation
   B. Withdraw the needle, raise her feet, and administer ammonia
   C. Discontinue the donation and provide a paper bag
   D. Tell her to sit upright and apply cold compresses to her forehead

Blood bank/.Select course of action/Donor processing/ Donor adverse reaction/3

12. A donor bag is half-filled during donation when the blood flow stops. Select the correct course of action:
   A. Closely observe the bag for at least 3 min; if blood flow does not resume, withdraw the needle
   B. Remove the needle immediately and discontinue the donation
   C. Check and reposition needle if necessary; if blood flow does not resume, withdraw the needle
   D. Withdraw the needle and perform a second venipuncture in the other arm

Blood bank/Select course of action/Collection/3

13. Who is the best candidate for a predeposit autologous donation?
   A. A 45-year-old man who is having elective surgery in 2 weeks; he has anti-k
   B. A 23-year-old female leukemia patient with a hemoglobin of 10 g/dL
   C. A 12-year-old boy who has hemophilia
   D. A 53-year-old woman who has a severe skin infection

Blood bank/Select course of action/Donor processing/Autologous donation/2

14. Can an autologous donor donate blood on Monday if he is having surgery on Friday?
   A. Yes, he can donate up to 72 hours before surgery
   B. No, he cannot donate within 7 days of surgery
   C. Yes, he can donate, but only half of a unit
   D. No, he cannot donate within 5 days of surgery

Blood bank/Apply knowledge of standard operating procedures/Autologous donation/2

15. Which of the following is an acceptable time in which a unit of whole blood is collected?
   A. 33 min
   B. 25 min
   C. 20 min
   D. 13 min

Blood bank/Apply knowledge of standard operating procedures/Collection/1

16. Which of the following is true regarding acute normo-volemic hemodilution?
   A. One or more units of blood are withdrawn from the patient and replaced with FFP
   B. Units removed may be stored in the operating room at room temperature for 8 hours
   C. Units removed may be stored in the operating room at room temperature for 24 hours
   D. Unused units can be added to the general donor blood inventory

Blood bank/Apply knowledge of standard operating procedures/Autologous donation/2

Answers to Questions 11–16

11. **C** This woman is hyperventilating; therefore, the donation should be discontinued. A paper bag should be provided for the donor to breathe into in order to increase the CO_2 in the donor's air.

12. **C** If blood flow has stopped, check needle first. If the blood flow does not resume after repositioning, then withdraw needle and discontinue the donation. Do not perform a second venipuncture on the donor.

13. **A** The 45-year-old man with anti-k is the best candidate for predeposit autologous donation because compatible blood will be hard to find if he needs blood after surgery. The other candidates may not be good choices for donation because the process may prove harmful to them.

14. **A** An autologous donor can donate up to 72 hours before expected surgery.

15. **D** A unit of whole blood should be collected within 15 minutes.

16. **B** In acute normovolemic hemodilution, one or more units of blood are removed from the donor and replaced with crystalloid or colloid just prior to surgery. Blood collected during anesthesia for this purpose may be stored at room temperature for up to 8 hours or at 1°–6°C for up to 24 hours. Bleeding during surgery results in less RBC loss after hemodilution, and the autologous red cells are infused after the bleeding stops. Such units are for autologous transfusion only.

17. All of the following apply to a double red cell unit apheresis collection, *except*:
   A. The Hct must be at least 38 mL/dL.
   B. The weight for a female is at least 130 lb
   C. The height for a male is at least 5 feet 3 inches
   D. The deferral period following collection is 16 weeks

Blood bank/Apply knowledge of standard operating procedures/Apheresis/1

18. Which of the following donors would be accepted for a Directed Donation?
   A. 37-year-old male currently taking etretinate (Tegison)
   B. A 17-year-old female with a hemoglobin of 12 g/dL
   C. A 24-year-old male who just received the hepatitis B vaccine prior to employment
   D. A 49-year-old male from the UK who is visiting the US for the first time

Blood bank/Select course of action/Donors/Directed donation/3

17. **A** The hematocrit for a donor giving a 2-unit red cell product should be at least 40% for both males and females.

18. **C** A directed donation must meet the same standards as any other nonautologous donation. The donor's Hgb must be 12.5 g/dL or higher (Hct 38% or higher). Etretinate is one of several drugs that is a cause for indefinite deferral because the drug may cause harm to the recipient. Others include finasteride (Propecia), isotretinoin (Accutane), dutasteride (Avodart), acitretin (Soriatane), bovine insulin made in the UK, and aspirin for platelet donors. There is no deferral for a donor who has recently been given the hepatitis B vaccine as long as he or she is asymptomatic.

1. **All of the following may be reasons for a positive DAT on cord cells of a newborn infant** *except*:
   A. High concentrations of Wharton's jelly on cord cells
   B. Immune anti-A from an O mother on the cells of an A baby
   C. Immune anti-D from an Rh-negative mother on the cells of an Rh-positive baby
   D. Immune anti-K from a K-negative mother on the cells of a K-negative baby

   Blood bank/Correlate clinical and laboratory data/Hemolytic disease of the newborn/DAT/2

2. **A fetal screen yielded negative results on a mother who is O-negative and infant who is O-positive. What course of action should be taken?**
   A. Perform a Kleihauer-Betke test
   B. Issue one vial of RhIg
   C. Perform a DAT on the infant
   D. Perform an antibody screen on the mother

   Blood bank/Select course of action/Hemolytic disease of the newborn/Rosette test/3

3. **What should be done when a woman who is 24 weeks pregnant has a positive antibody screen?**
   A. Perform an antibody identification panel; titer if necessary
   B. No need to do anything until 30 weeks of pregnancy
   C. Administer Rh immune globulin (RhIg) prophylactically
   D. Adsorb the antibody onto antigen-positive cells

   Blood bank/Apply knowledge of standard operating procedures/Hemolytic disease of the newborn/Antibody testing/2

4. **All of the following are interventions for fetal distress caused by maternal antibodies attacking fetal cells** *except*:
   A. Intrauterine transfusion
   B. Plasmapheresis on the mother
   C. Transfusion of antigen-positive cells to the mother
   D. Early induction of labor

   Blood bank/Apply knowledge of standard operating procedures/Hemolytic disease of the newborn/Clinical intervention/2

5. **Cord cells are washed six times and the DAT and negative control are still positive. What should be done next?**
   A. Obtain a heelstick sample
   B. Record the DAT as positive
   C. Obtain another cord sample
   D. Perform an elution on the cord cells

   Blood bank/Select course of action/Hemolytic disease of the newborn/DAT/3

Answers to Questions 1–5

1. **D** Immune anti-K from the mother would not coat the baby's red cells if they did not contain the K antigen; therefore, the DAT would be negative.

2. **B** If the fetal screen or rosette test is negative, indicating the fetal maternal blood is negligible in a possible RhIg candidate, standard practice is to issue one vial of RhIg.

3. **A** The identification of the antibody is very important at this stage of the pregnancy. If the antibody is determined to be clinically significant, then a titer may determine the strength of the antibody and the need for clinical intervention.

4. **C** Transfusion of antigen-positive cells to the mother who already has an antibody might cause a transfusion reaction and/or evoke an even stronger antibody response, possibly causing more harm to the fetus.

5. **A** If the cord cells contain excessive Wharton's jelly, then further washing or obtaining another cord sample will not solve the problem. A heelstick sample will not contain Wharton's jelly and should give a valid DAT result.

6. What may be done if HDN is caused by maternal anti-K?

A. Give Kell immune globulin

B. Monitor the mother's antibody level

C. Prevent formation of K-positive cells in the fetus

D. Not a problem; anti-K is not known to cause HDN

Blood bank/Apply principles of special procedures/
Hemolytic disease of the newborn/Antibody formation/2

7. Should an O-negative mother receive Rh immune globulin (RhIg) if a positive DAT on the newborn is caused by immune anti-A?

A. No, the mother is not a candidate for RhIg because of the positive DAT

B. Yes, but only if the baby's type is Rh-negative

C. Yes, but only if the baby's type is Rh-positive

D. No, the baby's problem is unrelated to Rh blood group antibodies

Blood bank/Correlate clinical and laboratory data/
Hemolytic disease of the newborn/RhIg/3

8. Should an A-negative woman who has just had a miscarriage receive RhIg?

A. Yes, but only if she does not already have anti-D from a previous pregnancy

B. No, the type of the baby is unknown

C. Yes, but only a minidose regardless of trimester

D. No, RhIg is given for term pregnancies only

Blood bank/Apply knowledge of standard operating
procedures/Hemotherapy/RhIg/2

9. A group O mother has given birth to an infant who appears, upon initial testing, to be group AB. What should be done next?

A. Nothing, report the result

B. Retype both using a different lot number of anti-A and anti-B antisera

C. Question the phlebotomist about the identity of the samples

D. Check all labels, repeat the tests, and obtain new samples if results are the same

Blood bank/Correlate clinical and laboratory data/
Hemolytic disease of the newborn/Genetics/3

10. Which of the following patients would be a candidate for RhIg?

A. B-positive mother; B-negative baby; first pregnancy; no anti-D in mother

B. O-negative mother; A-positive baby; second pregnancy; no anti-D in mother

C. A-negative mother; O-negative baby; fourth pregnancy; anti-D in mother

D. AB-negative mother; B-positive baby; second pregnancy; anti-D in mother

Blood bank/Correlate clinical and laboratory data/
Hemolytic disease of the newborn/RhIg/2

11. A Kleihauer-Betke acid elution test identifies 40 fetal red cells in 2000 maternal red cells. How many doses of RhIg are indicated?

A. 1

B. 2

C. 3

D. 4

Blood bank/Calculate/Hemolytic disease of the
newborn/RhIg/2

Answers to Questions 6–11

6. **B** Anti-D is the only antibody for which prevention of HDN is possible. If a pregnant woman develops anti-K, she will be monitored to determine if the antibody level and signs of fetal distress necessitate clinical intervention.

7. **C** RhIg is immune anti-D and is given to Rh-negative mothers who give birth to Rh-positive babies and who do not have anti-D already formed from previous pregnancies or transfusion.

8. **A** When the fetus is Rh-positive or the Rh status of the fetus is unknown, termination of the pregnancy from any cause presents a situation in which the patient should receive RhIg. A minidose is used if the pregnancy is terminated in the first trimester.

9. **D** A clerical, sampling, or testing error may have occurred because an O mother cannot have a group AB infant. Repeating the tests will determine whether a testing error has occurred. If not, new samples should be collected after making a positive identification of both the mother and infant.

10. **B** An O-negative mother who gives birth to an A-positive baby and has no anti-D formed from a previous pregnancy would be a candidate for RhIg. A mother who already has active anti-D or a mother who gives birth to an Rh-negative baby is not a candidate for RhIg. Anti-D formation via active immunization typically has a titer >4, compared with passive administration of anti-D, which has a titer <4.

11. **D** To calculate the number of vials of RhIg to infuse, divide 40 by 2000 and multiply by 5000, which is the estimated total blood volume of the mother. Divide this number by 30 to arrive at the number of doses. When the number to the right of the decimal point is less than 5, round down and add one dose of RhIg. Conversely, when the number to the right of the decimal point is 5 or greater, round up and add one dose of RhIg. In this example, the number of doses is 3.3. Rounding down and adding 1 vial gives an answer of 4 vials of RhIg.

12. Kernicterus is caused by the effects of:
A. Anemia
B. Unconjugated bilirubin
C. Antibody specificity
D. Antibody titer

Blood bank/Apply knowledge of biological principles/Hemolytic disease of the newborn/1

13. Anti-E is detected in the serum of a woman in the first trimester of pregnancy. The first titer for anti-E is 32. Two weeks later, the antibody titer is 64 and then 128 after another 2 weeks. Clinically, there are beginning signs of fetal distress. What may be done?
A. Induce labor for early delivery
B. Perform plasmapheresis to remove anti-E from the mother
C. Administer RhIg to the mother
D. Perform intrauterine transfusion using E-negative cells

Blood bank/Correlate clinical and laboratory data/Hemolytic disease of the newborn/2

14. What testing is done for exchange transfusion when the mother's serum contains an alloantibody?
A. Complete crossmatch and antibody screen
B. ABO, Rh, antibody screen, and crossmatch
C. ABO, Rh, antibody screen
D. ABO and Rh only

Blood bank/Apply knowledge of standard operating procedures/Hemolytic disease of the newborn/Hemotherapy/1

15. Which blood type may be transfused to an AB-positive baby who has HDN caused by anti-D?
A. AB-negative or O-negative
B. AB-positive or O-positive
C. AB-negative only
D. O-negative only

Blood bank/Select course of action/Hemolytic disease of the newborn/Hemotherapy/2

16. All of the following tests are routinely performed on a cord blood sample *except*:
A. Forward typing ABO
B. Antibody screen
C. Rh typing
D. DAT

Blood bank/Apply knowledge of laboratory operations/Hemolytic disease of the newborn/Cord blood/1

17. What test should be performed on blood that will be transfused to an acidotic or hypoxic infant?
A. Cytomegalovirus (CMV)
B. Hemoglobin S (Hgb S)
C. Epstein-Barr virus (EBV)
D. HLA

Blood bank/Apply knowledge of standard operating procedures/Hemolytic disease of the newborn/Exchange transfusion/2

Answers to Questions 12–17

12. B Kernicterus occurs because of high levels of unconjugated bilirubin. High levels of this pigment cross into the central nervous system causing brain damage to the infant.

13. B Plasmapheresis removes excess anti-E from the mother and provides a temporary solution to the problem until the fetus is mature enough to be delivered. The procedure may need to be performed several times, depending upon how quickly and how high the levels of anti-E are formed by the mother. Administration of RhIg (anti-D) would not contribute to solving this problem caused by anti-E. Intrauterine transfusion would not be performed before week 20 and would be considered only if there is evidence of severe hemolytic disease.

14. B ABO (forward) and Rh are required. An antibody screen using either the neonatal serum or maternal serum is required. A crossmatch is necessary as long as maternal antibody persists in the infant's blood.

15. A Either AB-negative or O-negative RBCs may be given to an AB-positive baby because both types are ABO-compatible and lack the D antigen.

16. B An antibody screen is not performed on a cord blood sample because a baby does not make antibodies until about 6 months of age. Any antibodies detected in a cord blood sample come from the mother.

17. B Hgb S testing should be performed on blood to be given in an exchange transfusion to an acidotic or hypoxic infant. If the blood is positive for Hgb S, the cells may sickle under conditions of low oxygen tension.

18. An O-negative mother gives birth to a B-positive infant. The mother has no history of antibodies or transfusion. This is her first child. The baby was mildly jaundiced and the DAT is weakly positive with polyspecific antisera. What is most likely causing the positive DAT?

A. Anti-D from the mother is coating infant cells

B. An alloantibody like anti-K is coating infant cells

C. A nonspecific protein is coating infant cells

D. Anti-A,B is coating infant cells

Blood bank/Correlate clinical and laboratory data/
Hemolytic disease of the newborn/DAT/3

Answer to Question 18

18. D Anti-A,B is an IgG antibody and can cross the placenta and attach to infant cells. Anti-D would not cause the problem in this case because this is the first pregnancy. If an alloantibody like anti-K were implicated her history would indicate past transfusion or a history of antibodies. A clinical finding of jaundice would not be consistent with a nonspecific protein coating infant cells.

1. Why is serological testing important for blood products?
   A. Some carriers of disease may be asymptomatic
   B. Diseases may have long incubation periods between initial infection and manifestation of disease symptoms
   C. To protect the health of the recipient
   D. All of the above

   Blood bank/Correlate clinical and laboratory data/ Processing/1

2. Currently nucleic acid amplification testing (NAT) is required to detect viral particles to what agents?
   A. HIV and HTLV-I
   B. HTLV-I/II
   C. HIV, HCV
   D. HIV, HBV, and WNV

   Blood bank/Apply knowledge of standard operating procedures/Processing/1

3. John comes into donate a unit of whole blood for the local blood supplier. The EIA screen is reactive for anti-HIV-1/2. The test is repeated in duplicate and is nonreactive. John is:
   A. Cleared for donation
   B. Deferred for 6 months
   C. Status is dependent on confirmatory test
   D. Deferred for 12 months

   Blood bank/Select course of action/Processing/3

4. What marker is the first to appear in hepatitis B infection?
   A. Anti-HBc (IgM)
   B. HbsAg
   C. Anti-HBs
   D. Anti-HBc (IgG)

   Blood bank/Apply knowledge of biological principles/ Processing/1

5. What HIV screening test(s) is(are) required for whole blood donors?
   A. Anti-HIV-1/2 by EIA and HIV-1 antigen
   B. Anti-HIV-1/2 by EIA and HIV-1 NAT testing
   C. Anti-HIV-1/2 by EIA
   D. Anti-HIV-1/2 by EIA, HIV-1 NAT, HIV-1/2 by Western blot

   Blood bank/Apply knowledge of standard operating procedures/Processing/1

Answers to Questions 1–5

1. **D** Serological testing is performed to protect the health of the recipient. Serological testing will identify most carriers of disease who are asymptomatic at the time of donation, and donors with infectious diseases that have a long incubation period, such as hepatitis B.

2. **C** According to AABB Standards NAT testing is required for viruses HIV-1, HCV.

3. **A** If the initial EIA screen for anti-HIV is reactive and the test is repeated in duplicate and found to be nonreactive, the blood components may be used.

4. **B** The first viral marker of hepatitis B to appear in the serum once exposed is the hepatitis B surface antigen, HbsAg, which appears in as few as 5 days.

5. **B** Current screening methods for HIV include detection of antibodies to HIV-1/2 and HIV-1 by NAT.

6. An EIA screening test for HTLV-I/II was performed on a whole blood donor. The results of the EIA were repeatedly reactive but the confirmatory test was negative. On the next donation the screening test was negative by two different EIA tests. The donor should be:
   A. Accepted
   B. Deferred
   C. Told that only plasma can be made from his donation
   D. Told to come back in 6 months

Blood bank/Select best course of action/Processing/3

7. A unit tests positive for syphilis using the rapid plasma reagin test (RPR). The microhemagglutination assay-*Treponema pallidum* (MHA-TP) on the same unit is negative. What is the disposition of the unit?
   A. The unit may be used to prepare components.
   B. The donor must be contacted and questioned further. If the RPR result is most likely a false-positive, then the unit may be used.
   C. The unit must be discarded.
   D. Cellular components may be prepared but must be irradiated before issue.

Blood bank/Apply knowledge of standard operating procedures/Processing/2

8. NAT testing involves what molecular technology?
   A. Western blot
   B. Southern blot
   C. Polymerase chain reaction
   D. Recombinant immunoblot assay

Blood bank/Apply knowledge of biological principles/Processing/1

9. All of the following are required tests on donor blood, *except*:
   A. HbsAg
   B. Anti-CMV
   C. Anti-HIV
   D. Anti-HTLV-I/II

Blood bank/Apply knowledge of standard operating procedures/Processing/1

10. Which of the following bands would constitute a positive Western blot test for HIV?
   A. p24, gp41, p17
   B. p55, gp120, p51
   C. Gp160, p31, p56
   D. p24, p30, p55

Blood bank/Apply knowledge of standard operating procedure/Processing/3

Answers to Questions 6–10

6. **A** If screening results are repeat reactive and the confirmatory test is negative for anti-HTLV and upon the next donation the EIA is negative by two different methods, the donor may be accepted.

7. **A** This is a case of false-positive results where the screening test (RPR) was reactive and the confirmatory test for treponemal antibodies was negative. The donor products are acceptable.

8. **C** NAT testing or nucleic acid amplification testing is most often based upon the polymerase chain reaction (PCR). The target sequence (DNA or RNA) is amplified using labeled primers that can be detected by fluorescent or enzymatic methods.

9. **B** Testing of donor blood for antibodies to CMV is not required. However, testing may be done on units intended for transfusion to low-birth-weight infants born to seronegative mothers or units used for intrauterine transfusion; units intended for immunocompromised patients who are seronegative; prospective transplant recipients who are seronegative; or transplant recipients who have received a seronegative organ. Leukoreduced and fresh frozen RBCs carry a reduced risk of transmitting CMV and are recommended for such patients when CMV testing has not been performed on donor units. The prevalence of anti-CMV in the population ranges from 40% to 90%.

10. **A** According to current FDA and CDC criteria, a sample is defined as anti-HIV positive if at least two of the following bands are present on a Western blot: p24, gp41, and/or GP120/160.

1. Is there a discrepancy between the following blood typing and secretor study results?

Blood typing results:

Anti-A	Anti-B	A$_1$ cell	B cell
4+	0	0	4+

Secretor Results: Anti-A + saliva + A$_1$ cells = 0
Anti-B + saliva + B cells = 4+
Anti-H + saliva + O cells = 0

A. No problem, the sample is from a group A secretor
B. Blood types as A and saliva types as B
C. Blood types as A, but secretor study is inconclusive
D. No problem, the sample is from a group A nonsecretor

Blood bank/Evaluate laboratory data to make identifications/Saliva neutralization/2

2. What is the best course of action given the following test result? (Assume the patient has not been recently transfused.)

Anti-A	Anti-B	A$_1$ cells	B cells
Mixed field	0	1+	4+

A. Nothing, typing is normal
B. Type patient cells with *Dolichos biflorus* and type serum with A$_2$ cells
C. Retype patient cells: type with anti-H and anti-A,B; use screen cells or A$_2$ cells on patient serum; run patient autocontrol
D. Wash patient cells four times with saline and repeat the forward type

Blood bank/Apply principles of special procedures/RBC/ABO discrepancy/3

3. The following results were obtained on a 41-year-old female:

Anti-A	Anti-B	A$_1$ cells	B cells
4+	0	1+	4+

Because of the discrepant reverse grouping, a panel was performed on patient serum, revealing the presence of anti-M. How can reverse grouping be resolved?

A. Repeat reverse grouping with a 10-min incubation at room temperature
B. Repeat reverse grouping using A$_1$ cells that are negative for M antigen

C. Repeat reverse grouping using A$_1$ cells that are positive for M antigen
D. No further work is necessary

Blood bank/Evaluate laboratory data to recognize problems/ABO discrepancy/3

Answers to Questions 1–3

1. **A** The blood typing result demonstrates A antigen on the red cells and anti-B in the serum. The secretor result reveals A substance in the saliva. The A substance neutralized the anti-A, preventing agglutination when A$_1$ cells were added. Each blood type (except a Bombay) contains some H antigen; therefore, the H substance in the saliva would be bound by the anti-H reagent. No agglutination would occur when the O cells are added.

2. **C** The mixed field reaction with anti-A suggests a subgroup of A, most likely A$_3$. The reverse grouping shows weak agglutination with A$_1$ cells, indicating Anti-A$_1$. A positive reaction with anti-A,B would help to differentiate an A subgroup from group O. If A$_2$ cells are not agglutinated by patient serum, the result would indicate the presence of anti-A$_1$. If the patient's serum agglutinates A$_2$ cells, then an alloantibody or autoantibody should be considered.

3. **B** There is an antibody in the patient serum directed toward the M antigen, and the M antigen happened to be on the A$_1$ cells used for reverse grouping. To resolve this discrepancy, find A$_1$ cells that are negative for the M antigen or enzyme-treat the A$_1$ reagent cells to destroy reactivity with anti-M.

4. When a patient's sample shows a discrepancy between forward and reverse grouping with missing or weak reactions, what can be done to enhance these reactions?

A. Nothing can be done to enhance weak ABO reactions

B. Incubate 15–30 min at room temperature or 4°C

C. Test with new reagents

D. Centrifuge the patient's serum to concentrate antibodies, and use a heavier suspension of the patient cells

Blood bank/Apply knowledge of fundamental biological characteristics/ABO discrepancy/2

5. The following results were obtained on a 51-year-old male with hepatitis C:

Anti-A	Anti-B	A₁ cells	B cells	Anti-D
4+	4+	0	0	3+

What should be done next?

A. The patient's sample must be retyped to confirm group AB positive

B. The Rh typing should be repeated

C. Run a saline control in forward grouping

D. Report patient as group AB, Rh-positive

Blood bank/Apply knowledge of routine laboratory procedures/ABO/2

6. An Rh phenotyping shows the following results:

Anti-D	Anti-C	Anti-E	Anti-c	Anti-e
4+	2+	0	0	3+

What is the most likely genotype?

A. R^1r'

B. R^0r

C. R^1R^1

D. R^1r

Blood bank/Apply knowledge of fundamental biological characteristics/Rh typing/3

7. An obstetric patient, 34 weeks pregnant, shows a positive antibody screen at the indirect antiglobulin phase of testing. She is group B, Rh-negative. This is her first pregnancy. She has no prior history of transfusion. What is the most likely explanation for the positive antibody screen?

A. She has developed an antibody to fetal red cells

B. She probably does not have antibodies because this is her first pregnancy, and she has not been transfused. Check for technical error

C. She received an antenatal dose of RhIg

D. Impossible to determine without further testing

Blood bank/Correlate clinical and laboratory data/HDN/3

8. A patient's serum contains a mixture of antibodies. One of the antibodies is identified as anti-D. Anti-Jkᵃ or anti-Fyᵃ and possibly another antibody are present. What technique(s) may be helpful to identify the other antibody(ies)?

A. Enzyme panel; select panel cell

B. Thiol reagents

C. Lowering the pH and increasing the incubation time

D. Using albumin as an enhancement medium in combination with selective adsorption

Blood bank/Apply principles of special procedures/Antibody ID/3

Answers to Questions 4–8

4. **B** Sometimes weak or missing reactions may be enhanced by incubation at room temperature or 4°C

5. **C** In the case of an AB positive person, a saline control must be run in forward grouping to obtain a negative reaction; this will ensure agglutination is specific in the other reactions.

6. **C** The most likely phenotype is R^1R^1. The possibilities are DCe/DCe or DCe/dCe, which translates to R^1R^1 or R^1r'. The former is more common.

7. **C** Because the patient has never been transfused or pregnant, she probably has not formed any atypical antibodies. Because she is Rh-negative, she would have received a dose of RhIg at 28 weeks (antenatal dose) if her prenatal antibody screen had been negative. Although technical error cannot be ruled out, it is far less likely than RhIg administration.

8. **A** An enzyme panel would help to distinguish between anti-Jkᵃ (reaction enhanced) and anti-Fyᵃ (destroyed). Anti-D, however, would also be enhanced and may mask reactions that may distinguish another antibody. A select panel of cells negative for D antigen may help to reveal an additional antibody or antibodies.

9. An anti-M reacts strongly through all phases of testing. Which of the following techniques would *not* contribute to removing this reactivity so that more clinically significant antibodies may be revealed?
  A. Acidifying the serum
  B. Prewarmed technique
  C. Adsorption with homozygous cells
  D. Testing with enzyme-treated red cells

Blood bank/Apply principles of special procedures/ Antibody ID/3

10. The reactivity of an unknown antibody could be anti-Jk^a, but the antibody identification panel does not fit this pattern conclusively. Which of the following would *not* be effective in determining if the specificity is anti-Jk^a?
  A. Testing with enzyme-treated cells
  B. Select panel of homozygous cells
  C. Testing with AET-treated cells
  D. Increased incubation time

Blood bank/Apply principles of special procedures/ Antibody ID/3

11. A cold-reacting antibody is found in the serum of a recently transfused patient and is suspected to be anti-I. The antibody identification panel shows reactions with all cells at room temperature, including the autocontrol. The reaction strength varies from 2+ to 4+. What procedure would help to distinguish this antibody from other cold-reacting antibodies?
  A. Autoadsorption technique
  B. Neutralization using saliva
  C. Autocontrol using ZZAP reagent-treated cells
  D. Reaction with cord cells

Blood bank/Apply principles of special procedures/ Antibody ID/3

12. An antibody identification panel reveals the presence of anti-Le^b and a possible second specificity. Saliva from which person would be best to neutralize this Le^b antibody?

	Lewis	ABO	Secretor
A.	Le	H	sese
B.	Le	hh	Se
C.	Le	H	Se
D.	lele	hh	sese

Blood bank/Apply principles of special procedures/ Antibody ID/3

9. **A** Lowering the pH will actually enhance reactivity of anti-M. Prewarming (anti-M is a cold-reacting antibody), cold adsorption with homozygous M cells, and testing the serum with enzyme-treated red cells (destroys M antigens) are all techniques to remove reactivity of anti-M.

10. **C** AET denatures Kell antigens and prevents the interference of Kell antibodies during testing for the presence of other antibodies. Because the detection of Kidd antibodies is subject to dosage effect, selection of cells homozygous for the Jk^a antigen (and longer incubation) would help to detect the presence of the corresponding antibody. Enzyme-treated red cells would also react more strongly in the presence of Kidd antibodies.

11. **D** Because RBCs contain variable amounts of I antigen, reactions with anti-I often vary in agglutination strength. However, because this patient was recently transfused, the variation in reaction strength may be the result of an antibody mixture. Although autoadsorption would remove the anti-I, this procedure does not confirm the antibody specificity and can result in removal of other antibodies as well. Cord cells express primarily i antigen with very little I antigen. Anti-I would react weakly or negatively with cord RBCs. ZZAP removes IgG antibodies from red cells. Because anti-I is usually IgM and always has an IgM component, the use of the ZZAP reagent would not be of value.

12. **C** Lewis antibodies are usually not clinically significant but may interfere with the testing for clinically significant antibodies. Lewis antibodies are most easily removed by neutralizing them with soluble Lewis substance. The Lewis antigens are secreted into saliva and plasma and are adsorbed onto the red cells. Le^b substance is made by adding an L-fucose to both the terminal and next to last sugar residue on the type 1 precursor chain. This requires the Le, H, and Se genes. Since some examples of anti-Le^b react only with group O or A$_2$ RBCs, neutralization is best achieved if the saliva comes from a person who is group O.

13. Which two blood group systems are similar in that the red-cell antigens are highly antigenic and may lead to the formation of clinically significant antibodies; the lack of normal antigens leads to damaged red cells and resultant anemic conditions; and there is usually no problem finding antigen-negative blood for patients with antibodies to the most common antigens of the systems?
   A. Rh and Kell
   B. P and I
   C. MNSs and Lewis
   D. Duffy and Kidd

Blood bank/Correlate clinical and laboratory data/Blood group antigens/2

14. A cord blood workup was ordered on baby boy Jones. The mother is O-negative. Results on the baby are as follows:

Anti-A	Anti-B	Anti-A, B	Anti-D	DAT (poly)
4+	0	4+	0	2+

The test for weak D was positive at AHG. Is the mother an RhIg candidate?
   A. No the baby is Rh-positive
   B. Yes, the baby's Rh type cannot be determined due to the positive DAT
   C. No, the baby is Rh-negative
   D. Yes, the mother is Rh-negative

Blood bank/Evaluate laboratory data/Rh type/3

15. Red cells from a recently transfused patient were DAT-positive when tested with anti-IgG. Screen cells and a panel performed on the patient's serum showed very weak reactions with inconclusive results. What procedure could help to identify the antibody?
   A. Elution followed by a panel on the eluate
   B. Adsorption followed by a panel on the adsorbed serum
   C. Enzyme panel
   D. Antigen typing the patient's red cells

Blood bank/Apply principles of special procedures/ Antibody identification/3

16. A patient types as O-positive. All three screen cells and red cells from two O-positive donor units show agglutination after incubation at 37°C and increase in reactivity at the IAT phase of testing. What action should be taken next?
   A. Perform an autocontrol and direct antiglobulin test on the patient
   B. Perform an enzyme panel

   C. Perform an elution
   D. Choose another two units and repeat the crossmatch

Blood bank/Select course of action/Incompatible crossmatch/3

Answers to Questions 13–16

13. **A** Rh and Kell systems are among the most antigenic of all blood group systems. Exposure to a small amount of antigen-positive cells in a negative recipient may invoke antibody production. K_{null} and Rh_{null} do not produce Kell and Rh red cell antigens, respectively, and the absence of these antigens leads to damaged cells. Damaged cells are removed by the spleen and anemic conditions may result from this action. K-negative and D-negative blood are easy to locate.

14. **B** The baby forward types as an A and the mother is O negative. It is possible that anti-A,B from the mother is attaching to baby's red cells causing a positive DAT. In the presence of a positive DAT, a weak test for D is not valid. Therefore, the baby's Rh type is unknown and the mother would be a candidate for RhIg.

15. **A** If the red cells show a positive DAT, then IgG or C3d antibody has coated incompatible, antigen-positive red cells. If screen cells and panel cells show missing or weak reactions, most of the antibody is on the red cells and would need to be eluted before it can be detected. An elution procedure followed by a panel performed on the eluate would help to identify the antibody.

16. **A** All screening cells and all units are positive at both 37°C and the IAT phase. This indicates the possibility of a high-frequency alloantibody or a warm autoantibody. An autocontrol would help to make this distinction. A positive autocontrol indicates an autoantibody is present; a negative autocontrol and positive screening cells indicates an alloantibody. A DAT would be performed to determine if an antibody has coated the patient's red cells and is directed against screening cells and donor cells.

17. Four units of blood are ordered for a patient. Blood bank records are checked and indicate that 5 years ago this patient had an anti-Jk^b. What is the next course of action?

A. Antigen type units for the Jk^b antigen and only crossmatch units positive for Jk^b

B. Antigen type units for the Jk^b antigen and only crossmatch units negative for Jk^b

C. Randomly pull four units of blood that are ABO-compatible and crossmatch

D. Perform an immediate spin crossmatch on 4 Jk^b-negative units

Blood bank/Apply principles of laboratory operations/Compatibility testing/3

18. A 56-year-old patient diagnosed with colon cancer demonstrates a positive antibody screen in all three screening cells at the antiglobulin phase. A panel study is done and shows 10 cells positive as well as the autocontrol at the antiglobulin phase. The reactions varied from 1+ to 3+. This patient had a history of receiving 2 units of blood approximately 1 month ago. What should be done next?

A. Perform a DAT on patient cells

B. Perform an autoabsorption

C. Perform an alloabsorption

D. Issue O-negative cells

Blood bank/Evaluate laboratory data to determine best course of action/Panel study/3

19. A cord cell typing appears to be AB-positive with a 2+ DAT. The baby was normal and the mother's type was O negative. Is there a problem here?

A. No problem, the positive DAT is due to an ABO incompatibility; the baby was not affected

B. No problem, the positive DAT is due to an antenatal dose of RhIg that coated the baby's cells in utero

C. A technical problem exists because the DAT should not have been positive; repeat the DAT with a negative autocontrol

D. A problem exists because an AB baby is not possible with an O mother; wash the cells and retype. Perform a negative control for the DAT

Blood bank/Evaluate laboratory data to determine possible inconsistent results/ABO/3

20. An O-negative mother with no record of any previous pregnancies gives birth to her first child, a B-positive baby. The DAT is weakly positive and the saline control is negative. The antibody screen is also negative. The baby appears healthy but develops mild jaundice after two days, which is treated with phototherapy. The baby goes home after 4 days in the hospital without complications. What is the most likely explanation for the weakly positive DAT?

A. A technical error

B. A low titer anti-D

C. Immune anti-B from the mother

D. A maternal antibody against a low-incidence antigen

Blood bank/Correlate clinical and laboratory data/HDN 2

21. Anti-K and anti-c were found in a patient with colon cancer. How many units of red cells would need to be screened to find two compatible units for surgery?

A. 5 units

B. 2 units

C. 7 units

D. 11 units

Blood bank/Immunohematology/Problem solving/Compatibility/3

Answers to Questions 17–21

17. **B** A patient with a history of a significant antibody like anti-Jk^b must receive blood that has been completely crossmatched and negative for the corresponding antigen; otherwise an anamnestic reaction may occur with subsequent lysis of donor cells.

18. **C** In this situation an allogeneic absorption must be performed to absorb out the autoantibody and leave potential alloantibodies in patient serum that will need to be identified before transfusion of blood to the patient. An autoabsorption cannot be performed because of the fact that any alloantibodies would be absorbed by circulating donor cells from a month prior.

19. **D** An O mother cannot give birth to an AB infant. The infant could not inherit an A or B gene from an O mother whose genotype must be O/O. The infant red cells may be agglutinating nonspecifically in the forward type and causing the positive DAT or maternal anti-A,B may be causing specific agglutination in the DAT. The best course of action is to wash the infant cells at least three times with saline and repeat the tests.

20. **C** In this case the maternal anti-A,B is probably coating the B cells of the infant causing a positive DAT and jaundice. Anti-A,B from an O person is a single entity that cannot be separated. The antibody is characterized as IgG and can cross the placenta. This antibody may attach to A, B, or AB red cells.

21. **D** To find two compatible units for this patient, the number of units desired for transfusion is divided by the product of the antigen negative frequency of K and c. The antigen negative frequency for K and c are 0.91 and 0.20, respectively. Therefore, 2 divided by 0.182 yields 11.

BIBLIOGRAPHY

1. American Association of Blood Banks Standards, ed 23. Bethesda, MD, 2004.
2. Brecher, M.E.: American Association of Blood Banks Technical Manual, ed 15. Bethesda, MD, 2005.
3. Harmening, D.: Modern Blood Banking and Transfusion Practices. FA Davis, Philadelphia, 2005.
4. Issitt, P.D.: Applied Blood Group Serology. Montgomery Scientific Publications, Miami, 1998.
5. Quinley, E.: Immunohematology: Principles and Practice. J.B. Lippincott, Philadelphia, 1998.
6. Rudmann, S.V.: Textbook of Blood Banking and Transfusion Medicine. W.B. Saunders, Philadelphia, 2005.
7. Turgeon, M.L.: Fundamentals of Immunohematology. Lea and Febiger, Philadelphia, 1995.

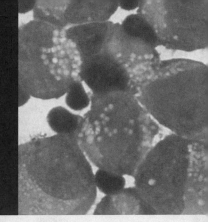

CHAPTER **5**

Clinical Chemistry

5.1   INSTRUMENTATION

5.2   BLOOD GASES, pH, AND ELECTROLYTES

5.3   GLUCOSE, HEMOGLOBIN, IRON, AND BILIRUBIN

5.4   CALCULATIONS, QUALITY CONTROL, AND STATISTICS

5.5   CREATININE, BUN, AMMONIA, AMINO ACIDS, AND URIC ACID

5.6   PROTEINS, ELECTROPHORESIS, AND LIPIDS

5.7   ENZYMES AND CARDIAC MARKERS

5.8   CLINICAL ENDOCRINOLOGY

5.9   TOXICOLOGY AND THERAPEUTIC DRUG MONITORING

5.10   TUMOR MARKERS

5.11   CLINICAL CHEMISTRY PROBLEM SOLVING

1. Which formula correctly describes the relationship between absorbance and %T?
   - **A.** $A = 2 - \log \%T$
   - **B.** $A = \log 1/T$
   - **C.** $A = -\log T$
   - **D.** All of the above

   Chemistry/Identify basic principle(s)/Instrumentation/2

2. A solution that has a transmittance of 1.0 %T would have an absorbance of:
   - **A.** 1.0
   - **B.** 2.0
   - **C.** 1%
   - **D.** 99%

   Chemistry/Calculate/Beer's law/2

3. In absorption spectrophotometry:
   - **A.** Absorbance is directly proportional to transmittance.
   - **B.** Percent transmittance is directly proportional to concentration.
   - **C.** Percent transmittance is directly proportional to the light path length.
   - **D.** Absorbance is directly proportional to concentration.

   Chemistry/Define fundamental characteristics/Beer's law/1

4. Which wavelength would be absorbed strongly by a red-colored solution?
   - **A.** 450 nm
   - **B.** 585 nm
   - **C.** 600 nm
   - **D.** 650 nm

   Chemistry/Define fundamental characteristics/ Spectrophotometry/2

Answers to Questions 1–4

1. **D** Absorbance is proportional to the inverse log of transmittance.

   $$A = -\log T = \log 1/T$$

   Multiplying the numerator and denominator by 100 gives:

   $$A = \log (100/100 \times T)$$

   $100 \times T = \%T$, substituting %T for $100 \times T$ gives:

   $$A = \log 100/\%T$$
   $$A = \log 100 - \log \%T$$
   $$A = 2 - \log \%T$$

   For example, if %$T = 10.0$, then

   $$A = 2 - \log 10.0$$
   $$\log 10.0 = 1.0$$
   $$A = 2 - 1 = 1.0$$

2. **B**

   $$A = 2 - \log \%T$$
   $$A = 2 - \log 1.0$$
   The log of $1.0 = 0$
   $$A = 2.0$$

3. **D** Beer's law states that $A = a \times b \times c$, where a is the absorbtivity coefficient (a constant), b is the path length, and c is concentration. Absorbance is directly proportional to both b and c. Doubling the path length results in incident light contacting twice the number of molecules in solution. This causes absorbance to double, the same effect as doubling the concentration of molecules.

4. **A** A solution transmits light corresponding in wavelength to its color and usually absorbs light of wavelengths complementary to its color. A red solution transmits light of 600–650 nm and strongly absorbs 400–500 nm light.

5. A green-colored solution would show highest transmittance at:
   A. 475 nm
   B. 525 nm
   C. 585 nm
   D. 620 nm

   Chemistry/Define fundamental characteristics/ Spectrophotometry/2

6. SITUATION: A technologist is performing an enzyme assay at 340 nm using a visible range spectrophotometer. After setting the wavelength and adjusting the readout to zero %T with the light path blocked, a cuvet with deionized water is inserted. With the light path fully open and the 100%T control at maximum, the instrument readout will not rise above 90%T. What is the most appropriate first course of action?
   A. Replace the source lamp
   B. Insert a wider cuvet into the light path
   C. Measure the voltage across the lamp terminals
   D. Replace the instrument fuse

   Chemistry/Select course of action/Spectrophotometry/3

7. Which type of monochromator produces the purest monochromatic light in the ultraviolet (UV) range?
   A. A diffraction grating and a fixed exit slit
   B. A sharp cutoff filter and a variable exit slit
   C. Interference filters and a variable exit slit
   D. A prism and a variable exit slit

   Chemistry/Select component/Spectrophotometry/2

8. Which monochromator specification is required in order to measure the true absorbance of a compound having a natural absorption bandwidth of 30 nm?
   A. A 50-nm bandpass
   B. A 25-nm bandpass
   C. A 15-nm bandpass
   D. A 5-nm bandpass

   Chemistry/Select component/Spectrophotometry/2

9. Which photodetector is most sensitive to low levels of light?
   A. Barrier layer cell
   B. Photodiode
   C. Diode array
   D. Photomultiplier tube

   Chemistry/Define fundamental characteristics/ Instrumentation/1

10. Which condition is a common cause of stray light?
   A. Unstable source lamp voltage
   B. Improper wavelength calibration
   C. Dispersion from second-order spectra
   D. Misaligned source lamp

   Chemistry/Identify source of error/Spectrophotometry/2

Answers to Questions 5–10

5. **B** Green light consists of wavelengths from 500–550 nm. A green-colored solution with a transmittance maximum of 525 nm and a 50-nm bandpass transmits light of 525 nm and absorbs light below 475 nm and above 575 nm. A solution that is green would be quantitated using a wavelength that it absorbs strongly, such as 450 nm.

6. **A** Visible spectrophotometers are usually supplied with a tungsten source lamp. Tungsten lamps produce a continuous range of wavelengths from about 320–1200 nm. Output increases as wavelength becomes longer and is poor below 400 nm. As the lamp envelope darkens with age, the amount of light reaching the photodetector at 340 nm becomes insufficient to set the blank reading to 100%T. Deuterium or hydrogen lamps produce UV-rich spectra optimal for UV work. Halogen, mercury vapor, and xenon give moderate visible and UV output.

7. **D** Diffraction gratings and prisms both produce a continuous range of wavelengths. A diffraction grating produces a uniform separation of wavelengths. A prism produces much better separation of high-frequency light because refraction is greater for higher energy wavelengths. Instruments using a prism and a variable exit slit can produce UV light of a very narrow bandpass. The adjustable slit is required in order to allow sufficient light to reach the detector to set 100%T.

8. **D** *Bandpass* refers to the range of wavelengths passing through the sample. The narrower the bandpass, the greater the photometric resolution. Bandpass can be made smaller by reducing the width of the exit slit. Accurate absorbance measurements require a bandpass less than one fifth the natural bandpass of the chromophore.

9. **D** The photomultiplier tube uses dynodes of increasing voltage to amplify the current produced by the photosensitive cathode. It is 10,000 times as sensitive as a barrier layer cell, which has no amplification. A photomultiplier tube requires a DC-regulated lamp because it responds to light fluctuations caused by the AC cycle.

10. **C** Stray light is caused by the presence of any light other than the wavelength of measurement reaching the detector. It is most often caused by second-order spectra, deteriorated optics, light dispersed by a darkened lamp envelope, or extraneous room light.

11. A linearity study is performed on a visible spectrophotometer at 650 nm and the following absorbance readings are obtained:

Concentration of Standard	Absorbance
10.0 mg/dL	0.20
20.0 mg/dL	0.41
30.0 mg/dL	0.62
40.0 mg/dL	0.79
50.0 mg/dL	0.92

The study was repeated using freshly prepared standards and reagents, but results were identical to those above. What is the most likely cause of these results?
A. Wrong wavelength used
B. Insufficient chromophore concentration
C. Matrix interference
D. Stray light

Chemistry/Evaluate source of error/Spectrophotometry/3

12. Which type of filter is best for measuring stray light?
A. Wratten
B. Didymium
C. Sharp cutoff
D. Neutral density

Chemistry/Evaluate source of error/Spectrophotometry/2

13. Which of the following materials is best suited for verifying the wavelength calibration of a spectrophotometer?
A. Neutral density filters
B. Potassium dichromate solutions traceable to the National Bureau of Standards reference
C. Wratten filters
D. Holmium oxide glass

Chemistry/Identify standard operating procedure/Spectrophotometry/2

14. Why do many optical systems in chemistry analyzers utilize a reference light path?
A. To increase the sensitivity of the measurement
B. To minimize error caused by source lamp fluctuation
C. To obviate the need for wavelength adjustment
D. To reduce stray light effects

Chemistry/Define fundamental characteristics/Spectrophotometry/2

Answers to Questions 11–14

11. **D** Stray light is the most common cause of loss of linearity at high-analyte concentrations. Transmitted incident light is lowest when absorption is highest. Therefore, stray light is a greater percentage of the detector response when sample concentration is high. Stray light is usually most significant when measurements are made at the extremes of the visible spectrum because lamp output and/or detector response are low.

12. **C** Sharp cutoff filters transmit almost all incident light until the cutoff wavelength is reached. At that point, they cease to transmit light. Because they give an "all or none effect," only stray light reaches the detector when the selected wavelength is beyond the cutoff.

13. **D** Wavelength accuracy is verified by determining the wavelength reading that gives the highest absorbance (or transmittance) when a substance with a narrow natural bandpass (sharp absorbance or transmittance peak) is scanned. For example, didymium glass has a sharp absorbance peak at 585 nm. Therefore, an instrument should give its highest absorbance reading when the wavelength dial is set at 585 nm. Holmium oxide produces a very narrow absorbance peak at 361 nm; likewise, the hydrogen lamp of a UV spectrophotometer produces a 656-nm emission line that can be used to verify wavelength. Neutral density filters and dichromate solutions are used to verify absorbance accuracy or linearity. A Wratten filter is a wide-bandpass filter made by placing a thin layer of colored gelatin between two glass plates and is unsuitable for spectrophotometric calibration.

14. **B** A reference beam is used to produce an electrical signal at the detector to which the measurement of light absorption by the sample is compared. This safeguards against measurement errors caused by power fluctuations that change the source lamp intensity. Although reference beams increase the accuracy of measurements, they do so at the expense of optical sensitivity because some of the incident light must be used to produce the reference beam.

15. Which component is required in a spectrophotometer in order to produce a spectral absorbance curve?
  A. Multiple monochromators
  B. A reference optical beam
  C. Photodiode array
  D. Laser light source

Chemistry/Define fundamental characteristics/Spectrophotometry/1

16. The half-band width of a monochromator is defined by:
  A. The range of wavelengths passed at 50% maximum transmittance
  B. One half the lowest wavelength of optical purity
  C. The wavelength of peak transmittance
  D. One half the wavelength of peak absorbance

Chemistry/Define fundamental characteristics/Spectrophotometry/1

17. The term *dark current* as used in spectrophotometry refers to:
  A. Drift in the 100%T reading of a spectrophotometer
  B. The %T reading when the reagent blank is measured
  C. The flow of current from a phototube caused by high gain on its anode
  D. Electron flow through the readout circuit induced by the magnetic field of the power supply transformer

Chemistry/Define fundamental characteristics/Spectrophotometry/1

18. The reagent blank corrects for absorbance caused by:
  A. The color of reagents
  B. Sample turbidity
  C. Bilirubin and hemolysis
  D. All of the above

Chemistry/Identify basic principle(s)/Reaction/2

19. Which instrument requires a highly regulated DC power supply?
  A. A spectrophotometer with a barrier layer cell
  B. A colorimeter with multilayer interference filters
  C. A spectrophotometer with a photomultiplier tube
  D. A densitometer with a photodiode detector

Chemistry/Select component/Spectrophotometry/2

Answers to Questions 15–19

15. **C** There are two ways to perform spectral scanning for compound identification. One is to use a stepping motor that continuously turns the monochromator so that the wavelength aligned with the exit slit changes at a constant rate. A more practical method is to use a diode array detector. This consists of a chip embedded with as many as several hundred photodiodes. Each photodiode is aligned with a narrow part of the spectrum produced by a diffraction grating and produces current proportional to the intensity of the band of light striking it (usually 1–5 nm in range). The diode signals are processed by a computer to create a spectral absorbance or transmittance curve.

16. **A** Half-band width is a measure of bandpass made using a solution or filter having a narrow natural bandpass (transmittance peak). The wavelength giving maximum transmittance is set to 100%T (or 0 A). Then, the wavelength dial is adjusted downward, until a readout of 50%T (0.301 A) is obtained. Next, the wavelength is adjusted upward until a readout of 50%T is obtained. The wavelength difference is the half-band width. The narrower the half-band width, the better the photometric resolution of the instrument.

17. **C** Dark current is the current generated by a detector when the light path is blocked to prevent incident light from striking it. Phototubes and photomultiplier tubes leak a small amount of current because electrons are drawn through the circuit by the high positive voltage applied to the anode or dynodes.

18. **A** When a spectrophotometer is set to 100%T with the reagent blank instead of water, the absorbance of reagents is automatically subtracted from each unknown reading. The reagent blank does not correct for absorbance caused by interfering chromogens in the sample such as bilirubin, hemolysis, or turbidity.

19. **C** When AC voltage regulators are used to isolate source lamp power, light output fluctuates as the voltage changes. Because this occurs at 60 Hz, it is not detected by the naked eye or slow-responding detectors. Photomultiplier tubes are sensitive enough to respond to the AC frequency and require a DC-regulated power supply.

20. Which statement regarding reflectometry is true?
   A. The relation between reflectance density and concentration is linear
   B. Single point calibration can be used to determine concentration
   C. 100% reflectance is set with an opaque film called a white reference
   D. The diode array is the photodetector of choice

Chemistry/Apply principles of special procedures/ Instrumentation/2

21. Bichromatic filter photometers can correct for interfering substances if:
   A. The contribution of the interferent to absorbance is the same at both wavelengths
   B. Both wavelengths pass through the sample simultaneously
   C. The side band is a harmonic of the primary wavelength
   D. The chromogen has the same absorbance at both wavelengths

Chemistry/Apply principles of special procedures/ Instrumentation/2

22. Which instrument requires a primary and secondary monochromator?
   A. Spectrophotometer
   B. Atomic absorption spectrophotometer
   C. Fluorometer
   D. Nephelometer

Chemistry/Apply principles of special procedures/ Instrumentation/1

23. Which of the following statements about fluorometry is accurate?
   A. Fluorometry is less sensitive than spectrophotometry
   B. Fluorometry is less specific than spectrophotometry
   C. Unsaturated cyclic molecules are often fluorescent
   D. Fluorescence is directly proportional to temperature

Chemistry/Apply principles of special procedures/ Instrumentation/2

24. Which of the following components is *not* needed in a chemiluminescent immunoassay analyzer?
   A. Source lamp
   B. Monochromator
   C. Photodetector
   D. Wash station

Chemistry/Define fundamental characteristics/ Instrumentation/1

Answers to Questions 20–24

20. **C** Reflectometry does not follow Beer's law, but the relationship between concentration and reflectance can be described by a logistic formula or algorithm that can be solved for concentration. For example, $K/S = (1 - R)^2/2R$, where K = Kubelka-Munk absorptivity constant, S = scattering coefficient, R = reflectance density. K/S is proportional to concentration. The white reference is analogous to the $100\%T$ setting in spectrophotometry and serves as a reference signal. $D_r = \log R_0/R_1$, where D_r is the reflectance density, R_0 is the white reference signal, and R_1 is the photodetector signal for the test sample.

21. **A** In bichromatic photometry, the absorbance of the sample is measured at two different wavelengths. The primary wavelength is at or near the absorbance maximum. An interfering substance having the same absorbance at both primary and secondary (side band) wavelengths does not affect the absorbance difference (Ad).

22. **C** A fluorometer uses a primary monochromator to isolate the wavelength for excitation and a secondary monochromator to isolate the wavelength emitted by the fluorochrome.

23. **C** Increasing temperature results in more random collision between molecules by increasing their motion. This causes energy to be dissipated as heat instead of fluorescence. Temperature is inversely proportional to fluorescence. Fluorescence is more sensitive than spectrophotometry because the detector signal can be amplified when dilute solutions are measured. It is also more specific than spectrophotometry because both the excitation and emission wavelengths are characteristics of the compound being measured.

24. **A** Chemiluminescence is the production of light following a chemical reaction. Immunoassays based upon chemiluminescence generate light when the chemiluminescent molecule becomes excited; therefore a light source is not used. In immunoassay platforms, chemiluminescent molecules such as acridinium can be used to label antigens or antibodies. Alternatively, chemiluminescent substrates such as luminol or dioxetane phosphate may be used. Light is emitted when an enzyme-labeled antibody reacts with the substrate. In such assays free and bound antigen separation is required and is usually accomplished using paramagnetic particles bound to either antibody or reagent antigen.

25. Which statement about fluorescence polarization immunoassay (FPIA) is true?
 A. Rotation of free antigen-conjugate is slower than that of antibody-bound conjugate
 B. Fluorescence by free antigen-conjugate is polarized
 C. Analyte concentration is related inversely to polarized fluorescence
 D. Source light does not have to be plane polarized

Chemistry/Apply principles of special procedures/ Instrumentation/2

26. Light scattering when wavelength is greater than ten times particle diameter is described by:
 A. Rayleigh's law
 B. The Beer-Lambert law
 C. Mie's law
 D. The Rayleigh-Debye law

Chemistry/Apply principles of special procedures/ Instrumentation/2

27. Which statement regarding nephelometry is true?
 A. Nephelometry is less sensitive than absorption spectrophotometry
 B. Nephelometry follows Beer's law
 C. The optical design is identical to a turbidimeter except that a helium neon (HeNe) laser light source is used
 D. The detector response is directly proportional to concentration

Chemistry/Apply principles of special procedures/ Instrumentation/2

28. The purpose of the nebulizer and atomizer in an atomic absorption spectrophotometer that uses a flame is to:
 A. Convert ions to atoms
 B. Cause ejection of an outer shell electron
 C. Reduce evaporation of the sample
 D. Burn off organic impurities

Chemistry/Apply principles of basic procedures/ Instrumentation/2

29. Internal standards are not needed in atomic absorption spectrophotometry because:
 A. Changes in aspiration have little effect on the number of ground state atoms
 B. Atomic absorption instruments have a stable light path
 C. The instrument measures only one atom at a time
 D. The instrument source lamp is used for a reference voltage

Chemistry/Apply principles of special procedures/ Instrumentation/2

25. **C** In FPIA, antigen in the patient's sample competes with antigen conjugated to a fluorochrome (tracer) for a limited number of antibodies. When antibody binds to the tracer, it slows its rotation. This increases the emission of plane polarized fluorescence. Polarized fluorescence is inversely related to concentration and can be measured without the need to separate free and antibody-bound tracer.

26. **A** Rayleigh's law states that when the incident wavelength is much longer than the particle diameter, there is maximum backscatter and minimum right-angle scatter. The Rayleigh-Debye law predicts maximum right-angle scatter when wavelength and particle diameter approach equality. In nephelometry, the relationship between wavelength and diameter determines the angle at which the detector is located.

27. **D** In nephelometry the detector output is proportional to concentration (as opposed to turbidimetry in which the detector is behind the cuvet). The detector(s) is(are) usually placed at an angle between 25° and 90° to the incident light, depending upon the application. Nephelometers, like fluorometers, are calibrated to read zero with the light path blocked, and sensitivity can be increased up to 1000 times by amplification of the detector output or photomultiplier tube gain.

28. **A** The atomizer of the atomic absorption spectrophotometer consists of either a nebulizer and flame or a graphite furnace. The nebulizer disperses the sample evenly into the flame. Heat is used to evaporate water and break the ionic bonds of salts, forming atoms. The flame also excites a small percentage of the atoms, which release a characteristic emission line.

29. **A** The steady state between ground state and excited atoms in a flame or graphite furnace favors the ground state by more than 10,000:1. Small fluctuations in aspiration rate or atomizer temperature have an insignificant effect on the number of ground state atoms but have a pronounced effect on the number excited.

30. A flameless atomic absorption spectrophotometer dehydrates and atomizes a sample using:
A. A graphite capillary furnace
B. An electron gun
C. A thermoelectric semiconductor
D. A thermospray platform

Chemistry/Apply principles of special procedures/Instrumentation/1

31. Interference in atomic absorption spectrophotometry caused by differences in viscosity is called:
A. Absorption interference
B. Matrix effect
C. Ionization interference
D. Quenching

Chemistry/Evaluate sources of error/Instrumentation/2

32. All of the following are required when measuring magnesium by atomic absorption spectrophotometry *except:*
A. A hollow cathode lamp with a magnesium cathode
B. A chopper to prevent optical interference from magnesium emission
C. A monochromator to isolate the magnesium emission line at 285 nm
D. A 285-nm reference beam to correct for background absorption

Chemistry/Select methods/Reagents/Media/Electrolytes/2

33. When measuring calcium by atomic absorption spectrophotometry, which is required?
A. An organic extraction reagent to deconjugate calcium from protein
B. An internal standard
C. A magnesium chelator
D. Lanthanum oxide to chelate phosphates

Chemistry/Select methods/Reagents/Media/Electrolytes/2

34. Ion-selective analyzers using *undiluted* samples have what advantage over analyzers that use a diluted sample?
A. They can measure over a wider range of concentration
B. They are not subject to pseudohyponatremia caused by high lipids
C. They do not require temperature equilibration
D. They require less maintenance

Chemistry/Apply knowledge to identify sources of error/Electrolytes/2

Answers to Questions 30–34

30. A Flameless atomic absorption uses a hollow tube of graphite with quartz ends. The tube is heated by current in order to char the sample, and argon is injected into the capillary to distribute the atoms. The furnace is more sensitive than a flame atomizer and more efficient in atomizing thermostable salts. However, it is prone to greater matrix interference and is slower than the flame atomizer because it must cool down before injection of the next sample.

31. B Significant differences in aspiration and atomization result when the matrix of sample and unknowns differ. Differences in viscosity and protein content are major causes of matrix error. Matrix effects can be reduced by using protein-based calibrators and diluting both standards and samples prior to assay.

32. D Atomic absorption requires a lamp with a cathode made from the metal to be assayed. The lamp emits the line spectrum of the metal, providing the wavelength that the atoms can absorb. The chopper pulses the source light, allowing it to be discriminated from light emitted by excited atoms. A monochromator eliminates light emitted by the ideal gas in the lamp. Wide bandpass light or Zeeman correction (splitting the incident light into side bands by a magnetic field) may be used to correct for background absorption.

33. D An acidic diluent such as hydrochloric acid (HCl) will displace calcium bound to albumin. However, calcium forms a thermostable bond with phosphate that causes chemical interference in atomic absorption. Lanthanum displaces calcium, forming lanthanum phosphate, and eliminates interference from phosphates. Unlike colorimetric methods for calcium (e.g., *o*-cresolphthalein complexone), magnesium does not interfere in atomic absorption since it does not absorb the 422.7-nm emission line from the calcium hollow cathode lamp.

34. B Ion-selective analyzers measure the electrolyte dissolved in the fluid phase of the sample in millimoles per liter of plasma water. When undiluted blood is assayed, the measurement is independent of colloids such as protein and lipid. Hyperlipemic samples cause falsely low sodium measurements when assayed by flame photometry and ion-selective analyzers requiring dilution because lipids displace plasma water containing the electrolytes. One drawback to undiluted or direct measuring systems is that the electrodes require more frequent deproteinization and usually have a shorter duty cycle.

35. Select the equation describing the potential that develops at the surface of an ion-selective electrode.
  A. Van Deemter's equation
  B. Van Slyke's equation
  C. Nernst's equation
  D. Henderson-Hasselbalch equation

Chemistry/Define fundamental characteristics/ Instrumentation/1

36. The reference potential of a silver-silver chloride electrode is determined by the:
  A. Concentration of the potassium chloride filling solution
  B. Surface area of the electrode
  C. Activity of total anion in the paste covering the electrode
  D. Concentration of silver in the paste covering the electrode

Chemistry/Define fundamental characteristics/ Instrumentation/1

37. The term RT/nF in the Nernst equation defines the:
  A. Potential at the ion-selective membrane
  B. Slope of the electrode
  C. Decomposition potential
  D. Isopotential point of the electrode

Chemistry/Define fundamental characteristics/ Instrumentation/1

38. The ion-selective membrane used to measure potassium is made of:
  A. High-borosilicate glass membrane
  B. Polyvinyl chloride dioctylphenyl phosphonate ion exchanger
  C. Valinomycin gel
  D. Calomel

Chemistry/Apply principles of basic laboratory procedures/Electrolytes/1

39. The response of a sodium electrode to a tenfold increase in sodium concentration should be:
  A. A tenfold drop in potential
  B. An increase in potential of approximately 60 mV
  C. An increase in potential of approximately 10 mV
  D. A decrease in potential of approximately 10 mV

Chemistry/Calculate/Electrolytes/2

35. C The Van Deemter equation describes the relation between the velocity of mobile phase to column efficiency in gas chromatography. The Henderson-Hasselbalch equation is used to determine the pH of a solution containing a weak acid and its salt. Van Slyke developed an apparatus to measure CO_2 and O_2 content using a manometer.

36. A The activity of any solid or ion in a saturated solution is unity. For a silver electrode covered with silver chloride paste, the Nernst equation is $E = E^o - RT/nF \times 2.3 \log_{10} [Ag^o \times Cl^-]/[AgCl]$. Because silver and silver chloride have an activity of 1.0, and all components except chloride are constants, the potential of the reference electrode is determined by the chloride concentration of the filling solution.

$$E = E^o - RT/nF \times 2.3 \log_{10}[Cl^-] = E^o - 59.2 \text{ mV} \times \log[Cl^-] \text{ (at room temperature)}.$$

37. B In the term RT/nF, R = the molar gas constant, T = temperature in degrees Kelvin, F = Faraday's constant, and n = the number of electrons donated per atom of reductant. The slope depends upon the temperature of the solution and the valence of the reductant. At room temperature, the slope is 59.2 mV for a univalent ion and 29.6 mV for a divalent ion.

38. C Valinomycin is an antibiotic with a highly selective reversible binding affinity for potassium ions. Sodium electrodes are usually composed of a glass membrane with a high content of aluminum silicate. Calcium and lithium ion-selective electrodes are made from organic liquid ion exchangers called neutral carrier ionophores. Calomel is made of mercury covered with a paste of mercurous chloride (Hg^o/Hg_2Cl_2) and is used as a reference electrode for pH.

39. B The Nernst equation predicts an increase of approximately 60 mV per tenfold increase in sodium activity. For sodium,

$$E = E^o + RT/nF \times 2.3 \log_{10}[Na^+]. \quad RT/nF \times 2.3 = 60 \text{ mV at } 37°C. \text{ Therefore, } E = E^o + 60 \text{ mV} \times \log_{10}[Na^+].$$

If sodium concentration is 10 mmol/L, then $E = E^o + 60 \text{ mV} \times \log_{10}[10] = E^o + 60 \text{ mV}$.

If sodium concentration increases from 10 mmol/L to 100 mmol/L, then $E = E^o + 60 \text{ mV} \times \log_{10}[100] = E^o + 60 \text{ mV} \times 2 = E^o + 120 \text{ mV}$.

40. Which of the electrodes below is a current-producing (amperometric) rather than a voltage-producing (potentiometric) electrode?
 A. The Clark electrode
 B. The Severinghaus electrode
 C. The pH electrode
 D. The ionized calcium electrode

Chemistry/Define fundamental characteristics/
Instrumentation/1

41. Which of the following would cause a "response" error from an ion-selective electrode for sodium when measuring serum but not calibrator?
 A. Interference from other electrolytes
 B. Protein coating the ion-selective membrane
 C. An over-range in sodium concentration
 D. Protein binding to sodium ions

Chemistry/Identify source of error/Electrolytes/2

42. In polarography, the voltage needed to cause depolarization of the cathode is called the:
 A. Half-wave potential
 B. Isopotential point
 C. Decomposition potential
 D. Polarization potential

Chemistry/Define fundamental characteristics/
Instrumentation/1

43. Persistent noise from an ion-selective electrode is most often caused by:
 A. Contamination of sample
 B. Blocked junction at the salt bridge
 C. Over-range from high concentration
 D. Improper calibration

Chemistry/Identify source of error/Electrolytes/2

44. Which element is reduced at the cathode of a Clark polarographic electrode?
 A. Silver
 B. Oxygen
 C. Chloride
 D. Potassium

Chemistry/Define fundamental characteristics/
Instrumentation/1

Answers to Questions 40–44

40. **A** The Clark electrode is composed of two half cells that generate current, not voltage. It is used to measure partial pressure of oxygen (P_{O_2}) and is based upon an amperometric method called polarography. When −0.8 V is applied to the cathode, O_2 is reduced, causing current to flow. Current is proportional to the P_{O_2} of the sample.

41. **B** Response is the time required for an electrode to reach maximum potential. Ion-selective analyzers use a microprocessor to monitor electrode response, slope, drift, and noise. When an electrode gives an acceptable response time when measuring aqueous calibrator but not when measuring serum, the cause is often protein build-up on the membrane.

42. **C** In polarography, a minimum negative voltage must be applied to the cathode to cause reduction of metal ions (or O_2) in solution. This is called the decomposition potential. It is concentration-dependent (dilute solutions require greater negative voltage) and can be determined using the Nernst equation.

43. **B** Electrode noise most often results from an unstable junction potential. Most reference electrodes contain a high concentration of KCl internal solution used to produce the reference potential. This forms a salt bridge with the measuring half-cell by contacting the sample but is kept from equilibrating via a barrier called a *junction*. When this junction becomes blocked by salt crystals, the reference potential becomes unstable, resulting in fluctuations in the analyzer readout.

44. **B** The Clark electrode is designed to measure oxygen. O_2 diffuses through a gas-permeable membrane covering the electrode. It is reduced at the cathode, which is usually made of platinum wire. Electrons are supplied by the anode, which is made of silver. The net reaction is:

$$4\,KCl + 2\,H_2O + O_2 + 4\,Ag^\circ \rightarrow 4\,AgCl + 4\,KOH.$$

45. Which of the following statements accurately characterizes the coulometric titration of chloride?
  A. The indicator electrodes generate voltage
  B. Constant current must be present across the generator electrodes
  C. Silver ions are formed at the generator cathode
  D. Chloride concentration is inversely proportional to titration time

Chemistry/Define fundamental characteristics/ Instrumentation/2

46. In the coulometric chloride titration:
  A. Acetic acid in the titrating solution furnishes the counter ion for reduction
  B. The endpoint is detected by amperometry
  C. The titrating reagent contains a phosphate buffer to keep pH constant
  D. Nitric acid (HNO_3) is used to lower the solubility of AgCl

Chemistry/Apply principles of special procedures/ Electrolytes/2

47. Which of the following compounds can interfere with the coulometric chloride assay?
  A. Bromide
  B. Ascorbate
  C. Acetoacetate
  D. Nitrate

Chemistry/Apply knowledge to identify sources of error/ Electrolytes/2

48. All of the following compounds contribute to the osmolality of plasma *except:*
  A. Lipids
  B. Creatinine
  C. Drug metabolites
  D. Glucose

Chemistry/Apply knowledge of fundamental biological characteristics/Osmolality/2

49. One mole per kilogram H_2O of any solute will cause all of the following *except:*
  A. Lower the freezing point by 1.86°C
  B. Raise vapor pressure by 0.3 mm Hg
  C. Raise the boiling point by 0.52°C
  D. Raise osmotic pressure by 22.4 atm

Chemistry/Apply knowledge of fundamental biological characteristics/Osmolality/2

50. What component of a freezing point osmometer measures the sample temperature?
  A. Thermistor
  B. Thermocouple
  C. Capacitor
  D. Electrode

Chemistry/Apply principles of special procedures/ Osmometry/1

45. **B** The Cotlove chloridometer is based upon the principle of coulometric titration with amperometric detection. Charge in the form of silver ions is generated by oxidation of silver wire at the generator anode. Silver ions react with chloride ions, forming insoluble silver chloride (AgCl). When all of the chloride is titrated, free silver ions are detected by reduction back to elemental silver, which causes an increase in current across the indicator electrodes (a pair of silver electrodes with a voltage difference of about 1.0 V DC). Charge or titration time is directly proportional to chloride concentration as long as the rate of oxidation remains constant at the generator anode.

46. **B** Reduction of Ag^+ back to Ag^o generates the current, which signals the endpoint. The titrating reagent contains HNO_3, acetic acid, H_2O, and either gelatin or polyvinyl alcohol. The HNO_3 furnishes nitrate, which is reduced at the generator cathode, forming ammonium ions. The ammonium becomes oxidized back to nitrate at the indicator anode. Gelatin or polyvinyl alcohol is needed to prevent pitting of the generator anode. Acetic acid lowers the solubility of AgCl, preventing dissociation back to Ag^+.

47. **A** Chloride assays based upon either coulometric or chemical titration are subject to positive interference from other anions and electronegative radicals that may be titrated instead of chloride ions. These include other halogens such as bromide, cyanide, and cysteine.

48. **A** Osmolality is the concentration (in moles) of dissolved solute per kilogram solvent. Proteins and lipids are not in solution and do not contribute to osmolality. The nonionized solutes such as glucose and urea contribute 1 osmole per mole per kilogram water, whereas dissociated salts contribute 1 osmole per mole of each dissociated ion or radical.

49. **B** Both freezing point and vapor pressure are lowered by increasing solute concentration. Boiling point and osmotic pressure are raised. Increasing solute concentration of a solution opposes a change in its physical state and lowers the concentration of H_2O molecules.

50. **A** A thermistor is a temperature-sensitive resistor. The resistance to current flow increases as temperature falls. The temperature at which a solution freezes can be determined by measuring the resistance of the thermistor. Resistance is directly proportional to the osmolality of the sample.

51. What type of measuring circuit is used in a freezing point osmometer?
- **A.** Electrometer
- **B.** Potentiometer
- **C.** Wheatstone bridge
- **D.** Thermal conductivity bridge

Chemistry/Apply principles of special procedures/ Osmometry/1

52. Which measurement principle is employed in a vapor pressure osmometer?
- **A.** Seebeck
- **B.** Peltier
- **C.** Hayden
- **D.** Darlington

Chemistry/Apply principles of special procedures/ Osmometry/1

53. The freezing point osmometer differs from the vapor pressure osmometer in that the freezing point osmometer only:
- **A.** Cools the sample
- **B.** Is sensitive to ethanol
- **C.** Requires a thermoelectric module
- **D.** Requires calibration with aqueous standards

Chemistry/Apply principles of special procedures/ Osmometry/2

54. The method for measuring iron by plating the metal and then oxidizing it is called:
- **A.** Polarography
- **B.** Coulometry
- **C.** Anodic stripping voltometry
- **D.** Amperometry

Chemistry/Apply principles of special procedures/ Instrumentation/1

55. The term isocratic is used in high-performance liquid chromatography (HPLC) to mean the:
- **A.** Mobile phase is at constant temperature
- **B.** Stationary phase is equilibrated with the mobile phase
- **C.** Mobile phase consists of a constant solvent composition
- **D.** Flow rate of the mobile phase is regulated

Chemistry/Apply principles of special procedures/High-performance liquid chromatography/1

56. The term reverse phase is used in HPLC to indicate that the mobile phase is:
- **A.** More polar than the stationary phase
- **B.** Liquid and the stationary phase is solid
- **C.** Organic and the stationary phase is aqueous
- **D.** A stronger solvent than the stationary phase

Chemistry/Apply principles of special procedures/High-performance liquid chromatography/1

Answers to Questions 51–56

51. C The resistance of the thermistor is measured using a network of resistors called a Wheatstone bridge. When the sample is frozen, the bridge is balanced using a calibrated variable resistor, so that no current flows to the readout. The resistance required to balance the meter is equal to the resistance of the thermistor.

52. A The Seebeck effect refers to the increase in voltage across the opposite ends of a thermocouple caused by decreasing temperature. Increasing osmolality lowers the dew point of a sample. When the sample is cooled to its dew point, the voltage change across the thermocouple is directly proportional to its osmolality.

53. B Alcohol enters the vapor phase so rapidly that it evaporates before the dew point of the sample is reached. Therefore, ethanol does not contribute to osmolality as measured using the vapor pressure osmometer. Freezing point osmometers measure alcohol and can be used in emergency room settings to estimate ethanol toxicity.

54. C Anodic stripping voltometry is used to measure lead and iron. The cation of the metal is plated onto a mercury cathode by applying a negative charge. The voltage of this electrode is reversed until the plated metal is oxidized back to a cation. Current produced by oxidation of the metal is proportional to concentration.

55. C An isocratic separation uses a single mobile phase of constant composition, pH, and polarity and requires a single pump. Some HPLC separations use a gradient mobile phase to increase distance between peaks. Gradients are made by mixing two or more solvents using a controller to change the proportions of solvent components.

56. A In reverse phase HPLC the separation takes place using a nonpolar sorbent (stationary phase) such as octadecylsilane (C18). Solutes that are nonpolar are retained longer than polar solutes. Most clinical separations of drugs, hormones, and metabolites use reverse phase HPLC because aqueous mobile phases are far less toxic and flammable.

57. What is the primary means of solute separation in HPLC using a C18 column?
- **A.** Anion exchange
- **B.** Size exclusion
- **C.** Partitioning
- **D.** Cation exchange

Chemistry/Apply principles of special procedures/High-performance liquid chromatography/1

58. The most commonly used detector for clinical gas-liquid chromatography (GLC) is based upon:
- **A.** UV light absorbance at 254 nm
- **B.** Flame ionization
- **C.** Refractive index
- **D.** Thermal conductance

Chemistry/Apply principles of special procedures/Gas chromatography/1

59. What type of detector is used in HPLC with electro-chemical detection (ECD)?
- **A.** Calomel electrode
- **B.** Conductivity electrode
- **C.** Glassy carbon electrode
- **D.** Polarographic electrode

Chemistry/Apply principles of special procedures/High-performance liquid chromatography/1

60. In gas chromatography the elution order of volatiles is usually based upon the:
- **A.** Boiling point
- **B.** Molecular size
- **C.** Carbon content
- **D.** Polarity

Chemistry/Apply principle of special procedures/Gas chromatography/2

61. Select the chemical that is used in most HPLC procedures to decrease solvent polarity.
- **A.** Hexane
- **B.** Nonane
- **C.** Chloroform
- **D.** Acetonitrile

Chemistry/Apply principles of special procedures/Biochemical/2

62. In thin-layer chromatography (TLC), the distance the solute migrates divided by the distance the solvent migrates is the:
- **A.** t_R
- **B.** K_d
- **C.** R_f
- **D.** pK

Chemistry/Apply principles of special procedures/High-performance liquid chromatography/1

57. **C** Stationary phases (column packings) used in HPLC separate solutes by multiple means, but in reverse phase HPLC the relative solubility between the mobile phase and the stationary phase is most important and depends upon solvent polarity, pH, and ionic strength.

58. **B** Volatile solutes can be detected in GLC using flame ionization, thermal conductivity, electron capture, and mass spectroscopy. In flame ionization, energy from a flame is used to excite the analytes as they elute from the column. The flame is made by igniting a mixture of hydrogen, carrier gas, and air. Current is produced when an outer shell electron is ejected from the excited analyte.

59. **C** HPLC-ECD uses a glassy carbon measuring electrode and a silver-silver chloride reference. The analyte is oxidized or reduced by holding the glassy carbon electrode at a positive voltage (oxidization) or negative voltage (reduction). The resulting current flow is directly proportional to concentration. Phenolic groups such as catecholamines can be measured by HPLC-ECD.

60. **A** The order of elution is dependent upon the velocity of the analyte. Usually the lower the boiling point of the compound, the greater its velocity or solubility in carrier gas.

61. **D** All the compounds mentioned have nonpolar properties. Because most HPLC is reverse phase (a polar solvent is used), hexane and nonane are too nonpolar. Acetonitrile is more polar and less toxic than chloroform and, along with methanol, is a common polarity modifier for HPLC.

62. **C** R_f is the distance migrated by the solute divided by the distance migrated by the solvent. The t_R refers to the retention time of the solute in HPLC or gas chromatography (GC). The K_d is the partition coefficient and is a measure of the relative affinity of solutes for the stationary phase. The solute with the greater K_d will be retained longer. The pK is the negative logarithm of K, the ionization constant, and is a measure of ionization.

63. Which reagent is used in TLC to extract cocaine metabolites from urine?
  A. Acid and sodium chloride
  B. Alkali and organic solvent
  C. Chloroform and sodium acetate
  D. Neutral solution of ethyl acetate

Chemistry/Apply principles of special procedures/ Biochemical/2

64. What is the purpose of an internal standard in HPLC and GC methods?
  A. It compensates for variation in extraction and injection
  B. It corrects for background absorbance
  C. It compensates for changes in flow rate
  D. It corrects for coelution of solutes

Chemistry/Apply principles of special procedures/ Chromatography/2

65. What is the confirmatory method for measuring drugs of abuse?
  A. HPLC
  B. Enzyme-multiplied immunoassay technique (EMIT)
  C. Gas chromatography with mass spectroscopy (GC-MS)
  D. TLC

Chemistry/Select instruments to perform test/Drugs of abuse/2

66. Which method is the most useful when screening for errors of amino and organic acid metabolism?
  A. Two-dimensional TLC
  B. Gas chromatography
  C. Electrospray ionization tandem mass spectroscopy
  D. Inductively charged coupled mass spectroscopy

Chemistry/Select instruments to perform test/Newborn Screening/2

67. Which component is needed for a thermal cycler to amplify DNA?
  A. Programmable heating and cooling unit
  B. Vacuum chamber with zero head space
  C. Sealed airtight constant temperature chamber
  D. Temperature controlled ionization chamber

Chemistry/Define fundamental characteristics/ Instrumentation/1

Answers to Questions 63–67

63. **B** Alkaline drugs such as cocaine, amphetamine, and morphine are extracted at alkaline pH. Ideally, the pH of the extracting solution should be 2 pH units greater than the negative log of dissociation constant (*pKa*) of the drug. More than 90% of the drug will be un-ionized and will extract in ethyl acetate or another organic solvent.

64. **A** Internal standards should have the same affinity as the analyte for the extraction reagents. Dividing peak height (or area) of all samples (standards and unknowns) by the peak height (or area) of the internal standard reduces error caused by variation in extraction recovery and injection volume.

65. **C** GC-MS determines the mass spectrum of the compounds eluting from the analytic column. Each substance has a unique and characteristic spectrum of mass fragments. This spectrum is compared to spectra in a library of standards to determine the percentage match. A match of greater than 95% is considered confirmatory.

66. **C** While two-dimensional TLC can separate both amino and organic acids, it is not sufficiently sensitive for newborn screening. Electrospray ionization allows a small alcohol-extracted whole blood sample to be analyzed by two mass spectrometers without prior separation by liquid or gas chromatography. Disorders of both organic and fatty acid metabolism are identified by the specific pattern of acylcarnitine ions produced. Amino acids are detected as amino species that have lost a carboxyl group during ionization, a process called neutral loss.

67. **A** The polymerase chain reaction for DNA amplification consists of three phases. Denaturation requires a temperature of 90°–94°C and separates the double stranded DNA. Annealing requires a temperature between 40°–65°C and allows the primers to bind to the target base sequence. Extension requires a temperature of 72°C and allows the heat-stable polymerase to add complementary bases to the primer in the 5′ to 3′ direction. A cycle consists of each temperature stage for a specific number of minutes and most procedures require 30 to 40 cycles to generate a detectable quantity of target DNA. Rapid heating and cooling are usually achieved using a thermoelectric block that is cooled by forced air flow.

68. In addition to velocity, what variable is needed to calculate the relative centrifugal force (g force) of a centrifuge?
    A. Head radius
    B. Angular velocity coefficient
    C. Diameter of the centrifuge tube
    D. Ambient temperature in degrees centigrade

    Chemistry/Define fundamental characteristics/Instrumentation/1

69. Which of the following situations is likely to cause an error when weighing with an electronic analytical balance?
    A. Failure to keep the knife edge clean
    B. Failure to close the doors of the balance before reading the weight
    C. Oxidation on the surface of the substitution weights
    D. Using the balance without allowing it to warm up for at least 10 minutes

    Chemistry/Identify source of error/Balances/3

70. When calibrating a semiautomatic pipette that has a fixed delivery of 10.0 μL using a gravimetric method, what should be the average weight of the deionized water transferred?
    A. 10.0 μg
    B. 100.0 μg
    C. 1.0 mg
    D. 10.0 mg

    Chemistry/Define fundamental characteristics/Instrumentation/1

Answers to Questions 68–70

68. **A** The relative centrifugal force (number times the force of gravity) is proportional to the square of the rotor speed in revolutions per minute and the radius in centimeters of the head (distance from the shaft to the end of the tube).

    $$RCF = s^2 \times r \times 1.118 \times 10^{-5}$$

    where s is the speed in RPM, r is the radius in cM, and 1.118×10^{-5} is a conversion constant.

69. **B** Electronic balances do not use substitution weights or knife edges to balance the weight on the pan. Instead, they measure the displacement of the pan by the weight on it using electromagnetic force to return it to its reference position. Regardless of the type of balance used, all weighing devices need to be located on a firm weighing table free of vibration. Doors must be closed to prevent air currents from influencing the weighing, and the pan and platform must be clean and free of dust and chemical residue.

70. **D** Gravimetric and spectrophotometric analysis are the two methods used to verify pipette volume accuracy and precision. Since spectrophotometric analysis involves dilution, gravimetric analysis is associated with greater certainty. At 20°C, the density of pure water is 0.99821 g/mL. Therefore each microliter weighs 1.0 mg.

BLOOD GASES, pH, AND ELECTROLYTES

1. Which of the following represents the Henderson-Hasselbalch equation as applied to blood pH?
   A. $pH = 6.1 + \log HCO_3^-/P_{CO_2}$
   B. $pH = 6.1 + \log HCO_3^-/(0.03 \times P_{CO_2})$
   C. $pH = 6.1 + \log dCO_2/HCO_3^-$
   D. $pH = 6.1 + \log (0.03 \times P_{CO_2})/HCO_3^-$

   Chemistry/Calculate/Acid-base/1

2. What is the P_{O_2} of calibration gas containing 20.0% O_2, when the barometric pressure is 30 in?
   A. 60 mm Hg
   B. 86 mm Hg
   C. 143 mm Hg
   D. 152 mm Hg

   Chemistry/Calculate/Blood gas/2

3. What is the blood pH when the partial pressure of carbon dioxide (P_{CO_2}) is 60 mm Hg and the bicarbonate level is 18 mmol/L?
   A. 6.89
   B. 7.00
   C. 7.10
   D. 7.30

   Chemistry/Calculate/Acid-base/2

4. Which of the following best represents the reference (normal) range for arterial pH?
   A. 7.35–7.45
   B. 7.42–7.52
   C. 7.38–7.68
   D. 6.85–7.56

   Chemistry/Apply knowledge of fundamental biological characteristics/Acid-base/1

5. What is the normal ratio of bicarbonate to dissolved carbon dioxide (HCO_3:dCO_2) in arterial blood?
   A. 1:10
   B. 10:1
   C. 20:1
   D. 30:1

   Chemistry/Apply knowledge of fundamental biological characteristics/Acid-base/1

Answers to Questions 1–5

1. **B** The Henderson-Hasselbalch equation describes the pH of a buffer made up of a weak acid and its salt. $pH = pK_a + \log salt/acid$, where pK_a is the negative logarithm of the dissociation constant of the acid.

2. **C** Convert barometric pressure in inches to mm Hg by multiplying by 25.4 (mm/in). Next, subtract the vapor pressure of H_2O at 37°C, 47 mm Hg, to give dry gas pressure. Multiply dry gas pressure by the %O_2:

   25.4 mm/in $\times$ 30 in = 762 mm Hg

   762 mm Hg – 47 mm Hg (vapor pressure) = 715 mm Hg (dry gas pressure)

   0.20×715 mm Hg = 143 mm Hg P_{O_2}

3. **C** Solve using the Henderson-Hasselbalch equation. $pH = pK' + \log HCO_3^-/(0.03 \times P_{CO})$, where pK', the negative logarithm of the combined hydration and dissociation constants for dissolved CO_2 and carbonic acid, is 6.1, and 0.03 is the solubility coefficient for CO_2 gas.

   $pH = 6.1 + \log 18/(0.03 \times 60) = 6.1 + \log 18/1.8$

   $pH = 6.1 + \log 10$. Because $\log 10 = 1$, $pH = 7.10$

4. **A** The reference range for arterial blood pH is 7.35–7.45 and is only 0.03 pH unit lower for venous blood owing to the buffering effects of hemoglobin (Hgb), known as the chloride-isohydric shift. Most laboratories consider lower than 7.20 and higher than 7.60 the critical values for pH.

5. **C** When the ratio of HCO_3:dCO_2 is 20:1, the log of salt/acid becomes 1.3. Substituting this in the Henderson-Hasselbalch equation and solving for pH gives $pH = 6.1 + \log 20$; $pH = 6.1 + 1.3 = 7.4$. Acidosis results when this ratio is decreased and alkalosis when it is increased.

6. What is the P_{CO_2} if the dco_2 is 1.8 mmol/L?
  A. 24 mm Hg
  B. 35 mm Hg
  C. 60 mm Hg
  D. 72 mm Hg

Chemistry/Calculate/Blood gas/2

7. In the Henderson-Hasselbalch expression pH = 6.1 + log HCO_3^-/dco_2 the 6.1 represents:
  A. The combined hydration and dissociation constants for CO_2 in blood at 37°C
  B. The solubility constant for CO_2 gas
  C. The dissociation constant of H_2O
  D. The ionization constant of sodium bicarbonate ($NaHCO_3$)

Chemistry/Apply knowledge of fundamental biological characteristics/Acid-base/1

8. Which of the following contributes the most to the serum total CO_2?
  A. P_{CO_2}
  B. dco_2
  C. HCO_3^-
  D. Carbonium ion

Chemistry/Apply knowledge of fundamental biological characteristics/Acid-base/2

9. What other measurement in addition to bicarbonate is needed to calculate buffer base?
  A. Hemoglobin concentration
  B. Dissolved O_2 concentration
  C. Inorganic phosphorus
  D. Total carbon dioxide

Chemistry/Apply knowledge of fundamental biological characteristics/Acid-base/2

10. Which of the following effects results from exposure of a normal arterial blood sample to room air?
  A. P_{O_2} increased P_{CO_2} decreased   pH increased
  B. P_{O_2} decreased P_{CO_2} increased   pH decreased
  C. P_{O_2} increased P_{CO_2} decreased   pH decreased
  D. P_{O_2} decreased P_{CO_2} decreased   pH decreased

Chemistry/Evaluate laboratory data to recognize problems/Blood gas/3

11. Which of the following formulas for O_2 content is correct?
  A. O_2 content = %O_2 saturation/100×Hgb g/dL × 1.34 mL/g + (0.003×P_{O_2})
  B. O_2 content = P_{O_2}×0.0306 mmol/L/mm
  C. O_2 content = O_2 saturation×Hgb g/dL×0.003 mL/g
  D. O_2 content = O_2 capacity×0.003 mL/g

Chemistry/Calculate/Blood gas/1

---

6. C Dissolved CO_2 is calculated from the measured P_{CO_2}×0.0306, the solubility coefficient for CO_2 gas in blood at 37°C.

dco_2 = P_{CO_2}×0.03

Therefore, P_{CO_2} = dco_2/0.03

P_{CO_2} = 1.8 mmol/L ÷ 0.03 = 60 mm Hg

7. A The equilibrium constant, K_h, for the hydration of CO_2 (dco_2 + H_2O → H_2CO_3), is only about $2.3×10^{-3}M$, making dco_2 far more prevalent than carbonic acid. The dissociation constant, K_d for the reaction H_2CO_3 →H^+ + HCO_3^- is about $2×10^{-4}M$. The product of these constants is the combined equilibrium constant, K'. The negative logarithm of K' is the pK', which is 6.103 in blood at 37°C.

8. C The total CO_2 is the sum of the dco_2, H_2CO_3 (carbonic acid or hydrated CO_2), and bicarbonate (as mainly $NaHCO_3$). When serum is used to measure total CO_2, the dco_2 is insignificant because all the CO_2 gas has escaped into the air. Therefore, serum total CO_2 is equivalent to the bicarbonate concentration. Total CO_2 is commonly measured by potentiometry. An organic acid is used to release CO_2 gas from bicarbonate and pco_2 is measured with a Severinghaus electrode. Alternately, bicarbonate can be measured by an enzymatic reaction using phosphoenolpyruvate carboxylase. The enzyme forms oxaloacetate and phosphate from phosphoenolpyruvate and bicarbonate. The oxaloacetate is reduced to malate by malate dehydrogenase and NADH is oxidized to NAD^+. The negative reaction rate is proportional to plasma bicarbonate concentration.

9. A Buffer base refers to all forms of base that will titrate hydrogen ions. The major blood buffers contributing to buffer base (in order of concentration) are bicarbonate, hemoglobin (Hgb), protein, and phosphate.

10. A The P_{O_2} of air at sea level (21% O_2) is about 150 mm Hg. The P_{CO_2} of air is only about 0.3 mm Hg. Consequently, blood releases CO_2 gas and gains O_2 when exposed to air. Loss of CO_2 shifts the equilibrium of the bicarbonate buffer system to the right, decreasing hydrogen ion concentration, and blood becomes more alkaline.

11. A Oxygen content is the sum of O_2 bound to Hgb and O_2 dissolved in the plasma. It is dependent upon the Hgb concentration and the percentage of Hgb bound to O_2 (O_2 saturation). Each gram of Hgb binds 1.34 mL of O_2. The dissolved O_2 is determined from the solubility coefficient of O_2 (0.003 mL/mm Hg) and the P_{O_2}. O_2 Content = % Sat/100×Hgb in g/dL×1.34 mL/g + (0.003×P_{O_2}).

12. The normal difference between alveolar and arterial P_{O_2} (P_{AO_2}–P_{aO_2} difference) is:
- **A.** 3 mm Hg
- **B.** 10 mm Hg
- **C.** 40 mm Hg
- **D.** 50 mm Hg

Chemistry/Apply knowledge of fundamental biological characteristics/Blood gas/2

13. A decreased P_{AO_2}–P_{aO_2} difference is found in:
- **A.** A/V (arteriovenous) shunting
- **B.** $\dot{V}/\dot{Q}$ (ventilation/perfusion) inequality
- **C.** Ventilation defects
- **D.** All of the above

Chemistry/Evaluate laboratory data to recognize health and disease states/Blood gas/2

14. Bichromatic measurement of oxyhemoglobin concentration is performed at:
- **A.** 577/548 nm
- **B.** 450/410 nm
- **C.** 340/380 nm
- **D.** 400/600 nm

Chemistry/Apply principles of special procedures/Hemoglobin/1

15. Correction of pH for a patient with a body temperature of 38°C would require:
- **A.** Subtraction of 0.015
- **B.** Subtraction of 0.01%
- **C.** Addition of 0.020
- **D.** Subtraction of 0.020

Chemistry/Calculate/Acid-base/2

16. Select the anticoagulant of choice for blood gas studies.
- **A.** Sodium citrate, 3.2%
- **B.** Lithium heparin, 100 U/mL blood
- **C.** Sodium citrate, 3.8%
- **D.** Ammonium oxalate, 5.0%

Chemistry/Apply knowledge of standard operating procedures/Specimen collection and handling/1

17. A patient's blood gas results are as follows: pH = 7.26; d_{CO_2} = 2.0 mmol/L; HCO_3^- = 29 mmol/L. These results would be classified as:
- **A.** Metabolic acidosis
- **B.** Metabolic alkalosis
- **C.** Respiratory acidosis
- **D.** Respiratory alkalosis

Chemistry/Evaluate laboratory data to recognize health and disease states/Acid-base/3

Answers to Questions 12–17

12. B The P_{AO_2}–P_{aO_2} difference results from the low ratio of ventilation to perfusion in the base of the lungs. This blood has a low O_2 saturation, causing it to take up O_2 from blood, leaving other well-ventilated areas of the lung.

13. C Patients with A/V shunts, $\dot{V}/\dot{Q}$ inequalities, and cardiac failure will have an increased P_{AO_2}–P_{aO_2} difference. However, patients with ventilation problems have low alveolar P_{O_2} owing to retention of CO_2. This reduces the P_{AO_2}–P_{aO_2} difference.

14. A Oxyhemoglobin is measured as an absorbance ratio, where the numerator represents a wavelength of high absorbance for oxyhemoglobin and the denominator an isosbestic wavelength (all Hgb pigments have the same absorptivity coefficient). The absorbance ratio increases linearly with increasing oxyhemoglobin concentration.

15. A The pH decreases by 0.015 for each degree Celsius above 37°C. Because the blood gas analyzer measures pH at 37°C, the in vivo pH would be 0.015 pH units below the measured pH.

16. B Heparin is the only anticoagulant that does not alter the pH of blood; heparin salts must be used for pH and blood gases. Solutions of heparin are air-equilibrated and must be used sparingly to prevent contamination of the sample by gas in the solution.

17. C Imbalances are classified as respiratory when the primary disturbance is with P_{CO_2} because P_{CO_2} is regulated by ventilation. P_{CO_2} = d_{CO_2}/0.03 or 60 mm Hg (normal 35–45 mm Hg). Increased d_{CO_2} increases hydrogen ion concentration, causing acidosis. Bicarbonate is moderately increased, but a primary increase in $NaHCO_3$ causes alkalosis. Thus, the cause of this acidosis is CO_2 retention (respiratory acidosis), and it is partially compensated for by renal retention of bicarbonate.

18. A patient's blood gas results are:

    pH = 7.50; P_{CO_2} = 55 mm Hg; HCO_3^- = 40 mmol/L

    These results indicate:
    A. Respiratory acidosis
    B. Metabolic alkalosis
    C. Respiratory alkalosis
    D. Metabolic acidosis

    Chemistry/Evaluate laboratory data to recognize health and disease states/Acid-base/3

19. Which set of results is consistent with uncompensated metabolic acidosis?
    A. pH 7.34 HCO_3 18 mmol/L P_{CO_2} 32 mm Hg
    B. pH 7.25 HCO_3 15 mmol/L P_{CO_2} 35 mm Hg
    C. pH 7.30 HCO_3 16 mmol/L P_{CO_2} 28 mm Hg
    D. pH 7.45 HCO_3 22 mmol/L P_{CO_2} 40 mm Hg

    Chemistry/Evaluate laboratory data to recognize health and disease states/Acid-base/3

20. Which of the following will shift the O_2 dissociation curve to the left?
    A. Anemia
    B. Hyperthermia
    C. Hypercapnia
    D. Alkalosis

    Chemistry/Calculate clinical and laboratory data/Blood gas/2

21. Which would be consistent with partially compensated respiratory acidosis?

	pH	P_{CO_2}	Bicarbonate
A.	increased	increased	increased
B.	increased	decreased	decreased
C.	decreased	decreased	decreased
D.	decreased	increased	increased

    Chemistry/Evaluate laboratory data to recognize health and disease states/3

22. Which condition results in metabolic acidosis with severe hypokalemia and chronic alkaline urine?
    A. Diabetic ketoacidosis
    B. Phenformin-induced acidosis
    C. Renal tubular acidosis
    D. Acidosis caused by starvation

    Chemistry/Correlate clinical and laboratory data/Acid-base and electrolytes/2

Answers to Questions 18–22

18. **B** A pH above 7.45 corresponds with alkalosis. Both bicarbonate and P_{CO_2} are elevated. Bicarbonate is the conjugate base and is under metabolic (renal) control, whereas P_{CO_2} is an acid and is under respiratory control. Increased bicarbonate (but not increased CO_2) results in alkalosis; therefore, the classification is metabolic alkalosis, partially compensated for by increased P_{CO_2}.

19. **B** Metabolic acidosis is caused by bicarbonate deficit. If uncompensated, the respiratory system is not excreting CO_2 at an increased rate; pH and bicarbonate are low, but P_{CO_2} is normal.

20. **D** A left shift in the oxyhemoglobin dissociation curve signifies an increase in the affinity of Hgb for O_2. This occurs in alkalosis, hypothermia, and in those hemoglobinopathies such as Hgb Chesapeake that increase the binding of O_2 to heme. A right shift in the oxyhemoglobin dissociation curve lowers the affinity of Hgb for O_2. This occurs in anemia caused by increased 2,3-diphosphoglycerate (2,3-DPG), with increased body temperature, increased hydrogen ion concentration, and hypercapnia (increased P_{CO_2}) and in some hemoglobinopathies, such as Hgb Kansas.

21. **D** Acidosis = low pH; respiratory = disturbance of P_{CO_2}; a low pH is caused by increased P_{CO_2}. In partially compensated respiratory acidosis, the metabolic component of the buffer system, bicarbonate, is retained. This helps to compensate for retention of P_{CO_2} by titrating hydrogen ions. The compensatory component always moves in the same direction as the cause of the acid-base disturbance.

22. **C** Metabolic acidosis can be caused by any condition that lowers bicarbonate. In nonrenal causes the kidneys will attempt to compensate by increased acid excretion. However, in renal tubular acidosis (RTA), an intrinsic defect in the tubules prevents bicarbonate reabsorption. This causes alkaline instead of acidic urine. Excretion of bicarbonate as potassium bicarbonate ($KHCO_3$) results in severe hypokalemia.

23. Which of the following mechanisms is responsible for metabolic acidosis?
    A. Bicarbonate deficiency
    B. Excessive retention of dissolved CO_2
    C. Accumulation of volatile acids
    D. Hyperaldosteronism

    Chemistry/Apply knowledge of fundamental biological characteristics/Acid-base/1

24. Which of the following disorders is associated with lactate acidosis?
    A. Diarrhea
    B. Renal tubular acidosis
    C. Hypoaldosteronism
    D. Alcoholism

    Chemistry/Correlate clinical and laboratory data/Acid-base/2

25. Which of the following is the primary mechanism of compensation for metabolic acidosis?
    A. Hyperventilation
    B. Release of epinephrine
    C. Aldosterone release
    D. Bicarbonate excretion

    Chemistry/Apply knowledge of fundamental biological characteristics/Acid-base/2

26. The conditions below are all causes of alkalosis. Which condition is associated with *respiratory* (rather than metabolic) alkalosis?
    A. Anxiety
    B. Hypovolemia
    C. Hyperaldosteronism
    D. Hypoparathyroidism

    Chemistry/Correlate clinical and laboratory data/Acid-base/2

27. Which of the following conditions is associated with both metabolic and respiratory alkalosis?
    A. Hyperchloremia
    B. Hypernatremia
    C. Hyperphosphatemia
    D. Hypokalemia

    Chemistry/Correlate clinical and laboratory data/Acid-base/2

28. In uncompensated metabolic acidosis, which of the following is normal?
    A. Plasma bicarbonate
    B. P_{CO_2}
    C. p50
    D. Total CO_2

    Chemistry/Correlate clinical and laboratory data/Acid-base/2

Answers to Questions 23–28

23. **A** Metabolic acidosis is caused by bicarbonate deficiency and metabolic alkalosis by bicarbonate excess. Respiratory acidosis is caused by P_{CO_2} retention (defective ventilation), and respiratory alkalosis is caused by P_{CO_2} loss (hyperventilation). Important causes of metabolic acidosis include renal failure, diabetic ketoacidosis, lactate acidosis, and diarrhea.

24. **D** Lactate acidosis often results from hypoxia, which causes a deficit of nicotinamide adenine dinucleotide, the oxidized form (NAD^+). This promotes the reduction of pyruvate to lactate, regenerating NAD^+ needed for glycolysis. In alcoholic acidosis, oxidation of ethanol to acetaldehyde consumes the NAD^+. In diabetes, lactate acidosis can result from depletion of Krebs cycle intermediates. Diarrhea and renal tubular acidosis result in metabolic acidosis via bicarbonate loss. Hypoaldosteronism causes metabolic acidosis via hydrogen and potassium ion retention.

25. **A** In metabolic acidosis the respiratory center is stimulated by chemoreceptors in the carotid sinus causing hyperventilation. This results in increased release of CO_2. Respiratory compensation begins almost immediately unless blocked by pulmonary disease or respiratory therapy. Hyperventilation can bring the P_{CO_2} down to approximately 10–15 mm Hg.

26. **A** Respiratory alkalosis is caused by hyperventilation, which leads to decreased P_{CO_2}. Anxiety and drugs such as epinephrine that stimulate the respiratory center are common causes of respiratory alkalosis. Excess aldosterone increases net acid excretion by the kidneys. Low parathyroid hormone causes increased bicarbonate reabsorption, resulting in alkalosis. Hypovolemia increases the relative concentration of bicarbonate. This is common and is termed dehydrational alkalosis, chloride responsive alkalosis, or alkalosis of sodium deficit.

27. **D** Hypokalemia is both a cause and result of alkalosis. In alkalosis hydrogen ions may move from the cells into the extracellular fluid and potassium into the cells. In hypokalemia caused by overproduction of aldosterone, hydrogen ions are secreted by the renal tubules. This increase in net acid excretion results in metabolic alkalosis.

28. **B** The normal compensatory mechanism for metabolic acidosis is respiratory hyperventilation. In uncompensated cases, the P_{CO_2} is not reduced, indicating a concomitant problem in respiratory control.

29. Which of the following conditions is classified as normochloremic acidosis?
A. Diabetic ketoacidosis
B. Chronic pulmonary obstruction
C. Uremic acidosis
D. Diarrhea

Chemistry/Correlate clinical and laboratory data/Acid-base/2

30. Which P_{CO_2} value would be seen in maximally compensated metabolic acidosis?
A. 15 mm Hg
B. 30 mm Hg
C. 40 mm Hg
D. 60 mm Hg

Chemistry/Evaluate laboratory data to recognize health and disease states/Blood gas/3

31. A patient has the following arterial blood gas results:

pH 7.56 P_{CO_2} 25 mm Hg P_{O_2} 100 mm Hg
HCO_3^- 22 mmol/L

These results are most likely the result of which condition?
A. Improper specimen collection
B. Prolonged storage
C. Hyperventilation
D. Hypokalemia

Chemistry/Evaluate laboratory data to recognize health and disease states/Acid-base/3

32. Why are three levels used for quality control of pH and blood gases?
A. Systematic errors can be detected earlier than with two controls
B. Analytical accuracy needs to be greater than for other analytes
C. High, normal, and low ranges must always be evaluated
D. A different level is needed for pH, P_{CO_2}, and P_{O_2}

Chemistry/Select appropriate controls/Acid-base/2

33. A single-point calibration is performed between each blood gas sample in order to:
A. Correct the electrode slope
B. Correct electrode and instrument drift
C. Compensate for temperature variance
D. Prevent contamination by the previous sample

Chemistry/Apply knowledge of standard operating procedures/Blood gas/2

34. In which condition would hypochloremia be expected?
A. Respiratory alkalosis
B. Metabolic acidosis
C. Metabolic alkalosis
D. All of the above

Chemistry/Correlate clinical and laboratory data/Blood gas electrolytes/2

Answers to Questions 29–34

29. **A** Bicarbonate deficit leads to hyperchloremia unless the bicarbonate is replaced by an unmeasured anion. In diabetic ketoacidosis, acetoacetate and other ketoacids replace bicarbonate. The chloride remains normal or low and there is an increased anion gap.

30. **A** In metabolic acidosis, hyperventilation increases the ratio of bicarbonate to dissolved CO_2. The extent of compensation is limited by the rate of both gas diffusion and diaphragm contraction. The lower limit is between 10 and 15 mm Hg P_{CO_2}, which is the maximum compensatory effect.

31. **C** The pH is alkaline (reference range 7.35–7.45), and this can be caused either by low P_{CO_2} or by increased bicarbonate levels. This patient has a normal bicarbonate reading (reference range 21–28 mmol/L) and a low P_{CO_2} (reference range 35–45 mm Hg). Low P_{CO_2} is always caused by hyperventilation, and therefore this is a case of uncompensated respiratory alkalosis. The acute stages of respiratory disorders are often uncompensated. Prolonged storage would cause the pH and P_{O_2} to fall and the P_{CO_2} to rise. Hypokalemia causes alkalosis, but it usually is associated with the retention of CO_2 as compensation.

32. **A** Error detection occurs sooner when more controls are used. Some errors, such as those resulting from temperature error and protein coating of electrodes, are not as pronounced near the calibration point, as in the acidosis and alkalosis range. The minimum requirement for blood gas quality control is one sample every 8 hours and three levels (acidosis, normal, alkalosis) every 24 hours. Three levels of control are also commonly used for therapeutic drug monitoring and hormone assays because precision differs significantly in the high and low ranges.

33. **B** Calibration using a single standard corrects the instrument for error at the labeled value of the calibrator but does not correct for analytic errors away from the set-point. A two-point calibration adjusts the slope response of the electrode, eliminating proportional error caused by poor electrode performance.

34. **C** Chloride is the major extracellular anion and is retained or lost to preserve electroneutrality. Low chloride levels occur in metabolic alkalosis because excess bicarbonate is retained. They also occur in partially compensated respiratory acidosis because the kidneys compensate by increased retention of bicarbonate.

35. Given the following serum electrolyte data, determine the anion gap.

$Na = 132$ mmol/L; $Cl = 90$ mmol/L; $HCO_3^- = 22$ mmol/L

A. 12 mmol/L
B. 20 mmol/L
C. 64 mmol/L
D. Cannot be determined from the information provided

Chemistry/Calculate/Electrolytes/2

36. Which of the following conditions will cause an increased anion gap?
A. Diarrhea
B. Hypoaldosteronism
C. Hyperkalemia
D. Renal failure

Chemistry/Correlate clinical and laboratory data/Electrolytes/2

37. Alcoholism, liver failure, and hypoxia induce acidosis by causing:
A. Depletion of cellular NAD$^+$
B. Increased excretion of bicarbonate
C. Increased retention of P_{CO_2}
D. Loss of carbonic anhydrase

Chemistry/Apply knowledge of fundamental biological characteristics/Acid-base/2

38. Which of the following is the primary mechanism causing respiratory alkalosis?
A. Hyperventilation
B. Deficient alveolar diffusion
C. Deficient pulmonary perfusion
D. Parasympathetic inhibition

Chemistry/Apply knowledge of fundamental biological characteristics/Acid-base/2

39. Excessive administration of oxygen can cause which of the following conditions?
A. Acidosis
B. O_2 saturation of Hgb approaching 100%
C. Optic nerve damage
D. All of the above

Chemistry/Correlate clinical and laboratory data/Blood gas/2

Answers to Questions 35–39

35. **B** The anion gap is defined as unmeasured anions minus unmeasured cations. It is calculated by subtracting the measured anions (bicarbonate and chloride) from the serum sodium (or sodium plus potassium). A normal anion gap is approximately 8–16 mmol/L.

Anion gap $= Na - (HCO_3 + Cl)$
Anion gap $= 132 - (90 + 22) = 20$ mmol/L

36. **D** An increased anion gap occurs when there is production or retention of anions other than bicarbonate or chloride (measured anions). For example, in renal failure retention of phosphates and sulfates (such as sodium salts) increases the anion gap. Other common causes of metabolic acidosis with an increased anion gap are diabetic ketoacidosis and lactate acidosis. The anion gap may also be increased in the absence of an acid-base disorder. Common causes include hypocalcemia, drug overdose, and laboratory error when measuring electrolytes.

37. **A** Oxygen debt and liver failure block oxidative phosphorylation, preventing nicotinamide adenine dinucleotide, the reduced form (NADH), from being oxidized back to NAD$^+$. Oxidation of ethanol to acetate results in accumulation of NADH. When NAD$^+$ is depleted, glycolysis cannot proceed. It is regenerated by reduction of pyruvate to lactate, causing lactic acidosis.

38. **A** Hyperventilation via stimulation of the respiratory center (or induced by a respirator) is the mechanism of respiratory alkalosis. Causes include low P_{O_2}, anxiety, fever, and drugs that stimulate the respiratory center. Acute respiratory alkalosis is often uncompensated for because renal compensation is not rapid. Uncompensated respiratory alkalosis is characterized by an elevated pH and a low P_{CO_2} with normal bicarbonate levels.

39. **D** When O_2 saturation of venous blood is greatly elevated, Hgb cannot release O_2. Oxyhemoglobin cannot bind CO_2 or hydrogen ions and acidosis results. Pure O_2 may cause neurological damage, leading to convulsions and blindness, especially in infants. It can induce respiratory failure by causing pulmonary hemorrhage, edema, and hyalinization.

40. Which of the following conditions is associated with an increase in ionized calcium (Ca_I) in the blood?
A. Alkalosis
B. Hypoparathyroidism
C. Hyperalbuminemia
D. Malignancy

Chemistry/Correlate clinical and laboratory data/ Electrolytes/2

41. Which of the following laboratory results is consistent with primary hypoparathyroidism?
A. Low calcium; high inorganic phosphorus (P_i)
B. Low calcium; low P_i
C. High calcium; high P_i
D. High calcium; low P_i

Chemistry/Correlate clinical and laboratory data/ Electrolytes/2

42. Which of the following conditions is associated with hypophosphatemia?
A. Rickets
B. Multiple myeloma
C. Renal failure
D. Hypervitaminosis D

Chemistry/Correlate laboratory data with physiological processes/Electrolytes/2

43. Which of the following test results is a specific marker for osteoporosis?
A. High urinary calcium
B. High serum P_i
C. Low serum calcium
D. High urine or serum N-telopeptide of type I collagen

Chemistry/Correlate laboratory data with physiological processes/Electrolytes/2

40. **D** Increased Ca_I occurs in hyperparathyroidism, malignancy, and acidosis. Ca_I is elevated in primary hyperparathyroidism as a result of resorption of calcium from bone. Many nonparathyroid malignancies create products called parathyroid hormone–related proteins that stimulate the parathyroid receptors of cells. Acidosis alters the equilibrium between bound and free calcium, favoring ionization. Hyperalbuminemia increases the total calcium by increasing the protein-bound fraction but does not affect the Ca_I.

41. **A** Parathyroid deficiency causes reduced resorption of calcium from bone, increased renal excretion of calcium, and decreased renal excretion of phosphorus. It is distinguished from other causes of hypocalcemia by Ca_I, which is reduced only by primary hypoparathyroidism and alkalosis.

42. **A** Rickets can result from dietary phosphate deficiency, vitamin D deficiency, or an inherited disorder of either vitamin D or phosphorus metabolism. Vitamin D–dependent rickets (VDDR) can be reversed by megadoses of vitamin D. Type I is caused by a deficiency in renal cells of 1-α-hydroxylase, an enzyme that converts 25 hydroxyvitamin D to the active form, 1,25 hydroxyvitamin D. Type II is caused by a deficiency in the vitamin D receptor of bone tissue. Vitamin D–resistant rickets (VDRR) is caused by a deficiency in the renal reabsorption of phosphate. Consequently, affected persons (usually men because it is most commonly X-linked) have a normal serum calcium level and a low P_i.

43. **D** Commonly used markers for other bone diseases such as serum or urinary calcium, P_i, alkaline phosphatase (ALP), and vitamin D are neither sensitive nor specific for osteoporosis. Calcium and phosphorus are usually within normal limits. Although estrogen deficiency reduces the formation of 1,25 hydroxyvitamin D (1,25 hydroxycholecalciferol), promoting postmenopausal osteoporosis, the 1,25 hydroxyvitamin D is low in only 30%–35% of cases, and low levels may be caused by other bone disorders. N-telopeptide of type 1 collagen or NTx (N-terminal cross-linked telopeptide of type 1 collagen) is released from bone during resorption. Serum markers for osteoporosis include both NTx and C-telopeptide of type 1 collagen or CTx (which is cross-linked at its C-terminus). These can be used to follow treatment with resorption antagonists (bisphosphonates) because they decrease significantly when therapy is successful.

44. The serum level of which of the following laboratory tests is decreased in both VDDR and VDRR?
   A. Vitamin D
   B. Calcium
   C. P_i
   D. Parathyroid hormone

Chemistry/Correlate laboratory data with physiological processes/Electrolytes/2

45. Which of the following is the most accurate measurement of P_i in serum?
   A. Rate of unreduced phosphomolybdate formation at 340 nm
   B. Measurement of phosphomolybdenum blue at 680 nm
   C. Use of aminonaptholsulfonic acid to reduce phosphomolybdate
   D. Formation of a complex with malachite green dye

Chemistry/Apply principles of basic laboratory procedures/Biochemical/2

46. What is the percentage of serum calcium that is ionized (Ca_I)?
   A. 30%
   B. 45%
   C. 60%
   D. 80%

Chemistry/Apply knowledge of fundamental biological characteristics/Electrolytes/1

47. Which of the following conditions will cause erroneous Ca_I results? Assume that the samples are collected and stored anaerobically, kept at 4°C until measurement, and stored for no longer than 1 hour.
   A. Slight hemolysis during venipuncture
   B. Assay of whole blood collected in sodium oxalate
   C. Analysis of serum in a barrier gel tube stored at 4°C until the clot has formed
   D. Analysis of whole blood collected in sodium heparin, 20 U/mL (low heparin tube)

Chemistry/Apply knowledge to recognize sources of error/Specimen collection and handling/3

48. Which of the following conditions is associated with a low serum magnesium determination?
   A. Addison's disease
   B. Hemolytic anemia
   C. Hyperparathyroidism
   D. Pancreatitis

Chemistry/Correlate clinical and laboratory data/ Electrolytes/2

44. **C** Persons with VDDR and VDRR have a low P_i. However, persons with VDDR have decreased calcium as well. Parathyroid hormone (PTH) is increased in persons with VDDR because calcium is the primary stimulus for PTH release but not in persons with VDRR. Vitamin D levels vary, depending upon the type of rickets and the vitamin D metabolite that is measured. 1,25-Hydroxyvitamin D (calcitriol) is the active form of vitamin D. It is low in type I but high in type II VDDR. It may be either normal or low in VDRR.

45. **A** The colorimetric method (Fiske and Subba-Row) used previously for P_i reacted ammonium molybdate with P_i, forming ammonium phosphomolybdate ($NH_4)_3[PMo_3O_{12}]$). A reducing agent, aminonaptholsulfonic acid (ANS), was added, forming phosphomolybdenum blue. The product was unstable and required sulfuric acid, making precipitation of protein a potential source of error. These problems are avoided by measuring the rate of formation of unreduced phosphomolybdate at 340 nm.

46. **B** Calcium exists in serum in three forms: protein-bound, ionized, and complexed (as undissociated salts). Only Ca_I is physiologically active. Protein-bound calcium and Ca_I each account for approximately 45% of total calcium, and the remaining 10% is complexed. The term "free" calcium refers to the sum of complexed and Ca_I.

47. **B** Unlike P_i, the intracellular calcium level is not significantly different from that of plasma calcium, and calcium is not greatly affected by diet. Whole blood collected with 5–20 U/mL heparin and stored on ice no longer than 2 hours is the sample of choice for Ca_I. Blood gas syringes prefilled with 100 U/mL heparin should not be used because the high heparin concentration causes low results. Citrate, oxalate, and ethylenediaminetetraacetic acid (EDTA) must not be used because they chelate calcium. Serum may be used provided that the sample is iced, kept capped while clotting, and assayed within 2 hours (barrier gel tubes may be stored longer).

48. **D** Low magnesium can be caused by gastrointestinal loss, as occurs in diarrhea and pancreatitis (loss of Mg and Ca as soaps). Hyperparathyroidism causes increased release of both calcium and magnesium from bone. Addison's disease (adrenocorticosteroid deficiency) may be associated with increased magnesium accompanying hyperkalemia. Hemolytic anemia causes increased release of magnesium as well as of potassium from damaged red blood cells (RBCs).

49. When measuring calcium with a complexometric dye, magnesium is kept from interfering by
- **A.** Using an alkaline pH
- **B.** Adding 8-hydroxyquinoline
- **C.** Measuring at 450 nm
- **D.** Complexing to EDTA

Chemistry/Apply principles of basic laboratory procedures/Biochemical/1

50. Which electrolyte measurement is *LEAST* affected by hemolysis?
- **A.** Potassium
- **B.** Calcium
- **C.** P_i
- **D.** Magnesium

Chemistry/Apply knowledge to recognize sources of error/Specimen collection and handling/2

51. Which of the following conditions is associated with hypokalemia?
- **A.** Addison's disease
- **B.** Hemolytic anemia
- **C.** Digoxin intoxication
- **D.** Alkalosis

Chemistry/Correlate clinical and laboratory data/Electrolytes/2

52. Which of the following conditions is most likely to produce an elevated plasma potassium level?
- **A.** Hypoparathyroidism
- **B.** Cushing's syndrome
- **C.** Diarrhea
- **D.** Digitalis overdose

Chemistry/Correlate clinical and laboratory data/Electrolytes/2

53. Which of the following values is the threshold critical value (alert or action level) for low plasma potassium?
- **A.** 1.5 mmol/L
- **B.** 2.0 mmol/L
- **C.** 2.5 mmol/L
- **D.** 3.5 mmol/L

Chemistry/Apply knowledge of fundamental biological characteristics/Electrolytes/1

Answers to Questions 49–53

49. **B** Complexometric dyes such as *o*-cresolphthalein complexone can be used to measure either magnesium or calcium. Interference in calcium assays is prevented by addition of 8-hydroxyquinoline, which chelates magnesium. When magnesium is measured, ethylene glycol tetraacetic acid (EGTA) or EDTA is used to chelate calcium. Dyes often used for both magnesium and calcium assay are calmagite and methylthymol blue. Arsenazo III dye is commonly used to measure calcium. It is more specific for Ca^{2+} than the others and does not require addition of an Mg^{2+} chelator.

50. **B** Potassium, phosphorus, and magnesium are the major intracellular ions, and even slight hemolysis will cause falsely elevated results. Serum samples with visible hemolysis (20 mg/dL free Hgb) should be redrawn.

51. **D** Addison's disease, adrenocortical insufficiency, results in low levels of adrenal corticosteroid hormones, including aldosterone and cortisol. Because these hormones promote reabsorption of sodium and secretion of potassium by the collecting tubules, patients with Addison's disease display hyperkalemia and hyponatremia. Hemolytic anemia and digoxin intoxication cause release of intracellular potassium. Alkalosis causes potassium to move from the extracellular fluid into the cells as hydrogen ions move from the cells into the extracellular fluid to compensate for alkalosis.

52. **D** Digitalis toxicity causes potassium to leave the cells and enter the extracellular fluid, resulting in hyperkalemia. Parathyroid disease affects calcium, phosphorus, and magnesium levels but not potassium. Cushing's syndrome (adrenal cortical hyperfunction) results in low potassium and elevated sodium levels. Diarrhea causes loss of sodium and potassium. Renal failure, hemolytic anemia, and Addison's disease are other frequent causes of hyperkalemia.

53. **C** The reference range for potassium is 3.6–5.4 mmol/L. However, values below 2.5 mmol/L require immediate intervention because there is a grave risk of cardiac arrhythmia, which can lead to cardiac arrest. The upper alert level for potassium is usually 6.5 mmol/L, except for neonatal and hemolyzed samples. Above this level there is danger of cardiac failure.

54. Which electrolyte is *LEAST* likely to be elevated in renal failure?
A. Potassium
B. Magnesium
C. Inorganic phosphorus
D. Sodium

Chemistry/Correlate clinical and laboratory data/ Electrolytes/2

55. Which of the following is the primary mechanism for vasopressin (ADH) release?
A. Hypovolemia
B. Hyperosmolar plasma
C. Renin release
D. Reduced renal blood flow

Chemistry/Apply knowledge of fundamental biological characteristics/Osmolality/2

56. Which of the following conditions is associated with hypernatremia?
A. Diabetes insipidus
B. Hypoaldosteronism
C. Burns
D. Diarrhea

Chemistry/Correlate clinical and laboratory data/ Electrolytes/2

57. Which of the following values is the threshold critical value (alert or action level) for high plasma sodium?
A. 150 mmol/L
B. 160 mmol/L
C. 170 mmol/L
D. 180 mmol/L

Chemistry/Apply knowledge of fundamental biological characteristics/Electrolytes/1

Answers to Questions 54–57

54. **D** Reduced glomerular filtration coupled with decreased tubular secretion causes accumulation of potassium, magnesium, and inorganic phosphorus. Poor tubular reabsorption of sodium offsets reduced glomerular filtration. Unfiltered sodium draws both chloride and water, causing osmotic equilibration between filtrate, serum, and the tissues. In renal disease, serum sodium is often normal, although total body sodium is increased as a result of fluid and salt retention.

55. **B** Antidiuretic hormone (ADH) is released by the posterior pituitary gland in response to increased plasma osmolality. Normally, this is triggered by release of aldosterone caused by ineffective arterial pressure in the kidney. Aldosterone causes sodium reabsorption, which raises plasma osmolality; release of ADH causes reabsorption of water, which increases blood volume and restores normal osmolality. A deficiency of ADH, diabetes insipidus, results in dehydration and hypernatremia. An excess of ADH, syndrome of inappropriate ADH release (SIADH), results in dilutional hyponatremia. This may be caused by regional hypovolemia, hypothyroidism, central nervous system injury, drugs, or malignancy.

56. **A** Diabetes insipidus results from failure to produce ADH. Because the collecting tubules are impermeable to water in the absence of ADH, severe hypovolemia and dehydration result. Hypovolemia stimulates aldosterone release, causing sodium reabsorption, which worsens the hypernatremia. Burns, hypoaldosteronism, diarrhea, and diuretic therapy are common causes of hyponatremia.

57. **B** The adult reference range for plasma sodium is approximately 135–145 mmol/L. Levels in excess of 160 mmol/L are associated with severe dehydration, hypovolemia, and circulatory and heart failure. The threshold for the low critical value for sodium is 120 mmol/L. This is associated with edema, hypervolemia, and circulatory overload. Alert levels must also be established for potassium, bicarbonate, calcium, pH, pO_2, glucose, bilirubin, hemoglobin, platelet count, and prothrombin time. When a sample result is below or above the low or high alert level, the physician must be notified immediately.

58. Which of the following conditions is more often associated with total body sodium excess than hypernatremia?

A. Renal failure

B. Hyperthyroidism

C. Hypoparathyroidism

D. Diabetic ketoacidosis

Chemistry/Correlate clinical and laboratory data/ Electrolytes/2

59. Which of the following conditions is associated with hyponatremia?

A. Diuretic therapy

B. Cushing's syndrome

C. Diabetes insipidus

D. Nephrotic syndrome

Chemistry/Correlate clinical and laboratory data/ Electrolytes/2

60. Which of the following conditions involving electrolytes is described correctly?

A. Pseudohyponatremia occurs only when undiluted samples are measured

B. Potassium levels are slightly higher in heparinized plasma than in serum

C. Hypoalbuminemia causes low total calcium but does not affect Ca_I

D. Hypercalcemia may be induced by low serum magnesium

Chemistry/Correlate clinical and laboratory data/ Electrolytes/2

58. **A** Total body sodium excess often occurs in persons with renal failure, congestive heart failure, and cirrhosis of the liver. When water is retained along with sodium, total body sodium excess results rather than hypernatremia. Heart failure causes sodium and water retention by reducing blood flow to the kidneys. Cirrhosis causes obstruction of hepatic lymphatics and portal veins leading to local hypertension and accumulation of ascites fluid. Renal failure results in poor glomerular filtration and isosmotic equilibration of salt and water.

59. **A** Diuretics lower blood pressure by promoting water loss. This is accomplished by causing sodium loss from the proximal tubule and/or loop. Addison's disease, SIADH, burns, diabetic ketoacidosis, hypopituitarism, vomiting, diarrhea, and cystic fibrosis also cause hyponatremia. Cushing's syndrome causes hypernatremia by promoting sodium reabsorption in the collecting tubule in exchange for potassium. Diabetes insipidus and nephrotic syndrome promote hypernatremia by causing water loss.

60. **C** When serum albumin is low, the equilibrium between bound and Ca_I is shifted, producing increased Ca_I. This inhibits release of parathyroid hormone (PTH) by negative feedback until the Ca_I level returns to normal. Potassium is released from platelets and leukocytes during coagulation, causing serum levels to be higher than plasma. Pseudohyponatremia is caused by the displacement of plasma water by fat and occurs whenever samples are diluted before measurement because the dilution is affected by the volume of fat in the sample. Only ion-selective electrodes that measure whole blood or undiluted serum are not affected. Magnesium is needed for release of PTH, and PTH causes release of calcium and magnesium from bone. Therefore, hypocalcemia can be associated with either magnesium deficiency or magnesium excess.

61. Which of the following laboratory results is usually associated with cystic fibrosis?
   A. Sweat chloride levels higher than 65 mmol/L
   B. Elevated serum sodium and chloride levels
   C. Elevated fecal trypsin activity
   D. Low glucose level

Chemistry/Evaluate laboratory data to recognize health and disease states/Electrolytes/2

62. When performing a sweat chloride collection, which of the following steps will result in analytical error?
   A. Using unweighed gauze soaked in pilocarpine nitrate on the inner surface of the forearm
   B. Using unweighed gauze soaked in saline on the outside of the arm
   C. Leaving the preweighed gauze on the inside of the arm exposed to air during collection
   D. Rinsing the collected sweat from the gauze pad using chloride titrating solution

Chemistry/Apply knowledge to recognize sources of error/Specimen collection and handling/3

63. Which electrolyte level best correlates with plasma osmolality?
   A. Sodium
   B. Chloride
   C. Bicarbonate
   D. Calcium

Chemistry/Apply knowledge of fundamental biological characteristics/Electrolytes/2

64. Which formula is most accurate in predicting plasma osmolality?
   A. $Na + 2(Cl) + BUN + glucose$
   B. $2(Na) + 2(Cl) + glucose + urea$
   C. $2(Na) + (glucose \div 18) + (BUN \div 2.8)$
   D. $Na + Cl + K + HCO_3$

Chemistry/Calculate/Osmolality/2

61. A Cystic fibrosis causes obstruction of the exocrine glands, including the sweat glands, mucus glands, and pancreas. Newborns with pancreatic involvement demonstrate fecal trypsin deficiency, which may be detected by a low fecal chymotrypsin or high blood immunoreactive trypsin result. However, these tests require confirmation. Serum sodium and chloride levels are low. More than 98% of affected infants have elevated sweat sodium and chloride and low serum levels. Sweat chloride levels in excess of 65 mmol/L confirm the clinical diagnosis. Some persons with the disease have insulin deficiency and elevated blood glucose levels. Genetic tests are now available to detect several mutations that occur at the cystic fibrosis transmembrane conductance regulator (CFTR) locus on chromosome 7.

62. C The sweat chloride procedure requires the application of pilocarpine to stimulate sweating, and the use of iontophoresis (application of 0.16-mA current for 5 minutes) to bring the sweat to the surface. The only gauze that needs to be preweighed is the pair of 2-in² pads that are applied to the skin after iontophoresis. During the 30-minute collection of sweat, the gauze must be completely covered to prevent contamination and loss of sweat by evaporation. The Gibson-Cooke reference method for sweat chloride uses the Schales and Schales method (titration by $Hg[NO_3]_2$ with diphenylcarbazone indicator) to assay 1.0 mL of sweat eluted from the gauze with 5 mL of water. A Cotlove chloridometer is often used to measure sweat chloride. The sweat is eluted from the gauze with the titrating solution to facilitate measurement. Alternatively, a macroduct collection system may be used that does not require weighing.

63. A Sodium and chloride are the major extracellular ions. Chloride passively follows sodium, making sodium the principal determinant of plasma osmolality.

64. C Calculated plasma osmolality is based on measurement of sodium, glucose, and urea. Because sodium associates with a counter ion, two times the sodium estimates the millimoles per liter of sodium and anions. Some laboratories multiply by 1.86 instead of 2 to correct for undissociated salts. Dividing glucose by 18 converts from milligrams per deciliter to millimoles per liter. Dividing blood urea nitrogen (BUN) by 2.8 converts from milligrams per deciliter BUN to millimoles per liter urea.

65. Which of the following conditions causes an increased osmolal gap?
  A. Diabetic ketoacidosis
  B. Drug overdose
  C. Renal failure
  D. All of the above

Chemistry/Correlate clinical and laboratory data/ Osmolality/2

65. D The osmolal gap is the difference between measured and calculated plasma osmolality. An osmolal gap exceeding 12 mOsm/kg is significant, and in emergency room settings it is a sensitive indicator of alcohol or drug overdose.

1. Which of the biochemical processes below is promoted by insulin?
   A. Glycogenolysis
   B. Gluconeogenesis
   C. Lipolysis
   D. Uptake of glucose by cells

   Chemistry/Apply knowledge of fundamental biological characteristics/Carbohydrate/1

2. Which of the following hormones promotes hyperglycemia?
   A. Calcitonin
   B. Growth hormone
   C. Aldosterone
   D. Renin

   Chemistry/Apply knowledge of fundamental biological characteristics/Carbohydrate/1

3. Which of the following is characteristic of type 1 diabetes mellitus?
   A. Requires an oral glucose tolerance test for diagnosis
   B. Is the most common form of diabetes mellitus
   C. Usually occurs after age 40
   D. Requires insulin replacement to prevent ketosis

   Chemistry/Correlate clinical and laboratory data/ Biological manifestation of disease/2

Answers to Questions 1–3

1. **D** Insulin reduces blood glucose levels by increasing glucose uptake by cells. It promotes lipid and glycogen production, induces synthesis of glycolytic enzymes, and inhibits the formation of glucose from pyruvate and Krebs cycle intermediates.

2. **B** Growth hormone and cortisol promote gluconeogenesis and epinephrine stimulates glycogenolysis. In addition to an excess of one of these three hormones, excess thyroid hormone also causes hyperglycemia by increasing insulin inactivation and glucagon (produced by some pancreatic tumors) by promoting both gluconeogenesis and glycogenolysis. All five may cause abnormal glucose tolerance. Calcitonin opposes the action of parathyroid hormone. Aldosterone is the primary mineralocorticoid hormone and stimulates sodium reabsorption and potassium secretion by the kidneys. Renin is released from the kidney as a result of ineffective arterial pressure and promotes aldosterone secretion and activation of angiotensinogen.

3. **D** Type 1 or juvenile diabetes is also termed insulin-dependent diabetes because patients must be given insulin to prevent ketosis. Type I accounts for only about 10%–20% of cases of diabetes mellitus and is usually diagnosed by a fasting plasma glucose level. Two consecutive results ≥ 126 mg/dL are diagnostic. Approximately 95% of patients produce autoantibodies against the β-cells of the pancreatic islets. Other autoantibodies may be produced against insulin, glutamate decarboxylase, and tyrosine phosphorylase IA2. There is genetic association between type I diabetes and human leukocyte antigens (HLA) DR3 and DR4.

4. Which of the following is characteristic of type 2 diabetes mellitus?

A. Insulin levels are consistently low

B. Most cases require a 3-hour oral glucose tolerance test to diagnose

C. Hyperglycemia is often controlled without insulin replacement

D. The condition is associated with unexplained weight loss

Chemistry/Correlate clinical and laboratory data/ Biological manifestation of disease/2

5. Which of the following results falls within the diagnostic criteria for diabetes mellitus?

A. Fasting plamsa glucose level of 120 mg/dL

B. Two-hour post-prandial plasma glucose of 160 mg/dL

C. Two-hour plasma glucose reading of 190 mg/dL following 75 g oral glucose challenge

D. Random plasma glucose of 250 mg/dL and presence of symptoms

Chemistry/Evaluate laboratory data to recognize health and disease states/Carbohydrate/2

6. Select the appropriate reference range for fasting blood glucose.

A. 40–100 mg/dL   (2.22–5.55 mmol/L)

B. 60–140 mg/dL   (3.33–7.77 mmol/L)

C. 65–99 mg/dL   (3.61–5.50 mmol/L)

D. 75–150 mg/dL   (4.16–8.32 mmol/L)

Chemistry/Apply knowledge of fundamental biological characteristics/Carbohydrate/1

7. When preparing a patient for an oral glucose tolerance test (OGTT), which of the following conditions will lead to erroneous results?

A. The patient remains ambulatory for 3 days prior to the test

B. Carbohydrate intake is restricted to below 150 g/day for 3 days prior to the test

C. No food, coffee, tea, or smoking is allowed 8 hours before and during the test

D. Administration of 75 g of glucose is given to an adult patient following a 10–12 hour fast

Chemistry/Apply knowledge to recognize sources of error/Glucose tolerance test/3

4. **C** Type 2 or *late-onset diabetes* is associated with a defect in the receptor site for insulin. Insulin levels may be low, normal, or high. The American Diabetes Association (ADA) recommends screening all adults over 45 years old for diabetes using the fasting glucose test every 3 years. Persons who exhibit major risk factors (family history, obesity, hypertension, abnormal blood lipids, impaired fasting glucose or glucose tolerance, gestational diabetes) should be screened starting at age 30 and tested more frequently. Patients do not require insulin to prevent ketosis, and hyperglycemia can be controlled in most patients by diet and drugs that promote insulin release. Patients are usually obese and over 40 years of age. Type 2 diabetes accounts for 80%–90% of all cases of diabetes mellitus.

5. **D** The American Diabetes Association recommends the following criteria for diagnosing diabetes mellitus: fasting glucose ≥126 mg/dL, casual (random) glucose ≥200 mg/dL in the presence of symptoms (polyuria, increased thirst, weight loss), glucose ≥200 mg/dL at 2 hours after an oral dose of 75 g of glucose. A diagnosis of diabetes mellitus is indicated if any one of these three criteria is met on more than a single occasion. The fasting plasma glucose test requires at least 8 hours with no food or drink except water. The 2-hour postloading test should be conducted according to the oral glucose tolerance guidelines currently recommended by the World Health Organization.

6. **C** Reference ranges vary slightly, depending upon method and specimen type. Enzymatic methods specific for glucose have an upper limit of normal no greater than 99 mg/dL. This is the cutoff value for impaired fasting plasma glucose (prediabetes) recommended by the American Diabetes Association. Although 65 mg/dL is considered the 2.5 percentile, a fasting level below 50 mg/dL is often seen without associated clinical hypoglycemia, and neonates have a lower limit of approximately 40 mg/dL because of maternal insulin.

7. **B** Standardized OGTTs require that patients receive at least 150 g of carbohydrate per day for 3 days prior to the test in order to stabilize the synthesis of inducible glycolytic enzymes. The 2-hour OGTT test is no longer recommended for screening and should be reserved for confirmation of diabetes in cases that are difficult to diagnose such as in persons who lack symptoms and signs of fasting hyperglycemia.

8. Which of the following 2-hour glucose challenge results would be classified as impaired glucose tolerance (IGT)?
Two-hour serum glucose

A. 130 mg/dL

B. 135 mg/dL

C. 150 mg/dL

D. 204 mg/dL

Chemistry/Evaluate laboratory data to recognize health and disease states/Glucose tolerance/2

9. Which statement regarding gestational diabetes mellitus (GDM) is correct?

A. It is diagnosed using the same oral glucose tolerance criteria as used in nonpregnancy

B. It converts to diabetes mellitus after pregnancy in 60%–75% of cases

C. It presents no increased health risk to the fetus

D. It is defined as glucose intolerance originating during pregnancy

Chemistry/Evaluate laboratory data to recognize health and disease states/Glucose tolerance test/2

10. Which of the following findings is characteristic of all forms of clinical hypoglycemia?

A. A fasting blood glucose value below 55 mg/dL

B. High fasting insulin levels

C. Neuroglycopenic symptoms at the time of low blood glucose values

D. Decreased serum C peptide

Chemistry/Correlate clinical and laboratory data/ Carbohydrate/2

11. Which statement regarding glycated (glycosylated) hemoglobin (G-Hgb) is true?

A. It has a sugar attached to the C-terminal end of the β-chain

B. It is a highly reversible aminoglycan

C. It reflects the extent of glucose regulation in the 8-to 12-week interval prior to sampling

D. It will be abnormal within 4 days following an episode of hyperglycemia

Chemistry/Correlate laboratory data with physiological processes/Carbohydrate/2

Answers to Questions 8–11

8. **C** With the exception of pregnant females, impaired glucose tolerance is defined by the ADA as a serum or plasma glucose of $\geq$140 mg/dL <200 mg/dL at 2 hours following a 75-g oral glucose load. Persons who have a fasting plasma glucose of $\geq$100 but < 126 mg/dL are classified as having impaired fasting glucose (IFG). Both IGT and IFG are risk factors for developing diabetes later in life.

9. **D** Control of GDM reduces perinatal complications such as respiratory distress syndrome, high birth weight, and neonatal jaundice. Women at risk are screened between 24 and 28 weeks' gestation. The screening test can be performed without fasting and consists of an oral 50 g glucose challenge followed by serum or plasma glucose measurement at one hour. A result of $\geq$140 mg/dL is followed by a 3-hour oral glucose tolerance test to confirm gestational diabetes. At least two of the following cutoff parameters must be exceeded: fasting, 105 mg/dL or higher; 1 hour, 190 mg/dL or higher; 2 hours, 165 mg/dL or higher; 3 hours, 145 mg/dL or higher. GDM converts to diabetes mellitus within 10 years in 30%–40% of cases.

10. **C** Clinical hypoglycemia can be caused by insulinoma, drugs, or reactive hypoglycemia. Reactive hypoglycemia is characterized by delayed or excessive insulin output after eating and is very rare. Fasting insulin is normal but postprandial levels are increased. High fasting insulin levels (usually >6 μg/L) are seen in insulinoma, and patients with insulinoma almost always display fasting hypoglycemia. C peptide is a subunit of proinsulin that is hydrolyzed when insulin is released. In hypoglycemia, low levels indicate an exogenous insulin source, whereas high levels indicate overproduction of insulin.

11. **C** G-Hgb results from the nonenzymatic attachment of a sugar such as glucose to the N-terminal valine of the β-chain. The reaction is nonreversible and is related to the time-averaged blood glucose concentration over the life span of the RBCs. There are three G-Hgb fractions designated A_{1a}, A_{1b}, and A_{1c}. Both total G-Hgb and A_{1c} are used to determine the adequacy of insulin therapy, since A_{1c} makes up about 80% of glycated hemoglobin. The time-averaged blood glucose is approximated by the formula (G-Hgb $\times$33.3) – 86 mg/dL, and insulin adjustments can be made to bring this level to within reference limits. Also, glycated protein assay (called fructosamine) provides similar data for the period between 2 and 4 weeks before sampling.

12. What is the American Diabetes Association's recommended cutoff value for adequate control of blood glucose as measured by glycated hemoglobin?
    A. 5%
    B. 7%
    C. 9%
    D. 11%

    Chemistry/Evaluate laboratory data to recognize health and disease states/Glucose/2

13. Which statement regarding measurement of G-Hgb is true?
    A. Levels do not need to be measured using fasting
    B. Affinity chromatography is more temperature-dependent than cation exchange
    C. Chromatography is the only technique that is clinically useful
    D. All methods measure the same G-Hgb fraction

    Chemistry/Apply knowledge to recognize sources of error/Carbohydrate/2

14. According to American Diabetes Association criteria, which result is consistent with a diagnosis of impaired fasting glucose?
    A. 99 mg/dL
    B. 117 mg/dL
    C. 126 mg/dL
    D. 135 mg/dL

    Chemistry/Evaluate laboratory data to recognize health and disease states/Glucose/2

15. What is the recommended cutoff for the early detection of chronic kidney disease in diabetics using the test for microalbuminuria?
    A. >30 mg/g creatinine
    B. >80 mg/g creatinine
    C. >200 mg/g creatinine
    D. >80 mg/L

    Chemistry/Evaluate laboratory data to recognize health and disease states/Glucose/2

16. Which testing situation is appropriate for the use of point-of-care whole blood glucose methods?
    A. Screening for type 2 diabetes mellitus
    B. Diagnosis of diabetes mellitus
    C. Monitoring of blood glucose control in types 1 and 2 diabetics
    D. Monitoring diabetics for hyperglycemic episodes only

    Chemistry/Select method/Carbohydrate/2

Answers to Questions 12–16

12. **B** The ADA recommends that 7% be used as the cutoff value for determining the adequacy of treatment for diabetes. A glycated hemoglobin test should be performed at the time of diagnosis and every 6 months thereafter if the result is ≤7%. If the result is greater than 8%, the treatment plan should be adjusted to achieve a lower level and the test performed every 3 months until control is improved.

13. **A** Since G-Hgb represents the average blood glucose 2–3 months prior to blood collection, the dietary status of the patient on the day of the test has no effect upon the results. G-Hgb can be assayed using cation exchange HPLC, weak affinity chromatography, immunoassay, or electrophoresis. The affinity column and HPLC methods are not subject to significant interference by temperature or the presence of abnormal hemoglobins. The affinity method uses aminophenylboronyl groups that form a diol bond with the glycated hemoglobins. The nonglycohemoglobins are washed from the column, and the total glycated hemoglobin is eluted with sorbitol.

14. **B** Impaired fasting glucose is defined as a plasma glucose ≥100 but <126 mg/dL. A fasting glucose of 126 or higher on two consecutive occasions indicates diabetes. A fasting glucose of 99 mg/dL is considered normal.

15. **A** Microalbuminuria is the excretion of small quantities of albumin in the urine. In diabetics, excretion of albumin that is within allowable limits for healthy persons may signal the onset of chronic kidney disease. The term microalbuminuria is defined as albumin excretion ≥ 30 mg/g creatinine but ≤ 300 mg/g creatinine. The use of the albumin to creatinine ratio is preferred to measures of albumin excretory rate (μg/min) because the latter is subject to error associated with timed specimen collection.

16. **C** The ADA does not recommend the use of whole blood glucose monitors for establishing a diagnosis of diabetes or screening persons for diabetes. The analytical measurement range of these devices varies greatly, and whole blood glucose is approximately 10% lower than serum or plasma glucose. In addition, analytical variance is greater and accuracy less than for laboratory instruments. Whole blood glucose meters should be used by diabetics and caregivers to monitor glucose control and can detect both hyper- and hypoglycemic states that result from too little or too much insulin replacement. Therefore, monitoring with such a device is recommended for all persons who receive insulin therapy.

17. Which of the following is the reference method for measuring serum glucose?
  A. Somogyi-Nelson
  B. Hexokinase
  C. Glucose oxidase
  D. Glucose dehydrogenase

Chemistry/Select method/Carbohydrate/2

18. Polarographic methods for glucose analysis are based upon which principle of measurement?
  A. Nonenzymatic oxidation of glucose
  B. The rate of O_2 depletion
  C. Chemiluminescence caused by the formation of adenosine triphosphate (ATP)
  D. The change in electrical potential as glucose is oxidized

Chemistry/Apply principles of basic laboratory procedures/Carbohydrate/2

19. Select the enzyme that is most specific for β-D-glucose.
  A. Hexokinase
  B. Glucose-6-phosphate dehydrogenase (G6PD)
  C. Phosphohexisomerase
  D. Glucose oxidase

Chemistry/Apply knowledge of fundamental biological characteristics/Biochemical/1

20. Select the coupling enzyme used in the hexokinase method for glucose.
  A. G6PD
  B. Peroxidase
  C. Glucose dehydrogenase
  D. Glucose-6-phosphatase

Chemistry/Apply knowledge of basic laboratory procedures/Carbohydrate/1

21. Which glucose method is subject to falsely low results caused by ascorbate?
  A. Hexokinase
  B. Glucose dehydrogenase
  C. Trinder glucose oxidase
  D. Polarography

Chemistry/Apply knowledge to recognize sources of error/Carbohydrate/2

Answers to Questions 17–21

17. **B** The hexokinase method is considered more accurate than glucose oxidase methods because the coupling reaction using G6PD is highly specific. The hexokinase method may be done on serum or plasma collected using heparin, EDTA, fluoride, oxalate, or citrate. The method can also be used for urine, cerebrospinal fluid, and serous fluids.

18. **B** Polarographic glucose electrodes measure the change in O_2 as glucose is oxidized. Glucose oxidase in the reagent catalyzes the oxidation of glucose by O_2 under first-order conditions, forming hydrogen peroxide (H_2O_2). The O_2-measuring electrode immersed in the reaction solution measures the decrease in O_2 in the solution. The hydrogen peroxide is prevented from re-forming O_2 by adding molybdate, iodide, catalase, and ethanol. Molybdate catalyzes the oxidation of iodide to iodine and water by peroxide. Catalase catalyzes the formation of acetaldehyde and water from peroxide and ethanol. As O_2 is consumed, the rate of current flow from the electrode decreases in proportion to glucose concentration. In other systems, the glucose oxidase is impregnated into the membrane covering the electrode. It reacts with glucose in the sample, forming H_2O_2. This diffuses across the membrane and breaks down forming O_2 and H_2O, which increase the current flow from the electrode.

19. **D** Glucose oxidase is the most specific enzyme reacting with only β-D-glucose. However, the peroxidase coupling reaction used in the glucose oxidase method is subject to positive and negative interference. Therefore, hexokinase is used in the reference method.

20. **A** The hexokinase reference method uses a protein-free filtrate prepared with barium hydroxide (BaOH) and zinc sulfate ($ZnSO_4$). Hexokinase catalyzes the phosphorylation of glucose in the filtrate using ATP as the phosphate donor. Glucose-6-phosphate (glucose-6-PO_4) is oxidized to 6-phosphogluconate, and NAD^+ is reduced to NADH using G6PD. The increase in absorbance at 340 nm is proportional to glucose concentration. Although hexokinase will phosphorylate some other hexoses, including mannose, fructose, and glucosamine, the coupling reaction is entirely specific for glucose-6-PO_4, eliminating interference from other sugars.

21. **C** Although glucose oxidase is specific for β-D-glucose, the coupling (indicator) reaction is prone to negative interference from ascorbate, uric acid, acetoacetic acid, and other reducing agents. These compete with dye (e.g., *o*-dianisidine) for peroxide, resulting in less dye being oxidized to chromophore.

22. Which of the following is a potential source of error in the hexokinase method?

A. Galactosemia

B. Hemolysis

C. Sample collected in fluoride

D. Ascorbic acid

Chemistry/Apply knowledge to recognize sources of error/Carbohydrate/2

23. Which statement about glucose in cerebrospinal fluid (CSF) is correct?

A. Levels below 40 mg/dL occur in septic meningitis, cancer, and multiple sclerosis

B. The CSF glucose level is normally the same as the plasma glucose level

C. Hyperglycorrhachia is caused by dehydration

D. In some clinical conditions, the CSF glucose level can be higher than the plasma glucose level

Chemistry/Correlate laboratory data with physiological processes/Cerebrospinal fluid/2

24. In peroxidase-coupled glucose methods, which reagent complexes with the chromogen?

A. Nitroprusside

B. Phenol

C. Tartrate

D. Hydroxide

Chemistry/Apply knowledge of basic laboratory procedures/Carbohydrate/1

25. Which of the following is classified as a mucopolysaccharide storage disease?

A. Pompe's disease

B. Von Gierke's disease

C. Hers' disease

D. Hurler's syndrome

Chemistry/Correlate clinical and laboratory data/Carbohydrates/1

26. Identify the enzyme deficiency responsible for type I glycogen storage disease (von Gierke's disease).

A. Glucose-6-phosphatase

B. Glycogen phosphorylase

C. Glycogen synthetase

D. β-Glucosidase

Chemistry/Correlate clinical and laboratory data/Carbohydrates/2

27. Which of the following abnormal laboratory results is found in von Gierke's disease?

A. Hyperglycemia

B. Increased glucose response to epinephrine administration

C. Metabolic alkalosis

D. Hyperlipidemia

Chemistry/Correlate clinical and laboratory data/Carbohydrate/2

22. **B** The hexokinase method can be performed on serum or plasma using heparin, EDTA, citrate, or oxalate. RBCs contain glucose-6-PO_4 and intracellular enzymes that generate NADH, causing positive interference. Therefore, hemolyzed samples require a serum blank correction (subtraction of the reaction rate with hexokinase omitted from the reagent).

23. **A** A high glucose value in CSF is a reflection of hyperglycemia and not central nervous system disease. The CSF glucose is usually 50%–65% of the plasma glucose. Low levels are significant and are most often associated with bacterial or fungal meningitis, malignancy in the central nervous system, and some cases of subarachnoid hemorrhage, rheumatoid meningitis, and multiple sclerosis.

24. **B** The coupling step in the Trinder glucose oxidase method uses peroxidase to catalyze the oxidation of a dye by H_2O_2. Dyes such as 4-aminophenozone or 4-aminoantipyrine are coupled to phenol to form a quinoneimine dye that is red and is measured at about 500 nm.

25. **D** Hurler's syndrome is an autosomal recessive disease resulting from a deficiency of iduronidase. Glycosaminoglycans (mucopolysaccharides) accumulate in the lysosomes. Multiple organ failure and mental retardation occur, resulting in early mortality. Excess heparin sulfate is excreted in urine. Other mucopolysaccharidoses (MPS storage diseases) are Hunter's, Scheie's, Sanfilippo's, and Morquio's syndromes.

26. **A** Type I glycogen storage disease, von Gierke's disease, is an autosomal recessive deficiency of glucose-6-phosphatase. Glycogen accumulates in tissues causing hypoglycemia, ketosis, and fatty liver. Pompe's disease (α-glucosidase deficiency) and Hers' disease (phosphorylase deficiency) are also forms of glycogenosis.

27. **D** Von Gierke's disease (type I glycogen storage disease) results from a deficiency of glucose-6-phosphatase. This blocks the hydrolysis of glucose-6-PO_4 to glucose and P_i, preventing degradation of glycogen to glucose. The disease is associated with increased triglyceride levels because fats are mobilized for energy and lactate acidosis caused by increased glycolysis. A presumptive diagnosis is made when intravenous galactose administration fails to increase serum glucose levels and can be confirmed by demonstrating glucose-6-phosphatase deficiency or decreased glucose production in response to epinephrine.

28. The D-xylose absorption test is used for the differential diagnosis of which two diseases?
    A. Pancreatic insufficiency from malabsorption
    B. Primary from secondary disorders of glycogen synthesis
    C. Type 1 and type 2 diabetes mellitus
    D. Generalized carbohydrate intolerance from specific carbohydrate intolerance

Chemistry/Correlate clinical and laboratory data/ D-xylose absorption/2

29. Which of the statements below about carbohydrate intolerance is true?
    A. Galactosemia results from deficiency of galactose-1-phosphate (galactose-1-PO_4) uridine diphosphate transferase
    B. Galactosemia results in a positive glucose oxidase test for glucose in urine
    C. Urinary galactose is seen in both galactosemia and lactase deficiency
    D. A galactose tolerance test is used to confirm a diagnosis of galactosemia

Chemistry/Correlate clinical and laboratory data/ Carbohydrate/2

30. Which of the statements below regarding iron metabolism is correct?
    A. The dietary requirement for adult men is about 1–2 mg/day
    B. Normally 40%–50% of ingested iron is absorbed
    C. The daily requirement is higher for pregnant and menstruating women
    D. Absorption increases with the amount of iron in the body stores

Chemistry/Apply knowledge of fundamental biological characteristics/Iron/1

31. Which of the processes below occurs when iron is in the oxidized (Fe^{3+}) state?
    A. Absorption by intestinal epithelium
    B. Binding to transferrin and incorporation into ferritin
    C. Incorporation into protoporphyrin IX to form functional heme
    D. Reaction with chromogens in colorimetric assays

Chemistry/Apply knowledge of fundamental biological characteristics/Iron/1

Answers to Questions 28–31

28. **A** Xylose is a pentose that is absorbed without the help of pancreatic enzymes and is not metabolized. In normal adults more than 25% of the dose is excreted into the urine after 5 hours. Low blood or urine levels are seen in malabsorption syndrome, sprue, Crohn's disease, and other intestinal disorders but not in pancreatitis.

29. **A** Galactose is metabolized to galactose-1-PO_4 by the action of galactokinase. Galactose-1-PO_4 uridine diphosphate (UDP) transferase converts galactose-1-PO_4 to glucose. Deficiency of either enzyme causes elevated blood and urine galactose. Lactase deficiency results in the presence of urinary lactose because it is not broken down to glucose and galactose. Tests for reducing sugars employing copper sulfate are used to screen for galactose, lactose, and fructose in urine. Nonglucose-reducing sugars are not detected by the glucose oxidase reaction. A positive test is followed by thin-layer chromatography (TLC) to identify the sugar and additional tests to demonstrate the enzyme deficiency in RBCs. The galactose tolerance test is used (rarely) to evaluate the extent of liver failure, since the liver is the site of galactose metabolism.

30. **C** For adult men and nonmenstruating women, approximately 1–2 mg/day of iron is needed to replace the small amount lost mainly by exfoliation of cells. Because 5%–10% of dietary iron is absorbed normally, the daily dietary requirement in this group is 10–20 mg/day. Menstruating women have an additional need of 1 mg/day and pregnant women 2 mg/day. Absorption efficiency increases in iron deficiency and decreases in iron overload. Iron absorption is enhanced by low gastric pH and is increased by alcohol ingestion.

31. **B** Intestinal absorption occurs only if the iron is in the reduced (Fe^{2+}) state. After absorption, Fe^{2+} is oxidized to Fe^{3+} by gut mucosal cells. Transferrin and ferritin bind iron efficiently only when in the oxidized state. Iron within Hgb binds to O_2 by coordinate bonding, which occurs only if the iron is in the reduced state. Likewise, in colorimetric methods, Fe^{2+} forms coordinate bonds with carbon and nitrogen atoms of the chromogen.

32. Which of the following is associated with low serum iron values and high total iron-binding capacity (TIBC)?
- **A.** Anemia associated with pregnancy
- **B.** Hepatitis
- **C.** Nephrosis
- **D.** Noniron deficiency anemias

Chemistry/Correlate clinical and laboratory data/Iron/2

33. Which condition is associated with the lowest percentage saturation of transferrin?
- **A.** Hemochromatosis
- **B.** Anemia of chronic infection
- **C.** Iron deficiency anemia
- **D.** Noniron deficiency anemia

Chemistry/Correlate clinical and laboratory data/Iron/2

34. Which condition is most often associated with a high serum iron level?
- **A.** Nephrosis
- **B.** Chronic infection or inflammation
- **C.** Polycythemia vera
- **D.** Noniron deficiency anemias

Chemistry/Correlate clinical and laboratory data/Iron/2

35. Which of the following is likely to occur first in iron deficiency anemia?
- **A.** Decreased serum iron
- **B.** Increased TIBC
- **C.** Decreased serum ferritin
- **D.** Increased transferrin

Chemistry/Correlate clinical and laboratory data/Iron/2

36. Which formula provides the best estimate of serum transferrin?
- **A.** Serum Fe/TIBC
- **B.** TIBC (μg/dL)$\times$0.70 = transferrin in mg/dL
- **C.** Percent iron saturation$\times$TIBC (μg/dL)/1.2 + 0.06 mg/dL
- **D.** Serum Fe (μg/dL)$\times$1.25 = transferrin (μg/dL)

Chemistry/Calculate/Iron/2

Answers to Questions 32–36

32. **A** Iron deficiency anemia is the principal cause of low serum iron and high TIBC because it promotes increased transferrin. Pregnancy without iron supplementation depletes maternal iron stores. Iron-supplemented pregnancy and use of contraceptives increase both iron and TIBC. Nephrosis causes low iron and TIBC owing to loss of both iron and transferrin by the kidneys. Hepatitis causes increased release of storage iron, resulting in high levels of iron and transferrin. Noniron deficiency anemias may cause high iron levels and usually show low TIBC and normal or high ferritin levels.

33. **C** Percent saturation = Serum Fe$\times$100/TIBC. Normally, transferrin is one-third saturated with iron. In iron-deficiency states, the serum iron level falls but transferrin rises. This causes the numerator and denominator to move in opposite directions, resulting in a very low percentage saturation (about 10%). The opposite occurs in hemochromatosis and sideroblastic anemia, resulting in an increased percent saturation.

34. **D** Anemia associated with chronic infection causes a low serum iron value, but unlike iron deficiency it causes a low (or normal) TIBC and does not cause low ferritin levels. Noniron deficiency anemias such as pernicious anemia and sideroblastic anemia produce high serum iron and low TIBC. Nephrosis causes iron loss by the kidneys. Polycythemia is associated with increased iron within the RBCs and depletion of iron stores.

35. **C** Body stores must be depleted of iron before serum iron falls. Thus, serum ferritin falls in the early stages of iron deficiency, making it a more sensitive test than serum iron in uncomplicated cases. Ferritin levels are low only in iron deficiency. However, concurrent illness such as malignancy, infection, and inflammation may promote ferritin release from the tissues, causing the serum ferritin to be normal in iron deficiency.

36. **B** Transferrin, a β-globulin, has a molecular size of about 77,000 daltons. Transferrin is the principal iron transport protein, and TIBC is determined by the serum transferrin concentration. The TIBC in micrograms per deciliter multiplied by 0.7 estimates transferrin concentration in milligrams per deciliter. This formula slightly overestimates transferrin because some of the iron added in the TIBC assay binds to other proteins.

37. Which statement regarding the diagnosis of iron deficiency is correct?
  A. Serum iron levels are always higher at night than during the day
  B. Serum iron levels begin to fall before the body stores become depleted
  C. A normal level of serum ferritin rules out iron deficiency
  D. A low serum ferritin level is diagnostic of iron deficiency

Chemistry/Correlate clinical and laboratory data/Iron/2

38. Which statement about iron methods is true?
  A. Interference from Hgb can be corrected by a serum blank
  B. Colorimetric methods measure binding of Fe^{2+} to a ligand such as ferrozine
  C. Atomic absorption is the method of choice for measurement of serum iron
  D. Serum iron can be measured by potentiometry

Chemistry/Apply principles of special procedures/Iron/2

39. Which of the statements below regarding the TIBC assay is correct?
  A. All TIBC methods require addition of excess iron to saturate transferrin
  B. All methods require the removal of unbound iron
  C. Measurement of TIBC is specific for transferrin-bound iron
  D. The chromogen used in the TIBC assay must be different from the one used for measuring serum iron

Chemistry/Apply principles of special procedures/Iron/2

40. Which of the statements below regarding the metabolism of bilirubin is true?
  A. It is formed by hydrolysis of the α-methene bridge of urobilinogen
  B. It is reduced to biliverdin prior to excretion
  C. It is a product of porphyrin metabolism
  D. It is produced from the destruction of RBCs

Chemistry/Apply knowledge of fundamental biological characteristics/Bilirubin/1

Answers to Questions 37–40

37. **D** Serum iron levels are falsely elevated by hemolysis and subject to diurnal variation. Levels are highest in the morning and lowest at night, but this pattern is reversed in persons who work at night. A low ferritin is specific for iron deficiency. However, only about 1% of ferritin is in the vascular system. Any disease that increases ferritin release may mask iron deficiency.

38. **B** Atomic absorption is not the method of choice for serum iron because matrix error and variation of iron recovered by extraction cause bias and poor precision. Most methods use HCl to deconjugate Fe^{3+} from transferrin, followed by reduction to Fe^{2+}. This reacts with a neutral ligand such as ferrozine, tripyridyltriazine (TPTZ), or bathophenanthroline to give a blue complex. Anodic stripping voltammetry can also be used to measure serum iron. Hemolysis must be avoided because RBCs contain a much higher concentration of iron than does plasma.

39. **A** All TIBC methods require addition of excess iron to saturate transferrin. Excess iron is removed by ion exchange or alumina gel columns or precipitation with $MgCO_3$, and the bound iron is measured by the same procedure as is used for serum iron. Alternatively, excess iron in the reduced state can be added at an alkaline pH. Under these conditions, transferrin will bind Fe^{2+} and the unbound Fe^{2+} can be measured directly. In this case, Fe^{2+} added – (minus) unbound (excess) Fe^{2+} = unsaturated iron binding capacity (UIBC). UIBC + serum iron = TIBC. In order to avoid bias in calculating percentage of iron saturation, the chromogen used for TIBC should be the same as that used for serum iron. Some of the iron added to serum in the TIBC assay binds to proteins other than transferrin, resulting in a slight overestimation of transferrin concentration. For this reason, some laboratories prefer to measure transferrin directly using an immunoassay and do not perform a TIBC.

40. **D** Synthesis of porphyrins results in production of heme, and metabolism of porphyrins other than protoporphyrin IX yields uroporphyrins and coproporphyrins, not bilirubin. Reticuloendothelial cells in the spleen digest Hgb and release the iron from heme. The tetrapyrrole ring is opened at the α-methene bridge by heme oxygenase, forming biliverdin. Bilirubin is formed by reduction of biliverdin at the γ-methene bridge. It is complexed to albumin and transported to the liver.

41. Bilirubin is transported from reticuloendothelial cells to the liver by:
   A. Albumin
   B. Bilirubin-binding globulin
   C. Haptoglobin
   D. Transferrin

Chemistry/Apply knowledge of fundamental biological characteristics/Bilirubin/1

42. In the liver, bilirubin is conjugated by addition of:
   A. Vinyl groups
   B. Methyl groups
   C. Hydroxyl groups
   D. Glucuronyl groups

Chemistry/Apply knowledge of fundamental biological characteristics/Bilirubin/1

43. Which enzyme is responsible for the conjugation of bilirubin?
   A. β-Glucuronidase
   B. Uridine diphosphate (UDP)-glucuronyl transferase
   C. Bilirubin oxidase
   D. Biliverdin reductase

Chemistry/Apply knowledge of fundamental biological characteristics/Bilirubin/1

44. The term δ-*bilirubin* refers to:
   A. Water-soluble bilirubin
   B. Free unconjugated bilirubin
   C. Bilirubin tightly bound to albumin
   D. Direct-reacting bilirubin

Chemistry/Apply knowledge of fundamental biological characteristics/Bilirubin/1

45. Which of the following processes is part of the normal metabolism of bilirubin?
   A. Both conjugated and unconjugated bilirubin are excreted into the bile
   B. Methene bridges of bilirubin are reduced by intestinal bacteria forming urobilinogens
   C. Most of the bilirubin delivered into the intestine is reabsorbed
   D. Bilirubin and urobilinogen reabsorbed from the intestine are mainly excreted by the kidneys

Chemistry/Apply knowledge of fundamental biological characteristics/Bilirubin/1

Answers to Questions 41–45

41. **A** Albumin transports bilirubin, haptoglobin transports free Hgb, and transferrin transports ferric iron. When albumin binding is exceeded, unbound bilirubin, called free bilirubin, increases. This may cross the blood-brain barrier, resulting in kernicterus.

42. **D** The esterification of glucuronic acid to the propionyl side chains of the inner pyrrole rings (I and II) makes bilirubin water-soluble. Conjugation is required before bilirubin can be excreted via the bile.

43. **B** UDP-glucuronyl transferase esterifies glucuronic acid to unconjugated bilirubin, making it water-soluble. Most conjugated bilirubin is diglucuronide; however, the liver makes a small amount of monoglucuronide and other glycosides. β-Glucuronidase hydrolyzes glucuronide from bilirubin, hormones, or drugs. It is used prior to organic extraction to deconjugate urinary metabolites (e.g., total cortisol). Biliverdin reductase forms bilirubin from biliverdin (and heme oxygenase forms biliverdin from heme). Bilirubin oxidase is used in an enzymatic bilirubin assay in which bilirubin is oxidized back to biliverdin, and the rate of biliverdin formation is measured at 410 nm.

44. **C** HPLC separates bilirubin into four fractions: α = unconjugated, β = monoglucuronide, γ = diglucuronide, δ = irreversibly albumin-bound. δ-Bilirubin is a separate fraction from the unconjugated bilirubin, which is bound loosely to albumin. δ-Bilirubin and conjugated bilirubin react with diazo reagent in the direct bilirubin assay.

45. **B** Most of the conjugated bilirubin delivered into the intestine is deconjugated by β-glucuronidase and then reduced by intestinal flora to form three different reduction products collectively called urobilinogens. The majority of bilirubin and urobilinogen in the intestine is not reabsorbed. Most of what is reabsorbed is re-excreted by the liver. The portal vein delivers blood from the bowel to the sinusoids. Hepatocytes take up about 90% of the returned bile pigments and secrete them again into the bile. This process is termed the *enterohepatic circulation.*

46. Which of the following is a characteristic of conjugated bilirubin?
- **A.** It is water-soluble
- **B.** It reacts more slowly than unconjugated bilirubin
- **C.** It is more stable than unconjugated bilirubin
- **D.** It has the same absorbance properties as unconjugated bilirubin

Chemistry/Apply knowledge of fundamental biological characteristics/Bilirubin/1

47. Which of the following statements regarding urobilinogen is true?
- **A.** It is formed in the intestines by bacterial reduction of bilirubin
- **B.** It consists of a single water-soluble bile pigment
- **C.** It is measured by its reaction with *p*-aminosalicylate
- **D.** In hemolytic anemia, it is decreased in urine and feces

Chemistry/Apply knowledge of fundamental biological characteristics/Bilirubin/1

48. Which statement regarding bilirubin metabolism is true?
- **A.** Bilirubin undergoes rapid photo-oxidation when exposed to daylight
- **B.** Bilirubin excretion is inhibited by barbiturates
- **C.** Bilirubin excretion is increased by chlorpromazine
- **D.** Bilirubin is excreted only as the diglucuronide

Chemistry/Evaluate laboratory data to recognize problems/Bilirubin/2

49. Which condition is caused by deficient secretion of bilirubin into the bile canaliculi?
- **A.** Gilbert's disease
- **B.** Neonatal hyperbilirubinemia
- **C.** Dubin-Johnson syndrome
- **D.** Crigler-Najjar syndrome

Chemistry/Correlate laboratory data with physiological processes/Bilirubin/2

50. In hepatitis the rise in serum conjugated bilirubin can be caused by:
- **A.** Secondary renal insufficiency
- **B.** Failure of the enterohepatic circulation
- **C.** Enzymatic conversion of urobilinogen to bilirubin
- **D.** Extrahepatic conjugation

Chemistry/Correlate laboratory data with physiological processes/Bilirubin/2

Answers to Questions 46–50

46. A Conjugated bilirubin refers to bilirubin mono- and diglucuronides. Conjugated bilirubin reacts almost immediately with the aqueous diazo reagent without need for a nonpolar solvent. Historically, conjugated bilirubin has been used synonymously with direct-reacting bilirubin, although the latter includes the δ-bilirubin fraction when measured by the Jendrassik-Grof method. Conjugated bilirubin is excreted in both bile and urine. It is easily photo-oxidized and has very limited stability. For this reason, bilirubin standards are usually prepared from unconjugated bilirubin, stabilized by the addition of alkali and albumin.

47. A Urobilinogen is a collective term given to the reduction products of bilirubin formed by the action of enteric bacteria. Urobilinogen excretion is increased in extravascular hemolytic anemias and decreased in obstructive jaundice (cholestatic disease). Urobilinogen is measured using Ehrlich's reagent, an acid solution of *p*-dimethylaminobenzaldehyde.

48. A Samples for bilirubin analysis must be protected from direct sunlight. Drugs may have a significant in vivo effect on bilirubin levels. Barbiturates lower serum bilirubin by increasing excretion. Other drugs such as chlorpromazine cause cholestasis and increase the serum bilirubin. Although most conjugated bilirubin is in the form of diglucuronide, some monoglucuronide and other glycosides are excreted. In glucuronyl transferase deficiency some bilirubin is excreted as sulfatides.

49. C Dubin-Johnson syndrome (type 2 hyperbilirubinemia) is inherited as an autosomal recessive condition producing mild jaundice from accumulation of conjugated bilirubin. Total and direct bilirubin levels are elevated, but other liver function is normal.

50. B Conjugated bilirubin is increased in hepatitis and other causes of hepatic necrosis because of failure to re-excrete conjugated bilirubin reabsorbed from the intestine. Increased direct bilirubin can also be attributed to accompanying intrahepatic obstruction, which blocks the flow of bile.

51. Which of the following is a characteristic of obstructive jaundice?

  A. The ratio of direct to total bilirubin is greater than 1:2

  B. Conjugated bilirubin is elevated, but unconjugated bilirubin is normal

  C. Urinary urobilinogen is increased

  D. Urinary bilirubin is normal

Chemistry/Correlate clinical and laboratory data/ Bilirubin/2

52. Which of the following would cause an increase in only the unconjugated bilirubin?

  A. Hemolytic anemia

  B. Obstructive jaundice

  C. Hepatitis

  D. Hepatic cirrhosis

Chemistry/Correlate clinical and laboratory data/ Bilirubin/2

53. Which form of hyperbilirubinemia is caused by an inherited absence of UDP-glucuronyl transferase?

  A. Gilbert's syndrome

  B. Rotor's syndrome

  C. Crigler-Najjar syndrome

  D. Dubin-Johnson syndrome

Chemistry/Correlate clinical and laboratory data/ Bilirubin/2

54. Which statement regarding total and direct bilirubin levels is true?

  A. Total bilirubin level is a less sensitive and specific marker of liver disease than the direct level

  B. Direct bilirubin level exceeds 3.5 mg/dL in most cases of hemolytic anemia

  C. Direct bilirubin is normal in cholestatic liver disease

  D. The ratio of direct to total bilirubin exceeds 0.40 in hemolytic anemia

Chemistry/Correlate clinical and laboratory data/ Bilirubin/2

Answers to Questions 51–54

51. **A** Obstruction prevents conjugated bilirubin from reaching the intestine, resulting in decreased production, excretion, and absorption of urobilinogen. Conjugated bilirubin regurgitates into sinusoidal blood and enters the general circulation via the hepatic vein. The level of serum direct bilirubin (conjugated) becomes greater than that of unconjugated bilirubin. The conjugated form is also increased because of accompanying necrosis, deconjugation, and inhibition of UDP-glucuronyl transferase.

52. **A** Conjugated bilirubin increases as a result of obstructive processes within the liver or biliary system or from failure of the enterohepatic circulation. Hemolytic anemia (prehepatic jaundice) presents a greater bilirubin load to a normal liver, resulting in increased bilirubin excretion. When the rate of bilirubin formation exceeds the rate of excretion, the unconjugated bilirubin rises.

53. **C** Crigler-Najjar syndrome is a rare condition that occurs in two forms. Type 1 is inherited as an autosomal recessive trait and causes a total deficiency of UDP-glucuronyl transferase. Life expectancy is less than 1 year. Type 2 is an autosomal dominant trait and is characterized by less severe jaundice and usually the absence of kernicterus. Bilirubin levels can be controlled with phenobarbital, which promotes bilirubin excretion. Gilbert's syndrome is an autosomal recessive condition characterized by decreased bilirubin uptake and decreased formation of bilirubin diglucuronide. Dubin-Johnson and Rotor's syndromes are autosomal recessive disorders associated with defective delivery of bilirubin into the biliary system.

54. **A** Direct bilirubin measurement is a sensitive and specific marker for hepatic and posthepatic jaundice because it is not elevated by hemolytic anemia. In hemolytic anemia, the total bilirubin does not exceed 3.5 mg/dL, and the ratio of direct to total is less than 0.20. Unconjugated bilirubin is the major fraction in necrotic liver disease because microsomal enzymes are lost. In cholestasis unconjugated bilirubin is elevated along with direct bilirubin because some necrosis takes place and some conjugated bilirubin is hydrolyzed back to unconjugated bilirubin.

55. Which statement best characterizes serum bilirubin levels in the first week following delivery?

  A. Serum bilirubin 24 hours after delivery should not exceed the upper reference limit for adults

  B. Jaundice is usually first seen 48–72 hours postpartum in neonatal hyperbilirubinemia

  C. Serum bilirubin above 5.0 mg/dL occurring 2–5 days after delivery indicates hemolytic or hepatic disease

  D. Conjugated bilirubin accounts for about 50% of the total bilirubin in neonates

Chemistry/Correlate clinical and laboratory data/ Bilirubin/2

56. A laboratory measures total bilirubin by the Jendrassik-Grof bilirubin method with sample blanking. What would be the effect of moderate hemolysis on the test result?

  A. Falsely increased due to optical interference

  B. Falsely increased due to release of bilirubin from RBCs

  C. Falsely low due to inhibition of the diazo reaction by hemoglobin

  D. No effect due to correction of positive interference by sample blanking

Chemistry/Apply knowledge to recognize sources of error/Bilirubin/2

57. Which reagent is used in the Jendrassik-Grof method to solubilize unconjugated bilirubin?

  A. 50% Methanol

  B. *N*-butanol

  C. Caffeine

  D. Acetic acid

Chemistry/Apply principles of basic laboratory procedures/Bilirubin/1

58. Which statement about colorimetric bilirubin methods is true?

  A. Direct bilirubin must react with diazo reagent under alkaline conditions

  B. Most methods are based upon reaction with diazotized sulfanilic acid

  C. Ascorbic acid can be used to eliminate interference caused by Hgb

  D. The color of the azobilirubin product is independent of pH

Chemistry/Apply principles of basic laboratory procedures/Bilirubin/1

Answers to Questions 55–58

55. **B** Bilirubin levels may reach as high as 2–3 mg/dL in the first 24 hours after birth owing to the trauma of delivery, such as resorption of a subdural hematoma. Neonatal hyperbilirubinemia occurs 2–3 days after birth as a result of increased hemolysis at birth and transient deficiency of the microsomal enzyme, UDP-glucuronyl transferase. Normally, levels rise to about 5–10 mg/dL but may be higher than 15 mg/dL, requiring therapy with UV light to photooxidize the bilirubin. Neonatal jaundice can last up to 1 week in a mature neonate and up to 2 weeks in premature babies. Neonatal bilirubin is almost exclusively unconjugated.

56. **C** The sample blank measures the absorbance of the sample and reagent in the absence of azobilirubin formation and corrects the measurement for optical interference caused by hemoglobin's absorbing the wavelength of measurement. However, hemoglobin is an inhibitor of the diazo reaction and will cause falsely low results in a blank corrected sample. For this reason, direct bichromatic spectrophotometric methods are preferred when measuring bilirubin in neonatal samples, which are often hemolyzed.

57. **C** A polarity modifier is required to make unconjugated bilirubin soluble in diazo reagent. The Malloy-Evelyn method uses 50% methanol to reduce the polarity of the diazo reagent. Caffeine is used in the Jendrassik-Grof method. This method is recommended because it is not falsely elevated by hemolysis and gives quantitative recovery of both conjugated and unconjugated bilirubin.

58. **B** Unconjugated bilirubin is poorly soluble in acid, and therefore direct bilirubin is assayed using diazotized sulfanilic acid diluted in weak HCl. The direct diazo reaction should be measured after no longer than 3 min to prevent reaction of unconjugated bilirubin, or the diazo group can be reduced using ascorbate or hydroxylamine, preventing any further reaction.

59. Which statement regarding the measurement of bilirubin by the Jendrassik-Grof method is correct?
   A. The same diluent is used for both total and direct assays to minimize differences in reactivity
   B. Positive interference by Hgb is prevented by the addition of HCl after the diazo reaction
   C. The color of the azobilirubin product is intensified by the addition of ascorbic acid
   D. Fehling's reagent is added after the diazo reaction to form a blue azobilirubin pigment

Chemistry/Apply principles of basic laboratory procedures/Bilirubin/2

60. A neonatal bilirubin assay performed at the nursery by bichromatic direct spectrophotometry is 4.0 mg/dL. Four hours later, a second sample assayed for total bilirubin by the Jendrassik-Grof method gives a result of 3.0 mg/dL. Both samples are reported to be hemolyzed. What is the most likely explanation of these results?
   A. Hgb interference in the second assay
   B. δ-Bilirubin contributing to the result of the first assay
   C. Falsely high results from the first assay caused by direct bilirubin
   D. Physiological variation due to premature hepatic microsomal enzymes

Chemistry/Apply knowledge to recognize sources of error/ Bilirubin/3

59. **D** The Jendrassik-Grof method uses HCl as the diluent for the measurement of direct bilirubin because unconjugated bilirubin is poorly soluble at a low pH. Total bilirubin is measured using an acetate buffer with caffeine added to increase the solubility of the unconjugated bilirubin. After addition of diazotized sulfanilic acid, the diazo group is reduced by ascorbic acid, and Fehling's reagent is added to alkalinize the diluent. At an alkaline pH the product changes from pink to blue, shifting the absorbance maximum to 600 nm, at which Hgb does not contribute significantly to absorbance.

60. **A** The Jendrassik-Grof method is based upon a diazo reaction that may be suppressed by Hgb. Because serum blanking and measurement at 600 nm correct for positive interference from Hgb, the results may be falsely low when significant hemolysis is present. Direct spectrophometric bilirubin methods employing bichromatic optics correct for the presence of Hgb. These are often called "neonatal bilirubin" tests. A commonly used approach is to measure absorbance at 454 nm and 540 nm. The absorbance contributed by Hgb at 540 nm is equal to the absorbance contributed by Hgb at 454 nm. Therefore, the absorbance difference will correct for free Hgb. Neonatal samples contain little or no direct or δ-bilirubin. They also lack carotene pigments that could interfere with the direct spectrophotometric measurement of bilirubin.

1. **How many grams of sodium hydroxide (NaOH) are required to prepare 150.0 mL of a 5.0% w/v solution?**
   A. 1.5 g
   B. 4.0 g
   C. 7.5 g
   D. 15.0 g

   Clinical chemistry/Calculate/Solutions/2

2. **How many milliliters of glacial acetic acid are needed to prepare 2.0 L of 10.0% v/v acetic acid?**
   A. 10.0 mL
   B. 20.0 mL
   C. 100.0 mL
   D. 200.0 mL

   Clinical chemistry/Calculate/Solutions/2

3. **A biuret reagent requires preparation of a stock solution containing 9.6 g of copper II sulfate ($CuSO_4$)/L. How many grams of $CuSO_4 \cdot 5H_2O$ are needed to prepare 1.0 L of the stock solution?**

   Atomic weights: H = 1.0; Cu = 63.6; O = 16.0; S = 32.1
   A. 5.4 g
   B. 6.1 g
   C. 15.0 g
   D. 17.0 g

   Clinical chemistry/Calculate/Reagent preparation/2

Answers to Questions 1–3

1. **C** A percent solution expressed in w/v (weight/volume) refers to grams of solute per 100.0 mL of solution. To calculate, multiply the percentage (as grams) by the volume needed (mL), then divide by 100.0 (mL).

   $$(5.0\ g \times 150.0\ mL) \div 100.0\ mL = 7.5\ g$$

   To prepare the solution, weigh 7.5 g of NaOH pellets and add to a 150.0-mL volumetric flask. Add sufficient deionized H_2O to dissolve the NaOH. After the solution cools, add deionized H_2O to the 150.0-mL line on the flask and mix again.

2. **D** The expression percent v/v refers to the volume of one liquid in mL present in 100.0 mL of solution. To calculate, multiply the percentage (as mL) by the volume required (mL), then divide by 100 (mL).

   $$(10.0\ mL \times 2000.0\ mL) \div 100.0\ mL = 200.0\ mL$$

   To prepare a 10.0% v/v solution of acetic acid, add approximately 1.0 L of deionized H_2O to a 2.0-L volumetric flask. Add 200.0 mL of glacial acetic acid and mix. Then add sufficient deionized H_2O to bring the meniscus to the 2.0-L line and mix again.

3. **C** Determine the mass of $CuSO_4 \cdot 5H_2O$ containing 9.6 g of anhydrous $CuSO_4$. First, calculate the percentage of $CuSO_4$ in the hydrate, then divide the amount needed (9.6 g) by the percentage.

   % $CuSO_4$ = molecular weight $CuSO_4$ ÷ molecular weight $CuSO_4 \cdot 5H_2O \times 100$

   $= (159.7 \div 249.7) \times 100$

   63.96%

   Grams $CuSO_4 \cdot 5H_2O$ = 9.6 g ÷ 0.6396

   = 15.0 g

   A convenient formula to use is:

   g hydrate = (MW hydrate ÷ MW anhydrous salt) × g anhydrous salt

4. How many milliliters of HNO_3 (purity 68.0%, specific gravity 1.42) are needed to prepare 1.0 L of a 2.0 N solution?

   Atomic weights: H = 1.0; N = 14.0; O = 16.0

   A. 89.5 mL
   B. 126.0 mL
   C. 130.5 mL
   D. 180.0 mL

   Clinical chemistry/Calculate/Reagent preparation/2

5. Convert 10.0 mg/dL calcium (atomic weight = 40.1) to comparable units in the International System of Units (SI).
   A. 0.25
   B. 0.40
   C. 2.5
   D. 0.4

   Clinical chemistry/Calculate/SI unit conversion/2

6. Convert 2.0 mEq/L magnesium (atomic weight = 24.3) to milligrams per deciliter.
   A. 0.8 mg/dL
   B. 1.2 mg/dL
   C. 2.4 mg/dL
   D. 4.9 mg/dL

   Clinical chemistry/Calculate/Unit conversion/2

Answers to Questions 4–6

4. **C** The molecular weight of HNO_3 is 63.0 g. Because the valence of the acid is 1 (1 mol of hydrogen is produced per mole of acid), the equivalent weight is also 63.0 g. The mass is calculated by multiplying the normality (2.0 N) by the equivalent weight (63.0 g) and volume (1.0 L); therefore, 126.0 g of acid are required.

   Because the purity is 68.0% and the specific gravity is 1.42, the amount of HNO_3 in grams per milliliter is 0.68×1.42 g/mL or 0.9656 g/mL. The volume required to give 126.0 g is calculated by dividing the mass needed (grams) by the grams per milliliter.

   mL HNO_3 = 126.0 g ÷ 0.9656 g/mL = 126.0 g × 1.0 mL/0.9656 g = 130.5 mL

5. **C** The SI unit is the recommended method of reporting clinical laboratory results. The SI unit for all electrolytes is millimoles per liter. To convert from milligrams per deciliter to millimoles per liter, multiply by 10 to convert to milligrams per liter, then divide by the atomic mass expressed in milligrams.

   10.0 mg/dL × 10.0 dL/1.0 L = 100.0 mg/L

   100.0 mg/L × 1.0 mmol/40.1 mg = 2.5 mmol/L

6. **C** To convert from milliequivalents per liter to milligrams per deciliter, first calculate the milliequivalent weight (equivalent weight expressed in milligrams), which is the atomic mass divided by the valence. Because magnesium is divalent, each mole has the charge equivalent of 2 mol of hydrogen. Then, multiply the milliequivalent per liter by the milliequivalent weight to convert to milligrams per liter. Next, divide by 10 to convert milligrams per liter to milligrams per deciliter.

   Milliequivalent weight Mg = 24.3 mg ÷ 2

   = 12.15 mg/mEq

   2.0 mEq/L × 12.15 mg/mEq = 24.3 mg/L

   24.3 mg/L × 1.0 L/10.0 dL = 2.4 mg/dL

7. How many milliliters of a 2000.0 mg/dL glucose stock solution are needed to prepare 100.0 mL of a 150.0 mg/dL glucose working standard?
A. 1.5 mL
B. 7.5 mL
C. 15.0 mL
D. 25.0 mL

Clinical chemistry/Calculate/Solutions/2

8. What is the pH of a solution of HNO_3, if the hydrogen ion concentration is 2.5×10^{-2} M?
A. 1.0
B. 1.6
C. 2.5
D. 2.8

Clinical chemistry/Calculate/pH/2

9. Calculate the pH of a solution of 1.5×10^{-5} M NH_4OH.
A. 4.2
B. 7.2
C. 9.2
D. 11.2

Clinical chemistry/Calculate/pH/2

10. How many significant figures should be reported when the pH of a 0.060 M solution of nitric acid is calculated?
A. 1
B. 2
C. 3
D. 4

Clinical chemistry/Calculate/Significant figures/2

Answers to Questions 7–10

7. B To calculate the volume of stock solution needed, divide the concentration of working standard by the concentration of stock standard, then multiply by the volume of working standard that is needed.
$$C_1\times V_1 = C_2\times V_2,$$
where C_1 = concentration of stock standard
V_1 = volume of stock standard
C_2 = concentration of working standard
V_2 = volume of working standard
2000.0 mg/dL$\times V_1$ = 150.0 mg/dL$\times$100.0 mL
V_1 = (150.0 ÷ 2000.0)$\times$100.0 mL
V_1 = 7.5 mL

8. B For a strong acid, the pH is equal to the negative logarithm of the hydrogen ion concentration.
pH = $-$Log H^+
pH = $-$Log 0.025
pH = 1.6

9. C First, calculate the pOH of the solution:
pOH = $-$Log [OH^-]
pOH = $-$Log 1.5×10^{-5} = 4.82
pH = 14 $-$ pOH
pH = 14 $-$ 4.8 = 9.2

10. B When zeros appear by themselves to the left of the decimal point, they are not significant. When they are to the left of the decimal point and are preceded by a number, they are significant. Zeros after the decimal point preceding a number are not significant. However, they are significant if they follow another number or are between two numbers. Therefore, 0.0<u>60</u> M has only two significant figures (the underlined digits). In laboratory practice, most analytes are reported with two significant figures. Routine analytes that are exceptions are pH, which includes three significant figures, and analytes with whole numbers above 100 such as sodium, cholesterol, triglycerides, and glucose.

11. What is the pH of a 0.05 M solution of acetic acid?
$K_a = 1.75 \times 10^{-5}$, $pK_a = 4.76$
A. 1.7
B. 3.0
C. 4.3
D. 4.6

Clinical chemistry/Calculate/pH/2

12. What is the pH of a buffer containing 40.0 mmol/L $NaHC_2O_4$ and 4.0 mmol/L $H_2C_2O_4$? ($pK_a = 1.25$)
A. 1.35
B. 2.25
C. 5.75
D. 6.12

Clinical chemistry/Calculate/pH/2

13. A solvent needed for HPLC requires a 20.0 mmol/L phosphoric acid buffer, pH 3.50, made by mixing KH_2PO_4 and H_3PO_4. How many grams of KH_2PO_4 are required to make 1.0 L of this buffer?

Formula weights: $KH_2PO_4 = 136.1$; $H_3PO_4 = 98.0$; pK_a $H_3PO_4 = 2.12$

A. 1.96 g
B. 2.61 g
C. 2.72 g
D. 19.2 g

Clinical chemisty/Calculate/Buffer/2

Answers to Questions 11–13

11. **B** Weak acids are not completely ionized, and pH must be calculated from the dissociation constant of the acid (in this case 1.75×10^{-5}).

$$Ka = \frac{[H^+] \times [Ac^-]}{[HAc]}$$

$$1.75 \times 10^{-5} = \frac{[H^+] \times [Ac^-]}{5.0 \times 10^{-2}}$$

Since $[H^+] = [Ac^-]$

$$X^2 = (1.75 \times 10^{-5}) \times (5.0 \times 10^{-2}) = 8.75 \times 10^{-7}$$
$$X = \sqrt{8.75 \times 10^{-7}} = [H^+] = 9.35 \times 10^{-4}\,M$$

$pH = -Log\ 9.35 \times 10^{-4}\,M = 3.0$

Alternatively, pH = ½ (pK_a − Log HA)

pH = ½ (4.7 − Log 5.0×10^{-2})
= ½ (4.76 + 1.30)
= 3.0

12. **B** The Henderson-Hasselbalch equation can be used to determine the pH of a buffer containing a weak acid and a salt of the acid.

$$pH = pKa + \log \frac{[salt]}{[acid]}$$

$$= 1.25 + \log \frac{40.0\ mmol/L}{4.0\ mmol/L}$$

$$= 1.25 + \log 10$$

$$= 2.25$$

13. **B** The Henderson-Hasselbalch equation is used to calculate the ratio of salt to acid needed to give a pH of 3.50.

$$pH = pKa + \log(salt/acid)$$

$$3.50 = 2.12 + \log (KH_2PO_4/H_3PO_4)$$

$$1.38 = \log (KH_2PO_4/H_3PO_4)$$

antilog 1.38 = KH_2PO_4/H_3PO_4

$$KH_2PO_4/H_3PO_4 = 23.99$$

Rearranging gives $KH_2PO_4 = 23.99 \times H_3PO_4$. Because the phosphate in the buffer is 20.0 mmol/L, then $H_3PO_4 + KH_2PO_4$ must equal 20. Because $KH_2PO_4 = 23.99 \times H_3PO_4$, then:

$$H_3PO_4 + (23.99 \times H_3PO_4) = 20.0\ mmol/L$$
$$24.99 \times H_3PO_4 = 20.0\ mmol/L$$
$$H_3PO_4 = 20.0/24.99 = 0.800\ mmol/L$$
$$KH_2PO_4 = 20.0 - 0.800 = 19.2\ mmol/L$$
(0.0192 M)

To determine the grams required, multiply the moles of KH_2PO_4 by the formula weight.

$$0.0192\ mol/L \times 136.1\ g/mol = 2.613\ g$$

14. A procedure for cholesterol is calibrated with a serum-based cholesterol standard that was determined by the Abell-Kendall method to be 200.0 mg/dL. Assuming the same volume of sample and reagent are used, calculate the cholesterol concentration in the patient's sample from the following results.

Standard Concentration	Absorbance of Reagent Blank	Absorbance of Standard	Absorbance of Patient Serum
200 mg/dL	0.00	0.860	0.740

  A. 123 mg/dL
  B. 172 mg/dL
  C. 232 mg/dL
  D. 314 mg/dL

Clinical chemistry/Calculate/Beer's law/2

15. A glycerol kinase method for triglyceride calls for a serum blank in which normal saline is substituted for lipase reagent in order to measure endogenous glycerol. Given the following results, and assuming the same volume of sample and reagent are used for each test, calculate the triglyceride concentration in the patient's sample.
  A. 119 mg/dL
  B. 131 mg/dL
  C. 156 mg/dL
  D. 180 mg/dL

Standard Concentration	Absorbance of Reagent Blank	Absorbance of Standard	Absorbance of Patient Serum	Absorbance of Serum Blank
125 mg/dL	0.000	0.62	0.750	0.100

Clinical chemistry/Calculate/Beer's law/2

16. A procedure for aspartate aminotransferase (AST) is performed manually because of a repeating error code for nonlinearity obtained on the laboratory's automated chemistry analyzer; 0.05 mL of serum and 1.0 mL of substrate are used. The reaction rate is measured at 30°C at 340 nm using a 1.0 cM light path, and the delta absorbance ($-\Delta A$) per minute is determined to be 0.382. Based upon a molar absorptivity coefficient for NADH at 340 nm of 6.22×10^3 M^{-1} cM^{-1} L^{-1}, calculate the enzyme activity in international units (IUs) per liter.
  A. 26 IU/L
  B. 326 IU/L
  C. 1228 IU/L
  D. 1290 IU/L

Clinical chemistry/Calculate/International units/2

14. **B** $Cu = A_u/A_s \times C_s$ where C_u = concentration of unknown, A_u = absorbance of unknown, A_s = absorbance of standard, and C_s = concentration of standard.

$$C_u = 0.74/0.86 \times 200 \text{ mg/dL}$$
$$= 172 \text{ mg/dL}$$

15. **B** The serum blank absorbance is subtracted from the result for the patient's serum before applying the ratiometric formula to calculate concentration.

$$C_u = [(A_u - A_{SB})/A_s] \times C_s \text{ where } A_{SB}$$
$$= \text{absorbance of serum blank}$$
$$= (0.750 - 0.100)/0.620 \times 125 \text{ mg/dL}$$
$$= 131 \text{ mg/dL}$$

16. **D** An IU is defined as 1 μmol of substrate consumed or product produced per minute. The micromoles of NADH consumed in this reaction are determined by dividing the change in absorbance per minute by the absorbance of 1 μmol of NADH. Because 1 mol/L/cm would have an absorbance of 6.22×10^3 absorbance units, then 1 μmol/mL/cm would produce an absorbance of 6.22. Therefore, dividing the ΔA per minute by 6.22 gives the micromoles of NADH consumed in the reaction. This is multiplied by the dilution of serum to determine the micromoles per milliliter and multiplied by 1000 to convert to micromoles per liter.

$$\text{IU/L} = \frac{\Delta A/\text{min} \times TV(\text{mL}) \times 1000 \text{ mL/L}}{6.22(A/\mu\text{mol/mL/cM}) \times 1 \text{ cm} \times SV \text{ (mL)}}$$

$$= \frac{\Delta A/\text{min} \times 1.05 \times 1000}{6.22 \times 0.05}$$

$$= \Delta A/\text{min} \times \frac{1050}{0.311}$$

$$= \Delta A/\text{min} \times 3376$$

$$= 0.382 \times 3376 = 1290 \text{ IU/L}$$

17. When referring to quality control (QC) results, what parameter usually determines the acceptable range?

 A. The 95% confidence interval for the mean
 B. The range that includes 50% of the results
 C. The central 68% of results
 D. The range encompassed by ±2.5 standard deviations

Chemistry/Evaluate laboratory data to assess validity/ Accuracy of procedures/Quality control/1

18. Which of the following QC rules would be broken 1 out of 20 times by chance alone?

 A. 1_{2S}
 B. 2_{2S}
 C. 1_{3S}
 D. 1_{4S}

Chemistry/Evaluate laboratory data to assess validity/Accuracy of procedures/Quality control/1

19. Which of the following conditions is cause for rejecting an analytical run?

 A. Two consecutive controls greater than 2 standard deviations above or below the mean
 B. Three consecutive controls greater than 1 standard deviation above the mean
 C. Four controls steadily increasing in value but less than ±1 standard deviation from the mean
 D. One control above +1 standard deviation and the other below −1 standard deviation from the mean

Chemistry/Select course of action/Quality control/3

20. One of two controls within a run is above + 2 standard deviations and the other control is below −2 standard deviations from the mean. What do these results indicate?

 A. Poor precision has led to random error (RE).
 B. A systematic error (SE) is present.
 C. Proportional error is present.
 D. QC material is contaminated.

Chemistry/Evaluate laboratory data to recognize problems/Quality control/2

21. Two consecutive controls are both beyond −2 standard deviations from the mean. How frequently would this occur on the basis of chance alone?

 A. 1:100
 B. 5:100
 C. 1:400
 D. 1:1600

Chemistry/Evaluate laboratory data to assess validity/Accuracy of procedures/Quality control/2

17. **A** The acceptable range for quality control results is usually set at the 95% confidence interval. This is defined as the range between -1.96 standard deviations and +1.96 standard deviations. This means that we can expect a QC result to fall within this range 95 out of 100 times. For practical purposes this is the same as ±2 standard deviations (95.5 out of 100 results should fall within ±2 standard deviations of the mean on the basis of chance).

18. **A** The notation 1_{2S} means that one control is outside ±2 standard deviation units. QC results follow the bell-shaped curve called the gaussian (normal) distribution. If a control is assayed 100 times, 68 out of 100 results would fall within +1 standard deviations and −1 standard deviations of the mean. Ninety-five (95.44) out of 100 results would fall within +2 standard deviations and −2 standard deviations. This leaves only 5 out of 100 results (1:20) that fall outside the ±2 standard deviations limit. Also, 99.7 out of 100 results fall within ±3 standard deviations of the mean.

19. **A** Rejecting a run when three consecutive controls fall between 1 and 2 standard deviations or when a trend of four increasing or decreasing control results occurs would lead to frequent rejection of valid analytical runs. Appropriate control limits are four consecutive controls above or below 1 standard deviation (4_{1S}) to detect a significant shift, and a cusum result exceeding the ±2.7 standard deviation limit to detect a significant trend. When controls deviate in opposite directions, the difference should exceed 4 standard deviations before the run is rejected.

20. **A** When control results deviate from the mean in opposite directions, the run is affected by random error (RE), which results from imprecision. An analytical run is rejected when two controls within the same run have an algebraic difference in excess of 4 standard deviations (R_{4S}). The R_{4S} rule is applied only to controls within a run (level 1–level 2), never across runs or days.

21. **D** QC results follow a gaussian or normal distribution. Ninety-five percent of the results fall within ±2 standard deviations of the mean; therefore, 2.5 out of 100 (1:40) are above +2 standard deviations and 2.5 out of 100 are below −2 standard deviations. The probability of two consecutive controls being beyond −2 standard deviations is the product of their individual probabilities. $1/40 \times 1/40 = 1/1600$ trials by chance.

22. The term R_{4S} means that:
  A. Four consecutive controls are greater than ± 1 standard deviation from the mean
  B. Two consecutive controls in the same run are greater than 4 standard deviation units apart
  C. Two consecutive controls in the same run are each greater than ± 4 standard deviations from the mean
  D. There is a shift above the mean for four consecutive controls

Chemistry/Evaluate laboratory data to assess validity/Accuracy of procedures/Quality control/2

23. A trend in QC results is most likely caused by:
  A. Deterioration of the reagent
  B. Miscalibration of the instrument
  C. Improper dilution of standards
  D. Electronic noise

Chemistry/Evaluate laboratory data to assess validity/Accuracy of procedures/Quality control/2

24. In most circumstances, when two controls within a run are both greater than ± 2 standard deviations from the mean, what action should be taken first?
  A. Recalibrate, then repeat controls followed by randomly selected patient samples if QC is acceptable
  B. Repeat the controls before taking any corrective action
  C. Change the reagent lot, then recalibrate
  D. Prepare fresh standards and recalibrate

Chemistry/Evaluate laboratory data to take corrective action according to predetermined criteria/Quality control/3

25. When establishing QC limits, which practice below is inappropriate?
  A. Using last month's QC data to determine current target limits
  B. Exclusion of any QC results greater than ± 2 standard deviations from the mean
  C. Using control results from all shifts on which the assay is performed
  D. Using limits determined by reference laboratories using the same method

Chemistry/Apply principles of laboratory operations/Quality control/2

26. Which of the following assays has the poorest precision?

	Analyte	Mean (mmol/L)	Standard Deviation
A.	Ca	2.5	0.3
B.	K	4.0	0.4
C.	Na	140	4.0
D.	Cl	100	2.5

Chemistry/Calculate/Coefficient of variation/3

22. **B** The R_{4S} rule is applied when two consecutive controls have an algebraic difference exceeding 4 standard deviations and only to controls within a run (level 1–level 2) and not across different runs. The R_{4S} rule detects random error (error due to poor precision).

23. **A** A trend occurs when six or more consecutive quality control results either increase or decrease in the same direction; however, this is not cause for rejection until a multirule is broken. Trends are systematic errors (affecting accuracy) linked to an unstable reagent, calibrator, or instrument condition. For example, loss of volatile acid from a reagent causes a steady pH increase, preventing separation of analyte from protein. This results in lower QC results each day.

24. **A** When a 2_{2S} rule is broken, a systematic error (SE) is present and corrective action is required (repeating just the QC will not correct the problem). If recalibration yields acceptable QC results, then at least three patient samples randomly chosen from the run must be repeated to determine the magnitude of the error. For example, if the average difference between results before and after recalibratiion is >2 standard deviations, then all samples should be repeated since the last acceptable QC. Both sets of QC results must be reported and the corrective action documented in the QC log.

25. **B** Data between ± 2 and ± 3 standard deviations must be included in calculations of the next month's acceptable range. Elimination of these values would continuously reduce the distribution of QC results, making "out-of-control" situations a frequent occurrence.

26. **A** Although calcium has the lowest standard deviation (s), it represents the assay with poorest precision. Relative precision between different analytes or different levels of the same analyte must be evaluated by the coefficient of variation (CV) because standard deviation is dependent upon the mean. $CV = s \times 100/\text{mean}$. This normalizes standard deviation to a mean of 100. The CV for calcium in the example is 12.0%.

27. Given the following data, calculate the coefficient of variation for glucose.

Analyte	Mean	Standard Deviation
Glucose	76 mg/dL	2.3

   A. 3.0%
   B. 4.6%
   C. 7.6%
   D. 33.0%

   Clinical chemistry/Calculate/Statistics/2

28. Which of the following plots is best for detecting all types of QC errors?
   A. Levy-Jennings
   B. Tonks-Youden
   C. Cusum
   D. Linear regression

   Chemistry/Evaluate laboratory data to recognize problems/Quality control/2

29. Which of the following plots is best for comparison of precision and accuracy among laboratories?
   A. Levy-Jennings
   B. Tonks-Youden
   C. Cusum
   D. Linear regression

   Chemistry/Evaluate laboratory data to recognize problems/Quality control/2

30. Which plot will give the earliest indication of a trend?
   A. Levy-Jennings
   B. Tonks-Youden
   C. Cusum
   D. Histogram

   Chemistry/Evaluate laboratory data to recognize problems/Quality control/2

31. All of the following are requirements for a QC material *except:*
   A. Long-term stability
   B. The matrix is similar to the specimens being tested
   C. The concentration of analytes reflects the clinical range
   D. Analyte concentration must be independent of the method of assay

   Chemistry/Apply principles of basic laboratory procedures/Quality control/2

Answers to Questions 27–31

27. **A** The coefficient of variation is calculated by dividing the standard deviation by the mean and multiplying by 100.

$$\% \text{ CV} = \frac{s}{\bar{x}} \times 100$$
$$= \frac{2.3}{76} \times 100 = 3.0\%$$

The CV is the most appropriate statistic to use when comparing the precision of samples that have different means. For example, when comparing the precision of the level 1 control to the level 2 control, the coefficient of variation normalizes the variance to be independent of the mean. The control with the lower CV is the one for which the analysis is more precise.

28. **A** The Levy-Jennings plot is a graph of all QC results with concentration plotted on the y axis and run number on the x axis. The mean is at the center of the y axis, and concentrations corresponding to -2 and $+2$ standard deviations are highlighted. Results are evaluated for multirule violations across both levels and runs. Corrective action for shifts and trends can be taken before QC rules are broken.

29. **B** The Tonks-Youden plot is used for interlaboratory comparison of monthly means. The method mean for level 1 is at the center of the y axis and the mean for level 2 is at the center of the x axis. Lines are drawn from the means of both levels across the graph, dividing it into four equal quadrants. If a laboratory's monthly means both plot in the lower left or upper right, then SE exists in its method.

30. **C** Cusum points are the algebraic sum of the difference between each QC result and the mean. The y axis is the sum of differences and the x axis is the run number. The center of the y axis is 0. Because QC results follow a random distribution, the points should distribute about the zero line. Results are out of control when the slope exceeds 45° or a decision limit (e.g., ± 2.7 standard deviations) is exceeded.

31. **D** Quality control materials are stable, made of the same components as the specimen, cover the dynamic linear range of the assay, and can be used for multiple analytes. The target mean for QC samples is determined from replicate assays by the user's method, not the "true" concentration of the analyte. Out-of-control results are linked to analytic performance rather than to the inherent accuracy of the method.

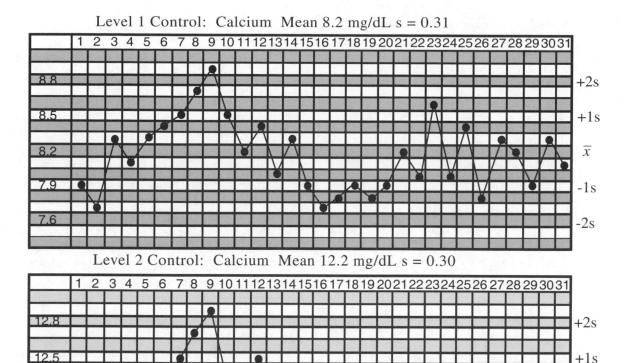

Level 1 Control: Calcium Mean 8.2 mg/dL s = 0.31

Level 2 Control: Calcium Mean 12.2 mg/dL s = 0.30

Questions 32–35 refer to the Levy-Jennings chart above.

32. Examine the Levy-Jennings chart and identify the QC problem that occurred during the first half of the month.
  A. Shift
  B. Trend
  C. Random error
  D. Kurtosis

Chemistry/Evaluate laboratory data to recognize problems/Quality control/3

33. Referring to the Levy-Jennings chart, what is the first day in the month when the run should be rejected and patient results should be repeated?
  A. Day 6
  B. Day 7
  C. Day 8
  D. Day 9

Chemistry/Evaluate laboratory data to recognize problems/Quality control/3

Answers to Questions 32–33

32. **B** A trend is characterized by six consecutive decreasing or increasing control results. The value for both controls becomes progressively higher from day 4 to day 9. Trends are caused by changes to the test system that increase over time, such as deterioration of reagents or calibrators, progressive changes in temperature, evaporation, light exposure, and bacterial contamination. A trend is a type of SE because all results are affected. Random error (RE) affects results in an unpredictable manner, resulting in isolated or sporadic control errors. Control rules affected by RE are 1_{3S} and R_{4S}.

33. **D** Although the trend is apparent across QC levels by day 7, the patient results would not be rejected until day 9 when the 2_{2S} and 4_{1S} rules are broken. An advantage to plotting control data is that trends can be identified before results are out of control and patient data must be rejected. In this case, corrective steps should have been implemented by day 7 to avoid the delay and expense associated with having to repeat the analysis of patient samples.

34. Referring to the Levy-Jennings chart, what analytical error is present during the second half of the month?

A. Shift
B. Trend
C. Random error
D. Kurtosis

Chemistry/Evaluate laboratory data to recognize problems/Quality control/3

35. What is the first day in the second half of the month that patient results would be rejected?

A. Day 16
B. Day 17
C. Day 18
D. Day 19

Chemistry/Evaluate laboratory data to recognize problems/Quality control/3

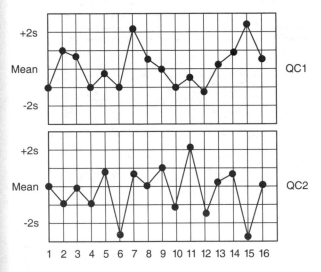

36. Given the QC chart shown above, identify the day in which a violation of the R_{4S} QC rule occurs.

A. Day 3
B. Day 8
C. Day 10
D. Day 15

Chemistry/Evaluate laboratory data to recognize problems/Quality control/3

37. What is the minimum requirement for performing QC for a total protein assay?

A. One level assayed every 8 hours
B. Two levels assayed within 8 hours
C. Two levels assayed within 24 hours
D. Three levels assayed within 24 hours

Chemistry/Apply principles of basic laboratory procedures/Quality control/2

38. Which of the following statistical tests is used to compare the means of two methods?

A. Student's *t* test
B. F distribution

C. Correlation coefficient (*r*)
D. Linear regression analysis

Chemistry/Evaluate laboratory data to assess the validity/Accuracy of procedures/Statistics/2

Answers to Questions 34–38

34. **A** A shift is characterized by six consecutive points lying on the same side of the mean. This occurs from day 15 to day 20. Shifts are caused by a change in the assay conditions that affect the accuracy of all results, such as a change in the concentration of the calibrator; a change in reagent; a new lot of reagent that differs in composition; or improper temperature setting, wavelength, or sample volume. The term *kurtosis* refers to the degree of flatness or sharpness in the peak of a set of values having a gaussian distribution.

35. **B** The 4_{1S} rule is broken across QC levels on day 17. This means that four consecutive controls are greater than ± 1 standard deviation from the mean. QC rules that are sensitive to SE are applied across both runs and levels to increase the probability of error detection. These are 2_{2S}, 4_{1S}, and $10\bar{x}$.

36. **D** An R_{4S} error is defined as the algebraic difference between two controls within the same run. In this Levy-Jennings plot, on day 15, level 1 is above the +2S limit (approximately +2.5 standard deviations) and level 2 is below the −2 standard deviations limit (approximately −2.5 standard deviations). These controls are approximately 5 standard deviations apart (+2.5 minus −2.5 = +5).

37. **C** The minimum requirement for frequency of quality control for a general chemistry analyte (based upon the Clinical Laboratory Improvement Act, 1988) is two levels of control assayed every 24 hours. Some laboratories prefer to assay two control levels every 8 hours or every 12 hours to increase the opportunity for error detection.

38. **A** Student's *t* test is the ratio of mean difference to the standard error of the mean difference (bias/random error) and tests for a significant difference in means. The F test is the ratio of variances and determines if one method is significantly less precise. The correlation coefficient is a measure of the association between two variables and should be high in any method comparison. An *r* value less than 0.90 in method comparisons usually occurs when the range of results is too narrow.

39. Two freezing point osmometers are compared by running 40 paired patient samples one time on each instrument, and the following results are obtained:

Instrument	Mean	Standard Deviation
Osmometer A	280 mOsm/kg	3.1
Osmometer B	294 mOsm/kg	2.8

If $F = 2.8$ at the 0.10 significance level (DF = 38), then what conclusion can be drawn regarding the precision of the two instruments?

A. There is no statistically significant difference in precision

B. Osmometer A demonstrates better precision that is statistically significant

C. Osmometer B demonstrates better precision that is statistically significant

D. Precision cannot be evaluated statistically when single measurements are made on samples

Chemistry/Evaluate laboratory data to assess the validity/Accuracy of procedures/Statistics/3

40. Two methods for total cholesterol are compared by running 40 paired patient samples one time on each instrument. The following results are obtained:

Instrument	Mean	Standard Deviation
Method x (reference method)	235 mg/dL	3.8
Method y (candidate method)	246 mg/dL	3.4

Assuming the samples are collected and stored in the same way and the analysis is done by a technologist who is familiar with both methods, what is the bias of method y?

A. 0.4

B. 7.2

C. 10.6

D. 11.0

Chemistry/Evaluate laboratory data to assess the validity/Accuracy of procedures/Statistics/2

Answers to Questions 39–40

39. A The F test determines whether there is a statistically significant difference in the variance of the two sampling distributions. Assuming the samples are collected and stored in the same way and the analysis is done by a technologist who is familiar with the instrument, differences in variance can be attributed to a difference in instrument precision. The F test is calculated by dividing the variance $(s_1)^2$ of the instrument having the higher standard deviation by the variance $(s_2)^2$ of the instrument having the smaller standard deviation.

$$F = (s_1)^2 \div (s_2)^2 = (3.1)^2 \div (2.8)^2 = 9.61 \div 7.84 = 1.22$$

If the value of F is smaller than the critical value at the 0.10 level of significance, then the hypothesis (there is no significant difference in the variance of the two instruments) is accepted.

40. D The bias is defined as the difference between the means of the two methods and is calculated using the formula: Bias $= \bar{y} - \bar{x}$. The bias is an estimate of SE. The student's t test is used to determine if bias is statistically significant. The t statistic is the ratio of bias to the standard error of the mean difference. The greater the bias, the higher the t score.

41. When the magnitude of error increases with increasing sample concentration it is called:
   A. Constant error
   B. Proportional error
   C. Random error
   D. Bias

Chemistry/Evaluate laboratory data to assess validity/Accuracy of procedures/Statistics/2

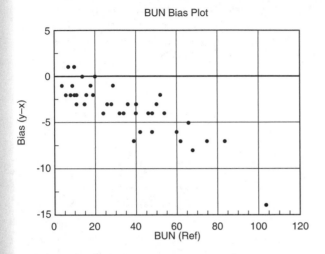

BUN Bias Plot

42. Which explanation is the best interpretation of the blood urea nitrogen (BUN) bias plot above?
   A. The new method consistently overestimates the BUN by a constant concentration
   B. The new method is greater than the reference method but not by a statistically significant margin
   C. The new method is lower than the reference method by 5 mg/dL
   D. The new method is lower than the reference method and the magnitude is concentration-dependent

Chemistry/Evaluate laboratory data to assess validity/Accuracy of procedures/Statistics/3

43. Serum samples collected from hospitalized patients over a 2-week period are split into two aliquots and analyzed for prostate-specific antigen (PSA) by two methods. Each sample was assayed by both methods within 30 minutes of collection by a technologist familiar with both methods. The reference method is method x (upper reference limit = 4.0 μg/L). Linear regression analysis was performed by the least squares method, and results are as follows:

Linear Regression	Correlation Coefficient (r)	Standard Error of Estimate ($s_{y/x}$)
$y = 2.10 + 1.01x$	0.984	0.23

Which statement best characterizes the relationship between the methods?
   A. There is a significant bias caused by constant error
   B. There is a significant proportional error
   C. There is no disagreement between the methods because the correlation coefficient approaches 1.0
   D. There are no SEs, but the RE of the new method is unacceptable

Chemistry/Evaluate laboratory data to assess the validity/Accuracy of procedures/Statistics/2

41. **B** Proportional error (slope or percent error) results in greater absolute error (deviation from the target value) at higher sample concentration. Constant error refers to a difference between the target value and the result, which is independent of sample concentration. For example, if both level 1 and level 2 controls for laboratory A average 5 mg/dL below the cumulative mean reported by all other laboratories using the same method, then laboratory A has a constant error of −5 mg/dL for that method.

42. **D** A bias plot compares the bias (candidate method minus reference method) to the result of the reference method. Ideally, points should be scattered equally on both sides of the zero line. When the majority of points is below the zero line, the candidate method is negatively biased (lower than the reference). In this case, the difference between the methods increases in proportion to the BUN concentration. This type of error occurs when the slope of the linear regression line is low.

43. **A** The linear regression analysis is the most useful statistic to compare paired patient results because it estimates the magnitude of specific errors. The y intercept of the regression line is a measure of constant error (bias), and the slope is a measure of proportional error. Together these represent the SE of the new method. The correlation coefficient is influenced by the range of the sample and the RE. Two methods that measure the same analyte will have a high correlation coefficient provided that the concentrations are measured over a wide range, and this statistic should not be used to judge the acceptability of the new method. The standard error of estimate is a measure of the closeness of data points to the regression line and is an expression of RE.

44. Which statement best summarizes the relationship between the new BUN method and the reference method based on the linear regression scatterplot shown below?

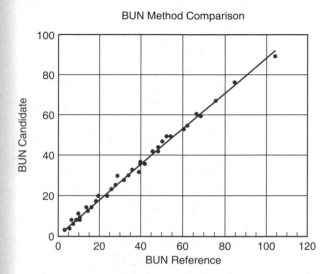

A. The methods agree very well but show a high standard error of estimate

B. There is little or no constant error but some proportional error

C. There will be a significant degree of uncertainty in the regression equation

D. There is significant constant and proportional error but little random error

Chemistry/Evaluate laboratory data to assess the validity/Accuracy of procedures/Statistics/3

45. A new method for BUN analysis is evaluated by comparing the results of 40 paired patient samples to the urease-UV method. Normal and high controls were run on each shift for 5 days, five times per day. The results are as follows:

Linear Regression	Low Control	High Control
y = –0.3 + 0.90x	x̄ = 14.2 mg/dL; s = 1.24	x̄ = 48.6 mg/dL; s = 1.12

What is the total analytical error estimate for a sample having a concentration of 50 mg/dL?

A. –2.2 mg/dL
B. –2.8 mg/dL
C. –7.5 mg/dL
D. –10.0 mg/dL

Chemistry/Calculate/Method comparison statistics/3

46. In addition to the number of true-negatives (TN), which of the following measurements is needed to calculate specificity?

A. True-positives
B. Prevalence
C. False-negatives
D. False-positives

Chemistry/Calculation/Specificity/2

44. **B** The scatterplot shows that each sample produces a coordinate (x corresponds to the reference result and y to the candidate method result) that is very close to the regression line. This means that the variance of regression is low and there is a high degree of certainty that the predicted value of y will be close to its measured value. Near zero concentration there is good agreement between methods; however, the higher the result, the greater the difference between x and y. The regression equation for this scatterplot is $y = -0.01 + 0.90 x$ indicating a proportional error of -10%.

45. **C** Linear regression analysis gives an estimate of SE, which is equal to $(y - x_c)$ where

x_c is the expected concentration and y is the value predicted by the linear regression equation.

SE = $[-0.3 + (0.9 \times 50 \text{ mg/dL})] - 50.0 \text{ mg/dL} = 44.7 - 50.0 = -5.3 \text{ mg/dL}$

The standard deviation of the new method for the high control is used to estimate the RE because the mean of this control is nearest to the expected concentration of 50 mg/dL. RE is estimated by $\pm 1.96 \times s$.

RE = $1.96 \times 1.12 = \pm 2.2 \text{ mg/dL}$

Total analytical error (TE) is equal to the sum of SE and RE.

TE = SE + RE = $-5.3 \text{ mg/dL} + (-2.2 \text{ mg/dL}) = -7.5 \text{ mg/dL}$

46. **D** The clinical specificity of a laboratory test is defined as the true-negatives (TNs) divided by the sum of TNs and false-positives (FPs).

$$\% \text{ Specificity} = \frac{TN \times 100}{TN + FP}$$

Specificity is defined as the percentage of disease-free people who have a negative test result. The probability of FPs is calculated from the specificity as:

$$1 - \frac{\% \text{ specificity}}{100}$$

47. A new tumor marker for ovarian cancer is evaluated for sensitivity by testing serum samples from patients who have been diagnosed by staging biopsy as having malignant or benign lesions. The following results were obtained:

Number of malignant patients who are positive for CA-125 = 21 out of 24

Number of benign patients who are negative for CA-125 = 61 out of 62

What is the sensitivity of the new CA-125 test?

A. 98.4%

B. 95.3%

C. 87.5%

D. 85.0%

Clinical chemistry/Calculate/Sensitivity/2

48. A new test for prostatic cancer is found to have a sensitivity of 80.0% and a specificity of 84.0%. If the prevalence of prostate cancer is 4.0% in men over 42 years old, what is the predictive value of a positive test result (PV+) in this group?

A. 96.0%

B. 86.0%

C. 32.4%

D. 17.2%

Chemistry/Calculate/Predictive value/2

49. What measurement in addition to TNs and prevalence is required to calculate the predictive value of a negative test result (PV−)?

A. FNs

B. Variance

C. TPs

D. FPs

Chemistry/Calculate/Predictive value/2

50. A laboratory is establishing a reference range for a new analyte and wants the range to be determined by the regional population of adults age 18 and older. The analyte concentration is known to be independent of race and gender. Which is the most appropriate process to follow?

A. Determine the mean and standard deviation of the analyte from 40 healthy adults and calculate the ± 2 standard deviation limit

B. Measure the analyte in 120 healthy adults and calculate the central 95th percentile

C. Measure the analyte in 120 healthy adults and use the lowest and highest as the reference range limits

D. Measure the analyte in 60 healthy adults and 60 adults with conditions that affect the analyte concentration. Calculate the concentration of least overlap

Chemistry/Select methods/Statistics/2

Answers to Questions 47–50

47. C Sensitivity is defined as the percentage of persons with the disease who have a positive test result. It is calculated as true-positives (TPs) divided by the sum of TPs and false-negatives (FNs).

$$\% \text{ Sensitivity} = \frac{TP \times 100}{TP + FN}$$

$$\text{Sensitivity} = (21 \times 100) \div (21 + 3) = 87.5\%$$

48. D The predictive value of a positive test is defined as the percentage of persons with a positive test result (PV+) who will have the disease or condition. It is dependent upon the sensitivity of the test and the prevalence of the disease in the population tested. PV+ is calculated by multiplying the TPs by 100, then dividing by the sum of TPs and FPs.

$$\% \, PV+ = \frac{TP \times 100}{TP+FP}$$

where TP equals (sensitivity × prevalence) and FP equals (1 − specificity) × (1 − prevalence)

$$= \frac{0.80 \times 0.04 \times 100}{(0.80 \times 0.04) + [(1-0.84) \times (1-0.04)]}$$

$$= \frac{0.032 \times 100}{0.032 + (0.16 \times 0.96)}$$

$$= 17.2\%$$

49. A The PV− is defined as the probability that a person with a negative test result is free of disease. A high PV− is a characteristic of a good screening test. The predictive value of a negative test is calculated by multiplying the TNs by 100, then dividing by the sum of the TNs and FNs.

$$\%PV- = \frac{TN \times 100}{(TN + FN)}$$

50. B Since the concentration of an analyte may not be normally distributed in a population, the reference range should not be determined from the standard deviation. It is more appropriate to determine the central 95th percentile (the range that encompasses 95% of the results). A minimum of 120 samples is needed for statistical significance. Results are rank ordered from lowest to highest. The third result is the lowest value and the 118th is the highest value in the reference range. The laboratory can verify a pre-existing reference range (e.g., as determined by the manufacturer's study) by testing 20 healthy persons. If no more than 10% fall outside the range, it can be considered valid for the patient population.

CREATININE, BUN, AMMONIA, AMINO ACIDS, AND URIC ACID

1. Creatinine is formed from the:
   A. Oxidation of creatine
   B. Oxidation of protein
   C. Deamination of dibasic amino acids
   D. Metabolism of purines

   Chemistry/Apply knowledge of fundamental biological characteristics/Biochemical/1

2. Creatinine is considered the substance of choice to measure endogenous renal clearance because:
   A. The rate of formation per day is independent of body size
   B. It is completely filtered by the glomeruli
   C. Plasma levels are highly dependent upon diet
   D. Clearance is the same for both men and women

   Chemistry/Apply knowledge of fundamental biological characteristics/Biochemical/1

3. Which statement regarding creatinine is true?
   A. Serum levels are elevated in early renal disease
   B. High serum levels result from reduced glomerular filtration rates
   C. Serum creatine has the same diagnostic utility as serum creatinine
   D. Serum creatinine is a more sensitive measure of renal function than creatinine clearance

   Chemistry/Calculate laboratory data with physiological processes/Biochemical/2

4. Which of the formulas below is the correct expression for creatinine clearance?
   A. Creatinine clearance = U/P×V×1.73/A
   B. Creatinine clearance = P/V×U×A/1.73
   C. Creatinine clearance = P/V×U×1.73/A
   D. Creatinine clearance = U/V×P×1.73/A

   Chemistry/Calculate/Creatinine clearance/1

Answers to Questions 1–4

1. **A** Creatinine is formed mainly in skeletal muscle from the oxidation of creatine. Creatinine is an anhydrous form of creatine formed at a rate of approximately 2% per day. Creatine can be converted to creatinine by addition of strong acid or alkali or by the enzyme creatine hydroxylase.

2. **B** Creatinine formation is dependent upon muscle mass and varies by less than 15% per day. It is not metabolized by the liver or dependent on diet and is 100% filtered by the glomeruli. It is not reabsorbed significantly but is secreted slightly, especially when filtrate flow is slow. Plasma creatinine and cystatin C are the two substances of choice for estimating the glomerular filtration rate.

3. **B** Serum creatinine is a specific but not a sensitive measure of glomerular function. About 60% of the filtration capacity of the kidneys is lost when serum creatinine becomes elevated. Because urine creatinine diminishes as serum creatinine increases in renal disease, the creatinine clearance is far more sensitive than serum creatinine in detecting glomerular disease. A creatinine clearance below 60 mL/min indicates loss of about 50% functional nephron capacity and is classified as moderate (stage 3) chronic kidney disease.

4. **A** Creatinine clearance is the volume of plasma that contains the same quantity of creatinine that is excreted in the urine in 1 minute. It is calculated as the ratio of urine creatinine to plasma creatinine in milligrams per deciliter. This is multiplied by the volume of urine produced per minute and corrected for lean body mass by multiplying by 1.73/*A*, where *A* is the patient's body surface area in square meters.

5. Which of the following conditions is most likely to cause a falsely high creatinine clearance result?
  A. The patient uses the midstream void procedure when collecting his or her urine
  B. The patient adds tap water to the urine container because he or she forgets to save one of the urine samples
  C. The patient does not empty his or her bladder at the conclusion of the test
  D. The patient empties his or her bladder at the start of the test and adds the urine to the collection

Chemistry/Identify source of error/Creatinine clearance/3

6. Given the following data, calculate the creatinine clearance. Serum creatinine = 1.2 mg/dL; urine creatinine = 120 mg/dL; urine volume = 1.75 L/day; surface area = 1.80 m^2
  A. Creatinine clearance = 16 mL/min
  B. Creatinine clearance = 117 mL/min
  C. Creatinine clearance = 126 mL/min
  D. Creatinine clearance = 168 mL/min

Chemistry/Calculate/Creatinine clearance/2

7. In the creatinine clearance formula the term 1.73/A is used to:
  A. Normalize clearance, making it independent of muscle mass
  B. Correct clearance for creatinine that is secreted by the renal tubules
  C. Make the clearance measurement independent of filtrate flow rate
  D. Adjust clearance so that it is equal to inulin clearance

Chemistry/Apply principles of special procedures/Creatinine clearance/1

8. As an alternative to clearance testing, the glomerular filtration rate can be estimated by which method?
  A. Determining 24-hour urinary protein concentration
  B. Calculation based upon plasma creatinine, age, race, and sex
  C. Measurement of 24-hour urinary urea nitrogen
  D. Measurement of 24-hour urinary sodium concentration

Chemistry/Apply knowledge of fundamental biological characteristics/Biochemical/1

5. D Urine in the bladder should be eliminated and not saved at the start of the test because it represents urine formed prior to the test period. The other conditions (choices A–C) will result in falsely low urine creatinine or volume and, therefore, falsely lower clearance results. Error is introduced by incomplete emptying of the bladder when short times are used to measure clearance. A minimum 4-hour timed urine specimen should be collected (a 24-hour timed urine is the specimen of choice). When filtrate flow falls below 2 mL/min, error is introduced because tubular function has a greater effect upon urine creatinine, and some urine is likely to be retained in the bladder. The patient must be kept well hydrated during the test to prevent this.

6. B Creatinine clearance = urine creatinine ÷ serum creatinine×1.75 L/day×1 day/1440 min×1000 mL/L×1.73 m^2/1.80 m^2

Creatinine clearance = 120 mg/dL ÷ 1.2 mg/dL×1700 mL/1400 min×1.73 m^2/1.80 m^2

Creatinine clearance = 117 mL/min

7. A The term *1.73/A* corrects the clearance for variation in muscle mass as it relates to body size (surface area). The greater the muscle mass, the greater the creatinine clearance. Reference ranges are established for men, women, and children because each has a different percentage of lean muscle mass.

8. B Since sample collection errors such as incomplete bladder emptying often lead to errors in determining creatinine clearance, the National Kidney Foundation guidelines recommend the use of a calculated estimate of glomerular filtration rate (eGFR) reported along with the serum or plasma creatinine as a means of screening patients for chronic kidney disease. One such equation (the abbreviated modification of diet in renal disease formula) is shown below:

eGFR (mL/min/1.73m^2) = 186×Plasma Cr$^{-1.154}$×Age$^{-.203}$×.742 (if female)×1.21 (if Afro-American)

 9. Which of the following enzymes allows creatinine
    to be measured by coupling the creatinine amidohy-
    drolase (creatininase) reaction to the peroxidase
    reaction?
    A. G6PD
    B. Creatinine iminohydrolase
    C. Sarcosine oxidase
    D. Creatine kinase

 *Chemistry/Apply principles of general laboratory proce-
 dures/Biochemical/1*

 10. Select the primary reagent used in the Jaffe method
    for creatinine.
    A. Alkaline copper II sulfate
    B. Saturated picric acid and NaOH
    C. Sodium nitroprusside and phenol
    D. Phosphotungstic acid

 *Chemistry/Apply principles of general laboratory proce-
 dures/Biochemical/1*

 11. Which of the statements below regarding creatinine
    methods is true?
    A. The reaction of creatinine with alkaline picrate is
      highly specific
    B. In persons with glomerular disease, enzymatic
      methods for creatinine are likely to give higher
      creatinine clearance results than the Jaffe
      method
    C. Enzymatic methods generally give higher results
      for serum creatinine than methods based on Jaffe's
      reaction
    D. When performing a creatinine clearance, the
      method used for serum should be enzymatic, and
      the method used for urine should be based upon
      Jaffe's reaction

 Chemistry/Identify source of error/Biochemical/3

 12. In which case would creatinine clearance likely give a
    more accurate measure of glomerular function than
    measurement of plasma cystatin C?
    A. In a diabetic patient
    B. In chronic renal failure
    C. In a postrenal transplant patient
    D. In renal failure secondary to systemic autoimmune
      disease

 Chemistry/Identify source of error/Biochemical/3

Answers to Questions 9–12

 9. C The peroxidase coupled enzymatic assay of crea-
    tinine is based upon the conversion of creatinine to
    creatine by creatinine amidohydrolase. The enzyme
    then hydrolyzes creatine to produce sarcosine and
    urea. The enzyme sarcosine oxidase converts sarco-
    sine to glycine, producing formaldehyde and hydro-
    gen peroxide. Peroxidase then catalyzes the
    oxidation of a dye (4-aminophenazone and phenol)
    by the peroxide, forming a red-colored product.
    This method is more specific than the Jaffe reaction,
    which tends to produce a falsely high creatinine
    value by about 5% in persons with normal renal
    function.

 10. B The Jaffe method reaction uses saturated picric
    acid, which oxidizes creatinine in alkali, forming
    creatinine picrate. The reaction is nonspecific;
    ketones, ascorbate, proteins, and other reducing
    agents contribute to the final color. Alkaline $CuSO_4$
    is used in the biuret method for protein and phos-
    photungstic acid is used to measure uric acid.

 11. B Enzymatic methods for creatinine are specific.
    The Jaffe reaction is nonspecific; proteins and other
    reducing substances such as pyruvate and ascorbate
    can cause positive interference. Some of this inter-
    ference is reduced by using a timed rate reaction
    (e.g., reading the absorbance difference 20–80 sec
    after mixing). When the serum creatinine is normal,
    the rate Jaffe method results in clearance values that
    compare well with inulin clearance because plasma
    creatinine is overestimated (interferents account for
    a greater share of the plasma value). The enzymatic
    methods tend to give higher clearance results than
    inulin clearance in normal persons because some
    creatinine is secreted by the tubules.

 12. C Cystatin C is a small protease inhibitor that is
    measured by enzyme immunoassay. It is produced
    at a constant rate, eliminated exclusively by
    glomerular filtration, and is not dependent on age,
    sex, or nutritional status. Plasma level increases
    when glomerular filtration decreases. It is more
    sensitive than creatinine clearance in detecting
    glomerular disease because it is subject to less phys-
    iological variation. However, it is affected by drugs
    currently used to prevent transplant rejection.

13. A sample of amniotic fluid collected for fetal lung maturity studies from a woman with a pregnancy compromised by hemolytic disease of the newborn (HDN) has a creatinine of 88 mg/dL. What is the most likely cause of this result?

A. The specimen is contaminated with blood

B. Bilirubin has interfered with the measurement of creatinine

C. A random error occurred when the absorbance signal was being processed by the analyzer

D. The fluid is urine from accidental puncture of the urinary bladder

Chemistry/Identify source of error/Biochemical/3

14. Which analyte should be reported as a ratio using creatinine concentration as a reference?

A. Urinary microalbumin

B. Urinary estriol

C. Urinary sodium

D. Urinary urea

Chemistry/Apply principles of general laboratory procedures/Creatinine/1

15. Urea is produced from:

A. The catabolism of proteins and amino acids

B. Oxidation of purines

C. Oxidation of pyrimidines

D. The breakdown of complex carbohydrates

Chemistry/Apply knowledge of fundamental biological characteristics/Biochemical/1

16. Urea concentration is calculated from the BUN by multiplying by a factor of:

A. 0.5

B. 2.14

C. 6.45

D. 14

Chemistry/Calculate/Biochemical/2

17. Which of the statements about serum urea is true?

A. Levels are independent of diet

B. Urea is not reabsorbed by the renal tubules

C. High BUN levels can result from necrotic liver disease

D. BUN is elevated in prenal as well as renal failure

Chemistry/Correlate laboratory data with physiological processes/Biochemical/2

Answers to Questions 13–17

13. D Creatinine levels in this range are found only in urine specimens. Adults usually excrete between 1.2 and 1.5 g of creatinine per day. For this reason, creatinine is routinely measured in 24-hour urine samples to determine the completeness of collection. A 24-hour urine sample with less than 0.8 g/day indicates that some of the urine was probably discarded. Creatinine is also used to evaluate fetal maturity. As gestation progresses, more creatinine is excreted into the amniotic fluid by the fetus. Although a level above 2 mg/dL is not a specific indicator of maturity, a level below 2 mg/dL indicates immaturity.

14. A Measurement of urinary microalbumin concentration should be reported as a ratio of albumin to creatinine (e.g., mg albumin per g creatinine). This eliminates the need for 24-hour collection in order to avoid variation caused by differences in fluid intake. A dry reagent strip test for creatinine is available that measures the ability of a creatinine-copper complex to break down H_2O_2, forming a colored complex. The strip uses buffered copper II sulfate, tetramethylbenzidine, and anhydrous peroxide. Binding of creatinine in urine to copper forms a peroxidase-like complex that results in oxidation of the benzidine compound. Also, 24-hour urinary metanephrines, vanillylmandelic acid, and homovanillic acid are reported per gram creatinine when measured in infants and children in order to compensate for differences in body size.

15. A Urea is generated by deamination of amino acids. Most is derived from the hepatic catabolism of proteins. Uric acid is produced by the catabolism of purines. Oxidation of pyrimidines produces orotic acid.

16. B BUN is multiplied by 2.14 to give the urea concentration in mg/dL.

$$BUN \ (mg/dL) = urea \times (\% \ N \ in \ urea \div 100)$$

$$Urea = BUN \times 1/(\% \ N \ in \ urea \div 100)$$

$$Urea = BUN \times (1/.467) = 2.14$$

17. D Urea is completely filtered by the glomeruli but reabsorbed by the renal tubules at a rate dependent on filtrate flow and tubular status. Urea levels are a sensitive indicator of renal disease, becoming elevated as a result of glomerular injury, tubular damage, or poor blood flow to the kidneys (prerenal failure). Serum urea (and BUN) levels are influenced by diet and are low in necrotic liver disease.

18. A patient's BUN is 60 mg/dL and serum creatinine is 3.0 mg/dL. These results suggest:
    A. Laboratory error measuring BUN
    B. Renal failure
    C. Prerenal failure
    D. Patient was not fasting

    Chemistry/Evaluate laboratory data to determine possible inconsistent results/Biochemical/3

19. Urinary urea measurements may be used for calculation of:
    A. Glomerular filtration
    B. Renal blood flow
    C. Nitrogen balance
    D. All of the above

    Chemistry/Correlate laboratory data with physiological processes/Biochemical/2

20. BUN is determined electrochemically by coupling the urease reaction to measurement of:
    A. Potential with a urea-selective electrode
    B. The timed rate of increase in conductivity
    C. The oxidation of ammonia
    D. Carbon dioxide

    Chemistry/Apply principles of special procedures/Biochemical/1

21. In the UV enzymatic method for BUN, the urease reaction is coupled to a second enzymatic reaction using:
    A. AST
    B. Glutamate dehydrogenase
    C. Glutamine synthetase
    D. Alanine aminotransferase (ALT)

    Chemistry/Apply principles of basic laboratory procedures/Biochemical/1

22. Which product is measured in the coupling step of the urease-UV method for BUN?
    A. CO_2
    B. Dinitrophenylhydrazine
    C. Diphenylcarbazone
    D. NAD^+

    Chemistry/Apply principles of basic laboratory procedures/Biochemical/1

Answers to Questions 18–22

18. **C** BUN is affected by renal blood flow as well as by glomerular and tubular function. When blood flow to the kidneys is diminished by circulatory insufficiency (prerenal failure), glomerular filtration decreases and tubular reabsorption increases owing to slower filtrate flow. Because urea is reabsorbed, BUN levels rise higher than those of creatinine. This causes the BUN:creatinine ratio to be greater than 10:1.

19. **C** Because BUN is handled by the tubules, serum levels are not specific for glomerular filtration rate. Urea clearance is influenced by diet and liver function as well as by renal function. Protein intake minus excretion determines nitrogen balance. A negative balance (excretion exceeds intake) occurs in stress, starvation, fever, cachexia, and chronic illness.

    Nitrogen balance = (protein intake in grams per day $\div$ 6.25) – (urine nitrogen in grams per day + 4)

20. **B** A conductivity electrode is used to measure the increase in conductance of the solution as urea is hydrolyzed by urease in the presence of sodium carbonate.

    $$\text{Urea} + H_2O \xrightarrow{\text{Urease}} 2NH_3 + CO_2$$
    $$2NH_3 + 2H_2O + Na_2CO_3 \rightarrow 2NH_4^+ + CO_3^{-2} + 2NaOH$$

    Ammonium ions increase the conductance of the solution. The timed rate of current increase is proportional to the BUN concentration. Alternatively, the ammonium ions produced can be measured using an ion selective electrode.

21. **B** BUN is most frequently measured by the urease-UV method in which the urease reaction is coupled to the glutamate dehydrogenase reaction, generating NAD^+.

    $$\text{Urea} + H_2O \xrightarrow{\text{Urease}} 2NH_3 + CO_2$$
    $$\text{2-Oxoglutarate} + NH_3 + NADH + H^+ \xrightarrow{\text{GLD}}$$
    $$\text{Glutamate} + NAD^+ + H_2O$$

    When the urease reaction is performed under first-order conditions, the decrease in absorbance at 340 nm is proportional to the urea concentration.

22. **D** In the urease-UV method, urease is used to hydrolyze urea, forming CO_2 and ammonia. Glutamate dehydrogenase catalyzes the oxidation of NADH, forming glutamate from 2-oxoglutarate and ammonia. The glutamate dehydrogenase reaction is used for measuring both BUN and ammonia.

23. Which enzyme deficiency is responsible for phenylke-tonuria (PKU)?
  A. Phenylalanine hydroxylase
  B. Tyrosine transaminase
  C. *p*-Hydroxyphenylpyruvic acid oxidase
  D. Homogentisic acid oxidase

Chemistry/Apply knowledge of fundamental biological characteristics/Aminoaciduria/1

24. Which of the following conditions is classified as a renal-type aminoaciduria?
  A. Fanconi's syndrome
  B. Wilson's disease
  C. Hepatitis
  D. Homocystinuria

Chemistry/Correlate clinical and laboratory data/ Aminoaciduria/2

25. Which aminoaciduria results in the overflow of branched chain amino acids?
  A. Hartnup's disease
  B. Alkaptonuria
  C. Homocystinuria
  D. Maple syrup urine disease

Chemistry/Apply knowledge of fundamental biological characteristics/Aminoaciduria/1

26. Which of the following best describes the Guthrie test?
  A. Bioassay for PKU dependent upon the phenylalanine requirement of *Bacillus subtilis*
  B. Ion exchange HPLC and postcolumn reaction with ninhydrin
  C. Two-dimensional TLC using ninhydrin staining
  D. Reaction of phenylpyruvic acid with ferric chloride to form a blue-green complex

Chemistry/Apply principles of special procedures/ Aminoaciduria/2

27. Of the methods used to measure amino acids, which is capable of measuring only phenylalanine?
  A. Tandem mass spectroscopy
  B. High-performance liquid chromatography
  C. Capillary electrophoresis
  D. Fluorometric analysis with ninhydrin

Chemistry/Apply principles of special procedures/ Biochemical/1

Answers to Questions 23–27

23. **A** PKU is an overflow aminoaciduria resulting from the accumulation of phenylalanine. It is caused by a deficiency of phenylalanine hydroxylase, which converts phenylalanine to tyrosine. Excess phenylalanine accumulates in blood. This is transaminated, forming phenylpyruvic acid, which is excreted in the urine.

24. **A** Fanconi's disease is an inherited syndrome of anemia, mental retardation, rickets, and aminoaciduria. Because the aminoaciduria results from a defect in the renal tubule, it is classified as a (secondary inherited) renal-type aminoaciduria. Wilson's disease, inherited ceruloplasmin deficiency, causes hepatic failure. It is classified as a secondary inherited overflow-type because the aminoaciduria results from urea cycle failure. Hepatitis is classified as a secondary acquired overflow-type aminoaciduria. Homocystinuria is a primary inherited overflow-type aminoaciduria and is caused by a deficiency of cystathionine synthase.

25. **D** Valine, leucine, and isoleucine accumulate as a result of branched chain decarboxylase deficiency in maple syrup urine disease. These are transaminated to ketoacids that are excreted, giving urine a maple sugar odor. Alkaptonuria is caused by homogentisic acid oxidase deficiency leading to homogentisic aciduria. Homocystinuria is a no-threshold-type aminoaciduria that usually results from cystathionine synthase deficiency.

26. **A** All the methods above may be used to screen for PKU, although the ferric chloride test is nonspecific and not sufficiently sensitive for newborns. The Guthrie test uses thienylalanine, which inhibits the growth of *B. subtilis* unless excess phenylalanine is present. Guthrie assays using specific amino acid inhibitors are used to screen for maple syrup urine disease, tyrosinemia, lysinemia, and homocystinuria. However, many states are now using thermospray ionization tandem mass spectroscopy (MS/MS), which can detect over 20 inborn errors of metabolism from a single blood spot.

27. **D** The first three methods along with two-dimensional TLC and gas chromatography are able to separate each amino acid (up to 40 species). Fluorometric analysis with ninhydrin is used to measure the concentration of phenylalanine. It is suitable as a quantitative test for phenylalanine, although there is slight interference from tyrosine and a few other amino acids. The other methods can be used to detect other inborn errors of amino acid metabolism.

28. Blood ammonia levels are usually measured in order to evaluate:
   A. Renal failure
   B. Acid-base status
   C. Hepatic coma
   D. Gastrointestinal malabsorption

Chemistry/Correlate clinical and laboratory data/Biochemical/2

29. Enzymatic measurement of ammonia requires which of the following substrates and coenzymes?

	Substrate	Coenzyme
A.	α-Ketoglutarate	NADH
B.	Glutamate	NADH
C.	Glutamine	ATP
D.	Glutamine	NAD⁺

Chemistry/Apply principles of basic laboratory procedures/Biochemical/1

30. Which statement about ammonia is true?
   A. Normally most of the plasma ammonia is derived from deamination of amino acids
   B. Ammonia-induced coma can result from salicylate poisoning
   C. Hepatic coma can result from Reye's syndrome
   D. High plasma ammonia is usually associated with respiratory alkalosis

Chemistry/Correlate clinical and laboratory data/ Biochemical/2

31. SITUATION: A sample for ammonia assay is taken from an intravenous line that had been capped and injected with lithium heparin (called a heparin lock). The sample is drawn in a syringe containing lithium heparin and immediately capped and iced. The plasma is separated and analyzed within 20 minutes of collection, and the result is 50 μg/dL higher than one measured 4 hours before. What is the most likely explanation of these results?
   A. Significantly greater physiological variation is seen with patients with systemic, hepatic, and gastrointestinal diseases
   B. The syringe was contaminated with ammonia
   C. One of the two samples was collected from the wrong patient
   D. Stasis of blood in the line caused increased ammonia

Chemistry/Evaluate sources of error/Specimen collection and handling/3

28. C Hepatic coma is caused by accumulation of ammonia in the brain as a result of liver failure. The ammonia increases central nervous system pH and is coupled to glutamate, a central nervous system neurotransmitter, forming glutamine. Blood and cerebrospinal fluid ammonia levels are used to distinguish encephalopathy caused by cirrhosis or other liver disease from nonhepatic causes and to monitor patients with hepatic coma.

29. A Enzymatic assays of ammonia utilize glutamate dehydrogenase (GLD). This enzyme forms glutamate from α-ketoglutarate (2-oxoglutarate) and ammonia, resulting in oxidation of NADH. The rate of absorbance decrease at 340 nm is proportional to ammonia concentration when the reaction rate is maintained under first-order conditions.

30. C Ammonia produced in the intestines from the breakdown of proteins by bacterial enzymes is the primary source of plasma ammonia. Most of the ammonia absorbed from the intestines is transported to the liver via the portal vein and converted to urea. Blood ammonia levels rise in any necrotic liver disease, including hepatitis, Reye's syndrome, and drug-induced injury such as acetaminophen poisoning. In hepatic cirrhosis, shunting of portal blood to the general circulation causes blood ammonia levels to rise. Ammonia crosses the brain-blood barrier, which accounts for the frequency of central nervous system complications and, if severe, causes hepatic coma.

31. D Falsely elevated blood ammonia levels are commonly caused by improper specimen collection. Venous stasis and prolonged storage cause peripheral deamination of amino acids, producing a falsely high ammonia level. Plasma is the sample of choice, since ammonia levels increase with storage. Lithium heparin and EDTA are acceptable anticoagulants; the anticoagulant used should be tested to make sure it is free of ammonia. A vacuum tube can be used if filled completely. Serum may be used provided that the tube is iced immediately and the serum is separated as soon as the sample clots. The patient should be fasting and must not have smoked for 8 hours because tobacco smoke can double the plasma ammonia level.

32. Uric acid is derived from the:
  A. Oxidation of proteins
  B. Catabolism of purines
  C. Oxidation of pyrimidines
  D. Reduction of catecholamines

Chemistry/Apply knowledge of fundamental biological characteristics/Biochemical/1

33. Which of the following conditions is associated with hyperuricemia?
  A. Renal failure
  B. Chronic liver disease
  C. Xanthine oxidase deficiency
  D. Paget's disease of the bone

Chemistry/Correlate clinical and laboratory data/Biochemical/2

34. Orders for uric acid are legitimate *stat* requests because:
  A. Levels above 10 mg/dL cause urinary tract calculi
  B. Uric acid is hepatotoxic
  C. High levels induce aplastic anemia
  D. High levels cause joint pain

Chemistry/Correlate clinical and laboratory data/Biochemical/2

35. Which uric acid method is associated with negative bias caused by reducing agents?
  A. Uricase coupled with the Trinder reaction
  B. UV uricase reaction coupled with catalase and alcohol dehydrogenase reactions
  C. Measurement of the negative rate at 290 nm after addition of uricase
  D. Phosphotungstic acid using a protein-free filtrate

Chemistry/Evaluate sources of error/Biochemical/2

32. **B** Uric acid is the principal product of purine (adenosine and guanosine) metabolism. Oxidation of proteins yields urea along with CO_2, H_2O, and inorganic acids. Catecholamines are oxidized, forming vanillylmandelic acid (VMA) and homovanillic acid (HVA).

33. **A** Excessive retention of uric acid results from renal failure and diuretics (or other drugs) that block uric acid excretion. Hyperuricemia may result from overproduction of uric acid in primary essential gout or excessive cell turnover associated with malignancy and chemotherapy. Overproduction of uric acid may also result from an enzyme deficiency in the pathway forming guanosine triphosphate (GTP) or adenosine monophosphate (AMP) (purine salvage). Hyperuricemia is also associated with ketoacidosis and lactate acidosis, hypertension, and hyperlipidemia. Xanthine oxidase converts xanthine to uric acid; therefore, a deficiency of this enzyme results in low serum levels of uric acid. Paget's disease of bone causes cyclic episodes of bone degeneration and regeneration and is associated with very high serum alkaline phosphatase and urinary calcium levels.

34. **A** Uric acid calculi form quickly when the serum uric acid level reaches 10 mg/dL. They are translucent compact stones that often lodge in the ureters and cause postrenal failure.

35. **A** The peroxidase-coupled uricase reaction is the most common method for measuring uric acid in serum or plasma. Uricase methods form allantoin, carbon dioxide, and hydrogen peroxide from the oxidation of uric acid. When peroxide is used to oxidize a Trinder dye (e.g., a phenol derivative and 4-aminoantipyrine), some negative bias may occur when high levels of ascorbate or other reducing agents are present. Rate UV methods are free from this interference. Reduction of phosphotungstic acid by uric acid forms tungsten blue. This colorimetric reaction is nonspecific, resulting in falsely elevated uric acid caused by proteins and many other reducing substances.

PROTEINS, ELECTROPHORESIS, AND LIPIDS

1. **Kjeldahl's procedure for total protein is based upon the premise that:**
   - **A.** Proteins are negatively charged
   - **B.** The pK_a of proteins is the same
   - **C.** The nitrogen content of proteins is constant
   - **D.** Proteins have similar tyrosine and tryptophan content

   Chemistry/Apply principles of special procedures/ Proteins and enzymes/1

2. **The term "biuret reaction" refers to:**
   - **A.** The reaction of phenolic groups with $CuSO_4$
   - **B.** Coordinate bonds between Cu^{2+} and carboxyl and amino groups of biuret
   - **C.** The protein error of indicator effect producing color when dyes bind protein
   - **D.** The reaction of phosphomolybdic acid with protein

   Chemistry/Apply principles of basic laboratory procedures/Proteins and enzymes/1

3. **Which statement about the biuret reaction for total protein is true?**
   - **A.** It is sensitive to protein levels below 0.1 mg/dL
   - **B.** It is suitable for urine, exudates, and transudates
   - **C.** Polypeptides and compounds with repeating imine groups react
   - **D.** Hemolysis will not interfere

   Chemistry/Apply knowledge to identify sources of error/Proteins and enzymes/2

4. **Which of the following protein methods has the highest analytical sensitivity?**
   - **A.** Refractometry
   - **B.** Folin-Lowry
   - **C.** Turbidimetry
   - **D.** Direct UV absorption

   Chemistry/Apply knowledge of special procedures/ Proteins and enzymes/2

Answers to Questions 1–4

1. **C** Kjeldahl's method measures the nitrogen content of proteins as ammonium ion by back titration following oxidation of proteins by sulfuric acid and heat. It assumes that proteins average 16% nitrogen by weight. Protein in grams per deciliter is calculated by multiplying protein nitrogen by 6.25. The Kjeldahl method is a reference method for total protein that is used to assign a protein assay value to calibrators.

2. **B** Biuret is a compound with two carbonyl groups and three amino groups and forms coordinate bonds with Cu^{2+} in the same manner as protein. Therefore, proteins and peptides are both measured in the biuret reaction. The biuret reagent consists of an alkaline solution of copper II sulfate. Tartrate salts are added to keep the copper in solution and potassium iodide to prevent oxidation.

3. **C** The biuret reaction is not sensitive to protein levels below 0.1 g/dL and, therefore, is not sensitive enough for assays of total protein in CSF, urine, or transudates. Slight hemolysis does not cause falsely high results, if the absorbance of the Cu^{2+}-protein complexes is measured bichromatically. However, frankly hemolyzed samples contain sufficient globin to cause positive interference.

4. **B** The Folin-Lowry (Lowry's) method uses both biuret reagent and phosphotungstic/molybdic acids to oxidize the aromatic side groups on proteins. The oxidized phenolic groups reduce the Cu^{2+} in the biuret reagent, greatly increasing sensitivity.

5. Which of the following statements regarding proteins is true?
  A. Total protein and albumin are about 10% higher in ambulatory patients
  B. Plasma total protein is about 15% higher than serum levels
  C. Albumin normally accounts for about 40% of cerebrospinal fluid total protein
  D. Transudative serous fluid protein is about two thirds of the serum level

Chemistry/Evaluate laboratory data to recognize health and disease states/Proteins and enzymes/2

6. Hyperalbuminemia is caused by:
  A. Dehydration syndromes
  B. Liver disease
  C. Burns
  D. Gastroenteropathy

Chemistry/Correlate clinical and laboratory data/ Proteins and enzymes/2

7. High serum total protein but low albumin is usually seen in:
  A. Multiple myeloma
  B. Hepatic cirrhosis
  C. Glomerulonephritis
  D. Nephrotic syndrome

Chemistry/Correlate clinical and laboratory data/ Proteins and enzymes/2

8. Which of the following conditions is most commonly associated with an elevated level of total protein?
  A. Glomerular disease
  B. Starvation
  C. Liver failure
  D. Malignancy

Chemistry/Correlate clinical and laboratory data/ Proteins and enzymes/2

9. Which of the following dyes is the most specific for measurement of albumin?
  A. Bromcresol green (BCG)
  B. Bromcresol purple (BCP)
  C. Tetrabromosulfophthalein
  D. Tetrabromphenol blue

Chemistry/Apply principles of basic laboratory procedures/Proteins and enzymes/1

Answers to Questions 5–9

5. **A** Water pools in the vascular bed in nonambulatory patients, lowering the total protein, albumin, hematocrit, and calcium. Plasma levels of total protein are about 0.2–0.4 g/dL higher than serum levels owing to fibrinogen. Cerebrospinal fluid albumin levels are normally 10–30 mg/dL, which is approximately two thirds of the CSF total protein. Transudates have a total protein below 3.0 g/dL and less than 50% of the serum total protein.

6. **A** A high serum albumin level is caused only by dehydration or administration of albumin. Liver disease, burns, gastroenteropathy, nephrosis, starvation, and malignancy cause hypoalbuminemia.

7. **A** In multiple myeloma, synthesis of large quantities of monoclonal immunoglobulin by plasma cells often results in decreased synthesis of albumin. In glomerulonephritis and nephrotic syndrome, both total protein and albumin are low owing to loss of proteins through the glomeruli. In hepatic cirrhosis, decreased hepatic production of protein results in low total protein and albumin.

8. **D** Malignant disease is usually associated with increased immunoglobulin and acute phase protein production. However, nutrients required for protein synthesis are consumed, causing reduced hepatic albumin production. Glomerular damage causes albumin and other low molecular weight proteins to be lost through the kidneys. Liver failure and starvation result in decreased protein synthesis.

9. **B** Tetrabromphenol blue and tetrabromosulfophthalein are dyes that change pK_a in the presence of protein. Although they have greater affinity for albumin than globulins, they are not sufficiently specific to apply to measurement of serum albumin. BCG and BCP are anionic dyes that undergo a spectral shift when they bind albumin at acid pH. BCP is more specific for albumin than BCG. Reaction of both dyes with globulins requires a longer incubation time than with albumin, and reaction times are kept at 30 seconds or less to increase specificity. Both dyes are free of interference from bilirubin. However, BCG is the method used most often. One reason for this is that renal dialysis patients produce an organic acid that competes with BCP for the binding site on albumin, causing a falsely low result.

10. Which of the following factors is most likely to cause a falsely low result when using the BCG dye-binding assay for albumin?

A. The presence of penicillin
B. An incubation time of 120 seconds
C. The presence of bilirubin
D. Lipemia

Chemistry/Apply knowledge to recognize source of error/Proteins and enzymes/2

11. At pH 8.6 proteins are _____ charged and migrate toward the _____.

A. Negatively   Anode
B. Positively   Cathode
C. Positively   Anode
D. Negatively   Cathode

Chemistry/Apply knowledge of fundamental biological characteristics/Electrophoresis/1

12. Electrophoretic movement of proteins toward the anode will be made to decrease by increasing the:

A. Buffer pH
B. Ionic strength of the buffer
C. Current
D. Voltage

Chemistry/Apply principles of basic laboratory procedures/Electrophoresis/2

13. At pH 8.6, the cathodal movement of γ globulins is caused by:

A. Electroendosmosis
B. Wick flow
C. A net positive charge
D. Cathodal sample application

Chemistry/Apply principles of basic laboratory procedures/Electrophoresis/2

14. Which of the conditions below will prevent any migration of proteins across an electrophoretic support medium such as agarose?

A. Using too high a voltage
B. Excessive current during the procedure
C. Loss of contact between a buffer chamber and the medium
D. Evaporation of solvent from the surface of the medium

Chemistry/Apply principles of basic laboratory procedures/Electrophoresis/2

Answers to Questions 10–14

10. A BCG and BCP are not significantly affected by bilirubin or hemolysis, although negative interference caused by free Hgb has been reported with some BCG methods. Lipemic samples may cause positive interference, which can be eliminated by serum blanking. Incubation times as long as 2 minutes result in positive interference from globulins, which react with the dye. Penicillin and some other anionic drugs bind to albumin at the same site as the dye, causing falsely low results.

11. A Proteins are amphoteric owing to ionization of acidic and basic side chains of amino acids. When the pH of the solution equals the isoelectric point (*pI*), the protein has no net charge and is insoluble. When the pH of the solution is above the *pI*, the protein has a net negative charge. Anions migrate toward the anode (positive electrode).

12. B *Electrophoresis* is the migration of charged molecules in an electric field. Increasing the strength of the field by increasing voltage (or current) increases migration. However, increasing ionic strength decreases the migration of proteins. Counterions (cations) in the buffer move with the proteins, reducing their electromagnetic attraction for the anode.

13. A Agarose and cellulose acetate contain fixed anions (e.g., acetate) that attract counterions when hydrated with buffer. When voltage is applied, the cations migrate to the cathode, creating an osmotic force that draws H_2O with them. This force, called *electroendosmosis*, opposes protein migration toward the anode and may cause some γ-globulins to be displaced toward the cathode.

14. C Movement of proteins is dependent upon the presence of a salt bridge that allows current to flow via transport of ions to the electrodes across the support medium. If the salt bridge is not intact, there will be no migration, even if voltage is maintained across the electrodes. For agarose and cellulose acetate, heat causes evaporation of solvent from the buffer. This increases the ionic strength, causing current to rise during the run. Excessive heat can damage the support medium and denature proteins. Power = E (voltage) $\times I$ (current) $\times t$ (time); since $E = I \times R$ (resistance), heat is proportional to the square of current ($P = I^2 \times R \times t$). Constant current mode is used for long runs to prevent heat damage.

15. Which of the proteins listed below has the highest pI?
   A. Albumin
   B. Transferrin
   C. Ceruloplasmin
   D. IgG

Chemistry/Apply knowledge of fundamental biological characteristics/Electrophoresis/1

16. Which of the proteins listed below migrates in the β region at pH 8.6?
   A. Haptoglobin
   B. Orosomucoprotein
   C. Antichymotrypsin
   D. Transferrin

Chemistry/Apply knowledge of fundamental biological characteristics/Electrophoresis/1

17. Which of the following is one advantage of high-resolution (HR) agarose electrophoresis over lower current electrophoresis?
   A. High-resolution procedures detect monoclonal and oligoclonal bands at a lower concentration
   B. A smaller sample volume is used
   C. Results are obtained more rapidly
   D. More samples can be applied to the support medium

Chemistry/Apply principles of special procedures/ Electrophoresis/2

18. Which of the following conditions is associated with "β-γ bridging"?
   A. Multiple myeloma
   B. Malignancy
   C. Hepatic cirrhosis
   D. Rheumatoid arthritis

Chemistry/Correlate clinical and laboratory data/ Electrophoresis/2

19. Which support medium can be used to determine the molecular weight of a protein?
   A. Cellulose acetate
   B. Polyacrylamide gel
   C. Agar gel
   D. Agarose gel

Chemistry/Apply principles of special procedures/ Electrophoresis/2

20. Which of the following stains is used for lipoprotein electrophoresis?
   A. Oil Red O
   B. Coomassie Brilliant Blue
   C. Amido Black
   D. Ponceau S

Chemistry/Select reagents/Media/Blood products/ Electrophoresis/1

15. **D** Albumin is the fastest migrating protein toward the anode at pH 8.6, followed by α_1-, α_2-, β-, and γ-globulins. Because albumin is fastest, it has the greatest net negative charge and lowest *pI* (about 4.6). γ-Globulins are predominantly immunoglobulins and have the highest *pI* (about 7.2).

16. **D** Transferrin, β-lipoprotein, C3, and C4 (fibrinogen if plasma is used) are the dominant proteins in the β-globulin region. Haptoglobin and α_2-macroglobulin are the principal proteins in the α_2-fraction. α_1-Antitrypsin, α_1-lipoprotein, and orosomucoprotein (α_1-acid glycoprotein) make up most of the α_1-fraction. Immunoglobulins dominate the γ region.

17. **A** HR agarose procedures use higher current and a cooling device to resolve 12 or more bands. Advantages include phenotyping of α_1-antitrypsin (detection of Z and S variants), detection of β_2-microglobulin in urine indicating tubular proteinuria (often associated with drug-induced nephrosis), and greater sensitivity in detecting monoclonal gammopathies, immune complexes, and oligoclonal bands in CSF that are associated with multiple sclerosis.

18. **C** Hepatic cirrhosis produces a polyclonal gammopathy associated with a high IgA level. This obliterates the valley between β and γ zones. Malignancy and rheumatoid arthritis produce polyclonal gammopathies classified as chronic inflammatory or delayed response patterns. Multiple myeloma produces a zone of restricted mobility usually in the γ- but sometimes in the β- or α_2-region.

19. **B** Polyacrylamide and starch gels separate by molecular sieving as well as charge. Sodium dodecyl sulfate (SDS) is a nonionic detergent that binds to proteins, neutralizing charge. Polyacrylamide gel with SDS added (SDS-PAGE) electrophoresis separates proteins on the basis of molecular size. The smaller proteins become trapped in the pores of the gel and migrate more slowly.

20. **A** Oil Red O and Sudan Black B stain neutral fats and are used to stain lipoproteins as well as fat in urine or stool. The other stains are used for proteins. Coomassie Brilliant Blue is more sensitive than Ponceau S or Amido Black, and all three stains have a slightly greater affinity for albumin than globulins. In addition, silver nitrate may be used to stain CSF proteins because it has far greater sensitivity than the other stains.

21. Which of the following serum protein electrophoresis results suggests an acute inflammatory process?

Globulins

	Albumin	α₁	α₂	β	γ
A.	Decreased	Increased	Decreased	Normal	Normal
B.	Normal	Increased	Normal	Increased	Increased
C.	Decreased	Increased	Increased	Normal	Normal
D.	Increased	Increased	Increased	Increased	Increased

Chemistry/Correlate clinical and laboratory data/ Electrophoresis/2

22. Which of the conditions below is usually associated with an acute inflammatory pattern?
A. Myocardial infarction (MI)
B. Malignancy
C. Rheumatoid arthritis
D. Hepatitis

Chemistry/Correlate clinical and laboratory data/ Electrophoresis/2

23. The electrophoretic pattern shown in the densitometric tracing below most likely indicates:
A. α₁-Antitrypsin deficiency
B. Infection
C. Nephrosis
D. Systemic sclerosis

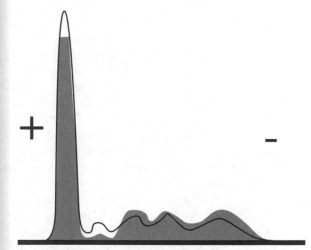

Chemistry/Evaluate laboratory data to recognize health and disease states/Proteins and enzymes/2

24. What is the clinical utility of testing for serum prealbumin?
A. Low levels are associated with increased free cortisol
B. High levels are an indicator of acute inflammation
C. Serial low levels indicate compromised nutritional status
D. Levels correlate with glomerular injury in patients with diabetes mellitus

Chemistry/Apply knowledge of fundamental biological characteristics/Nutrition markers/1

Answers to Questions 21–24

21. **C** Acute inflammation is characterized by increased production of acute phase proteins. These include α₁-antitrypsin, α₁-acid glycoprotein, α₁-antichymotrypsin, and haptoglobin. Albumin is slightly decreased; γ- and β-fractions are normal.

22. **A** MI produces a pattern of acute inflammation usually associated with tissue injury. This pattern results from production of acute phase proteins, including α₁-antitrypsin, α₁-antichymotrypsin, and haptoglobin. It is also seen in early infection, pregnancy, and early nephritis. Malignancy, rheumatoid arthritis, and hepatitis are associated with a chronic inflammatory pattern. This differs from the acute pattern by the addition of a polyclonal gammopathy.

23. **A** This pattern shows a marked decrease in the α₁-globulin (slightly less than one fifth of the expected peak area). Staining of the α₁-globulin fraction is predominantly determined by the α₁-antitrypsin level. A value of less than 20% of normal (0.2–0.4 g/dL) is usually caused by homozygous α₁-antitrypsin deficiency. There is a slight decrease in albumin and increase in the α₂-fraction. Patients with α₁-antitrypsin deficiency often display elevations in the α₂-globulin and γ-globulin fraction because the condition is associated with chronic emphysema and hepatic cirrhosis.

24. **C** Prealbumin (also called transthyretin) is a small protein with a half-life of only 2 days. Serum levels fall rapidly in patients with deficient protein nutrition. As a result, prealbumin is used to detect malnutrition and to measure the patient's response to dietary supplementation. The cutpoint used to identify nutritional deficiency in elderly patients is usually 11 mg/dL.

25. Which serum protein should be measured in a patient suspected of having Wilson's disease?
   A. Hemopexin
   B. α_1-Antitrypsin
   C. Haptoglobin
   D. Ceruloplasmin

   Chemistry/Apply knowledge of fundamental biological characteristics/Proteins/2

26. A patient with hemolytic-uremic syndrome associated with septicemia has a normal haptoglobin level although the plasma free hemoglobin is elevated and hemoglobinuria is present. Which test would be more appropriate than haptoglobin to measure this patient's hemolytic episode?
   A. Hemopexin
   B. α_1-Antitrypsin
   C. C-reactive protein
   D. Transferrin

   Chemistry/Apply knowledge to recognize inconsistent laboratory results/Proteins/3

27. Quantitative determination of Hgb A_2 is best performed by:
   A. Column chromatography
   B. Alkali denaturation
   C. Electrophoresis
   D. Direct bichromatic spectrophotometry

   Chemistry/Apply principles of basic laboratory procedures/Hemoglobin/1

28. Hgb F concentration is usually measured by:
   A. Alkali denaturation of Hgb A and Hgb A_2
   B. Specific Hgb F peroxidase reaction
   C. Turbidimetric assay of Hgb F after precipitation with ammonium sulfate
   D. Gas chromatography

   Chemistry/Apply principles of special procedures/Hemoglobin/1

Answers to Questions 25–28

25. D α_1-Antitrypsin, haptoglobin, and ceruloplasmin are acute phase proteins and are increased in inflammatory diseases. Ceruloplasmin is an α-2 globulin that binds the majority of the serum copper. Levels are low in almost all patients with Wilson's disease, an autosomal recessive disorder caused by accumulation of copper in the liver, brain, kidney, and other tissues. Low ceruloplasmin may occur in patients with nephrosis, malnutrition, and hepatobiliary disease. Therefore, the diagnosis of Wilson's disease is made by demonstrating decreased ceruloplasmin, increased serum and urinary copper, and the presence of Kayser-Fleischer rings (brown deposits at the edge of the cornea).

26. A Hemopexin is a small β-globulin that binds to free heme. Haptoglobin is an α-2 globulin that binds to free hemoglobin and disappears from the serum when intravascular hemolysis produces more than 3 g of free plasma hemoglobin. However, haptoglobin is an acute phase protein, and hepatic production and release are increased in response to acute infections. The normal serum haptoglobin is most likely the result of increased synthesis and would not accurately estimate the hemolytic episode in this patient.

27. A Hgb A_2 is most often measured by anion exchange column chromatography. Because Hgbs A and F have a greater negative charge than Hgb A_2, they are retained on the column after Hgb A_2 is eluted using glycine and potassium cyanide. The Hgb elutes as cyanmethemoglobin and is measured at 415 nm. Hgb F is measured by alkali denaturation. Ammonium sulfate precipitates Hgb A and Hgb A_2 but Hgb F remains soluble. High performance liquid chromatography is used by laboratories that screen a high volume of samples for abnormal hemoglobins to measure both Hgb A_2 and Hgb F. The procedure uses a cation exchange column to separate the hemoglobins, which are eluted from the column in order of increasing positive charge using a sodium phosphate buffer to produce a gradient of increasing ionic strength.

28. A Hgb is reacted with Drabkin's reagent to form cyanmethemoglobin. The cyanmethemoglobin derivatives of Hgb A and Hgb A_2 are denatured by NaOH and then precipitated using 40% ammonium sulfate. Hgb F is alkali-resistant and remains in solution. The absorbance of the supernatant is measured at 540 nm.

29. Select the correct order of Hgb migration on agarose or cellulose acetate at pH 8.6.
A. − C→F→S→A +
B. − S→C→A→F +
C. − C→S→F→A +
D. − S→F→A→C +

Chemistry/Apply principles of special procedures/Electrophoresis/2

30. Which of the following abnormal Hgbs migrates to the same position as Hgb S on agarose or cellulose acetate at pH 8.6?
A. Hgb C
B. Hgb D$_{Punjab}$
C. Hgb O
D. Hgb E

Chemistry/Apply principles of special procedures/Electrophoresis/2

31. Which Hgb is a β-δ chain hybrid and migrates to the same position as Hgb S at pH 8.6?
A. Hgb C$_{Harlem}$
B. Hgb$_{Lepore}$
C. Hgb G$_{Philadelphia}$
D. Hgb D$_{Punjab}$

Chemistry/Apply principles of special procedures/Electrophoresis/2

32. Select the correct order of Hgb migration on citrate agar at pH 6.2.
A. − F → S → C → A +
B. − F → A → S → C +
C. − A → S → F → C +
D. − A → C → S → F +

Chemistry/Apply principles of special procedures/Electrophoresis/2

33. Which Hgb separates from Hgb S on citrate (acid) agar but *not* on agarose or cellulose acetate?
A. Hgb D$_{Punjab}$
B. Hgb E
C. Hgb C$_{Harlem}$ (Georgetown)
D. Hgb O

Chemistry/Evaluate laboratory data to verify test results/Electrophoresis/2

34. In double immunodiffusion reactions the precipitin band is:
A. Invisible before the equivalence point is reached
B. Concave to the protein of greatest molecular weight
C. Closest to the well containing the highest level of antigen
D. Located in an area of antibody excess

Chemistry/Apply knowledge of special procedures/Immunodiffusion/1

Answers to Questions 29–34

29. C Hgb A$_2$ is the slowest of the normal Hgbs, and Hgb A is the fastest. Hgb F migrates just behind Hgb A. Hgb S migrates midway between Hgb A$_2$ and Hgb A. Hgbs C, C$_{Harlem}$ (Georgetown), O, and E migrate with Hgb A$_2$. Hgbs G and D$_{Punjab}$ and Hgb$_{Lepore}$ migrate with Hgb S.

30. B Hgb D migrates with Hgb S on cellulose acetate or agarose at pH 8.6–9.2. Hgb C, E, O, and C$_{Harlem}$ migrate to the same position as Hgb A$_2$ on cellulose acetate or agarose at pH 8.6–9.2. Hgb S may be differentiated from Hgb D using citrate (acid) agar at pH 6.2. Using this technique, Hgb S migrates further toward the anode than Hgb D.

31. B Hgb$_{Lepore}$ results from translocation of β and δ globin genes, resulting in a polypeptide chain that migrates midway between Hgb A$_2$ and Hgb A. The chain is transcribed more slowly than the β polypeptide chain, causing the quantity of Hgb$_{Lepore}$ to be less than 15%. Hgb$_{Lepore}$ is suspected when Hgb migrating in the "S" zone comprises less than 20% of the total Hgb. In Hgb S trait, the AS phenotype produces 20%–40% Hgb S.

32. B In an acid buffer, the hemoglobins are expected to migrate to the cathode with hemoglobin A being the slowest because it has the weakest net positive charge. However, Hgb C and Hgb S bind to sulfated pectins in the agar gel, forming a complex that is negatively charged and causing them to migrate toward the anode. Hgb C migrates furthest toward the anode, followed by Hgb S. Hgb F migrates furthest toward the cathode. Hgbs A, A$_2$, E, G, and$_{Lepore}$ migrate slightly toward the cathode.

33. A Hgbs O, E, and C$_{Harlem}$ migrate to the same position as Hgbs A$_2$ and C on agarose (or cellulose acetate) at pH 8.6. Hgb D$_{Punjab}$ migrates to the same position as Hgb S on agarose but moves with Hgb A on citrate agar. Agarose is a purified form of agar; it lacks the sulfated pectins required to separate Hgbs D and G from Hgb S, and Hgbs E, C$_{Harlem}$, and O from Hgb C. Hgb C$_{Harlem}$ is a sickling Hgb and it migrates to the same position as Hgb S on citrate (acid) agar.

34. B In double immunodiffusion (Ouchterlony), the molecules of lower molecular weight move fastest through the gel, causing a visible precipitin arc when antigen and antibody approach equivalence. At equivalence the precipitin arc remains stationary. If the concentration of antisera is constant, the distance of the precipitin arc from the antigen well is proportional to antigen concentration.

35. Which statement best describes immunofixation electrophoresis (IEF)?

  A. Proteins are separated by electrophoresis followed by overlay of monospecific anti-immunoglobulins

  B. Proteins react with monospecific antisera followed by electrophoresis

  C. Antisera are electrophoresed, then diffused against patient's serum

  D. Serum is electrophoresed; the separated immunoglobulins diffuse against specific antisera placed into troughs

Chemistry/Apply knowledge of special procedures/ Immunoelectrophoresis/2

36. Which of the following statements regarding the identification of monoclonal proteins by IFE is true?

  A. The monoclonal band must be present in the γ region

  B. When testing for a monoclonal gammopathy, both serum and urine must be examined

  C. A diagnosis of monoclonal gammopathy is based upon quantitation of IgG, IgA, and IgM

  D. A monoclonal band always indicates a malignant disorder

Chemistry/Correlate clinical and laboratory data/ Immunoelectrophoresis/2

37. Which statement regarding IFE is true?

  A. Serum containing a monoclonal protein should have a κ:λ ratio of 0.5

  B. A monoclonal band seen with monospecific antiserum should not be visible in the lane where polyvalent antiserum or sulfosalicylic acid was added

  C. CSF should be concentrated 50- to100-fold before performing IFE

  D. When oligoclonal bands are seen in the CSF, they must also be present in serum to indicate multiple sclerosis

Chemistry/Apply knowledge of special procedures/ Immunoelectrophoresis/2

35. **A** Immunofixation electrophoresis (IFE) is a rapid alternative to immunoelectrophoresis to identify monoclonal bands in serum or urine. Electrophoresis is performed on the serum or urine sample in the same manner as for protein electrophoresis except that six lanes are used for the same sample. After the proteins are separated, a different monospecific antiserum is applied across the surface of each lane. After incubating, the gel is washed to remove soluble proteins, and the immune complexes that remain are stained. Monoclonal bands are seen only in those lanes where the immunoglobulins were recognized by the corresponding antiserum.

36. **B** Quantitation of IgG, IgA, IgM, or IgD indicates the concentration of each class of immunoglobulin but does not distinguish monoclonal from polyclonal gammopathies. Monoclonal characteristics are determined by demonstrating restricted electrophoretic mobility, indicating that all immunoglobulins in the band are of the same amino acid sequence. Monoclonal light chains are seen in about 40% of monoclonal gammopathies. In up to 25% of multiple myeloma patients, a heavy chain gene deletion results in production of monoclonal light chains only. Because these are filtered by the glomerulus, the procedure must be performed on urine as well as serum. Some patients with a monoclonal protein fail to develop malignant plasma cell proliferation. This state is referred to as a monoclonal gammopathy of undetermined significance (MGUS). Within 10–15 years, 15%–20% of persons with MGUS develop some form of lymphoproliferative disease.

37. **C** Any monoclonal precipitin band formed when heavy- or light-chain specific antiserum reacts with sample should also be found in the same position when sample is fixed with sulfosalicylic acid or reacted with polyvalent antihuman Ig. Normally, immunoglobulins with κ light chains outnumber those with λ chains 2:1. In a monoclonal gammopathy, this ratio always heavily favors the light chain type of M protein. A diagnosis of multiple sclerosis is usually confirmed by demonstration of oligoclonal banding in the CSF, which is *not* present in the serum. CSF is usually concentrated 50–100 times to increase sensitivity.

38. Which of the following statements regarding IFE is true?
  A. Oligoclonal banding is seen in the CSF of more than 90% of multiple sclerosis cases
  B. The Bence-Jones protein heat test is confirmatory for monoclonal light chains
  C. Light chains found in urine are always derived from monoclonal protein
  D. The IgA band is usually cathodal to the IgG precipitin band

*Chemistry/Correlate clinical and laboratory data/
Immunoelectrophoresis/2*

39. Detection of isoenzyme bands following electrophoresis is facilitated by:
  A. Adding substrates to the gel and measuring catalytic activity
  B. Precipitation using antisera against the polypeptide chains of the enzyme
  C. Staining with a dye specific for the isoenzymes
  D. Elution of other proteins from the gel followed by precipitation with sulfosalicylic acid

*Chemistry/Apply principles of special procedures/
Electrophoresis/1*

40. Which isoenzyme of creatine kinase (CK) has the fastest electrophoretic mobility at pH 8.6?
  A. MM
  B. MB
  C. BB
  D. Macro CK

*Chemistry/Apply principles of special procedures/
Electrophoresis/1*

41. Capillary electrophoresis differs from agarose gel electrophoresis in which respect?
  A. A stationary support is not used
  B. An acidic buffer is used
  C. A low voltage is used
  D. Electroendosmosis does not occur

*Chemistry/Apply principles of special procedures/
Electrophoresis/1*

Answers to Questions 38–41

38. **A** The α-heavy chain is more acidic than γ or μ chains, giving IgA a greater net negative charge at alkaline pH. The IgA precipitin band is anodal to the IgG or IgM band. In hepatic cirrhosis the β-γ bridging observed on serum protein electrophoresis results from increased IgA. Light chains in the form of Fab fragments are often found in increased amounts in the urine of patients with polyclonal gammopathies, especially from patients with an autoimmune disease. These can cause a positive Bence-Jones test and will produce a polyclonal (spread-out) appearance on IFE gels.

39. **A** Quantitation of isoenzymes such as alkaline phosphatase, amylase, and creatine kinase is made after electrophoresis by saturating the pores of agarose or other support medium with substrate and incubating at 37°-45°C. Bands form on the gel where the isoenzymes are located on the medium. Densitometric scanning allows relative (%) concentration to be calculated.

40. **C** CK isoenzymes are dimers composed of M and B subunits. The B subunit is more acidic, resulting in CK-1 (BB) migrating the furthest toward the anode followed by CK-2 (MB), then CK-3 (MM). CK-1 migrates in the prealbumin zone, CK-2 after albumin, and CK-3 between the beta and gamma zones. When electrophoresis is used to measure CK isoenzymes, the fluorescence of NADH is measured. Measuring the fluorescence of NADH permits detection equivalent to about 2–3 IU/L enzyme activity. It is important to recognize the yellow fluorescence of albumin so that it is not confused with CK-1.

41. **A** Capillary electrophoresis is a rapid automated procedure for separating serum or body fluid proteins. Instead of a stationary support, the proteins migrate based upon their charge/mass ratio inside a small bore silica capillary tube (20–200 μm). The cations in the buffer are attracted to the negatively charged silicates and migrate to the cathode rapidly when voltage is applied. The electroendosmotic force created moves the proteins toward the cathode, and they are detected by an in-line UV photometer that measures their absorbance. High voltage (e.g., 9000 volts) is used to effect separation of serum proteins in an 8–10 minute run, giving about the same resolution as high resolution agarose gel electrophoresis.

42. Select the order of mobility of lipoproteins electrophoresed on cellulose acetate or agarose at pH 8.6.
A. – Chylomicrons→pre-β→β→α +
B. – β→pre-β→α→chylomicrons +
C. – Chylomicrons→β→pre-β→α +
D. – α→β→pre-β→chylomicrons +

Chemistry/Apply principles of special procedures/Electrophoresis/1

43. Following ultracentrifugation of plasma, which fraction correlates with pre-β lipoprotein?
A. Very low-density lipoprotein (VLDL)
B. Low-density lipoprotein (LDL)
C. High-density lipoprotein (HDL)
D. Chylomicrons

Chemistry/Apply principles of special procedures/Lipoproteins/2

44. Select the lipoprotein fraction that carries most of the endogenous triglycerides.
A. VLDL
B. LDL
C. HDL
D. Chylomicrons

Chemistry/Correlate laboratory data with physiological processes/Lipoproteins/2

45. The protein composition of HDL is what percentage by weight?
A. Less than 2%
B. 25%
C. 50%
D. 90%

Chemistry/Correlate laboratory data with physiological processes/Lipoproteins/1

46. Which apoprotein is inversely related to risk for coronary heart disease?
A. Apoprotein A-I
B. Apoprotein B
C. Apoprotein C-II
D. Apoprotein E-IV

Chemistry/Correlate clinical and laboratory data/Lipoproteins/2

47. Broad (floating) β-lipoprotein occurs in familial β-dyslipoproteinemia (type III hyperlipopoteinemia) and consists of _____.
A. Chylomicrons
B. VLDL
C. IDL
D. VLDL

Chemistry/Correlate clinical and laboratory data/Lipoproteins/2

42. **C** Although pre-β lipoprotein is lower in density than β-lipoprotein, it migrates faster on agarose or cellulose acetate owing to its more negative apoprotein composition. When lipoproteins are separated on polyacrylamide gel, pre-β moves more slowly than β lipoprotein. Molecular sieving causes migration to correlate with lipoprotein density when PAGE is used.

43. **A** The VLDL migrates in the pre-β zone. VLDL and most of the LDL are made in the liver. Enzymatic cleavage of VLDL results in formation of intermediate density lipoprotein (IDL) and remnant lipoproteins containing mostly apoprotein C and triglycerides. IDL is further degraded, forming LDL, which contains much of the remaining cholesterol, and apo B-100 and remnant lipoproteins, which contain most of the triglyceride and other apoproteins (including some apo B-100 that is atherogenic). The VLDL is about 50% triglyceride, but LDL is only 10% triglyceride by weight. The LDL is more dense than VLDL but is less negatively charged, causing it to migrate in the beta region when agarose is used.

44. **A** The VLDL is formed in the liver largely from chylomicron remnants and hepatic-derived triglycerides. Therefore, the VLDL transports the majority of endogenous triglycerides, while the triglycerides of chylomicrons are derived entirely from dietary absorption.

45. **C** About 50% of the weight of HDL is protein, largely apo A-I and apo A-II. The HDL is about 30% phospholipid and 20% cholesterol by weight. The HDL binds and esterifies free cholesterol from cells and transports it to the liver, where it can be eliminated in the bile.

46. **A** Apoprotein A-I and apo A-II are the principal apoproteins of HDL, and low apo A-I has a high correlation with atherosclerosis. Conversely, apo-B100 is the principal apoprotein of LDL, and an elevated level is a major risk factor in developing coronary heart disease. Apoprotein assays are not recommended as screening tests because they are not as well standardized as cholesterol assays.

47. **C** Floating β is a rare hyperlipoproteinemia inherited as an autosomal recessive trait. It results from a failure to convert VLDL to LDL, causing IDL to accumulate. Defective clearance of IDL is thought to result from deficiency of apo E-III. The IDL has a density of about 1.006–1.020, causing it to float on the 1.063 density potassium bromide solution used to recover LDL by ultracentrifugation.

48. Which of the following mechanisms accounts for the elevated plasma level of β-lipoproteins seen in familial hypercholesterolemia (type II hyperlipoproteinemia)?
   A. Hyperinsulinemia
   B. ApoB-100 receptor defect
   C. ApoC-II activated lipase deficiency
   D. ApoE-III deficiency

Chemistry/Apply knowledge of fundamental biological characteristics/Lipoproteins/2

49. Which enzyme deficiency is most commonly associated with familial hypertriglyceridemia, which is associated with fasting plasma chylomicrons (type I hyperlipoproteinemia)?
   A. β-Glucocerebrosidase deficiency
   B. Postheparin activated lipoprotein lipase deficiency
   C. Apo-B deficiency
   D. ApoC-III deficiency

Chemistry/Correlate clinical and laboratory data/ Lipoproteins/2

50. Which of the following conditions is most consistently associated with secondary hypercholesterolemia (type II lipoproteinemia)?
   A. Hypothyroidism
   B. Pancreatitis
   C. Oral contraceptive therapy
   D. Diabetes mellitus

Chemistry/Correlate clinical and laboratory data/ Lipoproteins/2

51. Which of the following is associated with Tangier's disease?
   A. Apoprotein C-II deficiency
   B. Heparin-activated capillary lipoprotein lipase deficiency
   C. Apoprotein C-II activated lipase
   D. Apoprotein A-I deficiency

Chemistry/Correlate clinical and laboratory data/ Lipoproteins/2

48. B The production of excess insulin leads to hypertriglyceridemia and is one mechanism responsible for familial hypertriglyceridemia. ApoC-II is an activator of lipoprotein lipase found in the capillary endothelium, and a deficiency causes chylomicronemia. ApoE-III deficiency results in accumulation of IDL, which results in a β-lipoprotein with decreased density (β-dyslipoproteinemia or type III hyperlipoproteinemia). Familial hypercholesterolemia is inherited as an autosomal dominant trait. Two forms have been described: a defective LDL receptor and a defect in the LDL molecule that lowers its affinity for the LDL receptor.

49. B Absence of lipoprotein lipase from capillary endothelium results in fasting chylomicronemia. β-Glucocerebrosidase deficiency results in accumulation of glycocerebrosides and is the cause of Gaucher's disease. ApoC-II deficiency results in decreased activity of peripheral and hepatic lipases and is associated with hypertriglyceridemia. Apo-B deficiency resulting from a point mutation in apo-B is responsible for hypobetalipoproteinemia and is inherited as an autosomal dominant trait. LDL levels are about half of normal in heterozygotes, and this reduces their risk of coronary artery disease. Abetalipoproteinemia results from defective hepatic transport of apo-B and is inherited as an autosomal recessive condition. LDL is absent, and the condition is associated with hemolytic anemia and central nervous system damage.

50. A The conditions listed are very commonly encountered causes of secondary hyperlipoproteinemia. Oral contraceptives, pregnancy, and estrogens may cause secondary hypertriglyceridemia (secondary type IV hyperlipoproteinemia) owing to increased VLDL and endogenous triglycerides. Hypothyroidism and obstructive hepatobiliary diseases are usually associated with secondary hypercholesterolemia (type II hyperlipoproteinemia) owing to high LDL. Diabetes mellitus and chronic pancreatitis may produce hypertriglyceridemia, chylomicronemia, or mixed hyperlipidemia.

51. D Deficiency of peripheral (blood) lipoprotein lipase is the cause of fasting chylomicronemia (type I hyperlipoproteinemia). Peripheral lipase is also known as postheparin-activated lipase and apo C-II-activated lipase. Deficiency of apo A-I is seen in Tangier's disease, a familial hypocholesterolemia with deficient or absent HDL. Tangier's disease is caused by a defect in the transport of HDL across the cell membrane rather than a defect in the production of apo-A1.

52. Which of the following formulas correctly estimates the VLDL cholesterol?
  A. Serum triglycerides divided by 5
  B. Total cholesterol minus HDL cholesterol
  C. Total cholesterol multiplied by 0.25
  D. LDL cholesterol multiplied by 0.25

Chemistry/Calculate/Lipoproteins/1

53. What is the screening procedure for adults recommended by the National Cholesterol Education Program (NCEP) to evaluate risk for atherosclerosis?
  A. Total cholesterol, fasting or nonfasting every year
  B. Total cholesterol, fasting, every 2 years
  C. Lipid profile, fasting, every 5 years
  D. HDL cholesterol, fasting or nonfasting every year

Chemistry/Apply knowledge of basic laboratory procedures/Lipids/1

54. What is the most appropriate fasting procedure when a lipid study of triglycerides, total cholesterol, HDL cholesterol, and LDL cholesterol tests are ordered?
  A. 8 hours, nothing but water allowed
  B. 10 hours, water, smoking, coffee, tea (no sugar or cream) allowed
  C. 12 hours, nothing but water allowed
  D. 16 hours, water, smoking, coffee, tea (no sugar or cream) allowed

Chemistry/Apply knowledge of basic laboratory procedures/Lipids/1

52. **A** In a patient without chylomicronemia, lipoprotein abnormalities, and a triglyceride level below 400 mg/dL, the serum triglycerides reflect the amount of plasma VLDL. Since the ratio of cholesterol to triglyceride in VLDL is between 1:5 and 1:6, the serum triglyceride divided by 5 estimates the cholesterol in VLDL. The Friedewald equation for calculation of LDL cholesterol is:

LDL cholesterol = Total cholesterol – (HDL cholesterol + TG/5)

In patients with hypertriglyceridemia, the LDL cholesterol should be measured rather than calculated. LDL cholesterol assays that require no sample pretreatment (direct LDL cholesterol) are most commonly used. The reference method for LDL cholesterol involves ultracentrifugation of plasma for 24 hours and measurement of the VLDL and HDL cholesterol fractions. These are subtracted from the total cholesterol to calculate the LDL cholesterol. Assays for LDL cholesterol are also available that use polyclonal antibodies bound to latex beads to precipitate lipoproteins containing apo-AI and apo-E, leaving the LDL fraction in the supernatant.

53. **C** Since LDL cholesterol, HDL cholesterol, VLDL cholesterol, and triglycerides are all risk factors for coronary artery disease, the NCEP recommends that a fasting lipid profile to include triglycerides, total cholesterol, HDL cholesterol, and LDL cholesterol be performed every 5 years beginning at age 20.

54. **C** Lipid orders that include triglyceride and LDL cholesterol should always be performed using a plasma or serum specimen collected after a 12–14 hour fast. The patient should be instructed to drink nothing but water during this period. Fasting specimens are preferred for total and HDL cholesterol as well, but nonfasting specimens may be used for initial screening purposes.

55. Select the cutpoint value for plasma or serum LDL cholesterol in a person with a history of coronary heart disease in whom therapeutic lifestyle changes should be initiated.

A. ≥ 80 mg/dL

B. ≥ 100 mg/dL

C. ≥ 120 mg/dL

D. ≥ 160 mg/dL

Chemistry/Evaluate laboratory data to recognize health and disease states/Lipids/1

56. What is the HDL cholesterol cutpoint recommend by NCEP?

A. < 30 mg/dL

B. < 40 mg/dL

C. < 30 mg/dL for males and < 40 mg/dL for females

D. < 45 mg/dL for males and < 50 mg/dL for females

Chemistry/Evaluate laboratory data to recognize health and disease states/Lipids/1

57. An EDTA blood sample is collected from a nonfasting person for a CBC. The physician collected the sample from the femoral vein because venipuncture from the arm was unsuccessful. He called the laboratory 15 minutes after the sample arrived and requested a lipid study, including triglycerides, total cholesterol, HDL cholesterol, and LDL cholesterol. Which test results should be used to evaluate the patient's risk for coronary artery disease?

A. Total cholesterol and LDL cholesterol

B. LDL cholesterol and triglyceride

C. Total cholesterol and HDL cholesterol

D. Total cholesterol and triglyceride

Chemistry/Apply knowledge of basic laboratory procedures/Lipids/3

58. Which of the following diseases is caused by a deficiency of sphingomyelinase?

A. Gaucher's disease

B. Fabry's disease

C. Niemann-Pick disease

D. Tay-Sachs disease

Chemistry/Correlate clinical and laboratory data/Lipids/2

Answers to Questions 55–58

55. B The NECP has identified LDL cholesterol as the target of therapy for reducing the risk of atherosclerosis because lowering of LDL cholesterol has proved to be an effective intervention. The greater the risk of coronary heart disease, the lower the cutpoint for intervention. For persons with a 10-year risk of more than 20%, the cutpoint is ≥100 mg/dL for initiation of therapeutic lifestyle changes (<100 mg/dL is considered optimal). More than 2 of 10 persons in this category will develop CHD within 10 years. Included are persons with a history of CHD, diabetes, peripheral artery disease, and abdominal aortic aneurysm. For persons with 2 or more risk factors and a 10-year risk of ≤20%, lifestyle changes are initiated at ≥130 mg/dL. For persons with no more than one risk factor, the cutoff point is ≥ 160 mg/dL.

56. B The HDL cholesterol cutpoint recommended by NCEP is <40 mg/dL regardless of sex. A result below 40 mg/dL counts as a risk factor for coronary artery disease. Conversely, if the HDL cholesterol is ≥60 mg/dL, then one risk factor is subtracted from the total number. The therapeutic goal for someone with low HDL cholesterol is still reduction of LDL cholesterol (if elevated), weight loss, and increased exercise.

57. C NCEP recommends a 12-hour fasting sample when screening persons for risk of coronary artery disease. However, if a fasting sample is unavailable, NCEP recommends performing the total cholesterol and HDL cholesterol because these tests are least affected by recent ingestion of food. If the total cholesterol is ≥200 mg/dL or the HDL cholesterol is <40 mg/dL, then testing for LDL cholesterol and triglycerides should be performed when a fasting sample can be obtained. An EDTA plasma sample is acceptable for most enzymatic cholesterol and triglyceride assays.

58. C The diseases mentioned result from inborn errors of lipid metabolism (lipidoses) caused by deficiency of an enzyme needed for lipid degradation. Specific lipids accumulate in the lysosomes. Niemann-Pick disease results from a deficiency of sphingomyelinase; Gaucher's disease from β-glucocerebrosidase; Fabry's disease (sex-linked) from α-galactosidase A; Tay-Sachs disease from *N*-acetylglucosaminidase A.

59. Which method is considered the candidate reference method for triglyceride measurement?

A. Glycerol kinase-ultraviolet

B. CDC modification of Van Handel and Zilversmit

C. Hantzsch condensation

D. Glycerol kinase coupled to peroxidase

Chemistry/Apply principles of basic laboratory procedures/Lipids/1

60. Which of the following enzymes is common to all enzymatic methods for triglyceride measurement?

A. Glycerol phosphate oxidase

B. Glycerol phosphate dehydrogenase

C. Glycerol kinase

D. Pyruvate kinase

Chemistry/Apply principles of basic laboratory procedures/Lipids/2

61. Select the reagent needed in the coupling enzyme reaction used to generate a colored product in the cholesterol oxidase method for cholesterol.

A. Cholestahexaene

B. H_2O_2

C. Phenol

D. Cholest-4-ene-3-one

Chemistry/Apply knowledge of basic laboratory procedures/Lipids/2

59. B Enzymatic methods for triglyceride measurement are widely used because they eliminate the need for extraction and saponification. However, they are subject to positive interference from endogenous glycerol and variations in the efficiency of lipase, which can result in under- or overestimation of triglycerides. The most accurate method for triglyceride assay is the nonenzymatic method based upon reaction of formaldehyde with chromotropic acid. In this method, extraction with silicic acid and chloroform separates triglycerides from lipoproteins, phospholipids, and glycerol. Saponification with alcoholic potassium hydroxide (KOH) produces glycerol, which is oxidized to formaldehyde by periodate. The formaldehyde reacts with chromotropic acid to form a pink product. The Centers for Disease Control and Prevention (CDC) method uses a 2:1 ratio of unsaturated (triolein) to saturated (tripalmitin) triglycerides to calibrate the assay because this represents the ratio normally found in serum.

60. C All enzymatic triglyceride methods require lipase to hydrolyze triglycerides and glycerol kinase to phosphorylate glycerol, forming glycerol-3-phosphate. The two most common methods measure the glycerol-3-phosphate produced.

1. Glycerol-3-phosphate + NAD^+ $\xrightarrow{GPD}$ dihydroxyacetone phosphate + NADH + H^+

2. Glycerol-3-phosphate + O_2 $\xrightarrow{GPO}$ dihydroxyacetone phosphate + H_2O_2

H_2O_2 + phenol + 4-aminophenazone $\xrightarrow{Px}$ quinoneimine dye + H_2O

GPD = Glycerol phosphate dehydrogenase

GPO = Glycerol phosphate oxidase

Px = Peroxidase

61. C In the cholesterol oxidase method, cholesterol ester hydrolase converts cholesterol esters to free cholesterol by hydrolyzing the fatty acid from the C3-OH group. Cholesterol oxidase catalyzes the oxidation of free cholesterol at the C3-OH group, forming cholest-4-ene-3-one and hydrogen peroxide. The peroxide is used in a peroxidase reaction to oxidize a dye (e.g., 4-aminophenazone), which couples to phenol, forming a red quinoneimine complex. The same coupling (indicator) reaction is used in the Trinder glucose oxidase method.

62. Which of the following methods for HDL cholesterol is the reference method?
   A. Manganese-heparin
   B. Magnesium-phosphotungstate
   C. Magnesium-dextran
   D. Ultracentrifugation

Chemistry/Apply knowledge of basic laboratory procedures/Lipids/1

63. Cholesterol esterase is used in enzymatic assays to:
   A. Oxidize cholesterol to form peroxide
   B. Hydrolyze fatty acids bound to the third carbon atom of cholesterol
   C. Separate cholesterol from apoproteins A-I and A-II by hydrolysis
   D. Reduce NAD^+ to NADH

Chemistry/Apply knowledge of basic laboratory procedures/Lipids/2

64. Which of the following reagents is used in the direct HDL cholesterol method?
   A. Sulfated cyclodextrin
   B. Magnesium sulfate and dextran sulfate
   C. Anti-ApoA-I
   D. Manganese heparin

Chemistry/Apply knowledge of basic laboratory procedures/Lipids/2

Answers to Questions 62–64

62. **D** Ultracentrifugation of plasma in a potassium bromide solution with a density of 1.063 is used to separate HDL from LDL and VLDL. The HDL fraction is transferred from the bottom of the tube and assayed for cholesterol content by the Abell-Kendall method. The remaining three methods rely upon selective precipitation or magnetic removal of lipoproteins containing apoprotein B using a polyanionic solution. Magnesium-dextran and magnesium-phosphotungstate tend to give slightly lower results than manganese-heparin because they precipitate some HDL. A "direct HDL" can also be performed using cholesterol esterase and oxidase enzymes that are conjugated to polyethylene glycol. In the presence of sulfated cyclodextrin, the polyethylene glycol (PEG)-modified enzymes display greatly reduced catalytic activity against the cholesterol of LDL, VLDL, and chylomicrons. Unlike polyanionic precipitation, the direct HDL cholesterol method is not subject to interference from high plasma triglycerides.

63. **B** Approximately two-thirds of the serum cholesterol has a fatty acid esterified to the hydroxyl group of the third carbon atom of the cholesterol molecule. Cholesterol esterase hydrolyzes fatty acids and is required because cholesterol oxidase cannot utilize esterified cholesterol as a substrate.

64. **A** The direct HDL method most commonly employed uses cholesterol esterase and oxidase enzymes conjugated to polyethylene glycol. In the presence of sulfated cyclodextrin, the enzymes react very poorly with non-HDL cholesterol molecules. Magnesium-dextran and manganese-heparin are polyanion salts that precipitate LDL and VLDL cholesterol. Anti-ApoA-I binds to HDL and is not used in HDL assays.

65. What do "direct" or homogenous methods for LDL cholesterol assay have in common?
  A. They are inaccurate when plasma triglyceride is above 250 mg/dL
  B. All use a detergent to facilitate selective reactivity with reagent enzymes
  C. All use monoclonal antibodies to Apo A1 and C.
  D. All are free of interference from abnormal lipoproteins

Chemistry/Apply knowledge of basic laboratory procedures/Lipids/2

66. What is the purpose of the saponification step used in the Abell-Kendall method for cholesterol measurement?
  A. Remove phospholipids
  B. Reduce sterol molecules structurally similar to those of cholesterol
  C. Convert cholesterol esters to free cholesterol
  D. Remove proteins that can interfere with color formation

Chemistry/Apply knowledge of basic laboratory procedures/Lipids/2

67. Lipoprotein (a), or Lp(a), is significant when elevated in serum because it:
  A. Is an independent risk factor for atherosclerosis
  B. Blocks the clearance of VLDLs
  C. Displaces Apo-A1 from HDLs
  D. Is linked closely to a gene for obesity

Chemistry/Apply knowledge of fundamental biological characteristics/Lipoproteins/1

68. Which type of dietary fatty acid is *not* associated with an increase in serum LDL cholesterol production?
  A. Monosaturated *trans*-fatty acids
  B. Saturated fatty acids
  C. Monosaturated *cis*-fatty acids
  D. Monosaturated *trans*-Ω-9 fatty acids

Chemistry/Apply knowledge of fundamental biological characteristics/Fatty acids/1 Chemistry/Correlate clinical and laboratory data/Lipids/2

Answers to Questions 65–68

65. **B** The direct LDL cholesterol assays are all detergent-based methods. One commonly used method employs a polyanionic detergent to release cholesterol from HDL, chylomicrons, and VLDL. The detergent binds to LDL and blocks its reaction with the esterase and oxidase enzymes in the reagent. Cholesterol oxidase oxidizes the non-LDL cholesterol, forming H_2O_2, and peroxidase catalyzes the oxidation of an electron donor by the H_2O_2, which does not result in color formation. A second nonionic detergent and chromogen are added. The second detergent removes the first from the LDL, allowing it to react with the enzymes. The resulting H_2O_2 reacts with the chromogen, forming a colored product. These methods are not subject to interference by triglycerides at a concentration below 700 mg/dL. They agree well with the reference method (ultracentrifugation) but are subject to interference by some abnormal lipoproteins.

66. **C** The Abell-Kendall method is the reference method for cholesterol assay because differences in esterase activity and interference in the peroxidase step are potential sources of error in enzymatic assays. Saponification is performed to hydrolyze the fatty acid esters of cholesterol, forming free cholesterol. This is required because the reagents react more intensely with cholesterol esters than with free cholesterol. Saponification is followed by extraction of cholesterol in petroleum ether to separate it from proteins and interfering substances. The extract is reacted with sulfuric acid, acetic anhydride, and acetic acid (Liebermann–Burchard reagent), which oxidizes the cholesterol, forming a colored product.

67. **A** Lp(a) is a complex of Apo B-100 and protein (a) formed by a disulfide bridge. The complex is structurally similar to that of plasminogen and is thought to promote coronary heart disease by interfering with the normal fibrinolytic process.

68. **C** Polyunsaturated and *cis* monosaturated fatty acids are not associated with increased production of LDL cholesterol. On the other hand, saturated and *trans*-monosaturated fatty acids are both associated with increased LDL. *Cis* fatty acids are those in which the H atoms belonging to the double-bonded carbons are on the same side of the molecule. Ω-9 (n-9) Fatty acids are those with a double bond located nine carbons from the terminal methyl group. Ω Fatty acids are associated with increased cholesterol, if the hydrogens attached to the double-bonded carbons are in the *trans* position.

69. **SITUATION:** A lipemic specimen collected from an adult after a 12-hour fast was assayed for total cholesterol, triglycerides, and HDL cholesterol using a direct HDL method. The results are shown below.

Total Cholesterol	HDL Cholesterol	Triglyceride
220 mg/dL	40 mg/dL	420 mg/dL

The physician requests an LDL cholesterol assay after receiving the results. How should the LDL cholesterol be determined?

A. Dilute the specimen 1:10 and repeat all tests; calculate LDL cholesterol using the Friedewald equation

B. Perform a direct LDL cholesterol assay

C. Ultracentrifuge the sample and repeat the HDL cholesterol on the infranatant. Use the new result to calculate the LDL cholesterol

D. Repeat the HDL cholesterol assay using the manganese heparin precipitation method. Use the new result to calculate the LDL cholsterol

Chemistry/Apply knowledge to recognize sources of error/Lipids/3

70. A person has a fasting triglyceride level of 240 mg/dL. The physician wishes to know the patient's non-HDL cholesterol level. What cholesterol fractions should be measured?

A. Total cholesterol and HDL cholesterol

B. Total cholesterol and LDL cholesterol

C. HDL cholesterol and LDL cholesterol

D. Total cholesterol and chylomicrons

Chemistry/Apply knowledge of special procedures/Lipids/3

Answers to Questions 69–70

69. **B** When the triglyceride level is ≥400 mg/dL the Friedewald equation for LDL cholesterol will result in an erroneously low value because of overestimation of the VLDL cholesterol. Although high triglycerides (≥400 mg/dL) can result in falsely elevated HDL cholesterol when precipitation methods are used, it does not cause significant error with either the direct HDL or direct LDL cholesterol methods. An accurate LDL cholesterol can be reported if the direct (detergent) method for LDL cholesterol is employed.

70. **A** When the HDL cholesterol is subtracted from the total cholesterol, the result is called the non-HDL cholesterol. This result, the sum of LDL cholesterol and VLDL cholesterol, represents the fraction with atherogenic remnant lipoproteins as well as LDL cholesterol. People who have a fasting triglyceride ≥200 mg/dL are at increased risk for coronary artery disease because of atherogenic VLDL remnants, and the treatment goal is to have a non-HDL cholesterol no more than 30 mg/dL greater than the LDL cholesterol.

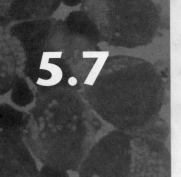

5.7 ENZYMES AND CARDIAC MARKERS

1. An International unit (IU) of enzyme activity is the quantity of enzyme that:
   A. Converts 1 μmol of substrate to product per liter
   B. Forms 1 mg of product per deciliter
   C. Converts 1 μmol of substrate to product per minute
   D. Forms 1 μmol of product per liter

   Chemistry/Apply principles of basic laboratory procedures/Enzymes/1

2. Which statement below describes a nonkinetic enzyme assay?
   A. Initial absorbance is measured, followed by a second reading after 5 minutes
   B. Absorbance is measured at 10-sec intervals for 100 sec
   C. Absorbance is monitored continuously for 1 min using a chart recorder
   D. Reflectance is measured from a xenon source lamp pulsing at 60 Hz

   Chemistry/Apply principles of basic laboratory procedures/Enzymes/2

3. Which of the following statements regarding enzymatic reactions is true?
   A. The enzyme shifts the equilibrium of the reaction to the right
   B. The enzyme alters the equilibrium constant of the reaction
   C. The enzyme increases the rate of the reaction
   D. The enzyme alters the energy difference between reactants and products

   Chemistry/Apply knowledge of fundamental biological characteristics/Enzymes/1

4. Which statement about enzymes is true?
   A. An enzyme alters the Gibb's free energy of the reaction
   B. Enzymes cause a reaction with a positive free energy to occur spontaneously

   C. An enzyme's natural substrate has the highest Michaelis-Menten constant (K_m)
   D. A competitive inhibitor will alter the apparent K_m of the reaction

   Chemistry/Apply knowledge of fundamental biological characteristics/Enzymes/2

Answers to Questions 1–4

1. **C** The IU is a rate expressed in micromoles per minute. Activity is reported as IUs per liter (IU/L) or mIU/mL. The SI unit for enzyme activity is the katal (1 katal converts 1 mol of substrate to product in 1 sec).

2. **A** A kinetic assay uses several evenly spaced absorbance measurements to calculate the change in absorbance per unit time. A constant change in absorbance per unit of time occurs only when the rate of the reaction is zero order (independent of substrate concentration). Enzyme activity is proportional to rate only under zero-order conditions.

3. **C** An enzyme accelerates the rate of a reaction, reducing the time required to reach equilibrium. The concentration of reactants and products at equilibrium is the same with or without the enzyme.

4. **D** Enzymes alter the energy of activation by forming a metastable intermediate, the enzyme substrate complex. Enzymes do not alter the free energy or direction of a reaction. Competitive inhibitors bind to the active site where the enzyme binds substrate and are overcome by increasing the substrate concentration.

5. Which substrate concentration is needed to achieve zero-order conditions?

A. $> \text{than } 99 \times K_m$
B. $[S] = K_m$
C. $< 10 \times K_m$
D. $[S] = 0$

Chemistry/Select reagents/Enzymes/3

6. Which statement is true?

A. Apoenzyme + prosthetic group = holoenzyme
B. A coenzyme is an inorganic molecule required for activity
C. Cofactors are as tightly bound to the enzyme as a prosthetic group
D. All enzymes have optimal activity at pH 7.00

Chemistry/Apply fundamental biological characteristics/Enzymes/2

7. Which of the following statements about enzymatic reactions is true?

A. NADH has absorbance maximums at 340 and 366 nm
B. Enzyme concentration must be in excess to achieve zero-order kinetics
C. Rate is proportional to substrate concentration in a zero-order reaction
D. Accumulation of the product increases the reaction rate

Chemistry/Apply principles of basic laboratory procedures/Enzymes/2

8. The increase in the level of serum enzymes used to detect cholestatic liver disease is caused mainly by:

A. Enzyme release from dead cells
B. Leakage from cells with altered membrane permeability
C. Decreased perfusion of the tissue
D. Increased production and secretion by cells

Chemistry/Correlate laboratory data with physiological processes/Enzymes/2

9. Which enzyme below is considered most tissue-specific?

A. CK
B. Amylase
C. Alkaline phosphatase
D. Alcohol dehydrogenase

Chemistry/Correlate clinical and laboratory data/Enzymes/2

Answers to Questions 5–9

5. **A** A zero-order reaction rate is independent of substrate concentration because there is sufficient substrate to saturate the enzyme. $V = V_{max} \times [S]/Km + [S]$ where V = velocity, V_{max} = maximum velocity, $[S]$ = substrate concentration, and Km = substrate concentration required to give $1/2\ V_{max}$. If $[S] >>> Km$, then the Km can be ignored. $V = V_{max} \times [S]/[S]$ or velocity approaches maximum and is independent of substrate concentration.

6. **A** A coenzyme is an organic molecule required for full enzyme activity. A prosthetic group is a coenzyme that is tightly bound to the apoenzyme and is required for activity. Cofactors are inorganic atoms or molecules needed for full catalytic activity. Pyridoxyl-5′-phosphate is a prosthetic group for ALT and AST. Consequently, patients with low levels of pyridoxal-5′-phosphate (P-5′-P) (vitamin B_6 deficiency) may have reduced transaminase activity in vitro. Enzymes can have diverse pH (and temperature) optimums.

7. **A** Most enzymes are measured by monitoring the rate of absorbance change at 340 nm as NADH is produced or consumed. This rate is proportional to enzyme activity when substrate is in excess. When the enzyme is present in excess, the initial reaction rate is proportional to substrate concentration. This condition, called a first-order reaction, is needed when the enzyme is used as a reagent to measure a specific analyte.

8. **D** The amount of enzyme in the serum can be increased by necrosis, altered permeability, secretion, or synthesis. It is also dependent upon tissue perfusion, enzyme half-life, molecular size, and location of the enzyme within the cell. Most enzymes are liberated by necrosis, but a few, such as ALP and γ-glutamyltransferase, are produced and secreted at a greater rate in obstructive liver disease.

9. **D** No enzyme is truly tissue-specific, and diagnostic accuracy depends upon recognizing the pattern of change produced by different diseases. This includes the quantity of enzyme released, characteristic rise and return to normal, the isoenzyme(s) released, and the concomitant changes of other enzymes. Alanine aminotransferase and alcohol dehydrogenase are primarily increased in necrotic liver disease.

10. Which of the following enzymes is activated by calcium ions?
    A. CK
    B. Amylase
    C. Alkaline phosphatase (ALP)
    D. Lactate dehydrogenase (LD)

    Chemistry/Apply knowledge of fundamental biological characteristics/Enzymes/2

11. Which of the following enzymes is a transferase?
    A. ALP
    B. CK
    C. Amylase
    D. LD

    Chemistry/Apply knowledge of fundamental biological characteristics/Enzymes/2

12. Which statement about methods for measuring LD is true?
    A. The formation of pyruvate from lactate (forward reaction) generates NAD$^+$
    B. The pyruvate to lactate reaction proceeds at about twice the rate as the forward reaction
    C. The lactate to pyruvate reaction is optimized at pH 7.4
    D. The negative rate reaction is preferred

    Chemistry/Apply principles of basic laboratory procedures/Lactate dehydrogenase/2

13. Which condition produces the highest elevation of serum lactate dehydrogenase?
    A. Pernicious anemia
    B. Myocardial infarction
    C. Acute hepatitis
    D. Muscular dystrophy

    Chemistry/Correlate clinical and laboratory data/Lactate dehydrogenase/2

14. In which condition is the LD most likely to be within normal limits?
    A. Hepatic carcinoma
    B. Pulmonary infarction
    C. Acute appendicitis
    D. Crush injury

    Chemistry/Correlate clinical and laboratory data/Lactate dehydrogenase/2

Answers to Questions 10–14

10. **B** Most enzymes require metals as activators or cofactors. CK and ALP require Mg^{2+} for full activity, and amylase requires Ca^{2+}. Metals required for activity should be components of the substrate used for enzyme analysis. The substrate must also contain anions required (e.g., Cl^- for amylase) and should not contain inhibiting cations or anions (e.g., Zn^{2+} and Mn^{2+} for CK).

11. **B** Enzymes are identified by a numeric system called the EC (Enzyme Commission) number. The first number refers to the class of the enzyme. There are six classes; in order these are oxidoreductases, transferases, hydrolases, lyases, isomerases, and ligases. Dehydrogenases are oxidoreductases, whereas kinases and transaminases are transferases. CK is EC number 2.7.3.2, which distinguishes it from other kinases.

12. **B** Although the rate of the reverse reaction (P → L) is faster, the L (→) P reaction is more popular because it produces a positive rate (generates NADH), is not subject to product inhibition, and is highly linear. The pH optimum for the forward reaction is approximately 8.8.

13. **A** Serum LD levels are highest in pernicious anemia, reaching 10–50 times the upper reference limit (URL) as a result of intramedullary hemolysis. Moderate elevations (3–10×URL) usually are seen in acute MI, necrotic liver disease, and muscular dystrophy. Slight increases (2–3×URL) are sometimes seen in obstructive liver disease.

14. **C** LD is increased slightly to moderately in most causes of liver disease. Smallest elevations are seen in obstructive jaundice and highest in hepatic carcinoma and toxic hepatitis, in which levels can reach 10-fold the upper reference limit. LD is also increased in crush injury and muscular dystrophies as a result of to skeletal muscle damage, and in pulmonary infarction because of embolism formation. Amylase is increased in a majority of patients with acute appendicitis but LD is not.

15. Following an acute MI, activity of LD usually peaks:
   A. Within 1 day postinfarction and returns to normal after 3 days
   B. Twenty-four to 36 hours postinfarction and returns to normal after 3 days
   C. Forty-eight hours postinfarction and returns to normal after 4 days
   D. Three days postinfarction and returns to normal after 1 week

Chemistry/Correlate clinical and laboratory data/ Creatine kinase/2

16. The LD pleural fluid:serum ratio for a transudative fluid is usually:
   A. 3:1 or higher
   B. 2:1
   C. 1:1
   D. 1:2 or less

Chemistry/Correlate clinical and laboratory data/Lactate dehydrogenase/2

17. In which type of liver disease would you expect the greatest elevation of LD?
   A. Toxic hepatitis
   B. Alcoholic hepatitis
   C. Cirrhosis
   D. Acute viral hepatitis

Chemistry/Correlate clinical and laboratory data/Lactate dehydrogenase/2

18. Which of the following conditions will interfere with the measurement of LD?
   A. Slight hemolysis during sample collection
   B. Storage at 4°C for 3 days
   C. Storage at room temperature for 16 hours
   D. Use of plasma collected in heparin

Chemistry/Apply knowledge to recognize sources of error/Lactate dehydrogenase/3

19. In the Oliver-Rosalki method, the reverse reaction is used to measure CK activity. The enzyme(s) used in the coupling reactions is (are):
   A. Hexokinase and G6PD
   B. Pyruvate kinase and LD
   C. Luciferase
   D. Adenylate kinase

Chemistry/Apply knowledge of basic laboratory procedures/Creatine kinase/2

Answers to Questions 15–19

15. **D** CK is the first enzyme to rise above the reference range after an acute MI, peaking at 18–36 hours and returning to normal within 3 days. AST follows, peaking at 24–48 hours postinfarction and returning to normal in 4–5 days. This pattern of CK ($\rightarrow$) AST ($\rightarrow$) LD is specific for acute MI but has been replaced by serial measurements of myoglobin, troponin I, and CK-MB, which usually can detect and confirm the acute MI within 6–8 hours. The troponins are three proteins (T, I, and C) that comprise the thin filaments of cardiac and skeletal muscle fibers. Both troponin I (TNI) and troponin T (TNT) have unique sequences that differ between cardiac and skeletal muscle. Antibodies specific for the cardiac isoforms can be used to measure their concentration in serum.

16. **D** The lactate dehydrogenase activity of body fluids is normally less than that of serum, and a fluid to serum LD ratio greater than 1:2 is highly suggestive of an exudative process. Elevated lactate dehydrogenase in chest fluid is often caused by lung malignancy, metastatic carcinoma, Hodgkin's disease, and leukemia.

17. **A** Liver disease produces elevated LD-4 and LD-5 levels. Levels may reach up to 10 times the upper reference limit (URL) in toxic hepatitis and in hepatoma. However, LD levels are lower in viral hepatitis (3–10×URL) and only slightly elevated in cirrhosis (2–3×URL).

18. **A** RBCs are rich in LD-1 and LD-2, and even slight hemolysis will falsely elevate results. Hemolytic, megaloblastic, and pernicious anemias are associated with LD levels of 10–50 times the URL. LD is stable for 2 days at room temperature or 1 week at 4°C; however, freezing causes deterioration of LD-5. The activity of LD is inhibited by EDTA, which binds divalent cations; serum or heparinized plasma should be used.

19. **A** The Oliver-Rosalki method for CK is based upon the formation of ATP from creatine phosphate. Hexokinase catalyzes the phosphorylation of glucose by ATP. This produces glucose-6-PO_4 and adenosine diphosphate (ADP). The glucose-6-PO_4 is oxidized to 6-phosphogluconate as $NADP^+$ is reduced to NADPH.

$$ATP + glucose \xrightarrow{\text{Hexokinase}} ADP + glucose\text{-}6\text{-}PO_4$$

$$glucose\text{-}6\text{-}PO_4 + NADP^+ \xrightarrow{\text{G-6-PD}} 6\text{-phosphogluconate} + NADPH + H^+$$

20. In the Oliver-Rosalki method for CK, adenosine monophosphate (AMP) is added to the substrate in order to:
  A. Inhibit adenylate kinase
  B. Block the oxidation of glutathione
  C. Increase the amount of ADP that is available
  D. Block the action of diadenosine pentaphosphate

Chemistry/Apply principles of basic laboratory procedures/Creatine kinase/2

21. Which substance is used in the CK assay to activate the enzyme?
  A. Flavin adenine dinucleotide (FAD)
  B. Imidazole
  C. *N*-acetylcysteine
  D. Pyridoxyl-5′-phosphate

Chemistry/Apply principles of basic laboratory procedures/Creatine kinase/2

22. SITUATION: A specimen for CK performed on an automated analyzer using an optimized Oliver-Rosalki method gives an error flag indicating substrate depletion. The sample is diluted 1:2 and 1:4 by the serial dilution technique and reassayed. After correcting for the dilution, the results are as follows:

  1:2 Dilution = 3000 IU/L; 1:4 Dilution = 3600 IU/L

Dilutions are made a second time and assayed again but give identical results. What is the most likely explanation?
  A. The serum became contaminated prior to making the 1:4 dilution
  B. The wrong pipette was used to make one of the dilutions
  C. An endogenous competitive inhibitor is present in the serum
  D. An error has been made in calculating the enzyme activity of one of the two dilutions

Chemistry/Apply knowledge to recognize sources of error/Creatine kinase/3

23. SITUATION: A physician calls to request a CK on a sample already sent to the laboratory for coagulation studies. The sample is 2-hour-old citrated blood and has been stored at 4°C. The plasma shows very slight hemolysis. What is the best course of action and the reason for it?
  A. Perform the CK assay on the sample because no interferent is present
  B. Reject the sample because it is slightly hemolyzed
  C. Reject the sample because it has been stored too long
  D. Reject the sample because the citrate will interfere

Chemistry/Apply knowledge to recognize sources of error/Creatine kinase/3

20. **A** Positive interference in the Oliver-Rosalki method can occur when adenylate kinase is present in the serum from hemolysis or damaged tissue. Adenylate kinase hydrolyzes ADP, forming AMP and ATP (2 ADP $\xrightarrow{\text{AK}}$ AMP + ATP). This reaction is inhibited by adding AMP and diadenosine pentaphosphate (Ap_5A) to the substrate.

21. **C** In addition to Mg^{2+}, CK requires a thiol compound to reduce interchain disulfide bridges and bind heavy metals that inactivate the enzyme. *N*-acetylcysteine is an activator of CK used for this purpose in the IFCC recommended method. Pyridoxyl-5′-phosphate is a prosthetic group of AST and ALT. FAD is a prosthetic group of glucose oxidase. Imidazole is used to buffer the CK reagent.

22. **C** When a competitive inhibitor is present in the serum, a dilution of the sample causes an increase in the reaction rate by reducing the concentration of the inhibitor. Dilution of serum frequently increases the activity of CK and amylase. The same effect occurs when a smaller volume of serum is used in the assay because less inhibitor is present in the reaction mixture.

23. **D** CK activity is lost with excessive storage, the most labile isoenzyme being CK-1. However, CK in serum is stable at room temperature for about 4 hours and up to 1 week at 4°C provided that an optimized method is used. Slight hemolysis does not interfere because CK is absent from RBCs. More significant hemolysis may cause positive interference by contributing ATP, glucose-6-PO_4, and adenylate kinase to the serum. Calcium chelators remove magnesium as well as calcium and should not be used.

24. Which of the statements below regarding total CK is true?
- **A.** Levels are unaffected by strenuous exercise
- **B.** Levels are unaffected by repeated intramuscular injections
- **C.** Highest levels are seen in Duchenne's muscular dystrophy
- **D.** The enzyme is highly specific for heart injury

Chemistry/Evaluate laboratory data to recognize health and disease states/Creatine kinase/2

25. Which of the following statements regarding the clinical use of CK-MB (CK-2) is true?
- **A.** CK-MB becomes elevated before myoglobin and troponin I (TnI) after an acute MI
- **B.** CK-MB levels are normal in cases of cardiac ischemia
- **C.** Mass unit assays are more sensitive than electrophoretic methods
- **D.** An elevated CK-MB level is always accompanied by an elevated total CK level

Chemistry/Correlate clinical and laboratory data/ Creatine kinase/2

26. Isoforms of CK are:
- **A.** Isoenzymes of CK formed from variants of the B subunit
- **B.** Formed in the circulation by hydrolysis of lysine from CK-MM and CK-MB
- **C.** Formed only when blood is collected in heparin
- **D.** Artifacts of electrophoresis caused by attachment to albumin

Chemistry/Apply knowledge of fundamental biological characteristics/Creatine kinase/2

27. A patient's CK-MB is reported as 18 μg/L and the total CK as 560 IU/L. What is the CK relative index (CKI)?
- **A.** 0.10%
- **B.** 3.2%
- **C.** 10.0%
- **D.** 30.0%

Chemistry/Correlate clinical and laboratory data/ Creatine kinase/2

28. In a nonmyocardial as opposed to a myocardial cause of an increased serum or plasma CK-MB, which would be expected?
- **A.** An increase in CK-MB that is persistent
- **B.** An increase in the percentage of CK-MB as well as the concentration
- **C.** The presence of increased troponin I
- **D.** A more modest increase in total CK than in CK-MB

Chemistry/Evaluate laboratory data to recognize health and disease states/Creatine kinase/2

24. **C** Total CK is neither sensitive nor specific for acute MI. An infarct can occur without causing an elevated total CK level. Exercise and intramuscular injections cause a significant increase in total CK. Crush injuries and muscular dystrophy can increase the total CK up to 50 times the URL.

25. **C** Serum myoglobin becomes abnormal within 3 hours after an acute MI before TnI and CK-MB. CK-MB becomes abnormal shortly after TnI when a cutoff of 6 μg/L is used, and both peak at around the same time following acute MI. TnI remains elevated for approximately 1 week after acute MI, is not increased in crush injury, and is not as likely to be elevated by renal failure as is CK-MB. Immunochemical methods for measuring CK-MB are more sensitive than electrophoresis (fluorescent densitometry). There is usually less than 5 μg/L CK-MB in the serum of healthy adults, whereas the total CK ranges from 10–110 U/L. Consequently, an abnormal CK-MB can occur in the absence of an elevated total CK.

26. **B** Isoforms are modified forms of isoenzymes and exist for CK-MM and MB. They result from the hydrolysis of lysine from the M peptide by carboxypeptidases in the plasma. Removal of lysine results in faster electrophoretic mobility. The isoforms of CK-MM are CK-MM1, CK-MM2, and CK-MM3. Isoforms of CK-MB are designated CK-MB1 and CK-MB2. CK-MM3 and CK-MB2 are the unmodified tissue isoforms and rise within 4 hours after acute MI.

27. **B** The CKI is an expression of the percentage of the total CK that is attributed to CK-MB.

$$CKI = \frac{CK\text{-}MB \text{ in } \mu g/L \text{ or } IU/L}{Total\ CK \text{ in } IU/L} \times 100$$

The reference range is 0%–2.5%. Values above 2.5% point to an increase in CK-MB from cardiac muscle.

28. **A** CK-MB rises 4–6 hours postinfarction, peaks in 16–20 hours, and usually returns to normal within 48 hours. In some noncardiac causes of elevated plasma CK-MB such as muscular dystrophy, there is a persistent elevation of both total CK and CK-MB. TnI (and TnT) are cardiac-specific markers. They become elevated slightly before CK-MB when a CK-MB cutoff of 6–10 μg/L is used, remain elevated for 7–10 days following an acute MI, and are not increased in muscular dystrophy, malignant hyperthermia, or crush injuries that are associated with an increase in the concentration of CK-MB. Absolute CK-MB increases are evaluated cautiously, when CK-MB is less than 2.5% of total enzyme because noncardiac sources may be responsible.

29. Which statement best describes the clinical utility of plasma or serum myoglobin?

A. Levels greater than 100 μg/L are diagnostic of acute MI

B. Levels below 100 μg/L on admission and 2-4 hours postadmission help to exclude a diagnosis of acute MI

C. Myoglobin peaks after the cardiac troponins but is more sensitive

D. The persistence of myoglobin >110 μg/L for 3 days following chest pain favors a diagnosis of acute MI

Chemistry/Evaluate laboratory data to recognize health and disease states/Cardiac markers/2

30. What is the typical time course for plasma myoglobin following an acute MI?

A. Abnormal before 1 hour; peaks within 3 hours; returns to normal in 8 hours

B. Abnormal within 3 hours; peaks within 6 hours; returns to normal in 18 hours

C. Abnormal within 3 hours; peaks within 12 hours; returns to normal in 36 hours

D. Abnormal within 6 hours; peaks within 24 hours; returns to normal in 72 hours

Chemistry/Evaluate laboratory data to recognize health and disease states/Cardiac markers/2

31. What is the typical time course for plasma TnI or TnT following an acute MI?

A. Abnormal within 3 hours; peaks within 12 hours; returns to normal in 24 hours

B. Abnormal within 4 hours; peaks within 18 hours; returns to normal in 48 hours

C. Abnormal within 4 hours; peaks within 24 hours; returns to normal in 1 week

D. Abnormal within 6 hours; peaks within 36 hours; returns to normal in 5 days

Chemistry/Evaluate laboratory data to recognize health and disease states/Cardiac markers/2

Answers to Questions 29–31

29. B Myoglobin is a heme-containing pigment in both skeletal and cardiac muscle cells. The upper limit of normal is approximately 90 μg/L for males and 75 μg/L for females. The plasma myoglobin is a sensitive marker for acute MI. Over 95% of affected persons have a value higher than the cutoff (typically >100 μg/L). However, specificity is approximately 75%–85% owing to skeletal muscle injury or renal insufficiency. For this reason, a plasma myoglobin below the cutoff on admission and within the first 3 hours following chest pain helps to rule out acute MI. A value above the cutoff must be confirmed using a cardiac specific assay such as TnI.

30. C After acute MI, myoglobin usually rises above the cutoff within 1–3 hours, peaks within 8–12 hours, and returns to normal within 36 hours. Typically, levels reach a peak concentration that is 10-fold the upper reference limit. Since myoglobin is the first marker to become abnormal after an acute MI, it should be measured on admission and, if negative, measured again 2–4 hours later. If both samples are below the cutoff, the probability of the occurrence of an acute MI is low. If the myoglobin is above the cutoff, a cardiac-specific marker such as TnI, TnT, or CK-MB must be performed at some point to confirm the diagnosis.

31. C Troponin is a complex of three polypeptides that function as a regulator of actin and myosin. The three subunits are designated TnC, TnI, and TnT. All are present in both cardiac and some skeletal muscles, but cardiac and skeletal isoforms of TnI and TnT can be differentiated by specific antiseras. TnI and TnT cardiac isoforms in plasma will at least double within 4–6 hours after MI, peak within 24 hours, and usually remain elevated for 7–10 days. Reference ranges for TnI and TnT are dependent on the antibody and calibrator used in the immunoassay, but plasma levels are normally less than 0.1 ng/mL (0.1 μg/L). This allows the cutpoint for AMI to be set somewhat lower than for CK-MB, resulting in detection slightly before CK-MB. Like CK-MB, TnI has a sensitivity >98% and a specificity of approximately 95% for acute MI. TnT has approximately the same sensitivity but slightly lower specificity owing to greater retention in renal failure and small elevations seen in unstable angina (chest pain while at rest).

32. Which of the following is the most effective serial sampling time for ruling out acute MI using both myoglobin and a cardiac-specific marker in an emergency department environment?

A. Admission and every hour for the next 3 hours or until positive

B. Admission, 2 hours, 4 hours, and 6 hours or until positive

C. Admission, 3 hours, 6 hours and a final sample within 12 hours

D. Admission and one sample every 8 hours for 48 hours

Chemistry/Apply knowledge of basic laboratory procedures/Cardiac markers/2

33. Which of the following cardiac markers is consistently increased in persons who exhibit unstable angina?

A. Troponin C

B. Troponin T

C. CK-MB

D. Myoglobin

Chemistry/Evaluate laboratory data to recognize health and disease states/Cardiac markers/2

34. A patient has a plasma myoglobin level of 10 μg/L at admission. Three hours later the myoglobin is 14 μg/L and the troponin I is 0.04 μg/L (reference range 0–0.04 μg/L). These results are consistent with which condition?

A. Skeletal muscle injury

B. Acute MI

C. Unstable angina

D. No evidence of myocardial or skeletal muscle injury

Chemistry/Evaluate laboratory data to recognize health and disease states/Cardiac markers/2

Answers to Questions 32–34

32. **C** Since the time between the onset of symptoms and arrival in the emergency room is often open to speculation, serial measurement of cardiac markers is required in order to rule out acute MI. Since myoglobin is the first marker to rise after acute MI, it should be measured on admission and at 3 hours postadmission. Since TnI, TnT, and CK-MB are more cardiac-specific, at least one should be measured starting at 3 hours postadmission and again at 6 hours postadmission. If all results are negative to this point, a final assay should be performed 6–12 hours postadmission to conclusively rule out the possibility of acute MI and evaluate its short-term risk.

33. **B** Persons with unstable angina (angina at rest) who have an elevated TnT are at about 8 times greater risk of having an MI within the next 6 months. This property is being used to identify short-term risk patients who should be considered for coronary angioplasty.

The reference range for TnT is very low (<0.1 ng/mL); persons with unstable angina usually have values between 0.2 and 2.0 ng/mL without evidence of acute MI, such as a positive test for CK-MB. TnI levels are not as sensitive as TnT in predicting the short-term (within 1 year) risk of acute MI in persons with unstable angina. Troponin C in cardiac and skeletal muscle is not differentiated by enzyme immunoassay. CK-MB and myoglobin have not been useful in identifying persons with unstable angina.

34. **D** This person displays very low plasma myoglobin (reference range for females is approximately 17–75 μg/L and detection limit is <10 μg/L for most assays). The TnI result is also within normal limits, based upon the reference range provided. These results are consistent with baseline levels and no evidence of cardiac or skeletal muscle injury. Reference ranges for TnI are quite variable, with chemiluminescent methods being lowest (approximately 0–0.04 μg/L). Cutpoints for acute MI are also dependent upon the method and may be higher than the upper limit of normal. Troponin results above the upper reference limit but below the cutpoint for acute MI may indicate myocardial injury and increased risk for acute MI.

35. A patient has a plasma CK-MB of 14 μg/L at admission and a total CK of 170 IU/L. Serum myoglobin is 130 μg/L and TnI is 1.6 μg/L. Three hours later, the CK-MB is 24 μg/L. Which statement best describes this situation?

A. This patient has had an acute MI and further testing is unnecessary

B. A second TnI and myoglobin test should have been performed at 3 hours postadmission to confirm an acute MI

C. These results are consistent with skeletal muscle damage associated with a crush injury that elevated the CK-MB levels

D. Further testing 6–12 hours postadmission is required to establish a diagnosis of acute MI

Chemistry/Evaluate laboratory data to recognize health and disease states/Cardiac markers/2

36. SITUATION: An EDTA sample for TnI assay gives a result of 0.07 ng/mL (reference range 0–0.04 ng/mL). The test is repeated 3 hours later on a new specimen, and the result is 0.06 ng/mL. A third sample collected 6 hours later gives a result of 0.07 ng/mL. What is the most likely explanation?

A. A false positive result occurred as a result of matrix interference

B. Heparin should have been used instead of EDTA, which causes false positive results

C. The patient had suffered cardiac injury, probably less severe than an MI

D. The patient suffered an MI

Chemistry/Evaluate laboratory data to recognize health and disease states/Cardiac markers/3

37. Which of the following laboratory tests is a marker for ischemic heart disease?

A. B-type natriuretic peptide

B. Myosin light chain 1

C. Albumin cobalt binding

D. Free fatty acid binding protein

Chemistry/Correlate clinical and laboratory data/ Cardiac markers/1

35. A Results on admission indicate strongly that the patient has suffered an MI. The 3-hour value confirms this and rules out the possibility of a sample collection or transcription error for the admission sample. Repeat testing of other cardiac markers at 3 hours was not necessary because admission results were significantly increased for all three markers. Skeletal muscle damage or crush injury does not cause an increase in cardiac TnI.

36. C EDTA is the additive of choice for TnI assays because it avoids microclots that can lead to false positive results when serum or heparinized plasma is used. Spurious false positives caused by matrix effects usually revert to normal when the test is repeated on a new sample. An MI will cause the TnI to increase in subsequent tests. Results between 0.05–0.10 ng/mL are often the result of cardiac injury and indicate an increased short-term risk of MI.

37. C When heart muscle suffers reversible damage as a result of oxygen deprivation, free radicals are released from the cells and bind to circulating albumin. The albumin is modified at the *N*-terminus, causing a reduced ability to bind certain metals. This *ischemia-modified albumin* can be measured by its inability to bind cobalt. An excess of cobalt is incubated with plasma, followed by the addition of dithiothreitol. The sulfhydryl compound complexes with the free cobalt, forming a colored complex. The absorbance of the reaction mixture is directly proportional to the ischemia-modified albumin concentration. In addition to ischemia-modified albumin, glycogen phosphorylase-BB is a marker for ischemia because it is released from heart muscle during an ischemic episode. Myosin light chains and fatty acid binding protein are released from necrotic heart tissue in the early stages of AMI. B-type natriuretic peptide is a hormone released by the ventricles in response to fluid overload and is a marker for congestive heart failure.

38. Which test provides the *earliest* warning of increased risk of coronary artery disease?
  A. Glycogen phosphorylase-BB
  B. TnT
  C. Ischemia modified albumin
  D. High-sensitivity C-reactive protein

Chemistry/Correlate laboratory data with physiological processes/Enzymes/2

39. Which statement best describes the clinical utility of B-type natriuretic peptide (BNP)?
  A. Levels ≥100 pg/mL are associated with the early stage of the acute coronary syndrome
  B. A positive test indicates prior myocardial damage caused by acute MI that occurred within the last 3 months
  C. A normal test result helps rule out congestive heart failure in persons with symptoms associated with coronary insufficiency
  D. A level above 100 pg/mL supports a diagnosis of unstable angina

Chemistry/Correlate clinical and laboratory data/Cardiac markers/2

38. **D** The acute coronary syndrome (ACS) refers to the evolution of coronary artery events that lead up to acute MI. Coronary artery disease (CAD) begins with the formation of a plaque made up of lipid from dead endothelium that proliferates into the artery lumen. The plaque becomes disrupted and the vessel wall inflamed in the asymptomatic stage of CAD. If platelet activation occurs and results in thrombosis, blood flow becomes significantly reduced, resulting in angina. This signals the transition to more advanced disease in which ischemia to heart muscle occurs and eventually to acute MI. Troponin, myoglobin, and CK-MB are not increased until the end stage of ACS. Glycogen phosphorylase-BB and albumin cobalt binding are increased by ischemia. Troponin T (and to a lesser extent TnI) may be increased slightly in unstable angina and ischemic injury, which indicates an increased risk for acute MI. High-sensitivity C-reactive protein (hs-CRP) is an ultrasensitive CRP assay that accurately measures CRP below 1 mg/L. CRP is an acute phase protein increased in inflammation. Levels of CRP at the upper end of the reference range (up to 10 mg/L) signal low-grade inflammation, which occurs in the asymptomatic phase of ACS. Such inflammation occurs when coronary artery plaques become disrupted, and therefore persons with CAD who have a mildly increased CRP are at high risk of disease progression.

39. **C** B-type natriuretic peptide is a hormone produced by the ventricles in response to increased intracardiac blood volume and hydrostatic pressure. It is formed in the heart from a precursor peptide (preproBNP) by enzymatic hydrolysis, first forming proBNP followed by BNP and NT (*N*-terminal) proBNP, which is not physiologically active. Both BNP and NT-proBNP are increased in persons with congestive heart failure (CHF). Levels are not increased in pulmonary obstruction, hypertension, edema associated with renal insufficiency, or other conditions that cause physical limitation and symptoms that overlap CHF. At a cutoff of <100 pg/mL the BNP test is effective in ruling out CHF. Diagnostic accuracy in distinguishing CHF from non-CHF ranges from 83%–95%. In addition, persons with ischemia who have an increased BNP are at greater risk for MI. The NTpro-BNP assay is similar in clinical value and can be used for persons being treated with nesiritide, a recombinant form of BNP used to treat CHF.

40. Which statement best describes the clinical utility of plasma homocysteine?
  A. Levels are directly related to the quantity of LDL cholesterol in plasma
  B. High plasma levels are associated with athero-sclerosis and increased risk of thrombosis
  C. Persons who have an elevated plasma homo-cysteine will also have an increased plasma Lp(a)
  D. Plasma levels are increased only when there is an inborn error of amino acid metabolism

Chemistry/Correlate clinical and laboratory data/ Cardiac markers/2

41. Which of the following statements about the amino-transferases (AST and ALT) is true?
  A. Isoenzymes of AST and ALT are not found in humans
  B. Both transfer an amino group to α-ketoglutarate
  C. Both require NADP$^+$ as a coenzyme
  D. Both utilize four carbon amino acids as substrates

Chemistry/Apply knowledge of fundamental biological characteristics/Aminotransferase/2

42. Select the products formed from the forward reaction of AST:
  A. Alanine and α-ketoglutarate
  B. Oxaloacetate and glutamate
  C. Aspartate and glutamine
  D. Glutamate and NADH

Chemistry/Apply knowledge of fundamental biological characteristics/Aminotransferase/1

43. Select the products formed from the forward reaction of ALT:
  A. Aspartate and alanine
  B. Alanine and α-ketoglutarate
  C. Pyruvate and glutamate
  D. Glutamine and NAD$^+$

Chemistry/Apply knowledge of fundamental biological characteristics/Aminotransferase/1

44. Which of the statements below regarding the methods of Henry for AST and ALT is correct?
  A. Hemolysis causes positive interference in both AST and ALT assays
  B. Loss of activity occurs if samples are frozen at −20°C
  C. The absorbance at the start of the reaction should not exceed 1.0A
  D. Reaction rates are unaffected by addition of P-5′-P to the substrate

Chemistry/Apply principles of basic laboratory proce-dures/Aminotransferase/2

Answers to Questions 40–44

40. B Homocysteine includes the monomeric amino acid as well as the dimers such as homocystine that contain homocysteine. Plasma levels are measured as an independent risk factor for coronary artery disease. High levels of homocysteine are toxic to vascular endothelium and promote inflammation and plaque formation. Plasma levels are independ-ent of LDL and other cholesterol fractions and help explain why approximately 35% of people with first time acute MI have LDL cholesterol levels <130 mg/dL.

41. B ALT catalyzes the transfer of an amino group from alanine, a three-carbon amino acid, to α-ketoglutarate (2-oxoglutarate), forming pyruvate. AST catalyzes the transfer of an amino group from aspartate (four carbons) to α-ketoglutarate, form-ing oxaloacetate. The reactions are highly reversible and regulate the flow of aspartate into the urea cycle. Both transaminases require P-5′-P as an intermediate amino acceptor (coenzyme). Cytoplasmic and mitochondrial isoenzymes are produced but are not differentiated in clinical practice.

42. B AST forms oxaloacetate and glutamate from aspartate and α-ketoglutarate (2-oxoglutarate). Both transaminases use α-ketoglutarate and gluta-mate as a common substrate and product pair. Both aspartate and alanine can be used to generate gluta-mate in the central nervous system, where it acts as a neurotransmitter.

43. C Because glutamate is a common product for transaminases, pyruvate (a three-carbon ketoacid) and glutamate would be generated from the transamination reaction between alanine and α-ketoglutarate.

44. A RBCs are rich in AST and to a lesser extent in ALT. Hemolysis causes positive interference in both assays, although the effect on AST is greater. Samples are stable for up to 24 hours at room tem-perature and up to 3 days at 4°C and should be frozen if kept longer. The starting absorbance should be at least 1.5A for both assays. Substrates with lower concentrations of NADH are subject to NADH depletion during the lag phase due to side reactions or high transaminase activity. When P-5′-P is added, a significant increase in activity sometimes occurs because some of the enzyme in the serum is in the inactive apoenzyme form.

45. Select the coupling enzyme used in the kinetic AST reaction of Henry:
  A. LD
  B. Malate dehydrogenase
  C. Glutamate dehydrogenase
  D. G6PD

Chemistry/Apply principles of basic laboratory procedures/Aminotransferase/1

46. What is the purpose of LD in the kinetic method of Henry for AST?
  A. Forms NADH, enabling the reaction to be monitored at 340 nm
  B. Rapidly exhausts endogenous pyruvate in the lag phase
  C. Reduces oxaloacetate, preventing product inhibition
  D. Generates lactate, which activates AST

Chemistry/Select reagents/Aminotransferase/2

47. Which statement regarding the naming of transaminases is true?
  A. Serum glutamic oxaloacetic transaminase (SGOT) is the older abbreviation for ALT
  B. Serum glutamic pyruvic transaminase (SGPT) is the older abbreviation for AST
  C. SGPT is the older abbreviation for ALT
  D. SGOT is the newer abbreviation for AST

Chemistry/Apply knowledge of fundamental biological characteristics/Aminotransferase/1

48. Which statement accurately describes serum transaminase levels in AMI?
  A. ALT is increased 5- to 10-fold after an acute MI
  B. AST peaks 24–48 hours after an acute MI and returns to normal within 4–6 days
  C. AST levels are usually 20–50 times the upper limit of normal after an acute MI
  D. Isoenzymes of AST are of greater diagnostic utility than the total enzyme level

Chemistry/Correlate clinical and laboratory data/Aminotransferase/2

49. Which condition gives rise to the highest serum level of transaminases?
  A. Acute hepatitis
  B. Alcoholic cirrhosis
  C. Obstructive biliary disease
  D. Diffuse intrahepatic cholestasis

Chemistry/Correlate clinical and laboratory data/Aminotransferase/2

45. B The method of Henry for AST uses malate dehydrogenase (MD) to reduce oxaloacetate to malate. The electrons come from NADH, forming NAD^+.

  Aspartate + α-ketoglutarate $\xrightarrow{\text{AST}}$ Oxaloacetate + Glutamate

  Oxaloacetate + NADH + H^+ $\xrightarrow{\text{MD}}$ Malate + NAD^+

46. B Patients with liver disease often have high levels of pyruvate and LD. The LD can catalyze the reaction of pyruvate with NADH in the substrate, forming NAD^+ and lactate. This would give a falsely high rate for AST because NAD^+ is the product measured. Adding LD to the substrate causes pyruvate to be depleted in the first 30 seconds, before AST and MD reactions reach steady state.

47. C SGOT (serum glutamic oxaloacetic transaminase) refers to the products measured in the in vitro reaction, and is more correctly named AST for the four-carbon amino acid substrate aspartate. SGPT is the older name referring to the products of the reaction for ALT. SGPT (serum glutamic pyruvic transaminase) is more correctly named ALT for the three-carbon amino acid substrate alanine.

48. B ALT may be slightly elevated after an acute MI. AST levels can reach up to 10 times the URL after AMI, but elevations of this range are also seen in patients with muscular dystrophy, crush injury, obstructive jaundice, pulmonary embolism, infectious mononucleosis, and cancer of the liver.

49. A The transaminases usually reach 20–50 times the URL in acute viral and toxic hepatitis. Both transaminases are moderately increased (5–10× URL) in infectious mononucleosis, diffuse intrahepatic obstruction, lymphoma, and cancer of the liver and slightly increased (2–5× URL) in cirrhosis and extrahepatic obstruction.

50. In which liver disease is the De Ritis ratio (ALT:AST) usually greater than 1.0?
A. Acute hepatitis
B. Chronic hepatitis
C. Hepatic cirrhosis
D. Hepatic carcinoma

Chemistry/Evaluate laboratory data to recognize health and disease states/Aminotransferase/2

51. Which of the following liver diseases produces the highest levels of transaminases?
A. Hepatic cirrhosis
B. Obstructive jaundice
C. Chronic hepatitis
D. Alcoholic hepatitis

Chemistry/Correlate clinical and laboratory data/Aminotransferase/2

52. Which of the following statements regarding transaminases is true?
A. ALT is often increased in muscular disease, pancreatitis, and lymphoma
B. ALT is increased in infectious mononucleosis, but AST is usually normal
C. ALT is far more specific for liver diseases than is AST
D. Substrate depletion seldom occurs in assays of serum from hepatitis cases

Chemistry/Correlate clinical and laboratory data/Aminotransaminases/2

53. Select the most sensitive marker for alcoholic liver disease.
A. GLD
B. ALT
C. AST
D. γ-Glutamyltransferase (GGT)

Chemistry/Correlate clinical and laboratory data/Enzymes/2

54. Which enzyme is *least* useful in differentiating necrotic from obstructive jaundice?
A. GGT
B. ALT
C. 5'- Nucleotidase
D. LD

Chemistry/Correlate clinical and laboratory data/Enzymes/2

55. Which of the statements below about the phosphatases is true?
A. They hydrolyze adenosine triphosphate and related compounds
B. They are divided into two classes based upon pH needed for activity

C. They exhibit a high specificity for substrate
D. They are activated by P_i

Chemistry/Apply knowledge of fundamental biological characteristics/Phosphatases/1

Answers to Questions 50–55

50. **A** ALT prevails over AST in acute hepatitis; however, AST is higher than ALT in chronic hepatitis, carcinoma, and cirrhosis of the liver.

51. **C** Elevation of transaminases is greatest in acute hepatitis (20–50×URL). Levels are moderately elevated (5–10×URL) in chronic hepatitis and hepatic cancer. They are slightly elevated (2–5×URL) in hepatic cirrhosis, alcoholic hepatitis, and obstructive jaundice.

52. **C** ALT is far more specific for liver disease than AST. High ALT levels may result from nonhepatic causes such as acute MI, muscle injury or disease, and severe hemolysis, but nonhepatic sources can be ruled out by a high direct bilirubin. Elevated ALT (e.g., >65 IU/L) is used along with immunological tests for hepatitis to disqualify blood donors. AST is increased in muscle disease, MI, pancreatitis, and lymphoma. Both transaminases are moderately increased in infectious mononucleosis.

53. **D** Although AST and ALT are elevated in alcoholic hepatitis, γ-glutamyltransferase (GGT) is a sensitive indicator of alcoholic liver disease. Levels of GGT can reach in excess of 25 times the URL in alcoholic hepatitis. It is also markedly elevated in obstructive jaundice; a high GGT level supports the inference that the liver is the tissue source of an elevated ALP.

54. **D** GGT and 5′- nucleotidase are markedly elevated in both intra- and posthepatic obstruction. ALT is slightly elevated in obstructive jaundice but is markedly elevated in necrotic jaundice. Although LD is usually greater in necrotic jaundice (3–10×N) than in obstructive jaundice (≤3×N), elevations in these ranges overlap frequently in hepatic disease and result from many other causes.

55. **B** Phosphatases are classified as either alkaline or acid, depending upon the pH needed for optimum activity. The phosphatases hydrolyze a wide range of monophosphoric acid esters. ALP is inhibited by phosphorus (product inhibition). The International Federation of Clinical Chemistry's (IFCC) recommended method employs 2-amino-2-methyl-1-propanol, a buffer that binds P_i.

56. Which of the following statements regarding ALP is true?
    A. In normal adults the primary tissue source is fast-twitch skeletal muscle
    B. Geriatric patients have a lower serum ALP than other adults
    C. Serum ALP levels are lower in children than in adults
    D. Pregnant women have a higher level of serum ALP than other adults

    Chemistry/Correlate clinical and laboratory data/ Phosphatases/2

57. Which isoenzymes of ALP are inhibited by L-phenylalanine?
    A. Intestinal and placental
    B. Bone and intestinal
    C. Liver and placental
    D. Renal and liver

    Chemistry/Apply principles of special procedures/ Phosphatases/1

58. Which isoenzyme of ALP is most heat-stable?
    A. Bone
    B. Liver
    C. Intestinal
    D. Placental

    Chemistry/Apply knowledge of fundamental biological characteristics/Phosphatases/1

59. Which isoenzyme of ALP migrates farthest toward the anode when electrophoresed at pH 8.6?
    A. Placental
    B. Bone
    C. Liver
    D. Intestinal

    Chemistry/Apply principles of special procedures/ Phosphatases/1

60. Which isoenzyme of ALP is inhibited by urea?
    A. Placental
    B. Bone
    C. Liver
    D. Intestinal

    Chemistry/Apply principles of special procedures/ Phosphatases/1

Answers to Questions 56–60

56. **D** ALP is higher in children than in adults as a result of bone growth. Children and geriatric patients have higher serum ALP values owing to increased bone isoenzyme. Serum ALP levels are often two- or threefold higher than the URL in the third term of pregnancy. In nonpregnant normal adults, serum ALP is derived from liver and bone. Liver, bone, placental, renal, and intestinal isoenzymes of ALP can be separated by electrophoresis, and many other ALP isoenzymes have been identified by isofocusing. RBCs, leukocytes, and the prostate are the primary sources of acid phosphatase isoenzymes.

57. **A** Liver and bone isoenzymes are difficult to separate by agarose gel electrophoresis, and many laboratories use heat stability and selective inhibitors to help identify the tissue source when ALP is elevated. Phenylalanine inhibits placental and intestinal forms; 3M urea inhibits bone ALP.

58. **D** Placental ALP and tumor-associated isoenzymes such as the Regan isoenzyme associated with lung cancer are the only isoenzymes that retain activity when serum is heated to 65° C for 10 minutes. Heat inactivation is used primarily to distinguish liver ALP from bone ALP. If less than 20% activity remains after heating serum to 56°C for 10 minutes, then bone ALP is most likely present.

59. **C** Liver ALP isoenzymes migrate farthest toward the anode, but fast and slow variants occur. The slow liver ALP band is difficult to distinguish from placental and bone ALP. The order from cathode to anode is:

    – Renal→Intestinal→Bone→Placental→Liver +

60. **B** Bone ALP isoenzyme is inhibited by urea, and placental and intestinal ALP are inhibited by phenylalanine. Bone ALP can be distinguished from liver ALP by coupling two methods. For example, loss of ALP activity by heating to 56°C for 10 minutes and by addition of 3M urea points to ALP derived from bone.

61. Which of the following statements regarding ALP is true?
- **A.** Isoenzymes of ALP are antigenically distinct and can be identified by specific antibodies
- **B.** Highest serum levels are seen in intrahepatic obstruction
- **C.** Elevated serum ALP levels seen with elevated GGT suggests a hepatic source
- **D.** When jaundice is present, an elevated ALP reading suggests acute hepatitis

Chemistry/Correlate clinical and laboratory data/ Phosphatases/2

62. In which condition would an elevated serum alkaline phosphatase be likely to occur?
- **A.** Squamous cell carcinoma
- **B.** Hemolytic anemia
- **C.** Prostate cancer
- **D.** Acute myocardial infarction

Chemistry/Correlate clinical and laboratory data/ Phosphatases/2

63. Which condition is *least* likely to be associated with increased serum ALP concentrations?
- **A.** Osteomalacia
- **B.** Pancreatic disease
- **C.** Hyperparathyroidism and hyperthyroidism
- **D.** Osteoporosis

Chemistry/Correlate clinical and laboratory data/ Phosphatases/2

64. Which substrate is used in the Bowers-McComb method for ALP?
- **A.** *p*-Nitrophenylphosphate
- **B.** β-Glycerophosphate
- **C.** Phenylphosphate
- **D.** α-Naphthylphosphate

Chemistry/Apply principles of basic laboratory procedures/Phosphatases/2

61. **C** ALP isoenzymes can result from different genes or from modification of a common gene product in the tissues. Some differ in carbohydrate content rather than protein content and cannot be identified by immunological methods. Highest levels of ALP are seen in Paget's disease of bone, in which ALP can be as high as 25 times the URL. GGT in serum is derived from the hepatobiliary system and is increased in alcoholic hepatitis and hepatobiliary obstruction. It is not increased in diseases of bone or in pregnancy. When the increase in GGT is twofold higher than the increase in ALP, the liver is assumed to be the source of the elevated ALP. Serum ALP is a sensitive marker for extrahepatic obstruction, which causes an increase of approximately 10 times the URL. A lesser increase is seen in intrahepatic obstruction. ALP is only mildly elevated in acute hepatitis as a result of accompanying obstruction.

62. **A** The primary diagnostic utility of ALP is to help differentiate necrotic jaundice (↑ALT) from obstructive jaundice (↑ALP). ALP is also increased in several bone diseases. Large increases are seen in Paget's disease, moderate increases in bone cancer, and slight increases in rickets. In addition to obstructive jaundice and bone diseases, alkaline phosphatase is a tumor marker. In most cases the alkaline phosphatase is the product of fetal gene activation and resembles placental ALP (e.g., hepatoma, squamous cell carcinoma of the lung, ovarian cancer). Leukemia and Hodgkin's disease may cause an elevated leukocyte or bone-derived ALP.

63. **D** ALP is elevated in osteomalacia (rickets), bone cancer, and bone disease secondary to hyperthyroidism and hyperparathyroidism, but it is high in less than 30% of osteoporosis patients. Pancreatic disease associated with biliary obstruction, such as cancer at the head of the pancreas, is associated with elevated ALP.

64. **A** The method of Bowers-McComb (Szasz modification) is the IFCC recommended method for ALP. This method uses 2-amino-2-methyl-1-propanol, pH 10.15, and measures the increase in absorbance at 405 nm as *p*-nitrophenylphosphate is hydrolyzed to *p*-nitrophenol.

65. Which of the following buffers is used in the IFCC recommended method for ALP?
   A. Glycine
   B. Phosphate
   C. 2-Amino-2-methyl-1-propanol
   D. Citrate

Chemistry/Apply principles of basic laboratory procedures/Phosphatases/2

66. **SITUATION:** Serum from a 50-year-old man was analyzed for both prostatic acid phosphatase (PAP) and prostate-specific antigen (PSA) following a digital rectal examination of the prostate. The PAP result is 6.0 μg/L (URL = 3.0 μg/L), and the PSA is 2.0 μg/L (URL = 4.0 μg/L). Both tests are repeated on the same sample, and the results remain unchanged. What is the most likely explanation?
   A. The PAP is falsely elevated by prostatic irritation
   B. The patient has benign prostatic hypertrophy
   C. The patient has an infection of the prostate
   D. The PSA is falsely low because it is not as sensitive as the PAP

Chemistry/Apply knowledge to identify sources of error/Phosphatases/3

67. Which definition best describes the catalytic activity of amylase?
   A. Hydrolyzes second α-1-4 glycosidic linkages of starch, glycogen, and other polyglucans
   B. Hydrolyzes all polyglucans completely to produce glucose
   C. Oxidatively degrades polysaccharides containing glucose
   D. Splits polysaccharides and disaccharides by addition of water

Chemistry/Apply knowledge of fundamental biological characteristics/Amylase/1

68. Which of the following amylase methods is typically based upon a rate reaction?
   A. Somogyi
   B. Dye-starch
   C. Starch-iodine
   D. Turbidimetric

Chemistry/Apply knowledge of basic laboratory procedures/Amylase/1

69. How soon following acute abdominal pain due to pancreatitis is the serum amylase level expected to rise?
   A. 1–2 hours
   B. 2–12 hours
   C. 3–4 days
   D. 5–6 days

Chemistry/Correlate clinical and laboratory data/Amylase/2

Answers to Questions 65–69

65. **C** The Szasz modification of the Bowers and McComb method measures the hydrolysis of *p*-nitrophenylphosphate and continuously monitors the formation of *p*-nitrophenol at 405 nm. AMP buffer chelates phosphorus, preventing product inhibition; Zn^{2+} and Mg^{2+} are added to the substrate to activate ALP. N-hydroxyethylethylenediaminetriacetic acid (HEDTA) is used to chelate the excess Zn^{2+}, which is inhibitory at high concentrations.

66. **A** Acid phosphatase is sometimes used along with PSA to monitor for recurrence of prostate cancer in patients who are being treated with antiandrogen therapy. The PSA test is clinically more sensitive than PAP in detecting stages A and B prostatic cancer. The PSA also has the advantage of being stable in storage and is not elevated by trauma associated with digital rectal examination. However, both PAP and PSA levels may be elevated in prostatic infections and benign prostatic hypertrophy. The primary clinical use of PAP is in the investigation of sexual assault. Acid phosphatase activity >50 IU/L establishes the presence of seminal fluid in the sample.

67. **A** Amylase in humans is a hydrolase that splits the second α-1-4 glycosidic bonds of polyglucans forming maltose. There are two major types of amylase, P-type derived from the pancreas and S-type derived from the salivary glands. These can be differentiated by both electrophoresis and immunoassay. In healthy persons the principal form in plasma is the salivary isoenzyme. There are several genetic variants of the salivary isoenzyme, which in part accounts for the broad reference range.

68. **D** The Somogyi method measures the formation of maltose after incubating serum and starch for 30 minutes at 37°C. Dye-starch or chromolytic methods measure the amount of dye released from starch after incubation with serum. The amount of dye released is determined by comparison to pure dye standards. Turbidimetric methods determine the clearing of starch as a negative rate reaction.

69. **B** Serum amylase usually peaks 2–12 hours following acute abdominal pain resulting from pancreatitis. Levels reach 2–6 times the URL and return to normal within 3–4 days. Urinary amylase peaks concurrently with serum but rises higher and remains elevated for up to 1 week.

70. Which of the statements below regarding the diagnosis of pancreatitis is correct?
  A. Amylase and lipase are as predictive in chronic as in acute pancreatitis
  B. Diagnostic sensitivity is increased by assaying both amylase and lipase
  C. Measuring the urinary amylase:creatinine ratio is useful only when patients have renal failure
  D. Serum lipase peaks several hours before amylase after an episode of acute pancreatitis

Chemistry/Correlate clinical and laboratory data/ Enzymes/2

71. Which of the following conditions is associated with a high level of S-type amylase?
  A. Mumps
  B. Intestinal obstruction
  C. Alcoholic liver disease
  D. Peptic ulcers

Chemistry/Correlate clinical and laboratory data/ Amylase/2

72. Which of the statements regarding amylase methods is true?
  A. Requires sulfhydryl compounds for full activity
  B. Activity will vary with the lot of starch if it is used as the substrate
  C. Amyloclastic methods measure the production of glucose
  D. Over-range samples are diluted in deionized water

Chemistry/Apply knowledge of basic laboratory procedures/Amylase/2

70.   B Amylase is not increased in all patients with pancreatitis and can be increased in several nonpancreatic conditions. Lipase adds both sensitivity and specificity to the diagnosis of acute pancreatitis. Plasma or serum lipase becomes abnormal within 6 hours, peaks at approximately 24 hours, and remains abnormal for about 1 week following an episode of acute pancreatitis. In acute pancreatitis the rate of urinary amylase excretion increases, and the urinary amylase:creatinine ratio or the amylase:creatinine (A:C) clearance ratio is helpful in diagnosing some cases of pancreatitis. The normal A:C clearance ratio is 1%–4%. In acute pancreatitis, the ratio is usually above 4% and can be as high as 15%. In chronic pancreatitis, acinar cell degeneration often occurs, resulting in loss of amylase and lipase production. This lowers the sensitivity of amylase and lipase in detecting chronic disease to below 50%. Patients with chronic disease have pancreatic insufficiency, giving rise to abnormal triolein, ^{131}I and β-carotene absorption, increased fecal fat, and decreased fecal trypsin.

71.   A Both salivary and pancreatic amylases designated S-type and P-type, respectively, are present in normal serum. High amylase occurs in mumps, ectopic pregnancy, biliary obstruction, peptic ulcers, alcoholism, malignancies, and other nonpancreatic diseases. Isoenzyme or immunoinhibition assay can be used to rule out mumps, malignancy, and ectopic pregnancy, which give rise to high S-type amylase.

72.   B Chloride and Ca^{2+} ions are required for amylase activity. Samples with high activity should be diluted with NaCl to prevent inactivation. Lipase and CK require sulfhydryl activators. Saccharogenic methods measure the production of glucose, while amyloclastic methods measure the degradation of starch. Starch is the natural substrate for amylase and is used in the reference method of Somogyi. Starch is a polymer of α-D-glucose subunits linked together by both α-1-4 and α-1-6 glycosidic bonds. Different lots may have more or less branching, depending on the number of α-1-6 bonds. Since amylase hydrolyzes at the α-1-4 sites only, the amount of product measured is influenced by the extent of branching.

73. Which of the following statements regarding amylase methods is true?
   A. Dilution of serum may result in lower than expected activity
   B. Methods generating NADH are preferred because they have higher sensitivity
   C. Synthetic substrates can be conjugated to *p*-nitrophenol (PNP) for a kinetic assay
   D. The reference range is consistent from method to method

   Chemistry/Apply knowledge to identify sources of error/Amylase/2

74. The reference method for lipase uses olive oil as the substrate because:
   A. Other esterases can hydrolyze triglyceride and synthetic diglycerides
   B. The reaction product can be coupled to NADH-generating reactions
   C. Synthetic substrates are less soluble than olive oil in aqueous reagents
   D. Triglyceride substrates cause product inhibition

   Chemistry/Apply knowledge of basic laboratory procedures/Lipase/2

75. Which statement about the clinical utility of plasma or serum lipase is true?
   A. Lipase is not increased in mumps, malignancy, or ectopic pregnancy
   B. Lipase is not increased as dramatically as amylase in acute pancreatitis
   C. Increased plasma or serum lipase is specific for pancreatitis
   D. Lipase levels are elevated in both acute and chronic pancreatitis

   Chemistry/Correlate clinical and laboratory data/Lipase/2

76. The reference method for serum lipase is based upon:
   A. Assay of triglycerides following incubation of serum with olive oil
   B. Rate turbidimetry
   C. Titration of fatty acids with dilute NaOH following controlled incubation of serum with olive oil
   D. Immunochemical assay

   Chemistry/Apply principles of basic laboratory procedures/Lipase/1

Answers to Questions 73–76

73. **C** Many endogenous inhibitors of amylase, such as wheat germ, are found in serum. Diluted samples often show higher than expected activity caused by dilution of the inhibitor. Units of amylase activity vary widely, depending upon the method of assay and calibration. Synthetic substrates such as maltotetrose or 4-nitrophenylmaltoheptoside can be used for kinetic assays. Maltotetrose is hydrolyzed to maltose by amylase, and the maltose is hydrolyzed by α-glucosidase or maltose phosphorylase, forming glucose or glucose-1-phosphate, respectively. These can be measured by coupling to NADH-generating reactions. A chromolytic method generating *p*-nitrophenol can be performed kinetically and is commonly used. The substrate, maltoheptoside esterified to *p*-nitrophenol, is "blocked" so that α-glucosidase will not hydrolyze it until after it is split by amylase, forming smaller oligosaccharides. The *p*-nitrophenol generated increases the absorbance at 410 nm in proportion to amylase activity.

74. **A** Triglycerides may be hydrolyzed by nonspecific esterases in serum as well as lipase. Lipase acts only at an interface of oil and H_2O and requires bile salts and colipase for activity. Colipase is a protein secreted by the pancreas.

75. **A** Lipase elevation is of greater magnitude ($2–50 \times N$) and duration than amylase in acute pancreatitis. When the lipase method is optimized by inclusion of colipase and bile salts, the test is more sensitive and specific than serum amylase for detection of acute pancreatitis. However, lipase is also increased in peptic ulcers, renal insufficiency, and intestinal obstruction. Lipase levels are usually low in chronic pancreatitis and are low in patients with cystic fibrosis.

76. **C** The reference method of Cherry and Crandall is based upon the titration of fatty acids formed by the hydrolysis of an emulsion of olive oil after incubation for 24 hours at 37°C. Because most of the activity occurs within the first 3 hours, the incubation time may be shortened to as little as 1 hour without loss of clinical utility.

77. The most commonly employed method of assay for plasma or serum lipase is based upon:
  A. Hydrolysis of olive oil
  B. Rate turbidimetry
  C. Immunoassay
  D. Peroxidase coupling

Chemistry/Apply principles of basic laboratory procedures/Lipase/1

78. Which of the following enzymes is usually depressed in liver disease?
  A. Leucine aminopeptidase (LAP)
  B. GLD
  C. Pseudocholinesterase
  D. Aldolase

Chemistry/Correlate clinical and laboratory data/Enzymes/2

79. A serum ALP level greater than twice the elevation of GGT suggests:
  A. Misidentification of the specimen
  B. Focal intrahepatic obstruction
  C. Acute alcoholic hepatitis
  D. Bone disease or malignancy

Chemistry/Evaluate laboratory data to recognize health and disease states/Enzymes/2

80. How many of the substances below would be needed to enable an early diagnosis of stroke?

D-dimer, von Willebrand's factor (VWF), matrix metalloproteinase-9 (MMP-9), S100β, brain naturetic peptide (BNP), vascular cell adhesion molecule (VCAM)
  A. D-dimer and VWF are the only two required
  B. MMP-9
  C. BNP, VCAM, and one other marker
  D. All six markers

Chemistry/Correlate clinical and laboratory data/Stroke markers/2

Answers to Questions 77–80

77. **D** Although all of the methods cited are available, the most commonly used method for lipase assay is based upon the hydrolysis of a synthetic diglyceride substrate yielding 2-monoglyceride. This is hydrolyzed, forming glycerol, which is phosphorylated forming glycerol-3-phosphate. This is oxidized by glycerophosphate oxidase, yielding hydrogen peroxide.

$$1,2 \text{ diglyceride} + H_2O$$
$$\downarrow \text{Lipase}$$
$$2\text{-monoglyceride} + \text{fatty acid}$$

$$2\text{- monoglyceride} + H_2O$$
$$\downarrow \text{Monoglyceride esterase}$$
$$\text{glycerol} + \text{fatty acid}$$

$$\text{glycerol} + ATP$$
$$\downarrow \text{Glycerol kinase}$$
$$\text{glycerol-3-phosphate} + ADP$$

$$\text{glycerol-3-}PO_4 + O_2$$
$$\downarrow \text{Glycerophosphate oxidase}$$
$$\text{dihydroxyacetone phosphate} + H_2O_2$$

$$H_2O_2 + 4\text{-aminoantipyrene} + TOOS$$
$$\downarrow \text{Peroxidase}$$
$$\text{quinoneimine dye} + H_2O$$

78. **C** Levels of pseudocholinesterase are decreased in patients with liver disease as a result of depressed synthesis. In cirrhosis and hepatoma, there is a 50%–70% reduction in serum level and a 30%–50% reduction in serum level in hepatitis. LAP is increased in both necrotic and obstructive jaundice. GLD is increased in necrotic jaundice, and aldolase is increased in necrotic jaundice and muscle disease.

79. **D** In obstructive jaundice, GGT is elevated more than ALP. A disproportionate increase in ALP points to a nonhepatic source of ALP, often bone disease. GGT is the most sensitive marker of acute alcoholic hepatitis, rising about fivefold higher than ALP or transaminases.

80. **D** Early detection of stroke (>90% specificity and sensitivity) requires a panel of four to six markers that signal inflammatory, thromboembolytic, and neural changes occurring within 6 hours of a stroke. MMP-9 and VCAM detect inflammation in the neurons. D-dimer and VWF signal a thromboembolytic event, and S100β detects glial cell activity. BNP is released in response to hypoxemia and necrosis. Other markers that are abnormal in stroke include CRP, CK-BB isoenzyme, neuron specific enolase, and caspase.

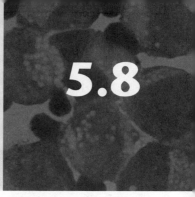

1. Which of the following hormones is often decreased by approximately 25% in the serum of pregnant women who have a fetus with Down's syndrome?
   A. Estriol (E_3)
   B. Human chorionic gonadotropin (hCG)
   C. Progesterone
   D. Estradiol (E_2)

   Chemistry/Correlate laboratory data with physiological processes/Endocrine/2

2. The syndrome of inappropriate antidiuretic hormone secretion (SIADH) causes:
   A. Low serum vasopressin
   B. Hypernatremia
   C. Urine osmolality to be lower than that of plasma
   D. Low serum electrolytes

   Chemistry/Correlate clinical and laboratory data/ Endocrine/2

3. Select the hormone that is associated with galactor-rhea, pituitary adenoma, and amenorrhea.
   A. E_2
   B. Progesterone
   C. Follicle-stimulating hormone (FSH)
   D. Prolactin

   Chemistry/Correlate clinical and laboratory data/ Endocrine/2

4. Zollinger-Ellison (Z-E) syndrome is characterized by great (e.g., 20-fold) elevation of:
   A. Gastrin
   B. Cholecystokinin
   C. Pepsin
   D. Glucagon

   Chemistry/Correlate clinical and laboratory data/ Gastric/2

Answers to Questions 1–4

1. **A** E_3 is produced in the placenta and fetal liver from dehydroepiandosterone derived from the mother and fetal liver. E_3 is the major estrogen produced during pregnancy, and levels rise throughout gestation. Serum free E_3 is often lower than expected for the gestational age in a pregnancy associated with Down's syndrome. The combination of low serum free estriol, low α-fetoprotein, high hCG, and high inhibin A is used as a screening test to detect Down's syndrome. When one of the four markers is abnormal, amniocentesis should be performed for the diagnosis of Down's syndrome by karyotyping or FISH. The four markers have a combined sensitivity (detection rate) of approximately 75%.

2. **D** SIADH results in excessive secretion of vaso-pressin (ADH) from the posterior pituitary, causing fluid retention and low plasma osmolality, sodium, potassium, and other electrolytes by hemodilution. It is suspected when urine osmolality is higher than that of plasma but urine sodium concentration is normal or increased. Patients with sodium deple-tion have a urine osmolality higher than that of plasma but low urine sodium levels.

3. **D** Serum prolactin may be increased from hypo-thalamic dysfunction or pituitary adenoma. When levels are greater than five times the URL, a pitu-itary tumor is suspected. Prolactin is measured by enzyme immunoassay (EIA).

4. **A** Z-E syndrome is caused by a pancreatic or intes-tinal tumor secreting gastrin (gastrinoma) and results in greatly increased gastric acid production. Basal acid output (BAO) and peak acid output (PAO) are greatly elevated, and the BAO/PAO exceeds 0.6.

5. Which statement about multiple endocrine neoplasia (MEN) is true?
  A. It is associated with hyperplasia or neoplasia of at least two endocrine organs
  B. Insulinoma is always present when the pituitary is involved
  C. It is inherited as an autosomal recessive disorder
  D. Plasma hormone levels from affected organs are elevated at least tenfold

Chemistry/Correlate clinical and laboratory data/ Endocrine/2

6. Select the main estrogen produced by the ovaries and used to evaluate ovarian function.
  A. Estriol (E_3)
  B. Estradiol (E_2)
  C. Epiestriol
  D. Hydroxyestrone

Chemistry/Apply knowledge of fundamental biological characteristics/Estrogen/1

7. Which statement best describes the relationship between luteinizing hormone (LH) and FSH in cases of dysmenorrhea?
  A. Both are usually increased when pituitary adenoma is present
  B. Increases in both hormones and a decrease in estrogen signal a pituitary cause of ovarian failure
  C. Both hormones normally peak 1–2 days before ovulation
  D. In menopause, the LH level at the midcycle peak is higher than the level of FSH

Chemistry/Correlate clinical and laboratory data/ Endocrine/2

8. When pituitary adenoma is the cause of decreased estrogen production, an increase of which hormone is most frequently responsible?
  A. Prolactin
  B. FSH
  C. LH
  D. Thyroid-stimulating hormone (TSH)

Chemistry/Correlate clinical and laboratory data/ Endocrine/2

Answers to Questions 5–8

5. **A** Multiple endocrine neoplasia syndrome is inherited as an autosomal dominant disease involving excess production of hormones from several endocrine glands. MEN I results from adenomas (usually benign) of at least two glands, including the pituitary, adrenal cortex, parathyroid, and pancreas. The parathyroid gland is the organ most commonly involved, and in those patients an elevated Ca_i is an early sign. The pancreas is the next most frequently involved organ, but the hormone most commonly oversecreted is gastrin (not insulin). MEN II usually results from pheochromocytoma and thyroid carcinoma. MEN II-B is a variant of MEN II showing the addition of neurofibroma.

6. **B** E_2 is the major estrogen produced by the ovaries and gives rise to both estrone (E_1) and E_3. E_2 is used to evaluate both ovarian function and menstrual cycle dysfunction.

7. **C** In women, serum or urine LH and FSH are measured along with estrogen and progesterone to evaluate the cause of menstrual cycle abnormalities and anovulation. Both hormones show a pronounced serum peak 1–2 days prior to ovulation and a urine peak 20–44 hours before ovulation. Normally, the LH peak is sharper and higher than the FSH peak; however, in menopause, the FSH usually becomes higher than LH. In patients with primary ovarian failure, the LH and FSH are elevated because low estrogen levels stimulate release of luteinizing hormone–releasing hormone (LHRH) from the hypothalamus. Conversely, in pituitary failure, levels of FSH and LH are reduced, and this reduction causes a deficiency of estrogen production by the ovaries.

8. **A** Prolactinoma can result in anovulation because high levels of prolactin suppress release of LHRH, causing suppression of growth hormone (GH), FSH, and estrogen. Prolactinoma is the most commonly occurring pituitary tumor accounting for 40%–60% of pituitary tumors. Adenomas producing FSH have a frequency of about 20%, whereas those pituitary tumors secreting LH and TSH are rare.

9. Which of the following statements is correct in assessing GH deficiency?
   A. Pituitary failure may involve one, several, or all adenohypophyseal hormones, but GH deficiency is usually found
   B. A normal random serum level of GH in a child under 6 years old rules out GH deficiency
   C. Administration of arginine, insulin, or glucagon suppresses GH release
   D. GH levels in the blood show little variation within a 24-hour period

   Chemistry/Apply knowledge of fundamental biological characteristics/Endocrine/2

10. Which statement best describes the level of GH in patients with pituitary adenoma associated with acromegaly?
    A. The fasting GH level is always elevated at least twofold
    B. Some patients require a glucose suppression test to establish a diagnosis
    C. A normal fasting GH level rules out acromegaly
    D. Patients produce a lower concentration of insulin-like growth factor I (IGF-1) than expected from their GH level

    Chemistry/Correlate clinical and laboratory data/ Endocrine/2

11. Hyperparathyroidism is most consistently associated with:
    A. Hypocalcemia
    B. Hypocalciuria
    C. Hypophosphatemia
    D. Metabolic alkalosis

    Chemistry/Correlate clinical and laboratory data/ Endocrine/2

Answers to Questions 9–11

9. **A** Because GH is the most abundant pituitary hormone, it may be used as a screening test for pituitary failure in adults. Pituitary hormone deficiencies are rare and are evaluated by measuring those hormones associated with the specific type of target organ dysfunction. GH secretion peaks during sleep, and pulsed increases are seen following exercise and meals. In adults, a deficiency of GH can be ruled out by demonstrating normal or high levels on two successive tests. In children, there is extensive overlap between normal and low GH levels, and a stimulation (provocative) test is usually needed to establish a diagnosis of deficiency. Exercise is often used to stimulate GH release. If GH levels are greater than 6 μg/L after vigorous exercise, deficiency is ruled out. In addition to exercise, drugs such as arginine, insulin, propranolol, and glucagon can be used to stimulate GH release. Deficiency is documented by registering a subnormal response to two stimulating agents.

10. **B** Approximately 90% of patients with acromegaly have an elevated fasting GH level, but 10% do not. In addition, a single measurement is not sufficient to establish a diagnosis of acromegaly because various metabolic and nutritional factors can cause an elevated serum GH in the absence of pituitary disease. The glucose suppression test is used to diagnose acromegaly. An oral dose of 100 g of glucose will suppress the serum GH level at 1 hour (postadministration) to below 1 μg/L in normal patients but not in patients with acromegaly. Patients with acromegaly also have high levels of insulin-like growth factor (IGF)-1, also called somatomedin C, which is overproduced by the liver in response to excess release of GH.

11. **C** Hyperparathyroidism causes increased resorption of calcium and decreased renal retention of phosphate. Increased serum calcium leads to increased urinary excretion. The distal collecting tubule of the nephron reabsorbs less bicarbonate as well as less phosphate, resulting in acidosis.

12. Which statement regarding the use of PTH is true?
    A. Determination of serum PTH level is the best screening test for disorders of calcium metabolism
    B. PTH levels differentiate primary and secondary causes of hypoparathyroidism
    C. PTH levels differentiate primary and secondary causes of hypocalcemia
    D. PTH levels are low in patients with pseudohypoparathyroidism

    Chemistry/Correlate clinical and laboratory data/ Endocrine/2

13. The best method of analysis for serum PTH involves using antibodies that detect:
    A. The amino-terminal fragment of PTH
    B. The carboxy-terminal end of PTH
    C. Both the amino-terminal fragment and intact PTH
    D. All fragments of PTH as well as intact hormone

    Chemistry/Apply principles of special procedures/ Hormone assays/1

14. Which of the following is most often elevated in hypercalcemia associated with malignancy?
    A. Parathyroid-derived PTH
    B. Ectopic PTH
    C. Parathyroid hormone-related protein (PTHRP)
    D. Calcitonin

    Chemistry/Apply principles of special procedures/ Hormone assays/1

Answers to Questions 12–14

12. **C** Serum Ca_i is the best screening test to determine if a disorder of calcium metabolism is present and will distinguish primary hyperparathyroidism (high Ca_i) and secondary hyperparathyroidism (low Ca_i). PTH levels are used to distinguish primary and secondary causes of hypocalcemia. Serum PTH is low in primary hypocalcemia (which results from parathyroid gland disease) but is high in secondary hypocalcemia (e.g., renal failure). Serum PTH is also used for the early diagnosis of secondary hypocalcemia because of its rise prior to a decrease in the serum Ca_i. Serum PTH is used to help distinguish primary hyperparathyroidism (high PTH) from hypercalcemia of malignancy (usually low PTH) and pseudohypoparathyroidism from primary hypoparathyroidism. Pseudohypoparathyroidism results from a deficient response to PTH and is associated with normal or elevated serum PTH.

13. **C** PTH is a polypeptide made up of 84 amino acids. The biological activity of the hormone resides in the N-terminal portion of the polypeptide, but the hormone is rapidly degraded producing N-terminal, middle, and C-terminal fragments. Fragments lacking the N-terminal portion are inactive. Immunoassays for PTH using antibodies to different portions of the polypeptide give different results. The assay of choice is a two-site double antibody sandwich method that measures only intact PTH and active fragments. Methods that use single antibodies may detect inactive as well as active PTH fragments and are not as specific for parathyroid disease.

14. **C** PTHRP is a peptide produced by many tissues and is normally present in the blood at a very low level. The peptide has an N-terminal sequence of eight amino acids that are the same as found in PTH and that will stimulate the PTH receptors of bone. Some malignancies (e.g., squamous, renal, bladder, and ovarian cancers) secrete PTHRP, causing hypercalcemia-associated malignancy. Because the region shared with PTH is small and poorly immunoreactive, the peptide does not cross-react in most assays for PTH. For this reason, and because tumors producing ectopic PTH are rare, almost all patients who have an elevated Ca_i and elevated PTH have primary hyperparathyroidism. The immunoassay for PTHRP is frequently elevated in patients who have not yet been diagnosed with malignancy but have an elevated Ca_i without an elevated serum PTH. Calcitonin is a hormone produced in the medulla of the thyroid that opposes the action of PTH. However, calcitonin levels do not greatly influence the serum calcium. Assay of calcitonin is used exclusively to diagnose medullary thyroid cancer, which produces very high serum levels.

15. Steroids with a dihydroxyacetone group at C17 are classified as:
    A. Androgens
    B. 17-Hydroxycorticosteroids
    C. 17-Ketosteroids
    D. Estrogens

    Chemistry/Apply knowledge of fundamental biological characteristics/Adrenal/1

16. Which statement below regarding adrenal cortical dysfunction is true?
    A. Patients with Cushing's syndrome usually have hyperkalemia
    B. Cushing's syndrome is associated with glucose intolerance
    C. Addison's disease is associated with hypernatremia
    D. Addison's disease is caused by elevated levels of cortisol

    Chemistry/Correlate clinical and laboratory data/ Adrenal/2

17. Which of the following statements about cortisol in Cushing's syndrome is true?
    A. Twenty-four-hour urinary free cortisol is a more sensitive test than plasma total cortisol
    B. Patients with Cushing's disease show pronounced diurnal variation in serum cortisol
    C. Urinary free cortisol is increased by a high serum cortisol–binding protein concentration
    D. An elevated serum total cortisol level is diagnostic of Cushing's syndrome

    Chemistry/Apply knowledge to identify sources of error/ Cortisol/2

18. Which of the following diseases is characterized by primary hyperaldosteronism caused by adrenal adenoma, carcinoma, or hyperplasia?
    A. Cushing's disease
    B. Addison's disease
    C. Conn's disease
    D. Pheochromocytoma

    Chemistry/Correlate clinical and laboratory data/ Endocrine/2

Answers to Questions 15–18

15. **B** The 17-hydroxycorticosteroids are defined as steroids with 21 carbons that have a dihydroxyacetone group at C17. The principal member of this group is cortisol, and plasma and urinary cortisol measurements are used to diagnose most types of adrenocortical dysfunction. The 17-ketosteroids are C19 steroids that have a dehydroxy (ketone) group at C17. Many of the androgens such as dehydroepiandrosterone are 17-ketosteroids (although testosterone, the principal androgen in males, is not). The three primary estrogens— estradiol, estriol, and estrone— are C18 steroid hormones that have a phenol A ring. All have a hydroxyl group at C3. Estradiol has a second hydroxyl group at C17 and estriol a third at C16.

16. **B** Patients with Cushing's syndrome have elevated levels of cortisol and other adrenal corticosteroids. This causes the characteristic cushingoid appearance that includes obesity, acne, and humpback posture. Osteoporosis, hypertension, hypokalemia, and glycosuria are characteristics. Addison's disease results from adrenal hypoplasia and produces the opposite symptoms, including hypotension, hyperkalemia, and hypoglycemia.

17. **A** Serum cortisol levels can be increased by factors such as stress, medications, and cortisol-binding protein, and the cortisol level of normal patients will overlap those seen in Cushing's syndrome because of pulse variation. When cortisol levels become elevated, cortisol-binding protein becomes saturated, and free (unbound) cortisol is filtered by the glomeruli. Most is reabsorbed, but a significant amount reaches the urine as free cortisol. Taking 24-hour urinary free cortisol readings avoids the diurnal variation that may affect plasma free cortisol levels and is a more sensitive test than serum total or free cortisol.

18. **C** Conn's syndrome is characterized by hypertension, hypokalemia, and hypernatremia with increased plasma and urine aldosterone and decreased renin. Cushing's syndrome results from excessive production of cortisol, and Addison's disease from deficient production of adrenal corticosteroids. Pheochromocytoma is a tumor of chromaffin cells (usually adrenal) that produces catecholamines.

19. Which of the following is the most common cause of Cushing's syndrome?
  A. Pituitary adenoma
  B. Adrenal hyperplasia
  C. Overuse of corticosteroids
  D. Ectopic adrenocorticotropic hormone (ACTH) production by tumors

  Chemistry/Correlate clinical and laboratory data/ Adrenal/2

20. Which of the following is the mechanism causing Cushing's disease?
  A. Excess secretion of pituitary ACTH
  B. Adrenal adenoma
  C. Treatment with corticosteroids
  D. Ectopic ACTH production by tumors

  Chemistry/Apply knowledge of fundamental biological characteristics/Adrenal/2

21. In which situation is the plasma or 24-hour urinary cortisol *not* consistent with the clinical picture?
  A. Evaluation of adrenal function in pregnancy
  B. In patients with a borderline positive overnight dexamethasone suppression test
  C. Evaluation of congenital adrenal hyperplasia
  D. Differentiation of Cushing's syndrome from disease

  Chemistry/Select course of action/Adrenal/2

22. Which test is used to distinguish Cushing's disease (pituitary Cushing's) from Cushing's syndrome caused by adrenal tumors?
  A. Overnight dexamethasone suppression
  B. Petrosal sinus sampling
  C. Serum ACTH
  D. Twenty-four-hour urinary free cortisol testing

  Chemistry/Select course of action/Adrenal/2

Answers to Questions 19–22

19. **C** The most common cause of Cushing's syndrome is the administration of medications with cortisol or glucocorticoid activity. Excluding iatrogenic causes, approximately 60%–70% of Cushing's syndrome cases result from hypothalamic-pituitary misregulation; this is called Cushing's disease. Adrenal adenoma or carcinoma (non-ACTH-mediated Cushing's syndrome) makes up about 20% of cases, and ectopic ACTH production accounts for 10%–20%.

20. **A** Cushing's disease refers to adrenal hyperplasia resulting from misregulation of the hypothalamic-pituitary axis. It is usually caused by small pituitary adenomas. Cushing's syndrome may be caused by Cushing's disease, adrenal adenoma or carcinoma, ectopic ACTH-producing tumors, or excessive corticosteroid administration. The causes of Cushing's syndrome can be differentiated using the ACTH and dexamethasone suppression tests.

21. **C** Congenital adrenal hyperplasia (adrenogenital syndrome) results from a deficiency of an enzyme required for synthesis of cortisol. Approximately 90% of cases are caused by a deficiency of 21-hydroxylase, which blocks conversion of 17-α-hydroxyprogesterone to 11-deoxycortisol. Most other cases are caused by 11-hydroxylase deficiency, which blocks conversion of 11-deoxycortisol to cortisol. Precursors of cortisol, usually either 17-α-hydroxyprogesterone or 11-deoxycortisol, are increased. This results in low serum cortisol levels but high levels of these intermediates (mainly 17-ketogenic steroids). The two most common features of CAH are salt wasting caused by low aldosterone and virilization resulting from increased androgens.

22. **C** Serum ACTH assays are very helpful in distinguishing the cause of Cushing's syndrome. Patients with adrenal tumors have values approaching zero. Patients with ectopic ACTH tumors have values higher than 200 pg/dL. Fifty percent of patients with Cushing's disease have high 8 a.m. ACTH levels (between 100–200 pg/dL). The high-dose dexamethasone suppression test is also used. Patients with pituitary Cushing's disease show more than 50% suppression of cortisol release after receiving an 8 mg dose of dexamethasone, but patients with adrenal tumors or ACTH-producing tumors do not.

23. Which is the most widely used screening test for Cushing's syndrome?
- **A.** Overnight dexamethasone suppression test
- **B.** Corticotropin-releasing hormone stimulation test
- **C.** Petrosal sinus sampling
- **D.** Metyrapone stimulation test

Chemistry/Select course of action/Adrenal/2

24. Which test is the most specific for establishing a diagnosis of Cushing's disease (pituitary Cushing's)?
- **A.** Low-dose dexamethasone suppression
- **B.** High-dose dexamethasone suppression
- **C.** Twenty-four-hour urinary free cortisol
- **D.** Petrosal sinus sampling following corticotropin-releasing hormone stimulation

Chemistry/Correlate clinical and laboratory data/ Adrenal/2

25. Which statement about the diagnosis of Addison's disease is true?
- **A.** Patients with primary Addison's disease show a normal response to ACTH stimulation
- **B.** Primary and secondary Addison's disease can often be differentiated by plasma ACTH
- **C.** Twenty-four-hour urinary free cortisol testing is normal in Addison's disease
- **D.** Pituitary ACTH reserves are normal in secondary Addison's disease

Chemistry/Correlate clinical and laboratory data/ Adrenal/2

26. Which of the statements below regarding the catecholamines is true?
- **A.** They are derived from tryptophan
- **B.** They are produced by the zona glomerulosa of the adrenal cortex
- **C.** Plasma levels show both diurnal and pulsed variation
- **D.** They are excreted in urine primarily as free catecholamines

Chemistry/Apply knowledge of fundamental biological characteristics/Catecholamines/2

Answers to Questions 23–26

23. A Dexamethasone is a synthetic corticosteroid that exhibits 30-fold greater negative feedback on the hypothalamus than cortisol. When an oral dose of 1 mg of the drug is given to a patient at 11 p.m., the 8 a.m. serum total cortisol level should be below 5.0 μg/dL. Patients with Cushing's syndrome almost always exceed this cutoff. Therefore, a normal response to dexamethasone excludes Cushing's syndrome with a sensitivity of about 98%. CRH stimulation and petrosal sinus sampling are confirmatory tests for Cushing's syndrome and are used when the dexamethasone suppression test is inconclusive. The metyrapone stimulation test measures the patient's ACTH reserve. Metyrapone blocks cortisol formation by inhibiting 11-β-hydroxylase. This causes an increase in ACTH output in normal patients. A subnormal ACTH response is seen in persons with Addison's disease caused by pituitary failure.

24. D Although dexamethasone suppression tests have a high sensitivity, some patients without Cushing's syndrome have indeterminate results (e.g., values between 5 and 10 μg/dL) or abnormal results owing to medications or other conditions. When corticotropin-releasing hormone is given intravenously, patients with pituitary Cushing's have an exaggerated ACTH response. Samples are drawn from the sinuses draining the pituitary gland and from the peripheral blood. In patients with pituitary tumors, the ACTH is several times higher in the sinus samples than in the peripheral blood samples.

25. B ACTH (Cortrosyn) stimulation is used as a screening test for Addison's disease. A 250-μg dose of Cortrosyn is given intravenously. Normal patients show a two to five times increase in serum cortisol levels. A subnormal response occurs in both primary and secondary Addison's disease. Plasma ACTH is high in primary but is low in secondary Addison's disease. Patients with secondary Addison's (pituitary failure) do not respond to metyrapone because the ACTH reserve is diminished.

26. C Catecholamines, epinephrine, and norepinephrine and dopamine are produced from the amino acid tyrosine by the chromaffin cells of the adrenal medulla. Plasma and urinary catecholamines are measured in order to diagnose pheochromocytoma. Symptoms include hypertension, headache, sweating, and other endocrine involvement. Plasma catecholamines are oxidized rapidly to metanephrines and VMA; only about 2% is excreted as free catecholamines. The zona glomerulosa is the outermost portion of the adrenal cortex where aldosterone is mainly produced.

27. Which assay using 24-hour urine is considered the best single screening test for pheochromocytoma?
  A. Total urinary catecholamines
  B. VMA
  C. Homovanillic acid (HVA)
  D. Metanephrines

Chemistry/Correlate clinical and laboratory data/ Catecholamines/2

28. Which metabolite is most often increased in carcinoid tumors of the intestine?
  A. 5-Hydroxyindolacetic acid (5-HIAA)
  B. 3-Methoxy-4-hydroxyphenylglycol (MHPG)
  C. 3-Methoxydopamine
  D. HVA

Chemistry/Correlate clinical and laboratory data/ Endocrine/1

29. Which statement regarding the measurement of urinary catecholamines is true?
  A. An increased excretion of total urinary catecholamines is specific for pheochromocytoma
  B. Twenty-four-hour urinary catecholamine assay avoids pulse variations associated with measurement of plasma catecholamines
  C. Total urinary catecholamine measurement provides greater specificity than measurement of urinary free catecholamines
  D. Total urinary catecholamines are not affected by exercise

Chemistry/Apply knowledge to identify sources of error/ Catecholamines/2

30. Which method used to measure catecholamines is the *LEAST* specific?
  A. Measurement of fluorescence following oxidation by potassium ferricyanide
  B. Measurement of free catecholamines by HPLC with electrochemical detection
  C. Measurement of radioactivity after conversion by catechol-*O*-methyltransferase (COMT) to tritiated metanephrines
  D. Production of N-acetylated and methylated derivatives followed by enzyme linked-immunosorbent assay

Chemistry/Apply principles of special procedures/ Catecholamines/2

Answers to Questions 27–30

27. D Catecholamines are metabolized to metanephrines and VMA. Urinary catecholamines are increased by exercise and dietary ingestion. Measurement of 24-hour urinary metanephrine is about 95% sensitive for pheochromocytoma and is the best single test. Specificity and sensitivity for detecting pheochromocytoma approach 100% when both VMA and metanephrines are measured.

28. A 5-HIAA is a product of serotonin catabolism. Excess levels are found in urine of patients with carcinoid tumors composed of argentaffin cells. Carcinoid tumors are usually found in the intestine or lung.

29. B Measurement of total urinary catecholamines is not a specific test for pheochromocytoma. Urine levels may be increased by exercise and in muscular diseases. Catecholamines in urine may also be derived from dietary sources rather than endogenous production. Most catecholamines are excreted as glucuronide, and the urinary free catecholamines increase only when there is increased secretion. Measurement of free hormone in urine is equal in clinical sensitivity and specificity to measurement of metanephrines. Twenty-four-hour urine is the sample of choice because plasma levels are subject to pulse variation and affected by the patient's psychological and metabolic condition at the time of sampling.

30. A Most laboratories measuring catecholamines use HPLC with electrochemical detection (ECD) because the trihydroxyindol reaction is not specific. HPLC-ECD separates catecholamines by reverse phase chromatography, then detects them by oxidizing the aromatic ring at +0.8 V to a quinone ring. Current is proportional to epinephrine and norepinephrine concentration. Fluorescent methods employing ferricyanide (trihydroxyindole method) or ethylenediamine (EDA method) show interference by methyldopa (Aldomet) and several other drugs. The radioenzymatic assay of catecholamines is a specific alternative to HPLC but requires a liquid scintillation counter. The method uses the enzyme COMT to transfer a tritiated methyl group from S-adenosyl methionine to the catecholamines. This results in the formation of radiolabeled metanephrines that are measured.

31. Which statement about sample collection for catecholamines and metabolites is true?
- **A.** Blood for catecholamines is collected in the usual manner following a 12-hour fast
- **B.** Twenty-four-hour urine samples for vanillylmandelic acid, catecholamines, or metanephrines are collected in 1 mL of boric acid
- **C.** Twenty-four hour urine creatinine should be measured with vanillylmandelic acid, homovanillic acid, or metanephrines
- **D.** There is no need to discontinue medications if a 24-hour-urine collection is used

Chemistry/Apply principles of special procedures/ Specimen collection and handling/2

32. Which statement below applies to both measurement of VMA and metanephrines in urine?
- **A.** Both can be oxidized to vanillin and measured at 360 nm without interference from dietary compounds
- **B.** Both can be measured immunochemically after hydrolysis and derivitization
- **C.** Both require acid hydrolysis prior to measurement
- **D.** Both can be measured by specific HPLC and GC-MS assays

Chemistry/Apply principles of special procedures/ Catecholamines/2

33. Urinary HVA is most often assayed to detect:
- **A.** Pheochromocytoma
- **B.** Neuroblastoma
- **C.** Adrenal medullary carcinoma
- **D.** Psychiatric disorders such as manic depressive

Chemistry/Correlate laboratory and clinical data/ Catecholamines/1

Answers to Questions 31–33

31. C Stress, exercise, and an upright position induce catecholamine elevation, and therefore patients must be resting supine for at least 30 minutes prior to blood collection. The preferred method of collection is catheterization, which eliminates the anxiety of venipuncture. A 4-hour fast is also recommended. Many drugs contain epinephrine, which may falsely elevate catecholamine measurements. In addition, many drugs inhibit monoamine oxidase, which is needed to convert metanephrines to VMA. Therefore, medications should be stopped prior to testing whenever possible. Twenty-four-hour urine samples are preserved with 10 mL of 6N HCl because catecholamines and their metabolites are rapidly oxidized when pH is higher than 2. Renal clearance affects excretion of catecholamine metabolites; it is preferable to report VMA, HVA, and metanephrines in μg/mg creatinine. The urinary creatinine measurement should be at least 0.8 g/day, to validate the completeness of the 24-hour urine sample.

32. D VMA and metanephrines can both be measured as vanillin after oxidation with periodate. However, these methods are affected by dietary sources of vanillin; coffee, chocolate, bananas, and vanilla must be excluded from the diet. For this reason, VMA is commonly measured by extraction with ethyl acetate and absorption onto a silica gel column that is washed with a 1:1 mixture of ethanol: ethyl acetate to remove interfering substances. The VMA is eluted with H_2O and reacted with a diazo reagent to produce a purple color. Metanephrines may be measured by competitive enzyme-linked immunosorbent assay (ELISA) after hydrolysis and conversion to an *N*-acylmetanephrine, which is immunoreactive. Metanephrines can be measured by HPLC using a fluorescence detector, and VMA (and HVA) can be measured by HPLC using an electrochemical detector. Both VMA and metanephrines can be measured by GC-MS.

33. B HVA is the major metabolite of dopa, and urinary HVA is elevated in more than 75% of neuroblastoma patients. MHPG is the major metabolite of norepinephrine in the central nervous system. Urinary levels of MHPG have been shown to correlate with manic-depressive status, being low in depression and elevated during the manic phase.

34. Thyroid hormones are derived from the amino acid:
  A. Phenylalanine
  B. Methionine
  C. Tyrosine
  D. Histidine

Chemistry/Apply knowledge of fundamental biological characteristics/Thyroid/1

35. Which statement regarding thyroid hormones is true?
  A. Circulating levels of T_3 and T_4 are about equal
  B. T_3 is about tenfold more active than T_4
  C. The rates of formation of monoiodotyrosine and diiodotyrosine are about equal
  D. Most of the T_3 present in plasma is from its direct release from thyroid storage sites

Chemistry/Apply knowledge of fundamental biological characteristics/Thyroid/2

36. Which of the statements below regarding thyroid hormones is true?
  A. Both protein-bound and free T_3 and T_4 are physiologically active
  B. Total T_3 and T_4 are influenced by the level of thyroxine-binding globulin
  C. Variation in thyroxine-binding protein levels affects both free T_3 and T_4
  D. An elevated serum total T_4 and T_3 is diagnostic of hyperthyroidism

Chemistry/Apply knowledge of fundamental biological characteristics/Thyroid/2

37. Which of the following conditions increases total T_4 by increasing thyroxine binding globulin (TBG) ?
  A. Acute illness
  B. Anabolic steroid use
  C. Nephrotic syndrome
  D. Pregnancy or estrogens

Chemistry/Correlate clinical and laboratory data/ Thyroid/2

38. Select the most appropriate single screening test for thyroid disease.
  A. Free thyroxine index
  B. Total T_3 assay
  C. Total T_4
  D. TSH assay

Chemistry/Correlate clinical and laboratory data/ Thyroid/2

39. The serum TSH level is decreased in:
  A. Primary hyperthyrodism
  B. Primary hypothyroidism
  C. Secondary hyperthyroidism
  D. Euthyroid sick syndrome

Chemistry/Correlate clinical and laboratory data/ Thyroid/1

34. C Thyroid hormones are derived from the enzymatic modification of tyrosine residues on thyroglobulin. Tyrosine is halogenated enzymatically with iodine, forming monoiodotyrosine (MIT) and diiodotyrosine (DIT). Enzymatic coupling of these residues form T_3 (3,5,3′-triiodothyronine) and T_4 (3,5,3′,5′-tetraiodothyronine). These are hydrolyzed from thyroglobulin, forming active hormones.

35. B The rate of DIT synthesis is twice that of MIT, and the rate of coupling favors formation of T_4. Levels of T_4 are about 50 times those of T_3, but T_3 is approximately 10 times more active physiologically. Eighty percent of circulating T_3 is derived from enzymatic conversion of T_4 by T_4 5′-deiodinase.

36. B Total serum T_4 and T_3 are dependent on both thyroid function and the amount of thyroxine-binding proteins such as thyroxine-binding globulin (TBG). Total T_4 or T_3 may be abnormal in a patient with normal thyroid function if the TBG level is abnormal. For this reason, free T_3 and T_4 are more specific indicators of thyroid function than are measurements of total hormone. Only free hormone is physiologically active.

37. D Pregnancy and estrogens are the most common causes of increased TBG. Other causes include hepatitis, morphine, and clofibrate therapy. Acute illness, anabolic steroids, and nephrotic syndrome decrease the level of TBG. Normal pregnancy causes an elevated serum total T_4 but does not affect free T_4 or thyroid status.

38. D TSH is produced by the anterior pituitary gland in response to low levels of free T_4 or T_3. A normal TSH rules out thyroid disease. TSH is low in primary hyperthyroidism and high in primary hypothyroidism.

39. A Low TSH and a high T_3 (and usually T_4) occur in primary hyperthyroidism. A high TSH and low T_4 occur in primary hypothyroidism but can also occur in an acutely ill patient without thyroid disease, called the euthyroid sick syndrome. Secondary hyperthyroidism is caused by pituitary hyperfunction resulting in increased serum TSH levels.

40. Which assay is the most specific and sensitive test for diagnosing thyroid disease?

A. Free T_3 assay

B. Free thyroxine index

C. Thyrotropin-releasing hormone (TRH) stimulation test

D. TBG assay

Chemistry/Correlate clinical and laboratory data/ Thyroid/2

41. Which of the following statements is true regarding reverse T_3 (rT_3)?

A. Formed in the blood by degradation of T_4

B. Physiologically active, but less than T_3

C. Decreased in euthyroid sick syndrome

D. Interferes with the measurement of serum T_3

Chemistry/Apply knowledge of fundamental biological characteristics/Thyroid/2

42. A patient has an elevated serum T_3 and free T_4 and a very low serum TSH. What is the most likely cause of these results?

A. Primary hyperthyroidism

B. Secondary hyperthyroidism

C. Euthyroid with increased thyroxine-binding proteins

D. Euthyroid sick syndrome

Chemistry/Correlate clinical and laboratory data/ Thyroid/3

43. A serum thyroid panel reveals an increase in total T_4, normal TSH, and normal free T_4. What is the most likely cause of these results?

A. Primary hyperthyroidism

B. Secondary hyperthyroidism

C. Euthyroid with increased thyroxine-binding protein

D. Subclinical hypothyroidisim

Chemistry/Correlate clinical and laboratory data/ Thyroid/3

Answers to Questions 40–43

40. **C** The TRH stimulation test is used to confirm borderline cases of abnormal thyroid function. In normal patients, intravenous injection of 500 μg of TRH causes a peak TSH response within 30 min. In patients with primary hypothyroidism, there is an exaggerated response (>30 U/L). Patients with hyperthyroidism do not show the expected rise in TSH after TRH stimulation.

41. **A** Reverse T_3 is formed from the deiodination of T_4 in the blood. It is an inactive isomer of T_3, (3,3′,5′-triiodothyronine). Reverse T_3 is increased in acute and chronic illness and is used to identify patients with euthyroid sick syndrome.

42. **A** A very low TSH is almost always caused by either primary hyperthyroidism (suppression via high free thyroid hormone) or secondary hypothyroidism (decreased pituitary function). In rare cases, it can be induced by medications. In this patient, high levels of T_3 and free T_4 are causing the low TSH, indicating primary hyperthyroidism. In secondary hyperthyroidism the TSH is elevated in addition to at least the T_3. Patients with an increased thyroxine-binding protein level have an increase in T_3 but not free T_4 or TSH and also have an increased unsaturated thyroxine–binding globulin (UTBG). Patients with euthyroid sick syndrome usually have a low T_3 or T_4 but a normal or slightly elevated TSH.

43. **C** Patients with a normal TSH are euthyroid, and most commonly an increase in total T_4 in these patients is caused by an increase in TBG. An increase in TBG causes an increase in total T_4 but not free T_4. Subclinical hypothyroidism is usually associated with a high TSH level but normal free T_3 and T_4 levels. When TSH is indeterminate, the diagnosis is made by demonstrating an exaggerated response to the TRH stimulation test.

44. Which statement about TSH and T_4 in early pregnancy is correct?

   A. TSH and thyroid hormone levels fall

   B. TSH falls and thyroid hormone levels rise

   C. TSH and thyroid hormone levels both rise

   D. TSH rises and thyroid hormone levels fall

*Chemistry/Correlate clinical and laboratory data/
Thyroid/3*

45. In which case might a very low plasma TSH result *not* correlate with thyroid status?

   A. Euthyroid sick syndrome

   B. Congenital hypothyroidism

   C. When TBG is elevated

   D. After high-dose corticosteroid treatment

*Chemistry/Correlate clinical and laboratory data/
Thyroid/3*

44. **B** Estrogens released in pregnancy cause an increase in TBG, which in turn produces an increase in total T_4 and T_3. In early pregnancy, the hCG produced by the placenta stimulates the thyroid, causing further production of thyroid hormones. This suppresses TSH production. In the second trimester, as hCG diminishes, free T_4 levels fall and may be lower than 0.8 ng/dL, the lower limit of the adult reference range as a result of expansion of the blood volume. Therefore, both TSH and free T_4 should be evaluated during pregnancy using trimester-specific reference ranges. In early pregnancy, a TSH above the first-trimester reference range should be followed up by free T_4 testing and thyroid peroxidase antibody levels to assess the need for thyroid treatment.

45. **D** In those with severe chronic diseases or who have hCG secreting tumors, TSH production may be suppressed. Some drugs, especially high doses of corticosteroids, suppress TSH production. Low TSH levels not matching thyroid status can also be seen in patients who have recently been treated for hyperthyroidism because there is a delay in the pituitary response. High-sensitivity TSH assays that can measure as little as 0.01 mIU/L and free T_4 and T_3 can help differentiate these conditions from clinical hyperthyroidism. If the TSH is below .05 mIU/L and the free hormone levels are increased, this points to hyperthyroidism. Laboratory values in euthyroid sick syndrome may mimic mild hypothyroidism. In euthyroid sick syndrome, thyroid function is normal but TSH is slightly increased owing to lower levels of free T_4.

TOXICOLOGY AND THERAPEUTIC DRUG MONITORING

1. **In which of the cases below is qualitative analysis of the drug usually adequate?**
   A. To determine whether the dose of a drug with a low therapeutic index is likely to be toxic
   B. To determine whether a patient is complying with the physician's instructions
   C. To adjust dose if individual differences or disease alter expected response
   D. To determine whether the patient has been taking amphetamines

   Chemistry/Apply knowledge of fundamental biological characteristics/Therapeutic drug monitoring/1

2. **The term pharmacokinetics refers to the:**
   A. Relationship between drug dose and the drug blood level
   B. Concentration of drug at its sites of action
   C. Relationship between blood concentration and therapeutic response
   D. The relationship between blood and tissue drug levels

   Chemistry/Apply knowledge of fundamental biological characteristics/1

3. **The term pharmacodynamics is an expression of the relationship between:**
   A. Dose and physiological effect
   B. Drug concentration at target sites and physiological effect
   C. Time and serum drug concentration
   D. Blood and tissue drug levels

   Chemistry/Apply knowledge of fundamental biological characteristics/Therapeutic drug monitoring/1

Answers to Questions 1–3

1. **D** The purpose of therapeutic drug monitoring is to achieve a therapeutic blood drug level rapidly and minimize the risk of drug toxicity caused by overdose. Therapeutic drug monitoring is a quantitative procedure performed for drugs with a narrow therapeutic index (ratio of the concentration producing the desired effect to the concentration producing toxicity). Drug groups that require monitoring because of high risk of toxicity include aminoglycoside antibiotics, anticonvulsants, antiarrhythmics, antiasthmatics, and psychoactive drugs. When testing for abuse substances the goal is usually to determine whether the drug is present or absent. The most common approach is to compare the result to a cutoff determined by measuring a standard containing the lowest level of drug that is considered significant.

2. **A** Pharmacokinetics is the mathematical expression of the relationship between drug dose and drug blood level. When the appropriate formula is applied to quantitative measures of drug dose, absorption, distribution, and elimination, the blood concentration can be accurately determined.

3. **B** Pharmacodynamics is the relationship between the drug concentration at the receptor site (tissue concentration) and the response of the tissue to that drug, e.g., the relationship between lidocaine concentration in the heart muscle and the duration of the action potential of Purkinje fibers.

4. The study of pharmacogenomics involves which type of testing?
  A. Family studies to determine the inheritance of drug resistance
  B. Testing drugs with cell cultures to determine the minimum toxic dosage
  C. Testing for single nucleotide polymorphisms known to affect drug metabolism
  D. Comparison of dose response curves among family members

Chemistry/Apply knowledge of fundamental biological characteristics/Therapeutic drug monitoring/1

5. Select the five pharmacological parameters that determine serum drug concentration.
  A. Absorption, anabolism, perfusion, bioactivation, excretion
  B. Liberation, equilibration, biotransformation, reabsorption, elimination
  C. Liberation, absorption, distribution, metabolism, excretion
  D. Ingestion, conjugation, integration, metabolism, elimination

Chemistry/Apply knowledge of fundamental biological characteristics/Therapeutic drug monitoring/1

6. Which route of administration is associated with 100% bioavailability?
  A. Sublingual
  B. Intramuscular
  C. Oral
  D. Intravenous

Chemistry/Apply knowledge of fundamental biological characteristics/Therapeutic drug monitoring/2

7. The phrase first-pass hepatic metabolism means that:
  A. 100% of a drug is excreted by the liver
  B. All drug is inactivated by hepatic enzymes after one pass through the liver
  C. Some drug is metabolized from the portal circulation, reducing bioavailability
  D. The drug must be metabolized in the liver to an active form

Chemistry/Apply knowledge of fundamental biological characteristics/Therapeutic drug monitoring/2

8. Which formula can be used to estimate dosage needed to give a desired steady-state blood level?
  A. Dose per hour = clearance (milligrams per hour) ×average concentration at steady state ÷ f
  B. Dose per day = fraction absorbed – fraction excreted
  C. Dose = fraction absorbed×(1/protein-bound fraction)
  D. Dose per day = half-life×log V_d (volume distribution)

Chemistry/Calculate/Therapeutic drug monitoring/2

Answers to Questions 4–8

4. **C** Pharmacogenomics refers to the study of genes that affect the performance of a drug in an individual. One method is to test for single nucleotide polymorphisms (SNPs) using DNA microarrays in genes such as those that code for the cytochrome P450 enzymes involved in the metabolism of many drugs. Genetic variations of one such enzyme may account for individual pharmacokinetic differences and can be used to predict the efficacy of the drug.

5. **C** *Liberation* is the release of the drug and *absorption* is the transport of drug from the site of administration to the blood. The percentage of drug absorption and the rate of absorption determine the bioavailable fraction, *f.* This is the fraction of the dose that reaches the blood. *Distribution* refers to the delivery of the drug to the tissues. It involves dilution and equilibration of the drug in various fluid compartments, including the blood, and is influenced by binding to proteins and blood cells. *Metabolism* is the process of chemical modification of the drug by cells. This results in production of metabolites with altered activity and solubility. *Excretion* is the process by which the drug and its metabolites are removed from the body.

6. **D** When a drug is administered intravenously, all the drug enters the bloodstream and therefore the bioavailable fraction is 1.0. All other routes of administration require absorption through cells, and this process reduces the bioavailable fraction. The bioavailable fraction for a drug given orally can be calculated by dividing the peak blood concentration after oral administration by the peak drug concentration after intravenous administration. A value of 0.7 or higher is desired for drugs given orally.

7. **C** Drugs given orally enter the blood via the portal circulation and are transported directly to the liver. Some drugs are excreted by the liver, and a fraction is lost by hepatic excretion before the drug reaches the general circulation. An example is propranolol, a β-blocker that reduces heart rate and hypertension. The bioavailable fraction is 0.2–0.4 when given orally because much of the drug is removed by first-pass hepatic metabolism.

8. **A** After a patient receives a loading dose to rapidly bring the drug level up to the desired therapeutic range, a maintenance dose must be given at consistent intervals to maintain the blood drug level at the desired concentration. The dose per hour is determined by multiplying the clearance per hour by the desired average steady-state concentration, then dividing by *f* (bioavailable fraction).

9. **Which statement is true regarding the V_d of a drug?**
   A. V_d is equal to the peak blood concentration divided by the dose given
   B. V_d is the theoretical volume in liters into which the drug distributes
   C. The higher the V_d, the lower the dose needed to reach the desired blood level of drug
   D. The V_d is the principal determinant of the dosing interval

   Chemistry/Apply knowledge of fundamental biological characteristics/Therapeutic drug monitoring/2

10. **For drugs with first-order elimination, which statement about drug clearance is true?**
    A. Clearance = elimination rate ÷ serum level
    B. It is most often performed by the liver
    C. It is directly related to half-life
    D. Clearance rate is independent of dose

    Chemistry/Apply knowledge of fundamental biological characteristics/Therapeutic drug monitoring/2

11. **Which statement about steady-state drug levels is true?**
    A. The absorbed drug must be greater than the amount excreted
    B. Steady state can be measured after two elimination half-lives
    C. Constant intravenous infusion gives the same minimums and maximums as an oral dose
    D. Oral dosing intervals result in peaks and troughs in the dose-response curve

    Chemistry/Apply knowledge of fundamental biological characteristics/Therapeutic drug monitoring/2

12. **If too small a peak-trough difference is seen for a drug given orally then:**
    A. The dose should be decreased
    B. Time between doses should be decreased
    C. Dose interval should be increased
    D. Dose per day and time between doses should be decreased

    Chemistry/Select course of action/Therapeutic drug monitoring/3

13. **If the peak level is appropriate but the trough level is too low at steady state, then the dose interval should:**
    A. Be lengthened without changing the dose per day
    B. Be lengthened and the dose rate decreased
    C. Not be changed but the dose per day increased
    D. Be shortened, but the dose per day not changed

    Chemistry/Select source of action/Therapeutic drug monitoring/3

9. **B** The V_d of a drug represents the dilution of the drug after it has been distributed in the body. The V_d is used to estimate the peak drug blood level expected after a loading dose is given. The peak blood level equals the dose multiplied by $f \div V_d$. The V_d can be calculated by dividing the dose, X_o, by the initial plasma drug concentration, C_o, ($V_d = X_o/C_o$) or by dividing the clearance rate by K, the elimination rate constant ($K = 0.693$ divided by drug half-life). The greater the V_d, the higher the dose that will be needed to achieve the desired blood concentration of drug. The V_d is the principal determinant of the dose, and the clearance rate is the principal determinant of the dosing interval.

10. **A** First-order elimination represents a linear relationship between the amount of drug eliminated per hour and the blood level of drug. For drugs following linear kinetics, clearance equals the elimination rate divided by the drug concentration in blood. When clearance (in milligrams per hour) and f are known, the dose per hour needed to give a desired average drug level at steady state can be calculated. Clearance is inversely related to the drug's half-life and is accomplished mainly by the kidneys.

11. **D** When drugs are infused intravenously, both the distribution and elimination rates are constant. This eliminates the peaks and troughs seen in the dose-response curve. Peak and trough levels are characteristics of intermittent dosing regimens. The steady state is reached when drug in the next dose is sufficient only to replace the drug eliminated since the last dose. Steady state can be measured after five drug half-lives because blood levels will have reached 97% of steady state.

12. **C** Increasing the dosing interval will reduce the trough concentration of the drug, and increasing the dose will increase the peak concentration of the drug, resulting in a greater peak-trough difference. The peak-trough ratio is usually adjusted to 2, with dose interval set to equal the drug half-life. Under these conditions both peak and trough levels often fall within the therapeutic range.

13. **D** Increasing the dose rate may result in peak drug levels in the toxic range. Decreasing the dosing interval raises the trough level so that it is maintained in the therapeutic range. The trough level is affected by the drug clearance rate. If clearance increases, then trough level decreases.

14. If the steady-state drug level is too high, the best course of action is to:
  A. Decrease the dose
  B. Decrease the dose interval
  C. Decrease the dose and decrease the dose interval
  D. Change the route of administration

Chemistry/Select course of action/Therapeutic drug monitoring/3

15. When should blood samples for trough drug levels be collected?
  A. 30 minutes after peak levels
  B. 45 minutes before the next dose
  C. 1–2 hours after the last dose
  D. Immediately before the next dose is given

Chemistry/Apply knowledge to recognize sources of error/ Sample collection and handling/1

16. Blood sample collection time for peak drug levels:
  A. Varies with the drug, depending on its rate of absorption
  B. Is independent of drug formulation
  C. Is independent of the route of administration
  D. Is 30 minutes after a bolus intravenous injection is completed

Chemistry/Apply knowledge to recognize sources of error/ Sample collection and handling/2

17. Which could account for drug toxicity following a normally prescribed dose?
  A. Decreased renal clearance caused by kidney disease
  B. Discontinuance of another drug
  C. Altered serum protein binding caused by disease
  D. All of the above

Chemistry/Apply knowledge of fundamental biological characteristics/Therapeutic drug monitoring/2

18. Select the elimination model that best describes most oral drugs.
  A. One compartment, linear first-order elimination
  B. Michaelis-Menten or concentration-dependent elimination
  C. Two compartments with a biphasic elimination curve
  D. Logarithmic elimination

Chemistry/Apply knowledge of fundamental biological characteristics/Therapeutic drug monitoring/2

19. Drugs rapidly infused intravenously usually follow which elimination model?
  A. One compartment, first order
  B. One compartment, logarithmic
  C. Biphasic or two compartment with serum level rapidly falling in the first phase
  D. Michaelis-Menten or concentration-dependent elimination

Chemistry/Apply knowledge of fundamental biological characteristics/Therapeutic drug monitoring/2

Answers to Questions 14–19

14. **A** Decreasing both dose and dosing interval has offsetting effects on peak and trough blood levels. The appropriate dose can be calculated if the clearance or V_d and f are known. For example, the initial dose is calculated by multiplying the desired peak blood drug concentration by the V_d.

15. **D** The trough concentration of a drug is the lowest concentration obtained in the dosing interval. This occurs immediately before the absorption of the next dose given. Trough levels are usually collected just before the next dose is given.

16. **A** The peak concentration of a drug is the highest concentration obtained in the dosing interval. For oral drugs the time of peak concentration is dependent on their rates of absorption and elimination and is determined by serial blood measurements. Peak levels for oral drugs are usually drawn 1–2 hours after administration of the dose. For drugs given intravenously, peak levels are measured immediately after the infusion is completed.

17. **D** Therapeutic drug monitoring is necessary for drugs that have a narrow therapeutic index. Individual differences alter pharmacokinetics, causing lack of correlation between dose and drug blood level. These include age, diet, ingestion with or without food, genetic factors, exercise, smoking, pregnancy, metabolism of other drugs, protein binding, and disease states.

18. **A** Most drugs given orally distribute uniformly through the tissues reaching rapid equilibrium, so both blood and tissues can be viewed as a single compartment. Elimination according to Michaelis-Menten kinetics is nonlinear because at high concentrations, the hepatic enzyme system becomes saturated, reducing the elimination efficiency.

19. **C** Drugs rapidly infused intravenously follow a two-compartment model of elimination. The central compartment is the blood and tissues that are well perfused. The second consists of tissues for which distribution of drug is time-dependent. In determining the loading dose the desired serum concentration should be multiplied by the volume of the central compartment to avoid toxic levels.

20. Which fact must be considered when evaluating a patient who displays signs of drug toxicity?
  A. Drug metabolites (e.g., *N*-acetylprocainamide) may need to be measured as well as the parent drug
  B. If the concentration of total drug is within therapeutic limits, the concentration of free drug cannot be toxic
  C. If the drug has a wide therapeutic index, then it will not be toxic
  D. A drug level cannot be toxic if the trough is within the published therapeutic range

Chemistry/Apply knowledge of fundamental biological characteristics/Therapeutic drug monitoring/2

21. When a therapeutic drug is suspected of causing toxicity, which specimen is the most appropriate for an initial investigation?
  A. Trough blood sample
  B. Peak blood sample
  C. Urine at the time of symptoms
  D. Gastric fluid at the time of symptoms

Chemistry/Select course of action/Therapeutic drug monitoring/3

22. For a drug that follows first-order pharmacokinetics, adjustment of dosage to achieve the desired blood level can be made using which formula?
  A. New dose = $\dfrac{\text{current dose}}{\text{concentration at steady state}} \times \text{desired concentration}$
  B. New dose = $\dfrac{\text{current dose}}{\text{desired concentration}} \times \text{concentration at steady state}$
  C. New dose = $\dfrac{\text{concentration at steady state}}{\text{desired concentration}} \times \text{half-life}$
  D. New dose = $\dfrac{\text{concentration at steady state}}{\text{current dose}} \times \text{desired concentration}$

Chemistry/Apply knowledge of fundamental biological characteristics/Therapeutic drug monitoring/2

23. For which drug group are both peak and trough measurements usually required?
  A. Antiarrhythmics
  B. Analgesics
  C. Tricyclic antidepressants
  D. Aminoglycoside antibiotics

Chemistry/Select course of action/Therapeutic drug monitoring/2

Answers to Questions 20–23

20. **A** Altered drug pharmacokinetics may result in toxicity even when the dose of drug is within the accepted therapeutic range. Two common causes of this are the presence of unmeasured metabolites that are physiologically active and the presence of a higher than expected concentration of free drug. Because only free drug is physiologically active, decreased binding protein or factors that shift the equilibrium favoring more unbound drug can result in toxicity when the total drug concentration is within the therapeutic range. Some drugs with a wide therapeutic index are potentially toxic because they may be ingested in great excess with little or no initial toxicity. For example, acetaminophen overdose does not usually become apparent until 3–5 days after the overdose. This creates the potential for hepatic damage to occur from continued use because the drug half-life is extended, especially in patients who have decreased hepatic or renal function.

21. **B** When a drug is suspected of toxicity, the peak blood sample (sample after absorption and distribution are complete) should be obtained because it is most likely to exceed the therapeutic limit. If the peak level is above the upper therapeutic limit, then toxicity is confirmed, and the drug dose is lowered. If the peak drug concentration is within the therapeutic range, toxicity is less likely but cannot be ruled out. A high concentration of free drug, the presence of active metabolites, and abnormal response to the drug are causes of drug toxicity that may occur when the blood drug level is within the published therapeutic range.

22. **A** Most drugs follow first-order pharmacokinetics, meaning the clearance of drug is linearly related to the drug dose. The dose of such drugs can be adjusted by multiplying the ratio of the current dose to blood concentration by the desired drug concentration provided the blood concentration is measured at steady state.

23. **D** Aminoglycoside antibiotics cause damage to the eighth cranial nerve at toxic levels, resulting in hearing loss. When given at subtherapeutic doses, they fail to resolve infection. Most drugs falling in the other classes have a narrow peak-trough difference but are highly toxic when blood levels exceed the therapeutic range. Usually, these can be safely monitored by measuring trough levels.

24. Which of the following statements about TLC for drug screening is true?
   A. Acidic drugs are extracted in an alkaline nonpolar solvent
   B. A drug is identified by comparing its R_f value and staining to standards
   C. Testing must be performed using a urine sample
   D. Opiates and other alkaloids are extracted at an acid pH

Chemistry/Apply principles of special procedures/ Chromatography/2

25. The EMIT for drugs of abuse uses an:
   A. Antibody conjugated to a drug
   B. Enzyme conjugated to an antibody
   C. Enzyme conjugated to a drug
   D. Antibody bound to a solid phase

Chemistry/Apply principles of special procedures/ Biochemical theory and principle/2

26. Which statement about EMIT is true?
   A. Enzyme activity is inversely proportional to drug level
   B. Formation of NADH is monitored at 340 nm
   C. ALP is the commonly used conjugate
   D. Assay use is restricted to serum

Chemistry/Apply principles of special procedures/ Biochemical theory and principle/2

27. Which statement below regarding FPIA is true?
   A. Plane-polarized fluorescence is directly related to the drug level
   B. β-Galactosidase is commonly used to label the antigen
   C. Separation of free and bound labeled antigen is not required
   D. Assays are based upon the double antibody sandwich method

Chemistry/Apply principles of special procedures/ Biochemical theory and principle/2

Answers to Questions 24–27

24. **B** TLC can be performed on urine, serum, or gastric fluid and qualitatively identifies most drugs. Each has a characteristic R_f, which is the ratio of the distance migrated by the drug to the solvent. The R_f of the sample must match the R_f of the drug standard. Extraction of drugs for TLC is highly pH-dependent. The pH must be adjusted to reduce the solubility (ionization) of the drug in the aqueous phase. Alkaline drugs (e.g., opiates) are extracted at pH 9.0 and acidic drugs (e.g., barbiturates) at pH 4.5.

25. **C** In EMIT, enzyme-labeled drug competes with drug in the sample for a limited amount of reagent antibodies. When antibody binds to the enzyme-drug conjugate, it blocks the catalytic site of the enzyme. Enzyme activity is directly proportional to sample drug concentration because the quantity of unbound drug-enzyme conjugate is highest when drug is present in the sample.

26. **B** EMIT is a homogeneous immunoassay, meaning that free antigen does not have to be separated from bound antigen. Most EMIT assays use a two-reagent system. Reagent A contains substrate (usually glucose-6-PO_4), coenzyme (NAD^+), and antibody to the drug. Reagent B contains enzyme-labeled drug (usually G6PD-drug) and buffer. The rate of NADH production is proportional to the drug concentration. EMIT assays are commonly used to test for drugs of abuse in urine. In such cases, the enzyme activity of the low calibrator (drug concentration equal to U.S. Substance Abuse and Mental Health Services Administration minimum for a positive test) is used as the cutoff.

27. **C** Fluorescein-labeled drug, serum, and antibody are mixed and placed in the light path of a fluorometer. When drug-fluorescein conjugate is bound by antibody, its rotation slows, causing plane polarized fluorescence. Unbound conjugate emits unpolarized green light, which is not detected. Antibody-bound conjugate (polarized fluorescence) is inversely related to serum drug concentration.

28. Quantitation of a drug by gas chromatography-mass spectroscopy (GC-MS) is usually performed in which mode?
    A. Total ion chromatography
    B. Selective ion monitoring
    C. Ion subtraction
    D. Selective reaction monitoring

    Chemistry/Apply principles of special procedures/ Chromatography/1

29. **SITUATION:** A urine sample is received in the laboratory with the appropriate custody control form and a request for drug of abuse screening. Which test result would be a cause for rejecting the sample?
    A. Temperature after collection 95°C
    B. pH of 5.0
    C. Specific gravity of 1.005
    D. Creatinine level of 5 mg/dL

    Chemistry/Evaluate laboratory data to detect sources of error/Toxicology/3

30. Which statement about the measurement of carboxy-hemoglobin is true?
    A. Treatment with alkaline dithionite is used to convert carboxyhemoglobin to oxyhemoglobin
    B. Oxyhemoglobin has no absorbance at 540 nm but carboxyhemoblogin does
    C. Bichromatic analysis is required in order to eliminate interference by oxyhemoglobin
    D. Carboxyhemoglobin can be measured by potentiometry

    Chemistry/Apply principles of special procedures/ Carboxyhemoglobin/2

Answers to Questions 28–30

28. **B** Most GC-MS instruments use an electron beam to split the drug emerging from the column into its component ions. These are drawn into the mass analyzer, usually a vacuum chamber containing two pairs of charged rods (a positive pair and a negative pair) called a quadrupole analyzer. By changing the polarity and radio frequency applied to the rods, the travel of ions will vary, depending on their mass to charge (m/z) ratio. As ions emerge from the mass filter, they are detected by an electron multiplier tube. CG-MS instruments can be operated in two modes, total ion chromatography and selective ion monitoring. A total ion chromatograph displays the retention time of all ions detected and their abundance. It is primarily used for identification of unknown compounds. Selective ion montoring (SIM) mode measures the abundance of a few principal ions that together provide sufficient specificity to eliminate potential interfering substances and greater quantitative sensitivity. For example, tetrahydrocannabinol (THC) can be quantitated by measuring ions m/z 371.3, 372.3, and 473.3.

29. **D** Approximately five per thousand urine samples received for DAU testing have been adulterated by dilution, substitution, or addition of substances such as glutaraldehyde that interfere with testing. The majority of these situations can be detected by determining temperature (90–100° C), pH (4.5–8.0), specific gravity (1.003–1.019), and creatinine ($\geq$ 20 mg/dL). All of the values above are within the limits of an acceptable sample with the exception of creatinine. Dry reagent strips are available that test for pH, specific gravity, creatinine, nitrite, bleach, pyridinium, and glutaraldehyde.

30. **C** The absorbance of hemoglobin pigments is overlapping and bichromatic analysis is required in order to accurately measure carboxyhemoglobin. Since oxyhemoglobin has a peak absorbance at 540 nm and carboxyhemoglobin at 541 nm, oxyhemoglobin must be removed before measurement. This is accomplished by treatment of the blood with alkaline sodium dithionite to reduce the oxyhemoglobin to deoxyhemoglobin, which has a significantly lower absorbance than carboxyhemoglobin at 541 nm. The ratio of absorbance at 541:555 nm is directly proportional to carboxyhemoglobin concentration. Percent carboxyhemoglobin can also be determined from simultaneous absorbance measurements at 548, 568, and 578 nm. Gas chromatography can also be used to measure carbon monoxide in blood after it is released from hemoglobin by adding potassium ferricyanide.

31. Which of the following statements about blood alcohol measurement is correct?
    A. Symptoms of intoxication usually begin when the level exceeds 0.05% w/v
    B. The skin puncture site should be disinfected with isopropanol
    C. The reference method is based upon enzymatic oxidation of ethanol by alcohol dehydrogenase
    D. Gas chromatography methods require extraction of ethanol from serum

    Chemistry/Apply principles of special procedures/ Ethanol/2

32. Which drug can be detected with ferric chloride in perchloric-nitric acids?
    A. Phenothiazines
    B. Acetaminophen
    C. Morphine
    D. Meprobamate

    Chemistry/Apply principles of special procedures/ Toxicology/1

33. Which specimen is the sample of choice for lead screening?
    A. Whole blood
    B. Hair
    C. Serum
    D. Urine

    Chemistry/Apply principles of special procedures/Lead/1

34. Which of the following enzymes can be used to measure plasma or serum salicylate?
    A. Peroxidase
    B. Salicylate esterase
    C. Salicylate hydroxylase
    D. *p*-Aminosalicylate oxidase

    Chemistry/Apply principles of special procedures/ Toxicology/1

Answers to Questions 31–34

31. **A** Alcohol dehydrogenase is not specific for ethanol, and in vitro interference can occur with some ADH methods when skin is disinfected with other alcohols. For this reason, and to avoid interference with the interpretation of chromatograms for volatiles, blood samples are collected after disinfecting the skin site with benzalkonium chloride or other nonalcohol antiseptic. GLC is the legally accepted method of ethanol analysis. The low boiling point of ethanol permits direct analysis on blood or plasma diluted with water containing 1-propanol or other suitable internal standard.

32. **A** Ferric ions react with phenothiazine tranquilizers, forming an intense purple complex. The reaction is nonspecific but useful as a screening test. Ferric ions react with many metabolites and drugs in urine, including salicylate (purple), phenylpyruvic acid (green), and acetoacetic acid (pink). Acetaminophen in urine is detected by boiling to form *p*-amphenol. This reacts with *o*-cresol, forming indophenol blue.

33. **A** Lead accumulates in RBCs, bones, and neural tissues, and whole blood, hair, and urine are suitable for demonstrating lead toxicity. Greatest sensitivity is obtained by using whole blood, which can detect exposure over time. Because lead is rapidly eliminated from plasma, serum or plasma should not be used to test for lead exposure. Lead binds to sulfhydryl groups of proteins such as delta-aminolevulinic acid (Δ-ALA), dehydratase, and ferrochelatase and interferes with heme synthesis. This results in increased free erythrocyte protoporphyrin, erythrocyte zinc protoporphyrin, urinary coproporphyrin III, and δ-aminolevulinic acid, which are also useful markers for lead poisoning. When screening for lead poisoning in children, the method of choice is graphite furnace atomic absorption spectrophotometry. This method has a sensitivity of 1.0 μg/dL, which is required to accurately demonstrate normal levels in children. The CDC cutoff for normal lead in children is less than 10.0 μg/dL.

34. **C** Salicylate can be measured colorimetrically using an acid solution of ferric nitrate, but related drugs also react. The enzymatic assay uses salicylate hydroxylase, which reduces salicylate with NADH forming catechol and NAD$^+$. Salicylate can also be measured by HPLC and various immunoassays such as EMIT and FPIA.

35. Which of the following tests is *LEAST* essential to the operation of an emergency room at a general hospital?
A. Carboxyhemoglobin
B. Osmolality
C. Salicylate
D. Lead

Chemistry/Select tests/Toxicology/2

35. D The vast majority of acute toxicology situations seen in the Emergency Department involve poisoning with alcohol, acetaminophen, salicylate, abuse substances, or carbon monoxide. Emergency departments should offer a minimum of these tests. In the absence of specific tests for abuse substances or a comprehensive drug screen, the serum osmolality measured by freezing point depression is a sensitive surrogate test for drug and alcohol overdose. In the ED environment a difference between measured and calculated osmolality greater than 10 mOsm/kg almost always indicates drug or alcohol poisoning. Toxicity from lead poisoning and most other trace metals is usually a chronic condition that does not often require immediate access to laboratory testing.

1. Which of the following tumor markers is classified as a tumor suppressor gene?
   A. BRCA-1
   B. Carcinoembryonic antigen (CEA)
   C. Human chorionic gonadotropin (hCG)
   D. Nuclear matrix protein

   Chemistry/Apply knowledge of fundamental biological characteristics/Tumor markers/1

2. In general, in which of the following situations is the analysis of a tumor marker most useful?
   A. Testing for recurrence
   B. Prognosis
   C. Screening
   D. Diagnosis

   Chemistry/Correlate clinical and laboratory data/Tumor markers/1

3. Which of the following enzymes is increased in persons with prostate and small cell lung cancer?
   A. Creatine kinase-1 (CK-1)
   B. Gamma glutamyl transferase (GGT)
   C. Amylase
   D. Lactate dehydrogenase

   Chemistry/Correlate clinical and laboratory data/Tumor markers/2

Answers to Questions 1–3

1. **A** Tumor markers may be enzymes, hormones, receptors, oncofetal (glycoprotein) antigens, or oncogenes. BRCA-1 is located on the long arm of chromosome 17 and carries an 85% lifetime risk of breast or ovarian cancer when present. Its product functions in DNA repair and slows cell proliferation.

2. **A** Most tumor markers are expressed at very low levels so that the concentration in early malignancy overlaps that seen in normal individuals. This makes them ineffective for screening. Three exceptions are hCG in males for testicular cancer, calcitonin for thyroid medullary cancer, and prostate-specific antigen (PSA) for prostate cancer. Most tumor markers are increased in nonmalignant disease, and this nonspecificity reduces their usefulness for diagnosis of malignancy. In addition to the three markers mentioned above, the hormones insulin (insulinoma), gastrin (gastrinoma), and prolactin (prolactinoma), and the catecholamines (pheochromocytoma) have some diagnostic utility. Some tumor markers are useful predictors of disease progression and response to treatment. These include BRCA-1, estrogen and progesterone receptors, cathepsin-D, and the Philadelphia chromosome. The major use of tumor markers is to monitor recurrence and therapy. Successful treatment reduces the concentration of the marker significantly or results in an undetectable level. A rise in level following treatment signals recurrence.

3. **A** CK-1 (CK-BB) is not normally found in plasma or serum except in neonates. It may be present in persons with central nervous system damage and some other disorders but its presence is often associated with various malignancies, especially prostate cancer and small cell carcinoma of the lung. Several other commonly measured enzymes are elevated by malignancy. ALP and LD are associated with various tumors. GGT levels are very high in hepatoma, and amylase is elevated in pancreatic cancer.

4. Which of the following is the best analyte to monitor for recurrence of ovarian cancer?

A. CA-15-3

B. CA-19-9

C. CA-125

D. CEA

Chemistry/Correlate clinical and laboratory data/Tumor markers/2

5. Which tumor marker is associated with cancer of the urinary bladder?

A. CA-19-9

B. CA-72-4

C. Nuclear matrix protein

D. Cathepsin-D

Chemistry/Correlate clinical and laboratory data/Tumor markers/2

6. A person presents with a Cushingoid appearance and an elevated 24-hour urinary cortisol level. The plasma adrenocotropic hormone (ACTH) is very elevated, and the physician suspects the cause is ectopic ACTH production. Which test would be most useful in substantiating this diagnosis?

A. Plasma cortisol

B. CA-50

C. Alkaline phosphatase isoenzymes

D. AFP

Chemistry/Evaluate laboratory and clinical data to specify additional tests/Tumor markers/3

4. **C** CA-125 is an oncofetal antigen, meaning that it is produced by genes that are active during fetal development but minimally active after birth except in malignant tissues. This group includes α-fetoprotein (AFP), CEA, PSA, and the carbohydrate-associated antigens (CA). CA-15-3 (which shares the same antigenic determinant as CA-27.29) is used mainly to monitor breast cancer treatment and recurrence. CA-19-9 (which shares the same antigenic determinant as CA-50) is a glycoprotein shed from the surface of gastric, pancreatic, and colorectal cancer cells.

5. **C** Nuclear matrix proteins (NMPs) are RNA-protein complexes. NMP-22 is shed into the urine in persons with bladder carcinoma and is about 25-fold higher than normal in this condition. It has a clinical sensitivity of about 70% but is likely to be negative when the tumor is low-grade. Other markers used for detection of bladder cancer include bladder tumor associated analytes (BTAs), a variant of the complement factor H protein; cytokeratin-20, a variant cytokeratin (fibrous protein) in the cytoplasm of malignant bladder epithelium; and telomerase, an enzyme that adds nucleotides to the ends of chromosomes, preventing telomere degradation. The specificity of these tests varies from approximately 75%–80%. Bladder cancer can also be detected by FISH because it is associated with a high incidence of ploidy and other chromosomal abnormalities that can be detected by fluorescent-labeled DNA probes. FISH specificity is over 94%, and like the immunoassays its sensitivity is higher for high-grade tumors (approximately 78% for grade 2 and 94% for grade 3 cancers).

6. **C** Most often ectopic ACTH production occurs in lung cancer. Tumors of the lung are often associated with the production of placental-like alkaline phosphatase, and a positive finding would support the diagnosis of an ectopic (nonpituitary) source of ACTH. Many other tumor markers, including neuron-specific enolase and parathyroid hormone-related protein, are also increased in lung cancers. CA-50 (along with CA-19-9) shares the same antigenic determinant as Lewis A and is a marker for recurrence and treatment of gastrointestinal and pancreatic cancers. AFP is the predominant protein produced by the fetus, and plasma levels are increased primarily in the yolk sac, liver, and testicular tumors.

7. Which of the following tumor markers is used to monitor persons with breast cancer for recurrence of disease?
  A. Cathepsin-D
  B. CA-15-3
  C. Retinoblastoma gene
  D. Estrogen receptor (ER)

Chemistry/Correlate clinical and laboratory data/Tumor markers/2

8. Which of the following statements regarding the Philadelphia chromosome is true?
  A. It is seen exclusively in chronic myelogenous leukemia
  B. It results from a translocation
  C. It appears as a short arm deletion of chromosome 21
  D. It is associated with a poor prognosis

Chemistry/Apply knowledge of fundamental biological characteristics/Tumor markers/1

9. What is the primary clinical utility of measuring CEA?
  A. Diagnosis of liver cancer
  B. Diagnosis of colorectal cancer
  C. Screening for cancers of endodermal origin
  D. Monitoring for recurrence of cancer

Chemistry/Apply knowledge of fundamental biological characteristics/Tumor markers/1

Answers to Questions 7–9

7. B CA-15-3 shares the same antigenic determinant as CA-27.29. Both are present on MUC1, a mucinous protein on the cell membrane of various tissues. The markers are used to monitor treatment and recurrence of breast cancer. However, abnormal plasma levels are seen in many nonmalignant conditions, and the test is not used for diagnostic purposes. CA-125 is a glycoprotein antigen shed by approximately 75% of ovarian cancers. It is an FDA-approved tumor marker for monitoring recurrence of ovarian cancer and evaluating the effectiveness of chemotherapy. Cathepsin-D and ER assays are performed to determine the prognosis of persons with breast cancer. Overexpression of cathepsin-D is associated with a higher relapse rate. Breast tissue that is negative for ER is poorly responsive to hormone suppression (tamoxifen) therapy. The retinoblastoma gene (RB) is a tumor suppressor gene found to be missing in persons with retinoblastoma. Various mutations of the gene have been reported in breast, lung, bladder, and other cancers.

8. B The Philadelphia chromosome (Ph[1]) is formed by translocation of the long arms of chromosomes 9 and 22. The result is that part of the ABL gene of chromosome 9 becomes inserted into the BCR gene of chromosome 22. The ABL gene is an oncogene and the product of the hybrid gene is a tyrosine kinase that is implicated in activating cell proliferation. The Ph[1] chromosome appears on karyotyping as a long arm deletion of chromosome 22 because only the terminal end of the long arm of chromosome 9 is exchanged for most of the long arm of chromosome 22. The BCR/ABL translocation can be detected using FISH hybridization probes. Approximately 95% of persons with chronic myelogenous leukemia have the Ph[1] chromosome. Those patients who do not demonstrate Ph[1] have a poorer prognosis. It is also present in the lymphocytes of up to 25% of adults with acute lymphocytic leukemia (ALL) and in a small number of children with ALL and persons with acute myelogenous leukemia.

9. D CEA is a glycoprotein that is secreted into plasma by various cancers of endodermal origin, including breast, lung, colorectal, and stomach cancer. However, it is present in only 40%–60% of such cancers, is present at low levels (<3.0 ng/mL) in normal adults, and is increased by causes other than cancer (e.g., smoking). Its clinical use is to detect recurrence and the need for second-look surgery in persons who have been treated and to evaluate the response to treatment.

10. Which tumor marker is used to determine the usefulness of trastuzumab (Herceptin) therapy for breast cancer?
   A. PR
   B. CEA
   C. HER-2/neu
   D. Myc

Chemistry/Apply knowledge of fundamental biological characteristics/Tumor markers/1

11. A person is suspected of having testicular cancer. Which type of hCG test would be most useful?
   A. Plasma immunoassay for intact hCG only
   B. Plasma immunoassay for intact hCG and the β-hCG subunit
   C. Plasma immunoassay for the free alpha and β-hCG subunits
   D. Urine assay for hCG β core

Chemistry/Apply knowledge of fundamental biological characteristics/Tumor markers/2

12. A patient treated for a germ cell tumor has a total and free β hCG assay performed prior to surgery. The result is 40,000 mIU/mL. One week following surgery, the hCG is 5000 mIU/mL. Chemotherapy is started, and the hCG is measured 1 week later and found to be 10,000 mIU/mL. What does this indicate?
   A. Recurrence of the tumor
   B. Falsely increased hCG owing to drug interference with the assay
   C. Analytical error with the test reported as 5000 mIU/mL
   D. Transient hCG increase caused by chemotherapy

Chemistry/Evaluate laboratory data to explain inconsistent results/Tumor markers/3

13. Which set of results for ER and PR is associated with the highest likelihood of a favorable response to treatment with estrogen suppression therapy (tamoxifen)?
   A. ER positive, PR positive
   B. ER positive, PR negative
   C. ER negative, PR positive
   D. ER negative, PR negative

Chemistry/Correlate clinical and laboratory data/Tumor markers/2

Answers to Questions 10–13

10. **C** Trastuzumab is an antibody to the HER-2/neu gene product, a tyrosine kinase receptor protein. HER-2/neu is an oncogene that is overexpressed in some breast cancers. Overexpression is associated with a more aggressive clinical course but responds to treatment with trastuzumab, which blocks the attachment of growth factor to the receptor. The progesterone receptor, like the ER, is used to identify persons with breast cancer who are more likely to respond to estrogen suppression therapy. Myc is a group of oncogenes that are activated in various cancers, including lung, breast, colon, stomach, leukemia, and lymphoma. HER-2/neu is measured in plasma by immunoassay. ER, PR, and myc are measured in tissue and not plasma using immunohistological stains or FISH.

11. **B** In addition to testicular cancer, hCG is produced by trophoblastic tumors and choriocarcinomas. In choriocarcinoma and testicular tumors other than seminoma, there is a high likelihood of the β-subunit's being present without intact hCG. This is especially true after treatment when hCG is used to monitor for recurrence. The use of an immunoassay that measures both the intact and free β hCG will have greater sensitivity than an assay for intact hCG or an assay for only free subunits. Free α hCG subunits may be produced in persons with urinary bladder (urothelial) cancer. Urinary β core (urinary gonadotropin peptide) is a metabolic product of the β subunit and has been used to monitor for persistence of trophoblastic disease and recurrence of some hCG producing tumors.

12. **D** Treatment of tumors with chemotherapy often causes a transient increase in the production of tumor markers as the drugs destroy tumor cells. The half-life of hCG is 24–36 hours; therefore the expected decline 1 week postsurgery was consistent with the result of 5000 mIU/mL. Initiation of chemotherapy probably caused the hCG to double in the following week. The hCG assay should be monitored at regular intervals for several months, since a failure for it to decline or an increased level would suggest recurrence.

13. **A** Both ER and PR receptor assays are performed on breast tissue biopsies to determine the probability of response to tamoxifen. The PR receptor is produced from the ER receptor and expression of both predicts a positive response to the drug. Less than 15% of persons who are ER negative and PR negative have a favorable response, whereas over 75% of those who are positive for both receptors have a favorable response to tamoxifen.

14. Which type of cancer is associated with the highest level of AFP?
   A. Hepatoma
   B. Ovarian cancer
   C. Testicular cancer
   D. Breast cancer

Chemistry/Correlate clinical and laboratory data/Tumor markers/1

15. Which of the following assays is recommended as a screening test for colorectal cancer in persons over 50 years old?
   A. CEA
   B. AFP
   C. Occult blood
   D. Fecal trypsin

Chemistry/Correlate clinical and laboratory data/Tumor markers/2

16. Which of the following substances is used to determine the risk of developing cancer?
   A. Epidermal growth factor receptor (EGF-R)
   B. Squamous cell carcinoma antigen (SCC)
   C. c-erb B-2 gene
   D. p53 gene

Chemistry/Apply knowledge of fundamental biological characteristics/Tumor markers 1

Answers to Questions 14–16

14. **A** AFP is increased in all persons with yolk sac tumors and over 80% of those with hepatoma. Levels above 1000 ng/mL are diagnostic of hepatoma. Ectopic AFP-secreting tumors are produced by ovarian, testicular, breast, GI, and bladder cancers, and these sources should be considered when tenfold or higher elevations are seen in the absence of abnormal liver function. AFP is used along with hCG to increase the diagnostic sensitivity of nonseminoma testicular tumors and to stage the disease. Approximately 42% of persons with nonseminoma testicular cancer are positive for hCG but over 70% are positive for both hCG or AFP.

15. **C** Bleeding in the gastrointestinal tract occurs during the early stages of colorectal cancer when treatment can be most effective. Although occult blood can be caused by many other GI problems, it is not associated with benign polyps and has a sensitivity of over 80% for detection of colorectal cancer. CEA is elevated in less than 60% of such cases. AFP is elevated in only about 5% of colon cancers. Fecal trypsin is not a marker for colorectal cancer, but fecal α_1-antitrypsin is produced by the majority of malignant colon tumors.

16. **D** The p53 gene (tumor suppressor gene) is located on chromosome 17 and produces a protein that down-regulates the cell cycle. A mutation of p53 is associated with an increased incidence of many cancers. The c-erb B-2 gene is the same as HER-2/neu; it codes for a growth factor receptor with tyrosine kinase activity on the cell membrane. EGF-R is a receptor for epithelial growth factor and its overexpression in breast tissue is associated with a poorer prognosis. SCC is a glycoprotein antigen found in the cytoplasm of tumors of squamous origin and is secreted in the plasma of persons with uterine cancer.

17. A person has an elevated 24-hour urinary homovanil-lic acid (HVA) and vanillymandelic acid (VMA). Urinary metanephrines, chromogranin A, and neuron-specific enolase are also elevated but 5-hydroxyindoleacetic acid is within the reference range. What is the most likely diagnosis?
    A. Carcinoid tumors of the intestine
    B. Pheochromocytoma
    C. Neuroblastoma
    D. Pancreatic cancer

    Chemistry/Correlate clinical and laboratory data/Tumor markers/2

18. In which of the following conditions is PSA *LEAST* likely to be increased?
    A. Precancerous lesions of the prostate
    B. Postprostate biopsy
    C. Benign prostatic hypertrophy
    D. Post–digital rectal examination

    Chemistry/Apply knowledge to recognize sources of error/Tumor marker/1

Answers to Questions 17–18

17. **C** Neuron-specific enolase is an isoenzyme containing two gamma polypeptides that are specific for nervous tissue and are found in neuroendocrine cells. Plasma levels are increased in neuroblastomas, carcinoid tumors, thyroid medullary carcinomas, and in some lung cancers and seminomas. Urinary VMA, catecholamines, and metanephrines are increased in both pheochromocytoma (a tumor of chromaffin cells) and neuroblastoma (also a tumor of neuroectodermal cells derived from the neural crest neuroblasts of the sympathetic ganglia). Urinary HVA is increased in about 75% of persons with neuroblastoma but is not usually increased in pheochromocytoma. Chromogranin A is a protein that inhibits release of catecholamines and is increased in pheochromocytoma, neuroblastoma, and carcinoid tumors. Urinary 5-hydroxyindoleacetic acid is increased in carcinoid tumors (endochromaffin tumors).

18. **D** PSA is a serine protease responsible for liquefaction of the seminal fluid. PSA has been used successfully to monitor for recurrence and follow the response of patients to androgen suppression therapy. Currently, it is one of the few FDA-approved tumor makers for cancer screening. Although digital rectal examination raises the prostatic acid phosphatase level, it does not increase the concentration of PSA in the plasma. In addition to prostate cancer, PSA may be increased in acute or chronic prostate inflammation, benign prostate hypertrophy, and after transurethral prostate resection or prostate biopsy. As a result the specificity of PSA is approximately 60% and the predictive value of a positive result approximately 30%.

19. Which of the following statements regarding PSA is true?

   A. Complexed PSA in plasma is normally less than free PSA

   B. Free PSA below 25% is associated with malignant disease

   C. A total PSA below 4 ng/mL rules out malignant disease

   D. A total PSA above 10 ng/mL is diagnostic of malignant disease

Chemistry/Correlate clinical and laboratory data/Tumor markers/2

20. A 55-year-old male with early stage prostate cancer diagnosed by biopsy had his prostate gland removed (simple prostatectomy). His PSA prior to surgery was 10.0 ng/mL. If the surgery was successful in completely removing the tumor cells, what would the PSA result be 1 month after surgery?

   A. Undetectable

   B. 1-3 ng/mL

   C. Less than 4 ng/mL

   D. Less than 10 ng/mL

Chemistry/Correlate clinical and laboratory data/Tumor markers/3

Answers to Questions 19–20

19. B In normal plasma 55%–95% of the PSA is bound to protease inhibitors, primarily α_1-antichymotrypsin, and the remainder is called free PSA. At a cutoff of 4 ng/mL commonly used for the upper reference limit, total PSA has a sensitivity of approximately 60%, and 22% of men with a PSA below 4 ng/mL have evidence of early prostate cancer on biopsy. For this reason, some laboratories prefer a cutoff of 2.5 ng/mL for total PSA. However, based upon this cutoff alone the number of false positive findings (unnecessary biopsies) would be extremely high. A PSA of 2.6 ng/mL that was 2.6 ng/mL the previous year would not likely be significant; however, a PSA of 2.6 ng/mL that was only 1.6 ng/mL the previous year would warrant further testing. In persons with a total PSA between 2.6 and 10.0 ng/mL, a low ratio of free PSA:total PSA ($<$25% fPSA) or a high level of complexed PSA (cPSA$>$2.7 ng/mL) increases the diagnostic sensitivity and specificity. Persons with a PSA between 2.6 and 10.0 ng/mL are selected for biopsy if either the fPSA is low or the cPSA is high. Initial studies also indicate that the incomplete cleavage of the proenzyme of PSA (proPSA) in persons with cancer results in a high ratio of proPSA to fPSA. This ratio was reported to have better diagnostic sensitivity and specificity than the percentage of fPSA alone. The probability of cancer when the total PSA is higher than 10 ng/mL is approximately 50%, and this necessitates a biopsy to determine if the prostate is malignant.

20. A If the tumor were confined to the prostate, the PSA would be undetectable 1 month following successful surgery, since there is no other tissue source of PSA. The half-life of PSA is 2.2–3.2 days, and the minimum detection limit of most assays is 0.2 ng/mL or lower. Therefore, it would require at least 2 weeks before the PSA level would be undetectable. The low minimum detection limit of the PSA assay, combined with the high tissue specificity of PSA, makes the test very sensitive in detecting recurrence.

1. **Which of the procedures below can be used to evaluate a new glucose method for proportional error?**
   A. Compare the standard deviation of 40 patient samples to the hexokinase method
   B. Measure a mixture made from equal parts of normal and high quality control sera
   C. Add 5.0 mg of glucose to 1.0 mL of a serum of known concentration and measure
   D. Compare the mean of 40 normal samples to the hexokinase method

   Chemistry/Select course of action/Method evaluation/3

2. **Which of two instruments can be assumed to have the narrower bandpass? Assume that wavelength is accurately calibrated.**
   A. The instrument giving the highest absorbance for a solution of 0.1 mmol/L NADH at 340 nm
   B. The instrument giving the lowest %T for a solution of nickel sulfate at 700 nm
   C. The instrument giving the highest %T reading for 1.0% v/v HCl at 350 nm
   D. The instrument giving the most linear plot of absorbance versus concentration

   Chemistry/Select course of action/Spectrophotometry/3

3. **A lipemic sample gives a sodium concentration of 130 mmol/L on an analyzer that uses a 1:50 dilution of serum or plasma before introducing it to the ion selective electrodes. The same sample gives a sodium value of 142 mmol/L using a direct (undiluted) ion selective electrode. Assuming acceptable quality control, which of the following is the most appropriate course of action?**

   A. Report a sodium result of 136 mmol/L
   B. Ultracentrifuge the sample and repeat by ion-selective electrode (ISE)
   C. Dilute the sample 1:4 and repeat by ISE
   D. Report the undiluted ISE result

   Chemistry/Select course of action/Electrolytes/3

Answers to Questions 1–3

1. **C** Proportional error is percentage deviation from the expected result and affects the slope of the calibration curve. It causes a greater absolute error (loss of accuracy) as concentration increases. It is measured by a recovery study in which a sample is spiked with known amounts of analyte. In the example, the concentration should increase by 500 mg/dL.

2. **A** Bandpass is defined by the range of wavelengths passed through the sample at the specified wavelength setting. It can be measured using any solution having a narrow absorbance peak (e.g., NADH at 340 nm). The instrument producing the purest monochromatic light has the highest absorbance reading.

3. **D** Lipemic samples give lower results for sodium (pseudohyponatremia) when diluted prior to measurment because the H_2O phase is mostly diluent, and a significant component of the sample volume is displaced by lipid. Direct ISEs measure sodium in the plasma water, more accurately reflecting patient status.

4. **SITUATION:** A 2_{2S} quality control error occurs for serum calcium by atomic absorption. Fresh standards prepared in 5.0% w/v albumin are found to be linear, but repeating the controls with fresh material does not improve the quality control results. Select the most likely cause of this problem.
   A. Matrix effect caused by a viscosity difference between the standards and quality control sera
   B. Chemical interference caused incomplete atomization
   C. Incomplete deconjugation of protein-bound calcium
   D. Ionization interference caused by excessive heat

   Chemistry/Evaluate laboratory data to recognize problems/Atomic absorption/3

5. **SITUATION:** A serum osmolality value measured in the emergency room is 326 mOsm/kg. Two hours later, chemistry results are:

   Na = 135 mmol/L; BUN = 18 mg/dL; glucose = 72 mg/dL; measured osmolality = 318 mOsm/kg

   What do these results suggest?

   A. Laboratory error in electrolyte or glucose measurement
   B. Drug or alcohol intoxication
   C. Specimen misidentification
   D. Successful rehydration of the patient

   Chemistry/Evaluate laboratory data to determine possible inconsistent results/Osmolality/3

6. When calibrating a pH meter, unstable readings occur for both pH 7.00 and 4.00 calibrators, although both can be set to within 0.1 pH unit. Select the most appropriate course of action.
   A. Measure the pH of the sample and report to the nearest 0.1 pH
   B. Replace both calibrators with unopened buffers and recalibrate
   C. Examine the reference electrode junction for salt crystals
   D. Move the electrodes to another pH meter and calibrate

   Chemistry/Select course of action/pH/3

7. A method calls for extracting an acidic drug from urine with an anion exchange column. The pK_a of the drug is 6.5. Extraction is enhanced by adjusting the sample pH to:
   A. 8.5
   B. 6.5

C. 5.5
D. 4.5

Chemistry/Select course of action/Chromatography/3

Answers to Questions 4–7

4. **B** Poor recovery of calcium by atomic absorption is often caused by failure to break thermostable bonds between calcium and phosphate (a form of chemical interference). This may be caused by failure to add lanthanum to the diluent or by low atomizer temperature. The use of 5.0% w/v albumin in the calibrator produces viscosity and protein binding characteristics similar to those of plasma.

5. **B** The *osmolal gap* is the difference between calculated and measured osmolality. Here the osmolal gap is 38 mOsm/kg. When the osmolal gap is greater than 12 mOsm/kg, an unmeasured solute is present or an analytical error occurred when measuring the osmolality, electrolytes, urea, or glucose. The reference range for serum osmolality is 280–295 mOsm/kg. Both measurements are above the URL. These results point to the presence of an unmeasured solute. A significant osmolal gap in samples from emergency room patients usually results from alcohol or drug consumption. The difference in osmolality between the two samples is 8 mOsm/kg and can be explained by alcohol metabolism during the 2 hours between samples.

6. **C** Noise in pH measurements often results from a blocked junction between the reservoir of the reference electrode and the test solution. This occurs when salt crystals collect at the junction or when KCl concentration in the reservoir increases due to evaporation of water. The fluid in the reference electrode should be replaced with warm deionized water. After the crystals have dissolved, the water is replaced with fresh reference electrolyte solution.

7. **A** Extraction of a negatively charged drug onto an anion exchange (positively charged) column is optimal when more than 99% of the drug is in the form of anion. The extraction pH should be 2 pH units above the pK_a of an acidic drug. When pH = pK_a, the drug will be 50% ionized, and when pH is greater than pK_a, the majority of drug is anionic.

8. **SITUATION:** A patient who has a positive urinalysis for glucose and ketones has a glycosylated Hgb of 4.0%. A fasting glucose performed the previous day was 180 mg/dL. Assuming acceptable quality control you would:
   A. Report the glycosylated Hgb
   B. Request a new specimen and repeat the glycosylated Hgb
   C. Perform an Hgb electrophoresis on the sample
   D. Perform a glucose measurement on the sample

   Chemistry/Evaluate laboratory data to determine possible inconsistent results/Glycosylated hemoglobin/3

9. A review of quality control results for uric acid is as follows:

   Expected Results

	Run 1	Run 2	Run 3	Run 4	Mean	s
QC1	3.5	3.8	4.1	4.2 mg/dL	3.6 mg/dL	0.40
QC2	6.8	7.2	7.4	7.5 mg/dL	7.0 mg/dL	0.25

   Results should have been reported from:
   A. Run 1 only
   B. Runs 1 and 2
   C. Runs 1, 2, and 3
   D. Runs 1, 2, 3, and 4

   Chemistry/Select course of action/Quality control/3

10. **SITUATION:** A peak blood level for orally administered theophylline (therapeutic range 8–20 mg/L) measured at 8 a.m. is 5.0 mg/L. The preceding trough level was 4.6 mg/L. What is the most likely explanation of these results?
    A. Laboratory error made on peak measurement
    B. Specimen for peak level was collected from wrong patient
    C. Blood for peak level was drawn too soon
    D. Elimination rate has reached maximum

    Chemistry/Apply knowledge to recognize sources of error/Therapeutic drug monitoring/3

11. **SITUATION:** A patient breathing room air has the following arterial blood gas and electrolyte results:

    pH = 7.54; P_{CO_2} = 18.5 mm Hg; P_{O_2} = 145 mm Hg; HCO_3 = 18 mmol/L

    Na = 135 mmol/L; K = 4.6 mmol/L; Cl = 98 mmol/L; TCO_2 = 20 mmol/L

    The best explanation for these results is:
    A. Blood for electrolytes was drawn above an intravenous catheter
    B. The serum sample was hemolyzed
    C. Venous blood was sampled for arterial blood gases
    D. The blood gas sample was exposed to air

    Chemistry/Evaluate laboratory data to determine possible inconsistent results/Blood gases/3

Answers to Questions 8–11

8. **B**   The glycosylated Hgb is within normal limits (2%–7%), but the fasting glucose indicates frank diabetes mellitus. Although the glycosylated Hgb reflects the average blood glucose 2–3 months earlier, the value reported is inconsistent with the other laboratory results. A high probability of sample misidentification or analytical error necessitates that the test be repeated.

9. **C**   Although no single result exceeds the 2s limit, the 4_{1S} rule is broken on Run 4. This means that both QC1 and QC2 exceeded +1s on Runs 3 and 4.

10. **C**   Sample collection time is critical for accurate therapeutic drug monitoring. Blood for trough levels must be collected immediately before the next dose. Blood collection time for peak levels must not occur prior to complete absorption and distribution of drug. This usually requires 1–2 hours for orally administered drugs. The therapeutic range for theophylline is 8–20 mg/L. These results are most consistent with a peak sample having been drawn prior to complete absorption of the drug.

11. **D**   A patient breathing room air cannot have an arterial P_{O_2} greater than 105 mm Hg because alveolar P_{O_2} is 110 mm Hg when $F_{O_2}(I)$ = 150 mm Hg. Exposure to air causes loss of CO_2 gas and increased pH.

12. SITUATION: The following laboratory results are reported. Which result is most likely to be erroneous?

Arterial blood gases:

pH	7.42	PCO_2	38.0 mm Hg
PO_2	90 mm Hg	HCO_3^-	24.0 mmol/L

Plasma electrolytes:

Na	135 mmol/L	Cl	98 mmol/L
K	4.6 mmol/L	TCO_2	33 mmol/L

A. pH
B. Na
C. K
D. TCO_2

Chemistry/Evaluate laboratory data to determine possible inconsistent results/Blood gases/3

13. SITUATION: Laboratory results on a patient from the emergency room are:

Glucose = 1100 mg/dL; Na = 155 mmol/L; K = 1.2 mmol/L; Cl = 115 mmol/L; TCO_2 = 3.0 mmol/L

What is the most likely explanation of these results?
A. Sample drawn above an intravenous catheter
B. Metabolic acidosis with increased anion gap
C. Diabetic ketoacidosis
D. Laboratory error measuring electrolytes caused by hyperglycemia

Chemistry/Evaluate laboratory data to recognize problems/Specimen collection/3

14. SITUATION: A plasma sample from a person in a coma as a result of an automobile accident gave the following results:

Total CK 380 IU/L   CK-MB (immunoinhibition) 100 IU/L

Myoglobin 600 μg/L   Troponin I 0.02 μg/L
CK-MB (sandwich immunoassay) 5.0 μg/L

Which result is erroneous?
A. CK-MB immunoinhibition
B. Troponin I
C. Myoglobin
D. CK-MB sandwich immunoassay

Chemistry/Evaluate laboratory data to assess validity/Accuracy of procedures/Cardiac markers/3

15. SITUATION: A patient has the following electrolyte results:

Na = 130 mmol/L; K = 4.8 mmol/L; Cl = 105 mmol/L; TCO_2 = 26 mmol/L

Assuming acceptable quality control, select the best course of action.
A. Report these results
B. Check the albumin, total protein, Ca, P, and Mg results; if normal, repeat the sodium test

C. Request a new sample
D. Recalibrate and repeat the potassium test

Chemistry/Evaluate laboratory data to check for sources of error/Anion gap/3

Answers to Questions 12–15

12. D The pH, PCO_2, and bicarbonate are normal and therefore agree. The electrolytes are normal also, but the TCO_2 is increased significantly. The reference range for venous TCO_2 is 22–28 mmol/L. Although TCO_2 is the sum of bicarbonate and dissolved CO_2, the venous TCO_2 is determined almost entirely by the bicarbonate, since dCO_2 is lost as CO_2 gas when the venous blood is exposed to air during processing. A TCO_2 value of 32 mmol/L would be expected in a person with metabolic alkalosis.

13. A These results are consistent with dilution of venous blood by intravenous fluid containing 5% dextrose and normal saline. The intravenous fluid is free of potassium and bicarbonate, accounting for the low level of these electrolytes (incompatible with life).

14. A The automobile accident caused both brain damage (coma) and muscle damage (myoglobin), resulting in the possible release of CK-BB from the central nervous system and/or myokinase from skeletal muscles. Both of these increase the result of CK-MB tests performed by immunoinhibition. This method utilizes an antibody, which blocks the catalytic activity of the M subunit of CK-MB but not the B subunit. The presence of CK-BB in this sample accounts for the very high activity seen. Note that the percent CK-MB is >25%, which is not possible from a cardiac muscle source since only the B subunit is active. The troponin I and CK-MB sandwich immunoassays are both within normal limits, indicating no evidence of a myocardial infarction at this time. The sandwich assay for MB uses antibodies to both the M and B subunits of CK-MB and therefore is not subject to interference from CK-BB, which does not react.

15. B The anion gap of this sample is only 6 mmol/L. This may result from laboratory error, retention of an unmeasured cation (e.g., calcium), or low level of unmeasured anion such as phosphorus or albumin. The sodium is inappropriately low for the chloride and bicarbonate and should be repeated if no biochemical cause is apparent.

16. A *stat* plasma lithium determined using an ion-selective electrode is measured at 14.0 mmol/L. Select the most appropriate course of action.
   A. Immediately report this result
   B. Check sample for hemolysis
   C. Call for a new specimen
   D. Rerun the lithium calibrators

Chemistry/Select course of action/Therapeutic drug monitoring/3

17. A chromatogram for blood alcohol (GC) gives broad trailing peaks and increased retention times for ethanol and internal standard. This is most likely caused by:
   A. A contaminated injection syringe
   B. Water contamination of the column packing
   C. Carrier gas flow rate that is too fast
   D. Oven temperature that is too high

Chemistry/Evaluate laboratory data to recognize problems/Gas chromatography/3

18. **SITUATION:** An amylase result is 550 U/L. A 1:4 dilution of the specimen in NaCl gives 180 U/L (before mathematical correction for dilution). The dilution is repeated with the same results. The technologist should:
   A. Report the amylase as 550 U/L
   B. Report the amylase as 720 U/L
   C. Report the amylase as 900 U/L
   D. Dilute the sample 1:10 in distilled water and repeat

Chemistry/Select course of action/Amylase/3

19. **SITUATION:** A patient's biochemistry results are:

   ALT = 55 IU/L; AST = 165 IU/L; glucose = 87 mg/dL; LD = 340 IU/L; Na = 142 mmol/L; K = 6.8 mmol/L; Ca = 8.4 mg/dL; P_i = 7.2 mg/dL

Select the best course of action.
   A. Report results along with an estimate of the degree of hemolysis
   B. Repeat LD but report all other results
   C. Request a new sample
   D. Dilute the serum 1:2 and repeat AST and LD assays

Chemistry/Select course of action/Hemolysis/3

20. A blood sample is left on a phlebotomy tray for 4 hours before it is delivered to the laboratory. Which group of tests could be performed?

   A. Glucose, Na, K, Cl, T_{CO_2}
   B. Uric acid, BUN, creatinine
   C. Total and direct bilirubin
   D. CK, ALT, ALP, ACP

Chemistry/Apply knowledge of fundamental biological characteristics/Sample collections and handling/3

Answers to Questions 16–20

16. **C** Lithium in excess of 2.0 mmol/L is toxic (in some laboratories 1.5 mmol/L is the upper therapeutic limit). A level of 14 mmol/L would not occur unless the sample were contaminated with lithium. This would most likely result from collection in a green-stoppered tube containing the lithium salt of heparin.

17. **B** Increased oven temperature or gas flow rate will shorten retention times and decrease peak widths. Syringe contamination may cause the appearance of ghost peaks. Water in a polyethylene glycol (PEG) column such as Carbowax used for measuring volatiles causes longer retention times and loss of resolution.

18. **B** A 1:4 dilution refers to one part serum and three parts diluent; the result is multiplied by 4 to determine the serum concentration. Serum may contain wheat germ gluten or other natural amylase inhibitors that, when diluted, result in increased enzyme activity. Serum for amylase should always be diluted with normal saline because chloride ions are needed for amylase activity.

19. **A** Results indicate a moderately hemolyzed sample. Because sodium, calcium, and glucose are not significantly affected, results should be reported along with an estimate of visible hemolysis. The physician may reorder affected tests of interest.

20. **B** Glucose in serum is metabolized by cells at a rate of about 7% per hour. Bilirubin levels will fall if the sample is exposed to sunlight. Hemolysis will adversely affect enzyme levels. Uric acid, BUN, and creatinine are least likely to be affected.

21. An HPLC assay for procainamide gives an internal standard peak that is 15% greater in area and height for sample 1 than sample 2. The technologist should suspect that:
  A. The column pressure increased while sample 2 was being analyzed
  B. Less recovery from sample 2 occurred in the extraction step
  C. The pH of the mobile phase increased during chromatography of sample 2
  D. There was more procainamide in sample 1 than sample 2

Chemistry/Apply principles of special procedures/Liquid chromatography/3

22. After staining a silica gel plate to determine the L/S ratio, the technologist notes that the lipid standards both migrated 1 cm faster than usual. The technologist should:
  A. Repeat the separation on a new silica gel plate
  B. Check the pH of the developing solvent
  C. Prepare fresh developing solvent and repeat the assay
  D. Reduce solvent migration time for all subsequent runs

Chemistry/Select course of action/Thin layer chromatography/3

23. A quantitative urine glucose level was determined to be 160 mg/dL by the Trinder glucose oxidase method. The sample was refrigerated overnight. The next day, the glucose was repeated and found to be 240 mg/dL using a polarographic method. What is the most likely cause of this discrepancy?
  A. Poor precision when performing one of the methods
  B. Contamination resulting from overnight storage
  C. High levels of reducing substances interfering with the Trinder reaction
  D. Positive interference in the polarographic method caused by hematuria

Chemistry/Evaluate laboratory data to determine possible inconsistent results/Glucose/3

24. **SITUATION:** Results of an iron profile are:

  Serum Fe = 40 μg/dL; TIBC = 400 μg/dL;
  ferritin = 40μg/L (reference range 15–200);
  transferrin = 310 mg/dL

These results indicate:
  A. Error in calculation of TIBC
  B. Serum iron falls before ferritin in iron deficiency
  C. A defect in iron transport and not Fe deficiency
  D. Excess release of ferritin caused by injury

Chemistry/Evaluate laboratory data to determine possible inconsistent results/Iron deficiency/3

25. **SITUATION:** Results of an iron profile are:

  Serum Fe = 40 μg/dL; TIBC = 400 μg/dL;
  ferritin = 50 μg/L

All of the following tests are useful in establishing a diagnosis of Fe deficiency *except*:
  A. Protein electrophoresis
  B. Erythrocyte zinc protoporphyrin
  C. Serum transferrin
  D. Hgb electrophoresis

Chemistry/Evaluate laboratory and clinical data to specify additional tests/Iron deficiency/3

Answers to Questions 21–25

21. **B** The internal standard compensates for variation in extraction, evaporation, reconstitution, and injection volume. The same amount of internal standard is added to all samples and standards prior to assay. Increased column pH or pressure usually alters retention time and may not affect peak quantitation.

22. **C** TLC plates migrate in solvent until the front comes to 1 cm of the top of the plate. Separation of lipids on silica gel is based upon adsorption. Higher R_f values indicate greater solubility of lipids in the developing solvent. This may be caused by evaporation of H_2O, lowering the polarity of the solvent.

23. **C** Urine often contains high levels of ascorbate and other reducing substances. These may cause significant negative bias when measuring glucose using a peroxidase-coupled method. The reductants compete with chromogen for H_2O_2.

24. **D** Serum ferritin levels fall before iron or TIBC in iron deficiency, and a low level of serum ferritin is diagnostic. However, low tissue levels of ferritin may be masked by increased release into the blood in liver disease, infection, and acute inflammation. Although this patient's serum ferritin is within reference limits, serum iron is low and percent saturation is only 10%. Note that the TIBC and transferrin results are both elevated and agree. Transferrin can be estimated by multiplying the TIBC by 0.7. These results point to iron deficiency.

25. **D** Electrophoresis may show an elevated β-globulin (transferrin) characteristic of iron deficiency, or inflammation that would help explain a normal ferritin. Zinc protoporphyrin is elevated in iron deficiency and in lead poisoning. Hemoglobinopathies and thalassemias are not associated with iron deficiency.

26. Serum protein and immunofixation electrophoresis are ordered on a patient. The former is performed, but there is no evidence of a monoclonal protein. Select the best course of action.
   A. Perform quantitative Ig G, A, and M
   B. Perform the immunofixation electrophoresis (IFE) on the serum
   C. Report the result; request a urine sample for protein electrophoresis
   D. Perform IFE on the serum and request a urine sample for IFE

   Chemistry/Evaluate laboratory data to recognize and report the need for additional tests/Immunofixation electrophoresis/3

27. **SITUATION:** Hgb electrophoresis is performed and all of the Hgbs have greater anodal mobility than usual. A fast Hgb (Hgb H) is at the edge of the gel and bands are blurred. The voltage is set correctly, but the current reading on the ammeter is too low. Select the course of action that would correct this problem.
   A. Reduce the voltage
   B. Dilute the buffer and adjust the pH
   C. Prepare fresh buffer and repeat the test
   D. Reduce the running time

   Chemistry/Select course of action/Electrophoresis/3

28. A technologist is asked to use the serum from a clot tube left over from a chemistry profile run at 8 a.m. for a *stat* ionized calcium (Ca_I) at 11 a.m. The technologist should:
   A. Perform the assay on the 8 a.m. sample
   B. Perform the test only if the serum container was tightly capped
   C. Perform the assay on the 8 a.m. sample only if it was refrigerated
   D. Request a new sample

   Chemistry/Select course of action/Ionized calcium/3

29. **SITUATION:** A patient's biochemistry results are:

   Na = 125 mmol/L; Cl = 106 mmol/L; K = 4.5 mmol/L; TCO_2 = 19 mmol/L; chol = 240 mg/dL; triglyceride = 640 mg/dL; glucose = 107 mg/dL; AST = 16 IU/L; ALT = 11 IU/L; amylase = 200 U/L

   Select the most likely cause of these results.
   A. The sample is hemolyzed
   B. Serum was not separated from cells in sufficient time
   C. Lipemia is causing in vitro interference
   D. The specimen is contaminated

   Chemistry/Evaluate laboratory data to recognize problems/Lipemia/3

30. A gastric fluid from a patient suspected of having taken an overdose of amphetamine is sent to the laboratory for analysis. The technologist should:
   A. Perform an EMIT assay for amphetamine
   B. Refuse the sample and request serum or urine
   C. Dilute 1:10 with H_2O and filter; perform TLC for amphetamines
   D. Titrate to pH 7.0, then follow procedure for measuring amphetamine in urine

   Chemistry/Select course of action/Toxicology/3

Answers to Questions 26–30

26. **C** An area of restricted mobility should be identified on serum protein electrophoresis before IFE is performed. About one out of four patients with multiple myeloma have monoclonal free λ or κ chains in urine only, and therefore urine electrophoresis should be included in initial testing.

27. **C** Increased mobility, decreased resolution, and low current result from low ionic strength. Reducing voltage will slow migration but will not improve resolution. Diluting the buffer will reduce the current, resulting in poorer resolution.

28. **D** Ca_I is pH-dependent. Heparinized blood is preferred because it can be assayed immediately. Serum may be used, but the specimen must remain tightly capped while clotting and centrifuging and analyzed as soon as possible.

29. **C** The triglyceride level is about five times normal, causing the sample to be lipemic. This will cause pseudohyponatremia (unbalanced electrolytes). Lipemia may cause a falsely high rate reaction when amylase is measured by turbidimetry; however, the high amylase level may be associated with pancreatitis, which results in hyperlipidemia.

30. **C** The gastric sample can be measured by TLC, but such a sample should not be used in place of serum or urine without documentation of acceptability by the reagent manufacturer or laboratory. A positive amphetamine result by a screening test such as TLC or immunoassay may be caused by a related drug that interferes with the result and therefore should be confirmed by GC-MS if there is a medicolegal implication.

31. **SITUATION:** Results of biochemistry tests are:

Na = 138 mmol/L; K = 4.2 mmol/L; Cl = 94 mmol/L; T_{CO_2} = 20 mmol/L; glucose = 100 mg/dL; T bili = 1.2 mg/dL; BUN = 6.8 mg/dL; creat = 1.0 mg/dL; albumin = 4.9 g/dL; T protein = 5.1 g/dL

What should be done next?
A. Request a new specimen
B. Repeat the total protein
C. Repeat all tests
D. Perform a protein electrophoresis

Chemistry/Evaluate laboratory data to determine possible inconsistent results/Total protein/3

32. The chart below compares the monthly total bilirubin mean of Laboratory A to the monthly mean of Laboratory B, which uses the same control materials, analyzer, and method.

	Level 1 Control		Level 2 Control	
	Mean	**CV**	**Mean**	**CV**
Lab A	1.1 mg/dL	2.1%	6.7 mg/dL	3.2%
Lab B	1.4 mg/dL	2.2%	7.0 mg/dL	3.6%

Both laboratories performed controls at the beginning of each shift using commercially prepared liquid quality control serum stored at –20°C. Which of the following conditions would explain these differences?
A. Improper handling of the control material by Laboratory A resulted in loss of bilirubin due to photodegradation
B. The laboratories used a different source of bilirubin calibrator
C. Laboratory B obtained higher results because its precision was poorer
D. Carryover from another reagent falsely elevated the results of Laboratory B

Chemistry/Evaluate data to determine possible sources of error/Quality Control/3

33. After installing a new analyzer and reviewing the results of patients for 1 month, the lead technologist notices a greater frequency of patients with abnormally high triglyceride results. Analysis of all chemistry profiles run the next day indicated that triglyceride results are abnormal whenever the test is run immediately after any sample that is measured for lipase. These observations point to which type of error?
A. Specificity of the triglyceride reagents
B. Precision in pipetting of lipemic samples
C. Bias caused by sequence of analysis
D. Reagent carryover

Chemistry/Evaluate data to determine possible sources of error/Automation/3

Answers to Questions 31–33

31. **B** All results are normal except for total protein. The albumin level cannot be 96% of the total protein, and a random error in total protein measurement should be assumed.

32. **B** Interlaboratory variation in bilirubin results is often caused by differences in the assigned value of the calibrator used. Bilirubin calibrators are either serum-based material that has been reference assayed or unconjugated bilirubin stabilized by addition of alkali and albumin. Calibrator differences result in systematic error and should be suspected if the laboratory's mean shows bias when compared to other laboratories reporting the same method. When this is the case, the molar absorptivity of the calibrator should be measured and the theoretical bilirubin calculated. Photodegradation generally results in a greater loss of bilirubin at higher concentrations and also contributes to random error. Note that the bias between Laboratory A and Laboratory B is constant and that Laboratory A has the lower CV.

33. **D** Carryover errors are usually attributed to interference caused by a sample with a very high concentration of analyte preceding a normal sample. However, reagent carryover may also occur on automated systems that use common reagent delivery lines or reusable cuvets. In the case of lipase methods, triglycerides used in the reagent may coat the reagent lines or cuvets, interfering with the triglyceride measurements that directly follow.

34. SITUATION: A digoxin result from a stable patient with a normal electrocardiogram (ECG) is reported as 7.4 ng/mL (URL 2.6 ng/mL) using an immunofluorescent method. Renal function tests were normal and the patient was not taking any other medications. The assay was repeated and results were the same. The sample was frozen and sent to a reference laboratory for confirmation. The result was 1.6 ng/mL measured by a competitive chemiluminescent procedure. Which best explains the discrepancy in results?

A. The fluorescent immunoassay was performed improperly

B. Digoxin was lower by the chemiluminescent method because it is less sensitive

C. An interfering substance was present that cross-reacted with the antibody in the fluorescent immunoassay

D. Freezing the specimen caused lower results by converting the digoxin to an inactive metabolite

Chemistry/Evaluate data to determine possible sources of error/Therapeutic drug monitoring/3

35. The following results are reported on an adult male patient being evaluated for chest pain:

	Myoglobin (Cutoff = 100 μg/L)	Troponin I (Cutoff = 0.04 μg/L)	CK-MB (Cutoff = 8 μg/L)
Admission	12 μg/L	1.1 μg/L	18 μg/L
3 hours postadmission	360 μg/L	1.8 μg/L	30 μg/L
6 hours postadmission	300 μg/L	2.4 μg/L	40 μg/L

What is the most likely cause of these results?

A. The wrong sample was assayed for the first myoglobin test

B. The patient did not suffer an MI until after admission

C. Hemolysis caused interference with the 3-hour and 6-hour myoglobin result

D. The patient is suffering from unstable angina

Chemistry/Evaluate data to determine possible sources of error/Cardiac markers/3

36. Analysis of normal and abnormal quality controls performed at the beginning of the evening shift revealed a 2_{2S} error across levels for triglyceride. Both controls were within the 3 standard deviation limit. The controls were assayed again, and one control was within the acceptable range and the other was slightly above the 2 standard deviation limit. No further action was taken, and the patient results that were part of the run were reported. Which statement best describes this situation?

A. Appropriate operating procedures were followed

B. Remedial evaluation should have been taken but otherwise the actions were appropriate

C. Remedial action should have been taken and controls repeated with a fresh aliquot; at least three of the patient samples should have been repeated

D. The controls should have been run twice before reporting results

Chemistry/Evaluate data to determine possible sources of error/Quality control/3

Answers to Questions 34–36

34. C An error was suspected because there was a discrepancy between the test result and the patient's clinical status (i.e., signs of digoxin toxicity such as ventricular arrhythmia were not present). Some substances termed DLIFs (digoxin-like immunological factors) can cross-react with antibodies used to measure digoxin. The extent of interference varies with the source of anti-digoxin used. In addition, falsely elevated digoxin results may occur from accidental ingestion of plant poisons such as oleandrin and from administration of Digibind, a Fab fragment that is used to reverse digoxin toxicity.

35. A Myoglobin is the first cardiac marker to rise outside the URL following an MI (2–3 hours) followed by TNI (4–6 hours) and CK-MB (4–8 hours). The admission TNI and CK-MB are both elevated, and they continue to rise in all three samples. Because TNI and CK-MB peak 8–16 hours post-MI and 12–18 hours post-MI, respectively, the infarction likely occurred within the last 8–12 hours. The myoglobin remains elevated for 24 hours post-MI and should have been elevated in the admission sample.

36. C Quality control limits are chosen to achieve a low probability of false rejection. For example, a 2_{2S} error occurs only once in 1600 occurrences by chance. Therefore, such an error can be assumed to be significant. However, this does not mean the error will occur if the controls are repeated again. The error detection rate (power function) of the 2_{2S} rule is only about 30% for a single run. This means that there is a greater chance that the repeated controls will be within range than outside acceptable limits. Therefore, when a systematic error is encountered controls should never be repeated until the test system is evaluated for the source of the error. Calibration should be performed before the controls are repeated using fresh materials. At least three samples chosen randomly (or the entire run if there are less than three samples) should also be repeated and the differences evaluated before releasing the results.

37. SITUATION: CK-MB is measured on an automated analyzer using a single antibody immunoinhibition method. The result is 12 µg/L (URL = 10 µg/L). The assay is repeated on the same sample using a double antibody immunoprecipitation method, and the result is 9 µg/L (URL = 10 µg/L). What is the most likely explanation for these results?

A. Deterioration of CK-MB during storage

B. Differences in the affinity of the antibody against the M subunit used in the tests

C. The immunoinhibition method has a higher variance

D. The presence of macro CK-1 in the sample

Chemistry/Evaluate data to determine possible sources of error/Cardiac markers/3

38. Which set of the following laboratory results is most likely from a patient who has suffered an acute MI? Reference intervals are in parenthesis.

	Total CK (10–110 U/L)	CK-MB (1–6 µg/L)	CK index (1%–2.5%)
A.	760 U/L	16 µg/L	2.1%
B.	170 U/L	14 µg/L	8.2%
C.	160 U/L	4 µg/L	2.5%
D.	80 U/L	2 µg/L	2.5%

Chemistry/Evaluate laboratory data to explain inconsistent results/Enzymes/3

37. D Single antibody immunoinhibition methods measure the activity of the B subunit of CK-MB after neutralizing the M subunit with anti-M. Macro CK-1 is the result of a complex between IgG and CK-1. Macro CK-2 is mitochondrial CK derived from liver cells and consists of polypeptides not related immunologically to either the M or B subunits of CK-MB. Both forms of macro CK may contribute to false positive results when immunoinhibition methods are used. Methods employing antibodies to both M and B subunits are specific for CK-MB because both antibodies must bind to generate a measurement signal. Single antibody assays are used as a screening test only. Results that are below the upper reference limit may be reported as normal. Results above the URL should be confirmed by a specific method for CK-MB or other specific biochemical marker for acute MI such as troponin I.

38. B Results shown in C and D can be excluded because the CK-MB is not increased. Results shown in A and B have CK-MB levels above the URL. However, patient A has a CK index under 2.5% and a five- to tenfold elevation of total CK. These results indicate release of a small of amount of CK-MB from skeletal muscle rather than from cardiac muscle. To maximize the sensitivity of CK-MB, some laboratories use an URL of 6µg/L. This cutoff can detect about two thirds of acute MI cases within 3 hours of the infarct but requires the use of a conservative CK index and other cardiac markers to avoid a high number of false positives.

Na	K	Cl	HCO$_3$	BUN	Glucose	Creatinine	Uric Acid
140 mmol/L	5.8 mmol/L	102 mmol/L	18 mmol/L	2.6 mg/dL	20 mg/dL	DL	DL
132 mmol/L	4.8 mmol/L	98 mmol/L	24 mmol/L	DL	DL	DL	DL

39. Hemoglobin electrophoresis performed on agarose at pH 8.8 gives the following results:

A$_2$ Position	S Position	F Position	A Position
35%	30%	5%	30%

All components of the Hgb C,S,F,A control hemolysate were within the acceptable range. What is the most likely cause of this patient's result?

A. Hgb $_{Lepore}$

B. Hgb S-β-thalassemia (Hgb S/β$^+$)

C. Hgb SC disease post-transfusion

D. Specimen contamination

Chemistry/Evaluate laboratory data to explain inconsistent results/Enzymes/3

40. Two consecutive serum samples give the results shown above for a metabolic function profile.

DL = Detection limit flag (absorbance below detectable limit)

The instrument is a random access analyzer that uses two sample probes. The first probe aspirates a variable amount of serum for the spectrophotometric chemistry tests and the second probe makes a 1:50 dilution of serum for electrolyte measurements. What is the most likely cause of these results?

A. Both patients have renal failure

B. There is an insufficient amount of sample in both serum tubes

C. There is a fibrin strand in the probe used for the spectrophotometric chemistry tests

D. The same patient's sample was accidentally run twice

Chemistry/Evaluate data to determine possible sources of error/Automation/3

Answers to Questions 39–40

39. **C** Hemoglobin $_{Lepore}$ results from a hybridization of the β and δ genes and produces a pattern that is similar to Hgb S trait (AS), except that the quantity of Hgb S is below 20%. Hemoglobin S-β-thalassemia minor results in an increase in Hgb A$_2$ (and possibly Hgb F) because there is reduced transcription of the structurally normal β chain. However, the Hgb S should be greater than the Hgb A, and the amount at the Hgb A$_2$ is far too high. The concentration of Hgb at the A$_2$ position is too high to result from contamination or to be considered as Hgb A$_2$. This pattern appears to express two abnormal Hgbs (Hgb S and C) as well as the normal adult Hgb A. Because inheritance of two abnormal β genes prohibits formation of normal Hgb A, this pattern would occur only if the patient has been transfused with normal RBCs. Hemoglobin SC disease usually produces almost equal amounts of Hgb C and S (and usually a slight increase in Hgb F) and is the most likely cause of these results. This could be confirmed by citrate agar electrophoresis or isofocusing to identify the abnormal Hgbs and review of the patient's medical record for evidence of recent blood transfusion.

40. **C** Electrolyte results for both patients are within the physiological range but are distinctly different. The first results indicate a high potassium and increased anion gap, and one would expect the BUN, uric acid, and creatinine to be elevated. However, the results for BUN and glucose are unlikely for any patient, and the creatinine and uric acid signals are below the detection limit of the analyzer, indicating that little or no sample was added because the sample probe is partially obstructed or the serum level is too low. The results for the second sample are below detection limits for all spectrophotometric tests, which may be the result of complete probe obstruction or the inability to generate a detectable signal with the trace quantity of serum that was added. Because all of the low or undetectable signals are for tests sampled by the first probe, the only explanation is that the probe is obstructed or malfunctioning.

41. SITUATION: A blood sample in a red-stoppered tube is delivered to the laboratory for electrolytes, calcium, and phosphorus analysis. The tube is approximately half full and is accompanied by a purple-stoppered tube ordered for a complete blood count that is approximately three quarters full. The chemistry results are as follows:

Na	K	Cl	HCO_3	Ca	InP
135 mmol/L	11.2 mmol/L	103 mmol/L	14 mmol/L	2.6 mg/dL	3.8 mg/dL

What is the most likely explanation of these results?
A. Severe hemolysis during sample collection
B. Laboratory error in the calcium measurement
C. The wrong order of draw was used for vacuum tube collection
D. Some anticoagulated blood was added to the red-stoppered tube

Chemistry/Evaluate data to determine possible sources of error/Electrolytes/3

42. SITUATION: A patient previously diagnosed with primary hypothyroidism and started on thyroxine replacement therapy is seen for follow-up testing after 2 weeks. The serum free T_4 is normal but the TSH is still elevated. What is the most likely explanation for these results?
A. Laboratory error in measurement of free T_4
B. Laboratory error in measurement of TSH
C. In vitro drug interference with the free T_4 assay
D. Results are consistent with a euthyroid patient in the early phase of therapy

Chemistry/Evaluate laboratory data to explain inconsistent results/Endocrinology/3

43. SITUATION: A 6-year-old being treated with phenytoin was recently placed on valproic acid for better control of seizures. After the patient displayed signs of phenytoin toxicity, including ataxia, a *stat* phenytoin was determined to be 15.0 mg/L (reference range 10–20 mg/L). A peak blood level drawn 5 hours after the last dose is 18.0 mg/L. The valproic acid measured at the same time is within therapeutic limits. Quality control is within acceptable limits for all tests, but the accuracy of the results is questioned by the physician. What is the most appropriate next course of action?
A. Repeat the valproic acid level using the last specimen
B. Repeat the phenytoin on both trough and peak samples using a different method
C. Recommend measurement of free phenytoin using the last specimen

D. Recommend that a second trough level be measured

Chemistry/Evaluate laboratory data to explain inconsistent results/TDM/3

41. **D** The potassium and the calcium results are above and below physiological limit values, respectively. Although hemolysis could explain the high potassium, hemolysis does not cause a significant change in serum calcium. The wrong order of draw could result in the falsely low calcium value but would not be sufficient to cause a result that is incompatible with life (and does not explain a grossly elevated potassium level). The results and the condition of the tubes indicate that blood from a full tube collected in K_3 EDTA was added to the clot tube, chelating the calcium and increasing the potassium.

42. **D** Results of thyroid tests (especially in hospitalized patients) may sometimes appear discrepant because medications and nonthyroid illnesses can affect test results. The pituitary is slow to respond to thyroxine replacement, and 6–8 weeks are usually required before TSH levels fall back to normal. In the early stage of therapy the patient should be monitored according to the free T_4 result. This patient's free T_4 is normal, indicating that replacement therapy is adequate. The high TSH value sometimes seen in treated patients is referred to as *pituitary lag*.

43. **C** Phenytoin levels must be monitored closely because toxic drug levels can occur unexpectedly as a result of changing pharmacokinetics. Phenytoin follows a nonlinear rate of elimination, which means that clearance decreases as blood levels increase. At high blood levels, saturation of the hepatic hydroxylating enzymes can occur, causing an abrupt increase in the blood level from a small increase in dose. The drug half-life estimated from the two drug levels is approximately 15 hours, which is within the range expected for children, so decreased clearance is probably not the problem. Valproic acid competes with phenytoin for binding sites on albumin. Free phenytoin is the physiologically active fraction and is normally very low, so small changes in protein binding can cause a large change in free drug. For example, a 5% fall in protein binding caused by valproic acid can increase the free phenytoin level by 50%. This patient's free phenytoin level should be measured, and the dose of phenytoin reduced to produce a free drug level that is within the therapeutic range.

Na	K	Cl	HCO$_3$	BUN	Glucose	Creatinine	Uric Acid
140 mmol/L	3.6 mmol/L	100 mmol/L	28 mmol/L	130 mg/dL	110 mg/dL	1.2 mg/dL	4.8 mg/dL
148 mmol/L	4.2 mmol/L	110 mmol/L	24 mmol/L	135 mg/dL	86 mg/dL	0.8 mg/dL	3.9 mg/dL
138 mmol/L	4.0 mmol/L	105 mmol/L	22 mmol/L	142 mg/dL	190 mg/dL	1.0 mg/dL	4.6 mg/dL

44. The results above are obtained from three consecutive serum samples using an automated random access analyzer that samples directly from a bar-coded tube. Calibration and quality control performed at the start of the shift are within the acceptable range, and no error codes are reported by the analyzer for any tests on the three samples. Upon verification of results, what is the most appropriate course of action?

A. Report the results and proceed with other tests, since no analytical problems are noted

B. Repeat the controls before continuing with further testing but report the results

C. Check sample identification prior to reporting

D. Do not report BUN results for these patients or continue BUN testing

Chemistry/Evaluate laboratory data to explain inconsistent results/Automation/3

45. An α-fetoprotein (AFP) measured on a 30-year-old pregnant woman at approximately 12 weeks' gestation is 2.5 multiples of the median (MOM). What course of action is most appropriate?

A. Repeat the serum AFP in 2 weeks

B. Recommend AFP assay on amniotic fluid

C. Repeat the AFP using the same sample by another method

D. Repeat the AFP using the sample by the same method

Chemistry/Select course of action/AFP/3

Answers to Questions 44–45

44. D BUN is elevated five- to tenfold for three consecutive patients in the absence of any other laboratory evidence of renal disease. The glucose results show conclusively that the samples are not from the same patient. Therefore, the BUN results must be caused by a systematic error and should not be reported. Further testing for BUN should cease until the analytical components of the BUN assay are completely evaluated and the cause of these results is identified and corrected. This is demonstrated by successful recalibration and performance of controls within acceptable limits. Following this, the BUN assay should be repeated on the three samples along with all other specimens with a spurious BUN result that have occurred since the start of the shift.

45. A The analytical sensitivity of immunochemical AFP tests is approximately 5 ng/mL. The maternal serum AFP at 12 weeks' gestation is barely above the analytical detection limit. Therefore, to achieve the needed sensitivity, the test should be repeated at 14 weeks. If the result is still equal to or greater than 2.5 MOM, then ultrasound should be performed to verify last menstrual period dating. AFP normally first becomes detectable in maternal serum at week 12 and increases by 15% per week through the 26th week. Levels of 2.5 MOM or higher are associated with spina bifida but also occur in ventral wall and abdominal wall defects, fetal death, Turner's syndrome, trisomy 13, congenital hypothyroidism, tyrosinemia, and several other fetal conditions. A positive serum test should always be repeated, and if positive again, followed by ultrasound. If ultrasound does not explain the elevation, amniotic fluid testing, including AFP and acetylcholinesterase, is usually recommended.

	AST U/L	ALT U/L	ALP U/L	LD U/L	CK U/L	GGT U/L	TP g/dL	ALB g/dL	TBIL mg/dL	GLU mg/dL	TG mg/dL	CA mg/dL	InP mg/dL	BUN mg/dL
Day 1	20	15	40	100	15	40	8.2	3.6	0.8	84	140	8.7	4.2	16
Day 2	22	14	65	90	20	36	8.3	3.8	1.0	128	190	8.8	5.2	26

46. SITUATION: Biochemistry tests are performed 24 hours apart on a patient and a δ-check flag is reported for inorganic phosphorus by the laboratory information system. Given the results above, identify the most likely cause.

A. Results suggest altered metabolic status caused by poor insulin control

B. The patient was not fasting when the sample was collected on day 2

C. The samples were drawn from two different patients

D. The δ-check limit is invalid when samples are collected 24 or more hours apart

Chemistry/Evaluate data to determine possible sources of error/Automation/3

47. A quantitative sandwich enzyme immunoassay for intact serum hCG was performed on week 4 and the result was 40,000 mIU/mL (reference range 10,000–80,000 mIU/mL). The physician suspected a molar pregnancy and requested that the laboratory repeat the test checking for the hook effect. Which process would identify this problem?

A. Obtain a new plasma specimen and heat inactivate before testing

B. Obtain a urine specimen and perform the assay

C. Perform a qualitative pregnancy test

D. Perform a serial dilution of the sample and repeat the test

Chemistry/Identify sources of error/Immunoassay/2

48. A patient presents to the Emergency Department with symptoms of intoxication, including impaired speech and movement. The plasma osmolality was measured and found to be 330 mOsm/kg. The osmolal gap was 40 mOsm/kg. A blood alcohol level was measured by the alcohol dehydrogenase method and found to be 0.15% w/v (150 mg/dL). Electrolyte results showed an increased anion gap. Ethylene glycol intoxication was suspected because the osmolal gap was greater than could be explained by ethanol alone, but gas chromatography was not available. Which of the following would be abnormal if this suspicion proved correct?

A. Arterial blood gases

B. Lactic acid

C. Urinary ketones

D. Glucose

Chemistry/Select course of action/Toxicology/3

Answers to Questions 46–48

46. B The δ check compares the difference of the patient's two most recent laboratory results within a 3-day period to a δ limit usually determined as a percentage difference. The purpose of the δ check is to detect sample identification errors. A δ-check flag can also be caused by random analytical errors and interfering substances such as hemolysis, icterus, and lipemia, and by metabolic changes associated with disease or treatment. Therefore, results should be carefully considered before determining the cause. In this case, hemolysis and icterus can be ruled out because enzymes sensitive to hemolysis interference (AST, ALT, and LD) and bilirubin are within normal limits. Tests showing a significant difference are P_i, ALP, triglycerides, and glucose. These four tests are elevated by diet (the ALP from postprandial secretion of intestinal ALP). All other tests show a high level of agreement between days, and the differences are attributable to normal physiological and analytical variation.

47. D The hook effect is the result of excessive antigen concentration and results in a dose response (calibration) curve that reverses direction at very high antigen concentrations. It occurs in two-site double antibody sandwich assays when both the capture antibody and the enzyme-conjugated antibody are incubated with the antigen at the same time. The excess antigen saturates both antibodies, preventing formation of a double antibody sandwich. The hook effect can cause results to be sufficiently low as to cause misdiagnosis. It can be detected by diluting the sample (antigen), in which case the assay result will be greater than in the undiluted sample. An alternative solution is to perform the test using a competitive binding assay or a sandwich assay in which the enzyme-labeled antibody is not added until after separation of free and bound antigen.

48. A Ethylene glycol is sometimes used as a substitute for ethanol by alcoholics. It is metabolized to formic acid and glycolic acid by the liver resulting in metabolic acidosis and an increased anion gap. Lactic acid, glucose, and urinary ketones would be useful in ruling out other causes of metabolic acidosis but would not be abnormal as a result of ethylene glycol intoxication.

49. Given the serum protein electrophoresis pattern shown, which transaminase results would you expect?

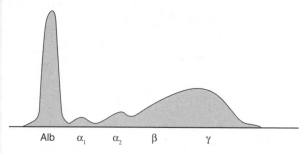

A. Within normal limits for both
B. Marked elevation of both (20- to 50-fold normal)
C. Mild elevations of both (two- to five-fold normal)
D. Marked increase of AST but normal ALT

Chemistry/Correlate laboratory results/Liver disease/2

50. Serial troponin I assays are ordered on a patient at admission and 3 and 6 hours afterwards. The samples were collected in heparinized plasma separator tubes. The results are shown below (reference range 0–0.04 μg/L)

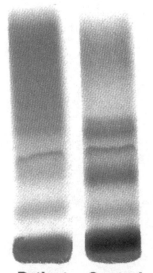

Admission	3 hours	6 hours
0.04 μg/L	0.07 μg/L	0.04 μg/L

These results indicate

A. A positive test for acute myocardial infarction
B. Unstable angina
C. Cardiac injury of severity less than myocardial infarction
D. Random error with the 3-hour sample

Chemistry/Identify sources of error/Immunoassay/2

Answers to Questions 49–50

49. **C** The protein electrophoresis and densitometric scan show a significantly reduced albumin and polyclonal gammopathy. The densitometric scan shows beta-gamma bridging that supports a diagnosis of hepatic cirrhosis. In this condition one would expect two- to fivefold increases of both transaminases with an ALT:AST ratio below 1.

50. **D** Troponin assays produce very little fluorescence or chemiluminescence when plasma levels are within the reference range and near the minimum detection limit of the assay. Fibrin, tube additives, and heterophile antibodies have been known to cause spurious elevations, and this result should be treated as a random error, since the result before and after are both normal.

BIBLIOGRAPHY

1. Anderson, S.C., and Cockayne, S: *Clinical Chemistry Concepts and Applications.* . McGraw Hill, New York, 2003.
2. Bennington, J.L. (ed): *Dictionary and Encyclopedia of Laboratory Medicine and Technology.* W.B. Saunders, Philadelphia. 1984.
3. Bishop, M.L., Duben-Engelkirk, J.L., and Fody, E.P: *Clinical Chemistry Principles, Procedures, and Correlations,* ed 5., Lippincott Williams and Wilkins, Philadelphia, 2005.
4. Burtis, C.A., Ashwood, E.R., and Burns, D. E. (eds): *Tietz Textbook of Clinical Chemistry* and Molecular Diagnostics, ed 4. Elsevier Saunders, St. Louis, 2006.
5. Henry, J.B. (ed): *Clinical Diagnosis and Management by Laboratory Methods,* ed 20. W. B. Saunders, Philadelphia, 2001.
6. Kaplan, L.A., and Pesce, A.J. (eds): *Clinical Chemistry Theory Analysis and Correlation,* ed 4. C.V. Mosby, St. Louis, 2003.

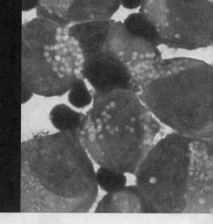

CHAPTER **6**

Urinalysis and Body Fluids

6.1   ROUTINE PHYSICAL AND BIOCHEMICAL URINE TESTS

6.2   URINE MICROSCOPY AND CLINICAL CORRELATIONS

6.3   CEREBROSPINAL, SEROUS, AND SYNOVIAL FLUIDS

6.4   AMNIOTIC, GASTROINTESTINAL, AND SEMINAL FLUIDS

6.5   BODY FLUIDS PROBLEM SOLVING

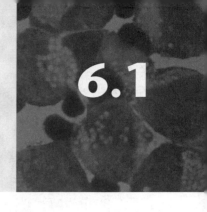

ROUTINE PHYSICAL AND BIOCHEMICAL URINE TESTS

6.1

1. **Which statement below regarding renal function is true?**
   A. Glomeruli are far more permeable to H_2O and salt than other capillaries
   B. The collecting tubule reabsorbs sodium and secretes potassium in response to antidiuretic hormone (ADH)
   C. The collecting tubule is permeable to H_2O only in the presence of aldosterone
   D. The thick ascending limb is highly permeable to H_2O and urea

   Body fluids/Apply knowledge of fundamental biological characteristics/Urine/1

2. **Which statement regarding normal salt and H_2O handling by the nephron is correct?**
   A. The ascending limb of the tubule is highly permeable to salt but not to H_2O
   B. The stimulus for ADH release is low arterial pressure in the afferent arteriole
   C. The descending limb of the tubule is impermeable to urea but highly permeable to salt
   D. Renin is released in response to high plasma osmolality

   Body fluids/Apply knowledge of fundamental biological characteristics/Urine/1

3. **Which statement concerning renal tubular function is true?**
   A. In salt deprivation the kidneys conserve sodium at the expense of potassium
   B. Potassium is not excreted when serum concentration is below 3.5 mmol/L
   C. No substance can be excreted into urine at a rate that exceeds the glomerular filtration rate
   D. When tubular function is lost, the specific gravity of urine will be below 1.005

   Body fluids/Correlate laboratory data with physiological processes/Urine electrolytes/2

Answers to Questions 1–3

1. **A** The formation of plasma ultrafiltrate depends upon high hydrostatic pressure and permeability of the glomeruli. Aldosterone is released when effective arterial pressure falls, and ADH when plasma osmolality becomes too high. The collecting tubule reabsorbs sodium and secretes potassium in response to aldosterone and is permeable to H_2O only in the presence of ADH. The thick ascending limb is permeable to salt but not to H_2O or urea.

2. **A** The tubules are able to concentrate the filtrate because the descending limb is highly permeable to H_2O and urea but not to salt and the ascending limb is permeable to salt. Salt leaving the ascending limb creates a hypertonic interstitium that forces H_2O from the descending limb. Renin is released in response to low hydrostatic pressure in the afferent arteriole, which stimulates the juxtaglomerular cells. ADH is released by the posterior pituitary in response to high plasma osmolality.

3. **A** Sodium is a threshold substance, meaning that no sodium will be excreted in the urine until the renal threshold (a plasma sodium concentration of approximately 120 mmol/L) is exceeded. Potassium is not a threshold substance and will be secreted by the tubules even when plasma potassium levels are low. Patients on diuretics or who have hypovolemia become hypokalemic for this reason. Some substances (e.g., penicillin) can be excreted at a rate exceeding glomerular filtration because the tubules secrete them. The tubules are responsible for concentrating the filtrate in conditions of water deprivation and diluting it in conditions of water excess. When tubular function is lost, salt and water equilibrate by passive diffusion and the specific gravity of the urine becomes the same as the plasma, approximately 1.010.

4. Which of the following is inappropriate when collecting urine for routine bacteriological culture?
  A. The container must be sterile
  B. The midstream void technique must be used
  C. The collected sample must be plated within 2 hours unless refrigerated
  D. The sample may be held at 2°C–8°C for up to 48 hours prior to plating

Body fluids/Apply knowledge to identify sources of error/Specimen collecting and handling/2

5. Which statement about sample collection for routine urinalysis is true?
  A. Preservative tablets should be used for collecting random urine specimens
  B. Containers may be washed and reused if rinsed in deionized H_2O
  C. Samples may be stored at room temperature for up to 2 hours
  D. Random samples are acceptable when renal disease is suspected

Body fluids/Apply knowledge to identify sources of error/Specimen collection and handling/2

6. Which urine color is correlated correctly with the pigment-producing substance?
  A. Smoky red urine with homogentisic acid
  B. Dark amber urine with myoglobin
  C. Deep yellow urine and yellow foam with bilirubin
  D. Red-brown urine with biliverdin

Body fluids/Correlate laboratory data with physiological processes/Urine color/2

7. Which of the following substances will cause urine to produce red fluorescence when examined with an ultraviolet lamp (360 nm)?
  A. Myoglobin
  B. Porphobilinogen (PBG)
  C. Urobilin
  D. Coproporphyrin

Body fluids/Correlate clinical and laboratory data/Urine porphyrins/2

8. Which of the conditions below is associated with normal urine color but produces red fluorescence when urine is examined with an ultraviolet (Wood's) lamp?
  A. Acute intermittent porphyria
  B. Lead poisoning
  C. Erythropoietic porphyria
  D. Porphyria cutanea tarda

Body fluids/Correlate clinical and laboratory data/Urine color/2

Answers to Questions 4–8

4. **D** Urine specimens should be plated and incubated within 2 hours of collection (some laboratories use a 1-hour time limit), and within 24 hours if the sample is refrigerated at 2°– 8°C immediately following collection. No additives are permitted when urine is collected for culture.

5. **D** The first morning voided sample is the most sensitive for screening purposes because formed elements are concentrated, but random samples are satisfactory because glomerular bleeding, albuminuria, and cast formation may occur at any time. Preservative tablets should be avoided because they may cause chemical interference with some dry reagent strip and turbidimetric protein tests. Samples should be refrigerated if not tested within 30 min of collection.

6. **C** Homogentisic acid causes a dark-brown or black-colored urine. Myoglobin causes a red to red-brown color in urine, and biliverdin causes a green or yellow-green color. In addition to metabolic diseases and renal disease, abnormal color can be caused by drugs (e.g., Gantrisin), dyes excreted by the kidneys (e.g., phenolsulfonphthalein [PSP]), and natural or artificial food coloring (e.g., beets).

7. **D** Myoglobin causes a positive test for blood but does not cause urine to fluoresce. PBG causes urine to become dark (orange to orange-brown) on standing but does not fluoresce. It reacts with *p*-dimethylaminobenzaldehyde (Watson-Schwartz test) and is not extracted into butanol or chloroform. Uroporphyrin and coproporphyrin produce red or orange-red fluorescence. Unlike hemoglobin, porphyrins lack peroxidase activity. Urobilin is an oxidation product of urobilinogen. It turns the urine orange to orange-brown but does not produce fluorescence.

8. **B** Lead poisoning blocks the synthesis of heme, causing accumulation of PBG and coproporphyrin III in urine. However, uroporphyrin levels are not sufficiently elevated to cause red pigmentation of the urine. There is sufficient coproporphyrin to cause a positive test for fluorescence. Acute intermittent porphyria is the most common inherited porphyria and produces increased urinary delta-aminolevulinic acid (Δ-ALA); and PBG. The PBG turns the urine orange to orange-brown on standing. Erythropoietic porphyria and porphyria cutanea tarda produce large amounts of uroporphyrin, causing the urine to turn red or port wine–colored.

9. A brown or black pigment in urine can be caused by:
  A. Gantrisin (Pyridium)
  B. Phenolsulfonphthalein
  C. Rifampin
  D. Melanin

Body fluids/Correlate clinical and laboratory data/Urine color/2

10. Urine that is dark red or port wine in color may be caused by:
  A. Lead poisoning
  B. Porphyria cutanea tarda
  C. Alkaptonuria
  D. Hemolytic anemia

Body fluids/Correlate clinical and laboratory data/Urine color/2

11. Which of the following tests is affected least by standing or improperly stored urine?
  A. Glucose
  B. Protein
  C. pH
  D. Bilirubin

Body fluids/Apply knowledge to identify sources of error/Urine/Specimen collection and handling/2

12. Which type of urine sample is needed for a D-xylose absorption test on an adult patient?
  A. 24-hour urine sample collected with 20 mL of 6 N HCl
  B. 2-hour timed postprandial urine preserved with boric acid
  C. 5-hour timed urine kept under refrigeration
  D. Random urine preserved with formalin

Body fluids/Apply principles of basic laboratory procedures/Urine/Specimen collection and handling/2

13. Which of the following is inappropriate when collecting a 24-hour urine sample for catecholamines?
  A. Urine in the bladder is voided and discarded at the start of the test
  B. At 24 hours any urine in the bladder is voided and added to the collection
  C. All urine should be collected in a single container that is kept refrigerated
  D. Hydrochloric acid (HCl) is added to the container after the 24-hour urine volume is measured

Body fluids/Apply knowledge to identify sources of error/Urinary catecholamines/2

14. Urine production of less than 400 mL/day is:
  A. Consistent with normal renal function and H_2O balance
  B. Termed isosthenuria
  C. Defined as oliguria
  D. Associated with diabetes mellitus

Body fluids/Correlate clinical and laboratory data/Urine volume/2

9. **D** Excretion of melanin in malignant melanoma and homogentisic acid in alkaptonuria causes the urine to turn black on standing. Other substances that may cause brown or black-colored urine are methemoglobin, PBG, porphobilin, and urobilin. Gantrisin, PSP dye, and rifampin are three examples of drugs that cause a red or orange-red color in urine.

10. **B** Porphyria cutanea tarda and erythropoietic porphyria produce sufficient uroporphyrins to cause dark-red urine. Acute intermittent porphyria produces large amounts of PBG, which may be oxidized to porphobilin, turning the urine orange to orange-brown.

11. **B** Standing urine may become alkaline as a result of loss of volatile acids and ammonia production. Bilirubin glucuronides may become hydrolyzed to unconjugated bilirubin or oxidized to biliverdin, resulting in a false-negative dry reagent strip test. Glucose can be consumed by glycolysis or oxidation by cells.

12. **C** The D-xylose absorption test is used to distinguish pancreatic insufficiency from intestinal malabsorption. The test requires a blood sample taken 2 hours after oral administration of 25 g of D-xylose and a 5-hour timed urine sample. D-xylose is absorbed without the aid of pancreatic enzymes and is not metabolized by the liver. Therefore, deficient absorption (denoted by a plasma level <25 mg/dL and urine excretion of <4g/5 hours) points to malabsorption syndrome. Tests requiring a 24-hour urine sample include catecholamines, vanillyl mandelic acid (VMA), metanephrines, cortisol, and estriol.

13. **D** When collecting a 24-hour urine sample, the bladder must be emptied of urine at the start of the test and discarded. The bladder must be emptied at the conclusion of the test and the urine added to the collection. In order to prevent degradation of catecholamines (also VMA, metanephrines, and cortisol) during storage, the urine should be kept at or below pH 2. HCl (10 mL of 6 N HCl) must be added to the container prior to the collection to prevent oxidative loss of these analytes.

14. **C** Normal daily urine excretion is usually 600–1600 mL/day. Isosthenuria refers to urine of constant specific gravity (SG) of 1.010, which is the SG of the glomerular filtrate. Glycosuria causes retention of H_2O within the tubule, resulting in dehydration and polyuria rather than oliguria.

15. Which of the following contributes to SG but not to osmolality?
  A. Protein
  B. Salt
  C. Urea
  D. Glucose

Body fluids/Evaluate laboratory data to determine possible inconsistent results/Specific gravity/2

16. Urine with a SG consistently between 1.002 and 1.003 indicates:
  A. Acute glomerulonephritis
  B. Renal tubular failure
  C. Diabetes insipidus
  D. Addison's disease

Body fluids/Evaluate laboratory data to recognize health and disease states/Specific gravity/2

17. In which of the following conditions is the urine SG likely to be below 1.025?
  A. Diabetes mellitus
  B. Drug overdose
  C. Chronic renal failure
  D. Prerenal failure

Body fluids/Evaluate data to recognize health and disease states/Specific gravity/2

18. Which statement below regarding methods for measuring SG is true?
  A. To correct a urinometer subtract 0.001 per each 3°C below 15.5°C
  B. Colorimetric SG tests are falsely elevated when a large quantity of glucose is present
  C. Colorimetric SG readings are falsely elevated when pH is alkaline
  D. Refractometry should be performed before the urine is centrifuged

Body fluids/Apply knowledge to identify sources of error/Specific gravity/2

19. What is the principle of the colorimetric reagent strip determination of SG in urine?
  A. Ionic strength alters the pK_a of a polyelectrolyte
  B. Sodium and other cations are chelated by a ligand that changes color
  C. Anions displace a pH indicator from a mordant, making it water-soluble
  D. Ionized solutes catalyze oxidation of an azo dye

Body fluids/Apply principles of basic laboratory procedures/Specific gravity/1

Answers to Questions 15–19

15. **A** All substances that dissolve in the urine contribute to osmotic pressure or osmolality. This includes nonionized solutes such as urea, uric acid, and glucose as well as salts but not colloids such as protein and lipids.

16. **C** In severe renal diseases the tubules fail to concentrate the filtrate. Salt and H_2O equilibrate by diffusion, causing an SG of about 1.010. If the SG of urine is below that of plasma, free H_2O is lost. This results from failure to produce ADH (diabetes insipidus) or scarring of the renal medulla, as occurs in chronic renal failure.

17. **C** Glucose and drug metabolites increase the SG of urine. In prerenal failure the tubules are undamaged. Ineffective arterial pressure stimulates aldosterone release. This increases sodium reabsorption, which stimulates ADH release. Water and salt are retained, and the urine-plasma osmolar ratio (U:P) exceeds 2:1. Chronic renal failure is associated with nocturia, polyuria, and low SG caused by scarring of the collecting tubules.

18. **A** The density of urine increases at low temperature, causing less fluid to be displaced by the urinometer. This causes the specific gravity to be falsely elevated unless corrected for the difference between the urine temperature and the calibration temperature (15.5°C). Cells and undissolved solutes refract light and cause a falsely high specific gravity reading by refractometry if urine is not centrifuged. Colorimetric specific gravity tests are less sensitive to nonionized compounds such as urea and glucose and are negatively biased when large quantities of nonelectrolytes are present. Colorimetric specific gravity readings are determined by a pH change on the test pad and are approximately 0.005 lower when pH is 6.5 or higher.

19. **A** A polyelectrolyte with malic acid residues will ionize in proportion to the ionic strength of urine. This causes the pH indicator, bromthymol blue, to react as if it were in a more acidic solution. The indicator is blue at low SG and green at higher SG.

20. Which statement below regarding urine pH is true?
- **A.** High-protein diets promote an alkaline urine pH
- **B.** pH tends to decrease as urine is stored
- **C.** Contamination should be suspected if urine pH is less than 4.5
- **D.** Bacteriuria is most often associated with a low urine pH

Body fluids/Correlate clinical and laboratory data/Urine pH/2

21. In renal tubular acidosis the pH of urine is:
- **A.** Consistently acid
- **B.** Consistently alkaline
- **C.** Neutral
- **D.** Variable, depending upon diet

Body fluids/Correlate clinical and laboratory data/Urine pH/2

22. The normal daily urine output for an adult is approximately:
- **A.** 0.2–0.5 L
- **B.** 0.6–1.6 L
- **C.** 2.7–3.0 L
- **D.** 3.2–3.5 L

Body fluids/Apply knowledge of fundamental biological characteristics/Urine/1

23. The SG of the filtrate in Bowman's space is approximately:
- **A.** 1.000–1.002
- **B.** 1.004–1.006
- **C.** 1.008–1.010
- **D.** 1.012–1.014

Body fluids/Apply knowledge of fundamental biological characteristics/Urine/1

24. A patient with partially compensated respiratory alkalosis would have a urine pH of:
- **A.** 4.5–5.5
- **B.** 5.5–6.5
- **C.** 6.5–7.5
- **D.** 7.5–8.5

Body fluids/Correlate clinical and laboratory data/Urine pH/2

25. Which of the following is most likely to cause a false-positive dry reagent strip test for protein?
- **A.** Urine of high SG
- **B.** Highly buffered alkaline urine
- **C.** Bence Jones proteinuria
- **D.** Salicylates

Body fluids/Apply knowledge to identify sources of error/Urinary protein/2

20. **C** Bacteriuria is usually associated with an alkaline pH caused by the production of ammonia from urea. Extended storage may result in loss of volatile acids, causing increased pH. A high-protein diet promotes excretion of inorganic acids. The tubular maximum for H^+ secretion occurs when urine pH reaches 4.5, the lowest urinary pH that the kidneys can produce.

21. **B** Renal tubular acidosis results from a defect in the renal tubular reabsorption of bicarbonate. Hydrogen ions are not secreted when bicarbonate ions are not reabsorbed. Wasting of sodium bicarbonate ($NaHCO_3$) and potassium bicarbonate ($KHCO_3$) results in alkaline urine and hypokalemia in association with acidosis.

22. **B** Under conditions of normal fluid intake, the reference range for urine volume is 0.6–1.6 L per day. Urine output varies widely with fluid intake. In cases of fluid deprivation, almost all filtrate is reabsorbed, resulting in daily excretion as low as 500 mL. When fluid intake is excessive, up to 2.0 L of urine may be voided. Urine output beyond these extremes is considered abnormal.

23. **C** The SG of the filtrate in Bowman's space approximates the SG of the plasma because sodium, chloride, glucose, urea, and other main solutes are completely filtered by the glomeruli. This corresponds to an osmolality of approximately 280 mOsm/kg.

24. **D** Urine pH is determined by diet, acid-base balance, water balance, and renal function. In partially compensated respiratory alkalosis, the kidneys reabsorb less bicarbonate, which results in lower net acid excretion. The loss of bicarbonate helps to compensate for alkalosis and causes urine pH to be alkaline.

25. **B** In addition to highly buffered alkaline urine, a false-positive dry reagent test may be caused by quaternary ammonium compounds that increase urine pH. Because the dry reagent strip tests are insensitive to globulins, a false-negative reaction is likely in the case of Bence Jones proteinuria. Positive interference by drugs is uncommon for dry reagent strip protein tests but is common for turbidimetric tests. High urinary SG suppresses the color reaction of the strip protein tests.

26. When testing for urinary protein with sulfosalicylic acid (SSA), which condition may produce a false-positive result?
    A. Highly buffered alkaline urine
    B. The presence of x-ray contrast media
    C. Increased urinary SG
    D. The presence of red blood cells (RBCs)

    Body fluids/Apply knowledge to identify sources of error/Urinary protein/2

27. A discrepancy between the urine SG determined by measuring refractive index and urine osmolality would be most likely to occur:
    A. After catheterization of the urinary tract
    B. In diabetes mellitus
    C. After an intravenous pyelogram (IVP)
    D. In uremia

    Body fluids/Evaluate data to determine possible inconsistent results/Specific gravity/2

28. Which of the following is likely to result in a false-negative dry reagent strip test for proteinuria?
    A. Penicillin
    B. Aspirin
    C. Amorphous phosphates
    D. Bence Jones protein

    Body fluids/Apply knowledge to identify sources of error/Urinary protein/1

29. Daily loss of protein in urine normally does not exceed:
    A. 30 mg
    B. 50 mg
    C. 100 mg
    D. 150 mg

    Body fluids/Apply knowledge of fundamental biological characteristics/Urinary protein/1

30. Which of the following is *LEAST* likely to cause a false-positive result with turbidimetric protein tests?
    A. Tolbutamide
    B. X-ray contrast media
    C. Penicillin or sulfa antibiotics
    D. Ascorbic acid

    Body fluids/Apply knowledge to identify sources of error/Urinary protein/2

Answers to Questions 26–30

26. **B** Turbidimetric assays are used to test urine suspected of giving a false-positive dry reagent strip test for albumin because the urine is highly alkaline (pH≥8.0) or contains pigmentation that interferes with reading the protein test pad. In addition, SSA tests are used when screening urine for an increased concentration of globulins because dry reagent strip tests are insensitive to globulins. SSA is less specific but more sensitive for albuminuria than dry reagent strip tests. Iodinated dyes, penicillin, salicylate, and tolbutamide may result in false-positive results. Trace turbidity is difficult to determine when urine is cloudy due to bacteriuria, mucus, or crystals. Alkaline urine may titrate SSA, reducing its sensitivity.

27. **C** The IVP dye contains iodine and is highly refractile. This increases the refractive index of urine, causing falsely high measurement of solute concentration. Refractive index is affected by the size and shape of solutes and undissolved solids such as protein. Osmolality is the most specific measure of total solute concentration because it is affected only by the number of dissolved solutes.

28. **D** Dry reagent strip tests using tetrabromphenol blue or tetrachlorophenol tetrabromosulfophthalein are insensitive to globulins and may not detect immunoglobulin light chains. Turbidimetric methods such as 3% SSA often detect Bence Jones protein but may give a false-positive reaction with penicillin, tolbutamide, salicylates, and x-ray contrast dyes containing iodine. Amorphous phosphates may precipitate in refrigerated urine, making interpretation of turbidimetric tests difficult.

29. **D** Small amounts of albumin and other low-molecular-weight proteins such as amylase, β-microglobulins, and immunoglobulin fragments are excreted in the urine. Proteinuria does not normally exceed 30 mg/dL or 150 mg/day. The detection limit of the SSA test to albumin is approximately 1.5 mg/dL and for dry reagent strip tests approximately 15 mg/dL. Therefore trace positives by either method may occur in the absence of renal disease.

30. **D** Ascorbic acid may reduce diazo salts used in the bilirubin and nitrite tests and react with hydrogen peroxide in peroxidase reactions. Therefore, persons taking megadoses of ascorbic acid (vitamin C) may show interference with tests for glucose, blood, bilirubin, and nitrite. Ascorbate does not cause either a false-negative or false-positive reaction for protein.

31. Which statement best describes the clinical utility of tests for microalbuminuria?
   A. Testing may detect early renal involvement in diabetes mellitus
   B. Microalbuminuria refers to a specific subfraction of albumin found only in persons with diabetic nephropathy
   C. A positive test result indicates the presence of orthostatic albuminuria
   D. Testing should be part of the routine urinalysis

Body fluids/Correlate clinical and laboratory data/Urinary protein/2

32. Dry reagent strip tests for microalbuminuria that compare albumin to creatinine determine the creatinine concentration based upon which principle?
   A. Creatinine binds to Cu^{2+}, forming a complex with peroxidase-like activity
   B. The sarcosine oxidase reaction coupled to the peroxidase reaction
   C. Reaction of creatinine with alkaline sodium picrate
   D. Change in pH as creatinine is converted to creatine

Body Fluids/Apply principles of special laboratory procedures/Urine protein/2

33. Which of the conditions below is *LEAST* likely to be detected by dry reagent strip tests for proteinuria?
   A. Orthostatic albuminuria
   B. Chronic renal failure
   C. Pyelonephritis
   D. Renal tubular proteinuria

Body fluids/Apply principles of basic laboratory procedures/Urine protein/2

34. The normal renal threshold for glucose is:
   A. 70–85 mg/dL
   B. 100–115 mg/dL
   C. 130–145 mg/dL
   D. 165–180 mg/dL

Body fluids/Apply knowledge of fundamental biological characteristics/Urine glucose/1

31. **A** The microalbumin test is an assay for measuring urinary albumin concentration that has an increased sensitivity (detection limit below 15 mg/dL), and is recommended for persons who are at risk for chronic renal disease, especially those with diabetes mellitus. In diabetes, an early sign of renal involvement is an increased rate of albumin excretion in the range of 20–200 µg/mL or in excess of 30 mg albumin per gram creatinine. Results in this range are significant in the at-risk population, even though the dry reagent strip test for protein may be negative. Consequently, dry reagent strip tests for microalbuminuria are too sensitive for use in routine urinalysis but are useful in screening persons with diabetes and hypertension for increased urinary albumin excretion.

32. **A** The dry reagent strip test for creatinine contains anhydrous buffered $CuIISO_4$, alcoholic tetramethylbenzidine, and diisopropyl benzene dihydroperoxide. In the presence of creatinine, a copper-creatinine complex forms. This catalyzes the oxidation of a benzidine derivative by an alcoholic peroxide, forming a blue color on the test pad. Color intensity is proportional to creatinine concentration. Negative interference occurs from ascorbate and EDTA (which chelates the copper). Positive interference occurs from hemoglobin and some drugs (e.g., nitrofurantoin antibiotics). The microalbumin concentration is determined by the protein error of indicator effect using a dye with increased sensitivity, bis-tetrabromosulfonepithalein.

33. **D** The detection limit (sensitivity) of dry reagent strip protein tests is approximately 15 mg/dL albumin and is sufficient to detect urinary albumin levels found in orthostatic albuminuria and renal diseases, with the exception of tubular proteinuria. Renal tubular proteinuria results from failure of damaged tubules to reabsorb β-microglobulin. Dry reagent strip tests for proteinuria are insensitive to globulins and do not detect small quantities of hemoglobin, myoglobin, or microglobulins. Protein electrophoresis is used to detect $β_2$-microglobulinuria.

34. **D** The renal threshold is the concentration of a substance (e.g., glucose) in blood that must be exceeded before it can be detected in the urine. Threshold substances require a carrier to transport them from the tubular lumen to the vasa recta. When the carrier becomes saturated the tubular maximum is reached, causing the substance to be excreted in the urine.

35. In which of the following conditions is glycosuria most likely?
  A. Addison's disease
  B. Hypothyroidism
  C. Pregnancy
  D. Hypopituitarism

Body fluids/Correlate clinical and laboratory data/Urine glucose/2

36. In addition to ascorbate, the glucose oxidase reaction may be inhibited by which substance?
  A. Acetoacetic acid (AAA)
  B. ε-Aminocaproic acid
  C. Creatinine
  D. Azopyridium

Body fluids/Apply knowledge to identify sources of error/Urine glucose/1

37. A positive glucose oxidase test and a negative test for reducing sugars indicate:
  A. True glycosuria
  B. False-positive reagent strip test
  C. False-negative reducing test caused by ascorbate
  D. Galactosuria

Body fluids/Evaluate laboratory data to determine possible inconsistent results/Urine glucose/2

38. A negative glucose oxidase test and a positive test for reducing sugars in urine indicate:
  A. True glycosuria
  B. A false-negative glucose oxidase reaction
  C. The presence of a nonglucose reducing sugar such as galactose
  D. A trace quantity of glucose

Body fluids/Evaluate laboratory data to determine possible inconsistent results/Urine glucose/2

39. In what condition may urinary ketone tests underestimate ketosis?
  A. Acidosis
  B. Hemolytic anemia
  C. Renal failure
  D. Excessive use of vitamin C

Body fluids/Apply knowledge to identify sources of error/Urinary ketones/2

40. AAA is detected in urine by reaction with:
  A. Sodium nitroprusside
  B. *o*-Toluidine
  C. *m*-Dinitrobenzene
  D. *m*-Dinitrophenylhydrazine

Body fluids/Apply principles of basic laboratory procedures/Urinary ketones/1

Answers to Questions 35–40

35. **C** In addition to diabetes mellitus, glycosuria may occur in other endocrine diseases, pregnancy, in response to drugs that affect glucose tolerance or renal threshold, and in several other conditions, especially those involving the liver or central nervous system (CNS). Cushing's disease and hyperthyroidism cause impaired glucose tolerance and cause hyperglycemia. Increased estrogens produced in pregnancy lower the renal threshold for glucose and may impair glucose tolerance. Hyperpituitarism causes hyperglycemia mediated by increased release of growth hormone.

36. **A** AAA and salicylates may inhibit the glucose oxidase reaction by the same mechanism as ascorbate. These reducing agents compete with the chromogen for hydrogen peroxide. Low SG may increase and high SG decrease the color reaction for glucose in urine.

37. **A** Glucose oxidase is specific for β-D-glucose. Therefore a positive reaction is always considered significant unless contamination is evident. A reducing test should not be used to confirm a positive glucose oxidase test because it is not as specific or as sensitive. Reducing sugar tests are used to screen infants for inborn errors of carbohydrate metabolism such as galactosuria but are not used to screen for glycosuria.

38. **C** Reducing tests utilize alkaline copper sulfate and heat to oxidize glucose. Other reducing substances, including several sugars and antibiotics, may react, making the test inappropriate as a screening test for glucose. A positive test for reducing sugars seen with a negative glucose oxidase test may occur in lactose, galactose, fructosuria, and other disorders of carbohydrate metabolism.

39. **A** Tests for urinary ketone bodies are sensitive to AAA. They react weakly with acetone and do not react with β-hydroxybutyric acid. Acidosis favors formation of β-hydroxybutyric acid and may cause a falsely low estimate of serum or urine ketones in diabetic ketoacidosis. Ketonuria has many causes other than diabetic ketoacidosis, such as pregnancy, fever, protein calorie malnutrition, and dietary carbohydrate restriction. Trace ketones tend to be more clinically significant when seen in urine with a low specific gravity.

40. **A** Urinary ketones are detected using alkaline sodium nitroprusside or nitroferricyanide. L-Dopa may cause a false-positive reaction with the former and phenylpyruvic acid (PKU) and some antibiotics with the latter.

41. Nondiabetic ketonuria can occur in all of the following *except*:
   A. Pregnancy
   B. Renal failure
   C. Starvation
   D. Lactate acidosis

Body fluids/Correlate clinical and laboratory data/ Urinary ketones/2

42. Which of the following statements regarding the tablet (Acetest) and classic nitroprusside reaction for ketones is true?
   A. The reaction is most sensitive to acetone
   B. Nitroprusside reacts with acetone, AAA, and β-hydroxybutyric acid
   C. It may be falsely positive in phenylketonuria
   D. The reaction is recommended for diagnosing ketoacidosis

Body fluids/Apply knowledge to identify sources of error/ Urinary ketones/2

43. Hemoglobin in urine can be differentiated from myoglobin using:
   A. 80% ammonium sulfate to precipitate hemoglobin
   B. Sodium dithionite to reduce hemoglobin
   C. *o*-Dianisidine instead of benzidine as the color indicator
   D. Microscopic examination

Body fluids/Select methods/Hemoglobinuria/2

44. Which of the following conditions is associated with a negative blood test and an increase in urine urobilinogen?
   A. Calculi of the kidney or bladder
   B. Malignancy of the kidney or urinary system
   C. Crush injury
   D. Extravascular hemolytic anemia

Body fluids/Correlate clinical and laboratory data/ Hematuria/2

45. Which statement about the dry reagent strip blood test is true?
   A. The test is based on the reaction of hemoglobin with peroxidase
   B. Abnormal color may be absent from the urine when the reaction is positive
   C. A nonhemolyzed trace is present when there are 1–2 RBCs per high power field
   D. Salicylates cause a false-positive reaction

Body Fluids/Apply principles of basic laboratory procedures/Hematuria/2

41. B Ketonuria results from excessive oxidation of fats forming acetyl coenzyme A (CoA). In addition to diabetes mellitus, ketonuria occurs in starvation, carbohydrate restriction, alkalosis, lactate acidosis, and von Gierke's disease (glycogen stores cannot be utilized). Ketonuria also occurs in pregnancy and is associated with increased vomiting and cyclic fever.

42. C The tablet nitroprusside test is sensitive to 5–10 mg/dL AAA. Both tablet and dry reagent strip tests for ketones are less sensitive to acetone than AAA and do not detect β-hydroxybutyric acid. High levels of phenylpyruvic acid (phenylketonuria) cause a false-positive reaction in the tablet and classic nitroprusside reactions but do not usually interfere with the dry reagent strip test for ketones. Serum ketones can be measured by gas chromatography, and β-hydroxybutyric acid can be measured enzymatically. The enzymatic assay for β-hydroxybutyrate in plasma is the recommended test for diagnosing ketoacidosis, since acidosis favors its formation.

43. A Both hemoglobin and myoglobin have peroxidase activity and cause a positive blood test. However, myoglobin is soluble in 80% w/v ammonium sulfate in urine, but hemoglobin precipitates. A positive blood reaction with supernatant after addition of ammonium sulfate and sodium hydroxide (NaOH) confirms the presence of myoglobin.

44. D A positive test for blood can occur from renal or lower urinary tract bleeding, intravascular hemolytic anemia, and transfusion reaction. Extravascular hemolysis results in increased bilirubin production rather than plasma hemoglobin. This may cause increased urobilinogen in urine but not a positive blood reaction.

45. B The blood reaction uses anhydrous peroxide and benzidine. Hemoglobin has peroxidase activity and catalyzes the oxidation of benzidine by peroxide. The reaction is sensitive to submilligram levels of free hemoglobin, whereas visible hemolysis does not occur unless free hemoglobin exceeds 20 mg/dL. The test detects approximately 4–5 intact RBCs per high power field as a nonhemolyzed trace. More than 3 RBCs/high power field is abnormal.

46. A moderate-positive blood test and trace protein test are seen on the dry reagent strip, and 11–20 red blood cells per high power field are seen in the microscopic examination. These results are most likely caused by which of the following?
- **A.** Transfusion reaction
- **B.** Myoglobinuria
- **C.** Intravascular hemolytic anemia
- **D.** Recent urinary tract catheterization

Body Fluids/Correlate clinical and laboratory data/ Hematuria/3

47. Which of the following results are discrepant?
- **A.** Small blood but negative protein
- **B.** Moderate blood but no RBCs in microscopic examination
- **C.** Negative blood but 6–10 RBCs/high power field
- **D.** Negative blood, positive protein

Body Fluids/Apply knowledge to recognize sources of error/Hematuria/3

48. Which of the following statements regarding the dry reagent strip test for bilirubin is true?
- **A.** A positive test is seen in prehepatic, hepatic, and posthepatic jaundice
- **B.** The test detects only conjugated bilirubin
- **C.** Standing urine may become falsely positive as a result of bacterial contamination
- **D.** High levels of ascorbate cause positive interference

Body fluids/Apply knowledge to recognize sources of error/Urine bilirubin/2

46. **D** The blood test detects intact RBCs, hemoglobinuria, and myoglobinuria. Causes of hemoglobinuria include intravascular hemolytic anemias, transfusion reactions, and lysis of RBCs in the filtrate or urine caused by alkaline or hypotonic conditions. Causes of hematuria include acute and chronic glomerulonephritis, pyelonephritis, polycystic kidney disease, renal calculi, bladder and renal cancer, and postcatheterization of the urinary tract.

47. **C** The blood test detects as little as 0.015 mg/dL free hemoglobin and 5 RBCs/μL. The protein test detects 15 mg/dL albumin but substantially more hemoglobin is required to give a positive test. Therefore, a small blood reaction (nonhemolyzed or moderately hemolyzed trace, trace, or small) usually occurs in the absence of a positive protein. A positive blood test often occurs in the absence of RBCs in the microscopic. This can result from intravascular hemolysis, myoglobinuria, or lysis of RBCs caused by alkaline or hypotonic urine. A positive test for protein and a negative blood test occur commonly in conditions such as orthostatic albuminuria, urinary tract infection, and diabetes mellitus. However, a negative blood test should not occur if more than 3–4 RBCs/high power field are seen in the microscopic examination. Either the blood test is falsely negative (a missed nonhemolyzed trace) or yeast has been mistaken for RBCs.

48. **B** Only the conjugated form of bilirubin is excreted into the urine. Urinary bilirubin is positive in necrotic and obstructive jaundice but not in prehepatic jaundice, which results in a high level of serum unconjugated bilirubin. The highest levels of urinary bilirubin occur in obstructive jaundice, which causes decreased urinary urobilinogen. Very few drugs have been reported to interfere with urine bilirubin tests, which are based on the formation of azobilirubin by reaction with a diazonium salt. Positive interference by rifampin and chlorpromazine has been reported. Urine must be fresh because sunlight destroys bilirubin. Bacteria may cause hydrolysis of glucuronides forming unconjugated bilirubin, which does not react with the diazonium reagent. Ascorbate inhibits the reaction by reducing the diazo reagent.

49. Which of the following reagents is used to detect uro-bilinogen in urine?
  A. *p*-Dinitrobenzene
  B. *p*-Aminosalicylate
  C. *p*-Dimethylaminobenzaldehyde
  D. *p*-Dichloroaniline

Body fluids/Apply principles of basic laboratory procedures/Urine urobilinogen/1

50. Which of the following statements regarding urinary urobilinogen is true?
  A. Diurnal variation occurs, with highest levels seen in the early morning
  B. High levels occurring with a positive bilirubin test indicate obstructive jaundice
  C. Dry reagent strip tests do not detect decreased levels
  D. False-positive results may occur if urine is stored for more than 2 hours

Body fluids/Correlate clinical and laboratory data/Urine bilirubin/2

51. Which statement about the Watson-Schwartz test is true?
  A. Urobilinogen is water-soluble and produces a pink color in the upper layer
  B. Urobilinogen is extracted in chloroform and gives a pink color in the lower layer
  C. PBG is extracted in n-butanol
  D. Dietary indoles cannot be separated from PBG

Body fluids/Apply principles of special procedures/Urine urobilinogen/2

52. Which of the following statements regarding the test for nitrite in urine is true?
  A. It detects more than 95% of clinically significant bacteriuria
  B. Formation of nitrite is unaffected by the urine pH
  C. The test is dependent upon an adequate dietary nitrate content
  D. A positive test differentiates bacteriuria from in vitro bacterial contamination

Body fluids/Apply knowledge to recognize sources of error/Nitrite/2

49. **C** Urobilinogen reacts with Ehrlich's aldehyde reagent (*p*-dimethylaminobenzaldehyde in HCl) to form a pink color. Dry reagent strips use either p-dimethylaminobenzaldehyde or 4-methoxybenzene diazonium tetrafluoroborate to detect urobilinogen. The former reagent may react with PBG, salicylate, and sulfonamides, giving falsely high results. False-positive results may occur in the presence of Pyridium and Gantrisin, which color the urine orange-red. Formalin may cause a false-negative reaction.

50. **C** Urobilinogen exhibits diurnal variation, and highest levels are seen in the afternoon. A 2-hour postprandial afternoon sample is the sample of choice for detecting increased urine urobilinogen. Urobilinogen is formed by bacterial reduction of conjugated bilirubin in the bowel. In obstructive jaundice, delivery of bilirubin into the intestine is blocked, resulting in decreased fecal, serum, and urine urobilinogen. However, the dry reagent strip tests are not sensitive enough to detect abnormally low levels. Urobilinogen is rapidly oxidized to urobilin, which does not react with dry reagent strip tests.

51. **B** The Watson-Schwartz test differentiates urobilinogen and indole derivatives from PBG. A pink color extracted by chloroform is found in the lower layer and is caused by the urobilinogen-aldehyde product. Dietary indoles may react and will extract in the chloroform layer. Melanogens and most drugs are extracted into n-butanol. PBG remains in the aqueous layer after extraction with both chloroform and n-butanol. A pink color forming in the aqueous phase that remains in the aqueous phase after addition of n-butanol is caused by PBG.

52. **C** The nitrite test is dependent upon the activity of bacterial reductase, and false-negative reactions have been reported when urine is highly acidic. Nitrite is formed by reduction of diet-derived nitrates and reacts with p-arsanilic acid or sulfanilamide to form a diazonium compound. This reacts with benzoquinoline to form a pink azo dye. False-negative reactions also occur in the presence of ascorbate, which reduces the diazonium product. Nitrite is positive in about 70% of clinically significant bacterial infections of the urinary tract. Sensitivity is limited by the requirements for dietary nitrate and 3–4 hour storage time in the bladder. In addition, the causative bacteria must be able to reduce nitrate.

53. Which statement about the dry reagent strip test for leukocytes is true?
- **A.** The test detects only intact white blood cells (WBCs)
- **B.** The reaction is based upon the hydrolysis of substrate by WBC esterases
- **C.** The presence of several antibiotics may give a false-positive reaction
- **D.** The test is sensitive to 2–3 WBCs per high power field

Body fluids/Apply principles of basic laboratory procedures/Leukocytes/2

54. Which of the following statements about creatinine clearance is correct?
- **A.** Dietary restrictions are required during the 24 hours preceding the test
- **B.** Fluid intake must be restricted to below 600 mL in the 6 hours preceding the test
- **C.** Creatinine clearance is mainly determined by renal tubular function
- **D.** Creatinine clearance is dependent on lean body mass

Body fluids/Apply knowledge of fundamental biological characteristics/Creatinine clearance/1

55. A male patient's creatinine clearance is 75 mL/min. This indicates:
- **A.** Normal glomerular filtration rate
- **B.** The patient is uremic and will be hyperkalemic
- **C.** Renal tubular dysfunction
- **D.** Reduced glomerular filtration without uremia

Body fluids/Correlate clinical and laboratory data/Creatinine clearance/2

56. Which of the following tests is a specific measure of glomerular filtration?
- **A.** *p*-Aminohippuric acid (PAH) clearance
- **B.** Fishberg's concentration test
- **C.** Mosenthal's dilution test
- **D.** Cystatin C

Body fluids/Correlate laboratory data with physiological processes/Renal function/1

Answers to Questions 53–56

53. **B** PMNs in urine are detected by the presence of esterases that hydrolyze an ester such as indoxylcarbonic acid. The product reacts with a diazonium salt to give a purple color. The test detects esterases in urine as well as intact WBCs but is not sensitive to less than 5–10 WBCs per high power field. Several antibiotics, high protein, and high SG inhibit the esterase reaction. Formalin may cause a false-positive result.

54. **D** Although some creatinine is derived from the diet, it is rapidly filtered by the glomeruli, and time variations are reduced by the collection of urine for at least 4 hours. Creatinine is produced from oxidation of creatine at a constant rate of about 2% per day. It is filtered completely and not significantly reabsorbed. However, creatinine secretion by the tubules is increased when filtrate flow is slow, and patients must be given at least 600 mL of H_2O at the start of the test and kept well hydrated throughout. Body size determines how much creatinine is produced, and clearance must be normalized to eliminate this variable.

55. **D** Normal creatinine clearance in men is 107–140 mL/min. Men have a slightly higher clearance than women (87–107 mL/min) as a result of greater lean body mass. Values below the lower reference limit but above 60 mL/min indicate glomerular damage but not of severity sufficient to cause uremia.

56. **D** Cystatin C is a small protease inhibitor that is produced at a constant rate, eliminated exclusively by glomerular filtration, and is not dependent on age, sex, or nutritional status. Plasma cystatin C is increased when the glomerular filtration rate is decreased. PAH is a substance that is completely filtered by the glomerulus and also secreted by the tubules. PAH clearance has been used rarely to measure renal blood flow. The other two tests are measures of tubular function but are used infrequently because they are associated with significant health risks. The Fishberg concentration test measures the ability to concentrate urine after deprivation of water. The Mosenthal test measures the ability to excrete free water after excessive water intake.

57. Which of the following statements regarding creatinine clearance is true?

  A. As renal failure progresses, the creatinine clearance more accurately reflects the true glomerular filtration rate

  B. Results are slightly higher than inulin clearance because of tubular secretion

  C. Creatinine clearance results are independent of the method of creatinine assay

  D. Creatinine clearance may be normal when serum creatinine is increased

Body fluids/Apply knowledge to recognize sources of error/Creatinine clearance/2

58. Which statement regarding urea is true?

  A. Urea is 100% filtered by the glomeruli

  B. Blood urea levels are independent of diet

  C. Urea is not significantly reabsorbed by the tubules

  D. Urea excretion is a specific measure of glomerular function

Body fluids/Correlate laboratory data with physiological processes/Urea/1

59. Given the following data, calculate the creatinine clearance.

  Serum creatinine = 1.5 mg/dL;
  urine creatinine = 102 mg/dL;
  urine volume = 1.7 mL/min;
  body surface area = 1.73 m^2

  A. 47 mL/min

  B. 97 mL/min

  C. 100 mL/min

  D. 116 mL/min

Body fluids/Calculate/Creatinine clearance/2

60. Given the following data, calculate the creatinine clearance.

  Serum creatinine = 2.4 mg/dL;
  urine creatinine = 105 mg/dL;
  urine volume = 1.4 L/day;
  surface area = 1.80 m^2

  A. 41 mL/min

  B. 78 mL/min

  C. 87 mL/min

  D. 110 mL/min

Body fluids/Calculate/Creatinine clearance/2

57. B Creatinine clearance tends to overestimate the glomerular filtration rate when compared to inulin clearance. When Jaffe's reaction is used to measure creatinine, the presence of nonspecific reactants in the serum tends to compensate for this, and results agree more closely than when creatinine is measured by an enzymatic method. However, as renal failure progresses, the relative contribution of nonspecific substances decreases. The tubules secrete more creatinine as glomerular filtration slows. These two factors combine to cause significant overestimation of the glomerular filtration rate as glomerular function deteriorates.

58. A BUN is a sensitive indicator of renal disease but is not specific for glomerular function. BUN levels are affected by diet, hepatic function, tubular function, and filtrate flow as well as the glomerular filtration rate. Although urea is completely filtered by the glomerulus, the tubules reabsorb 30%–40% of the filtered urea, and this is why BUN concentration is higher than plasma creatinine. In prerenal failure up to 70% of the filtered urea can be reabsorbed because of the slow movement of filtrate through the tubules. This causes BUN to rise much more than plasma creatinine in this condition. A BUN:creatinine ratio of 20:1 is highly suggestive of prerenal failure.

59. D The clearance formula is U ÷ P × V × 1.73/A, where U = urine creatinine (mg/dL), P = plasma creatinine (mg/dL), V = urine volume (mL/min), and 1.73 = mean body surface area (m^2)

  102 mg/dL ÷ 1.5 mg/dL × 1.7 mL/min × (1.73 m^2 ÷ 1.73 m^2) = 115.6 mL/min

60. A Convert volume in liters per day to milliliters per minute by multiplying 1000/1440.

  1.4 L/day × 1000 mL/L × 1 day/24 hr × 1 hr/60 min = 1400 mL/1440 min = 1 mL/min

  Creatinine clearance = 105 mg/dL ÷ 2.4 mg/dL × 1 mL/min × (1.73 m^2 ÷ 1.8 m^2) = 41 mL/min

1. Which of the following dyes are used in the Sternheimer-Malbin stain?
   A. Hematoxylin and eosin
   B. Crystal violet and safranin
   C. Methylene blue and eosin
   D. Methylene blue and safranin

   Body fluids/Apply principles of basic laboratory procedures/Staining/1

2. Which of the following statements regarding WBCs in urinary sediment is true?
   A. "Glitter cells" seen in the urinary sediment are a sign of renal disease
   B. Bacteriuria in the absence of WBCs indicates lower urinary tract infection (UTI)
   C. WBCs other than PMNs are not found in urinary sediment
   D. WBC casts indicate that pyuria is of renal rather than lower urinary origin

   Body fluids/Correlate clinical and laboratory data/ Urinary sediment/2

Answers to Questions 1–2

1. **B** Sternheimer-Malbin is a supravital stain used to help differentiate renal tubular epithelium from transitional cells and polymorphonuclear neutrophils (PMNs). The mononuclear cells are clearly distinguished from both live and dead PMNs. Transitional cells appear mostly blue, but renal cells take up both dyes, resulting in an azurophilic appearance (orange-purple cytoplasm and dark purple nucleus).

2. **D** The majority of WBCs in the urinary sediment are PMNs. Eosinophils and monocuncular WBCs are occasionally seen. High numbers of eosinophils often indicate an allergic drug reaction causing inflammation in the medullary interstitium and tubules. Mononuclear cells are especially likely in patients with chronic inflammatory diseases and in renal transplant rejection patients, where they may account for as many as 30% of the WBCs. Glitter cells are PMNs with highly refractile granules exhibiting brownian movement. They are seen only when urine SG is below 1.020. These cells resist staining with Sternheimer-Malbin stain and are considered to be living (fresh) WBCs. When seen in large numbers, they indicate urinary tract injury (with pseudopod extensions they point to infection). The presence of bacteria in urine in the absence of PMNs usually results from contamination by vaginal or skin flora that multiply in vitro, especially in unrefrigerated specimens. The presence of WBC casts is always significant, and when associated with pyuria and bacteriuria, indicates renal involvement in the infection.

3. Which description of sediment staining with the Sternheimer-Malbin stain is correct?

   A. Transitional epithelium: cytoplasm pale blue, nucleus dark blue

   B. Renal epithelium: cytoplasm light blue, nucleus dark purple

   C. Glitter cells: cytoplasm dark blue, nucleus dark purple

   D. Squamous epithelium: cytoplasm pink, nucleus pale blue

Body fluids/Apply knowledge of fundamental biological characteristics/Staining/2

4. SITUATION: A 5-mL urine specimen is submitted for routine urinalysis and analyzed immediately. The SG of the sample is 1.012 and the pH is 6.5. The dry reagent strip test for blood is a large positive (3+) and the microscopic examination shows 11–20 RBCs per high power field. The leukocyte esterase reaction is a small positive (1+), and the microscopic examination shows 0–5 WBCs per high power field. What is the most likely cause of these results?

   A. Myoglobin is present in the sample

   B. Free hemoglobin is present

   C. Insufficient volume is causing microscopic results to be underestimated

   D. Some WBCs have been misidentified as RBCs

Body fluids/Apply knowledge to identify sources of error/Urinalysis/3

5. Which of the following statements regarding epithelial cells in the urinary system is correct?

   A. Caudate epithelial cells originate from the upper urethra

   B. Transitional cells originate from the upper urethra, ureters, bladder, or renal pelvis

   C. Cells from the proximal renal tubule are usually round in shape

   D. Squamous epithelium lines the vagina, urethra, and wall of the urinary bladder

Body fluids/Apply knowledge of fundamental biological characteristics/Urine sediment/2

6. Which of the statements regarding examination of unstained sediment is true?

   A. Renal cells can be differentiated reliably from WBCs

   B. Large numbers of transitional cells are often seen after catheterization

   C. Neoplastic cells from the bladder are not found in urinary sediment

   D. RBCs are easily differentiated from nonbudding yeasts

Body fluids/Correlate clinical and laboratory data/Urine sediment/2

Answers to Questions 3–6

3. A After staining with Sternheimer-Malbin stain, transitional epithelial cells are readily differentiated from renal tubular cells and WBCs because their cytoplasm is pale blue. Live WBCs exclude Sternheimer-Malbin stain, whereas dead cells stain with a deep blue-purple nucleus and pale orange-blue cytoplasm. Renal epithelial cells have an orange-purple cytoplasm and dark purple nucleus. Squamous epithelium has a blue or purple cytoplasm and an orange-purple nucleus. Red cells stain very pale pink or not at all and hyaline casts stain faintly pink.

4. C Given the SG and pH, most RBCs and WBCs are intact. Both the RBC and WBC counts are lower than expected from the dry reagent strip results. Myoglobin or free hemoglobin may account for the poor correlation between the blood reaction and the RBC count but does not explain the lower than expected WBC count. Microscopic reference ranges are based upon concentrating a uniform volume of sediment from 12 mL of urine. When less urine is used, falsely low results are obtained unless corrective action is taken. The specimen should be diluted with normal saline to 12 mL, then centrifuged at $450 \times g$ for 5 min. Sediment should be prepared according to the established procedure and the results multiplied by the dilution factor (in this case, $12 \div 5$ or 2.4).

5. B Caudate cells are transitional epithelium that have a sawtooth-shaped tail and are found in the urinary bladder and the pelvis of the kidney. Transitional epithelium line the upper two thirds of the urethra and the ureters as well as the urinary bladder and renal pelvis. Renal tubular cells may be columnar, polyhedral, or oval, depending upon the portion of the tubule from which they originate. Cells from the proximal tubule are columnar and have a distinctive brush border. Squamous epithelium lines the vagina and lower third of the urethra.

6. B Renal cells and PMNs are about the same size and can be confused in unstained sediment. Catheterization often releases large clumps or sheets of transitional and squamous cells. These should be distinguished from neoplastic cells derived from the urinary bladder. When cells appear atypical (e.g., large cells in metaphase), they should be referred to a pathologist for cytological examination. Nonbudding yeast cells are approximately the same in size and appearance as RBCs. When RBCs are initially seen in the absence of a positive blood test, the probability of a falsely positive microscopic examination is very high. The microscopic examination should be reviewed for the presence of yeast.

7. Which of the following statements regarding cells found in urinary sediment is true?
   A. Transitional cells resist swelling in hypotonic urine
   B. Renal tubular cells are often polyhedral and have an eccentric round nucleus
   C. Trichomonads have an oval shape with a prominent nucleus and a single anterior flagellum
   D. Clumps of bacteria are frequently mistaken for blood casts

Body fluids/Apply knowledge of fundamental biological characteristics/Urine sediment/2

8. Which of the following statements regarding RBCs in the urinary sediment is true?
   A. Yeast cells will lyse in dilute acetic acid but RBCs will not
   B. RBCs are often swollen in hypertonic urine
   C. RBCs of glomerular origin often appear dysmorphic
   D. Yeast cells will tumble when the coverglass is touched but RBCs will not

Body fluids/Apply knowledge of fundamental biological characteristics/Urine sediment/2

9. Renal tubular epithelial cells are shed into the urine in largest numbers in which condition?
   A. Malignant renal disease
   B. Acute glomerulonephritis
   C. Nephrotic syndrome
   D. Cytomegalovirus (CMV) infection of the kidney

Body fluids/Evaluate laboratory data to recognize health and disease states/Urinary sediment/2

10. The ova of which parasite may be found in the urinary sediment?
   A. *T. vaginalis*
   B. *Entamoeba histolytica*
   C. *Schistosoma haematobium*
   D. *Trichuris trichiura*

Body fluids/Apply knowledge of fundamental biological characteristics/Urinary sediment/1

11. Oval fat bodies are often seen in:
   A. Chronic glomerulonephritis
   B. Nephrotic syndrome
   C. Acute tubular nephrosis
   D. Renal failure of any cause

Body fluids/Correlate clinical and laboratory data/Urine sediment/2

Answers to Questions 7–11

7. B Transitional epithelial cells readily take up H_2O and appear much larger than renal cells or WBCs when urine is hypotonic. Transitional cells are considered a normal component of the sediment unless present in large numbers and associated with signs of inflammation such as mucus and PMNs or presenting features of malignant cells. In contrast, renal cells are significant when seen conclusively in the sediment. They are often teardrop, polyhedral, or elongated cells with a round eccentric nucleus. Conclusive identification requires staining. *Trichomonas vaginalis* displays an indistinct nucleus and two pairs of prominent anterior flagella. Amorphous urate crystals deposited on the slide may be mistaken for granular or blood casts.

8. C RBCs are difficult to distinguish from nonbudding yeasts in unstained sediment. RBCs tumble when the coverglass is touched and will lyse when the sediment is reconstituted in normal saline containing 2% v/v acetic acid. A nonhemolyzed trace blood reaction confirms the presence of RBCs. RBCs have a granular appearance in hypertonic urine due to crenation. The RBC membrane becomes distorted when passing through the glomerulus, often appearing scalloped, serrated, or invaginated. Such cells are termed dysmorphic RBCs and are associated with glomerulonephritis.

9. D Although seen in glomerulonephritis and pyelonephritis, the largest numbers of renal tubular cells appear in urine in association with viral infections of the kidney. Renal epithelium may show characteristic viral inclusions associated with CMV and rubella. High numbers of renal epithelium are also found in the sediment of patients with drug-induced tubular nephrosis and some cases of heavy metal poisoning. Renal tumors do not usually shed cells into the urine.

10. C Ova of *S. haematobium* are most often recovered from urine because the adult trematodes colonize the blood vessels of the urinary bladder. The eggs are approximately 150×60 μm and are nonoperculated. They are yellowish and have a prominent terminal spine.

11. B Oval fat bodies are degenerated renal tubular epithelium that have reabsorbed cholesterol from the filtrate. Although they can occur in any inflammatory disease of the tubules, they are commonly seen in the nephrotic syndrome, which is characterized by marked proteinuria and hyperlipidemia.

12. All of the following statements regarding urinary casts are true *except*:
  A. Many hyaline casts may appear in sediment after jogging or exercise
  B. An occasional granular cast may be seen in a normal sediment
  C. Casts can be seen in significant numbers even when protein tests are negative
  D. Hyaline casts dissolve readily in alkaline urine

Body fluids/Apply knowledge to recognize sources of error/Urine casts/2

13. Which condition promotes the formation of casts in the urine?
  A. Chronic production of alkaline urine
  B. Polyuria
  C. Reduced filtrate formation
  D. Low urine SG

Body fluids/Apply knowledge of fundamental characteristics/Urine casts/2

14. The mucoprotein that forms the matrix of a hyaline cast is called:
  A. Bence Jones protein
  B. β-Microglobulin
  C. Tamm-Horsfall protein
  D. Arginine-rich glycoprotein

Body fluids/Apply knowledge of fundamental biological characteristics/Urine casts/1

15. "Pseudocasts" are often caused by:
  A. A dirty coverglass or slide
  B. Bacterial contamination
  C. Amorphous urates
  D. Mucus in the urine

Body fluids/Apply knowledge to identify sources of error/Urine casts/2

16. Which of the following statements regarding urinary casts is correct?
  A. Fine granular casts are more significant than coarse granular casts
  B. Cylindruria is always clinically significant
  C. The appearance of cylindroids signals the onset of end-stage renal disease
  D. Broad casts are associated with severe renal tubular obstruction

Body fluids/Apply knowledge of fundamental biological characteristics/Urine casts/2

17. A sediment with moderate hematuria and RBC casts most likely results from:
  A. Chronic pyelonephritis
  B. Nephrotic syndrome
  C. Acute glomerulonephritis
  D. Lower urinary tract obstruction

Body fluids/Correlate clinical and laboratory data/Urine sediment/2

Answers to Questions 12–17

12. **C** Proteinuria accompanies cylindruria because protein is the principal component of casts. After strenuous exercise, hyaline casts may be present in the sediment in significant numbers but disappear after resting for at least 24 hours.

13. **C** Cast formation is promoted by an acid filtrate, high solute concentration, slow movement of filtrate, and reduced filtrate formation. The appearance of a cast is dependent on the location and time spent in the tubule as well as the chemical and cellular composition of the filtrate.

14. **C** Hyaline casts are composed of a mucoprotein called Tamm-Horsfall protein. In addition, casts may contain cells, immunoglobulins, light chains, cellular proteins, fat, bacteria, and crystalloids.

15. **C** Pseudocasts are formed by amorphous urates that may deposit in uniform cylindrical shapes as the sediment settles under the coverglass. They may be mistaken for granular or blood casts. However, they are highly refractile and lack the well-defined borders of true casts.

16. **D** There is no clinical difference between fine and coarse granular casts. Granular casts may form by degeneration of cellular casts, but some show no evidence of cellular origin. Granular casts may form from inclusion of urinary calculi, but some are of unknown etiology. Cylindruria refers to the presence of casts in the urine. Hyaline casts may be seen in small numbers in normal patients and in large numbers following strenuous exercise and long-distance running. Hyaline casts may also be increased in patients taking certain drugs such as diuretics. Broad casts form in dilated or distal tubules and indicate chronic renal failure or severe obstruction. Waxy casts form when there is prolonged stasis in the tubules and signal end-stage renal failure. Cylindroids are casts with tails and have no special clinical significance.

17. **C** Red-cell casts indicate the renal orgin of hematuria. Urinary obstruction may be associated with hematuria from ruptured vessels, but not casts. WBCs and WBC casts predominate in pyelonephritis. Sediment in chronic glomerulonephritis is variable but usually exhibits moderate to severe intermittent hematuria. In addition, pyuria and cylindruria (with granular, blood, waxy, and epithelial casts) are frequent. In nephrotic syndrome the sediment may be unremarkable except for the presence of oval fat bodies and hyaline casts. In some cases, fatty, waxy, and epithelial cell casts may also be found.

18. Urine sediment characterized by pyuria with bacterial and WBC casts indicates:
   A. Nephrotic syndrome
   B. Pyelonephritis
   C. Polycystic kidney disease
   D. Cystitis

Body fluids/Correlate clinical and laboratory data/Urine sediment/2

19. Which type of casts signals the presence of chronic renal failure?
   A. Blood casts
   B. Fine granular casts
   C. Waxy casts
   D. Fatty casts

Body fluids/Apply knowledge of fundamental biological characteristics/Urine casts/2

20. **SITUATION:** Urinalysis of a sample from a patient suspected of having a transfusion reaction reveals small yellow-brown crystals in the microscopic examination. Dry reagent strip tests are normal with the exception of a positive blood reaction (moderate) and trace positive protein. The pH of the urine is 6.5. What test should be performed to positively identify the crystals?
   A. Confirmatory test for bilirubin
   B. Cyanide-nitroprusside test
   C. Polarizing microscopy
   D. Prussian blue stain

Body fluids/Select course of action/Urine sediment/3

21. When examining urinary sediment, which of the following is considered an abnormal finding?
   A. 0–2 RBCs per high power field
   B. 0–1 hyaline casts per low power field
   C. 0–1 renal cell casts per low power field
   D. 2–5 WBCs per high power field

Body fluids/Evaluate laboratory data to recognize health and disease states/Urinary sediment/2

22. **SITUATION:** A urine sample with a pH of 6.0 produces an abundance of pink sediment after centrifugation that appears as densely packed yellow-brown granules under the microscope. The crystals are so dense that no other formed elements can be evaluated. What is the best course of action?
   A. Request a new urine specimen
   B. Suspend the sediment in prewarmed saline, then repeat centrifugation
   C. Acidify a 12-mL aliquot with three drops of glacial acetic acid and heat to 56°C for 5 min before centrifuging
   D. Add five drops of 1 N HCl to the sediment and examine

Body fluids/Select course of action/Urine sediment/3

Answers to Questions 18–22

18. **B** Pyelonephritis results from bacterial infection of the renal pelvis and interstitium. It is characterized by polyuria resulting from failure of the tubules to reabsorb fluid. Obstruction of tubules and compression by WBCs may reduce glomerular filtration as well as H_2O reabsorption. The finding of WBC casts helps to differentiate pyelonephritis from urinary tract infection.

19. **C** Waxy casts form from the degeneration of cellular casts. Because the casts must remain lodged in the tubule long enough for the granular protein matrix to waxify, they are associated with chronic or end-stage renal failure. Both waxy and broad casts form in chronic renal failure when there is severe stasis, and they are associated with a poor prognosis.

20. **D** A positive blood test and trace protein occurring with a normal test for urobilinogen and an absence of RBCs are consistent with an intravascular transfusion reaction. Small yellow-brown granular crystals at an acid pH may be uric acid, bilirubin, or hemosiderin. Bilirubin crystals are ruled out by the negative dry reagent strip test for bilirubin. Potassium ferrocyanide is used in the Prussian blue staining reaction to detect hemosiderin deposits in urinary sediment. Hemosiderin is associated with hemochromatosis and increased RBC destruction. Causes of urinary hemosiderin include transfusion reaction, hemolytic anemia, and pernicious anemia.

21. **C** Epithelial casts are rarely seen but indicate a disease process affecting the renal tubules. They are associated with diseases causing necrosis of the tubules such as hepatitis, CMV, and other viral infections and mercury and ethylene glycol toxicity. Even a rare cellular cast is considered clinically significant.

22. **B** Urates are yellow-brown granules and form in acid or neutral urine. They often form following refrigeration of urine and can be dissolved by addition of warm saline or dilute NaOH. Amorphous phosphates are colorless and form in neutral or alkaline urine. They dissolve in dilute acetic acid but precipitate if heated.

23. How can hexagonal uric acid crystals can be distinguished from cystine crystals?

A. Cystine is insoluble in hydrochloric acid but uric acid is soluble

B. Cystine gives a positive nitroprusside test after reduction with sodium cyanide

C. Cystine crystals are more highly pigmented

D. Cystine crystals form at neutral or alkaline pH, uric acid at neutral to acidic pH

Body fluids/Apply principles of special procedures/Urine crystals/2

24. The presence of tyrosine and leucine crystals together in a urine sediment usually indicates:

A. Renal failure

B. Chronic liver disease

C. Hemolytic anemia

D. Hartnup's disease

Body fluids/Correlate clinical and laboratory data/Urine crystals/2

25. Which of the following crystals is considered non-pathological?

A. Hemosiderin

B. Bilirubin

C. Ammonium biurate

D. Cholesterol

Body fluids/Evaluate laboratory data to recognize health and disease states/Urine crystals/2

26. At which pH are ammonium biurate crystals usually found in urine?

A. Acid urine only

B. Acid or neutral urine

C. Neutral or alkaline urine

D. Alkaline urine only

Body fluids/Correlate laboratory data with physiological processes/Urine crystals/2

27. Which of the following crystals is seen commonly in alkaline and neutral urine?

A. Calcium oxalate

B. Uric acid

C. Magnesium ammonium phosphate

D. Cholesterol

Body fluids/Correlate laboratory data with physiological processes/Urine crystals/1

28. Which crystal appears in urine as a long, thin hexagonal plate and is linked to ingestion of large amounts of benzoic acid?

A. Cystine

B. Hippuric acid

C. Oxalic acid

D. Uric acid

Body fluids/Correlate laboratory data with physiological processes/Urine crystals/2

Answers to Questions 23–28

23. **B** Flat six-sided uric acid crystals may be mistaken for cystine crystals. Both crystals form at an acid to neutral pH. Cystine transmits polarized light and is soluble in dilute HCl. Uric acid is insoluble in HCl and is less anisotropic. Cystine is reduced by NaCN, forming cysteine. The –SH group of cysteine reacts with nitroprusside to form a red color. Cystine crystals are colorless, whereas uric acid crystals are pigmented (yellow, reddish brown).

24. **B** Tyrosine crystals may occur in tyrosinemia, an inborn error of tyrosine metabolism caused by a deficiency of fumarylacetoacetate hydrolase, p-hydroxyphenylpyruvic acid oxidase, or tyrosine aminotransferase, causing tyrosinuria. However, when seen along with leucine crystals, the cause is chronic liver disease, usually cirrhosis of the liver. Tyrosine usually forms fine brown or yellow needles, and leucine forms yellow spheres with concentric rings.

25. **C** Abnormal crystals are those that result from a pathological process. Hemosiderin crystals result from intravascular RBC destruction. Bilirubin crystals are found in severe necrotic and obstructive liver diseases, and cholesterol crystals are found in nephrotic syndrome, diabetes mellitus, and hypercholesterolemia.

26. **D** Ammonium biurate is often called a "thornapple" crystal because it forms a dark brown spiny sphere. Calcium carbonate is another common crystal that is seen only in alkaline urine. Sodium urate and uric acid form in acid or neutral urine.

27. **C** Magnesium ammonium phosphate, also called triple phosphate, may be present in neutral or alkaline urine. Most commonly, triple phosphate crystals are six-sided plates that resemble a coffin lid. Crystals containing phosphates do not occur in acid urine.

28. **B** Hippuric acid forms long, flat six-sided plates. It results from the metabolism of benzoic acid and resembles the "coffin lid" appearance of triple phosphate. It may occur normally as a result of ingestion of vegetables preserved with benzoic acid.

29. Small yellow needles are seen in the sediment of a urine sample with a pH of 6.0. Which of the following crystals can be ruled out?
  A. Sulfa crystals
  B. Bilirubin crystals
  C. Uric acid crystals
  D. Cholesterol crystals

Body fluids/Apply knowledge of fundamental biological characteristics/Urine crystals/2

30. Oval fat bodies are derived from:
  A. Renal tubular epithelium
  B. Transitional epithelium
  C. Degenerated WBCs
  D. Mucoprotein matrix

Body fluids/Apply knowledge of fundamental biological characteristics/Urine sediment/1

31. Oval fat bodies are often associated with:
  A. Lipoid nephrosis
  B. Acute glomerulonephritis
  C. Aminoaciduria
  D. Pyelonephritis

Body fluids/Correlate clinical and laboratory data/Urine sediment/2

32. Urine of constant low SG ranging from 1.008 to 1.010 most likely indicates:
  A. Addison's disease
  B. Renal tubular failure
  C. Prerenal failure
  D. Diabetes insipidus

Body fluids/Evaluate laboratory data to recognize health and disease states/Specific gravity/2

33. Which of the following characterizes prerenal failure and helps to differentiate it from acute renal failure caused by renal disease?
  A. BUN:creatinine ratio of 20:1 or higher
  B. Urine:plasma osmolal ratio less than 2:1
  C. Excess loss of sodium in the urine
  D. Dehydration

Body fluids/Correlate clinical and laboratory data/Renal disease/2

34. Which of the following conditions characterizes chronic glomerulonephritis and helps to differentiate it from acute glomerulonephritis?
  A. Hematuria
  B. Polyuria
  C. Hypertension
  D. Azotemia

Body fluids/Correlate clinical and laboratory data/Renal disease/2

Answers to Questions 29–34

29. **D** Cholesterol crystals are colorless rectangular plates that often have a notched corner and appear stacked in a stair-step arrangement. Cholesterol crystals are highly anisotropic and can be positively identified using a polarizing microscope. Bilirubin, sulfa, or uric acid crystals may occur as small yellow or yellow-brown needles or rods in neutral or acid urine. Bilirubin crystals should be suspected when the dry reagent strip test for bilirubin is positive, and cells in the sediment are dark yellow (bile-stained). Sulfa crystals are soluble in acetone, concentrated HCl, and NaOH. They can be confirmed by the lignin test in which one drop of sediment and one drop of 10% HCl react with newsprint to produce a yellow-orange color.

30. **A** Oval fat bodies form from degenerated renal epithelial cells that have reabsorbed cholesterol from the filtrate. They stain with Oil Red O or Sudan III. The fat globules within the cells give a Maltese cross effect when examined under polarized light.

31. **A** The term lipoid nephrosis is a synonym for idiopathic nephrotic syndrome. Like other causes of nephrotic syndrome, it is associated with gross proteinuria, edema, and hyperlipidemia; however, the idiopathic form is also associated with hematuria.

32. **B** The SG of the filtrate in Bowman's space is approximately 1.010. Urine produced consistently with a SG of 1.010 has the same osmolality of the plasma and results from failure of the tubules to modify the filtrate.

33. **A** Prerenal failure is caused by deficient renal blood flow. The tubules are undamaged and reabsorb more BUN than normal because filtrate flow is slow. Under the influence of aldosterone they reabsorb sodium and concentrate the urine. The BUN:creatinine ratio and U:P osmolal ratio are very high and sodium output is low. In renal disease, the BUN:creatinine ratio is 10 or less, the U:P osmolal ratio approaches 1.0, and the daily sodium excretion is high.

34. **B** Acute glomerulonephritis results in severe compression of the glomerular vessels. This reduces filtration, causing a progression from oliguria to anuria. In contrast, polyuria is associated with chronic glomerulonephritis, which causes scarring of the collecting tubules. Both acute and chronic glomerulonephritis cause low urine osmolality, azotemia, acidosis, hypertension, proteinuria, and hematuria.

35. Which of the following conditions is seen in acute renal failure and helps to differentiate it from prerenal failure?

A. Hyperkalemia and uremia

B. Oliguria and edema

C. Low creatinine clearance

D. Abnormal urinary sediment

Body fluids/Correlate clinical and laboratory data/Renal disease/2

36. Which of the following conditions characterizes acute renal failure and helps to differentiate it from chronic renal failure?

A. Hyperkalemia

B. Hematuria

C. Cylindruria

D. Proteinuria

Body fluids/Correlate clinical and laboratory data/Renal disease/2

37. The serum concentration of which analyte is likely to be decreased in untreated cases of acute renal failure?

A. Hydrogen ions

B. Inorganic phosphorus

C. Calcium

D. Uric acid

Body fluids/Correlate clinical and laboratory data/Renal disease/2

38. Which condition below is associated with the greatest proteinuria?

A. Acute glomerulonephritis

B. Chronic glomerulonephritis

C. Nephrotic syndrome

D. Acute pyelonephritis

Body fluids/Correlate clinical and laboratory data/Renal disease/2

Answers to Questions 35–38

35. **D** Reduced glomerular filtration as evidenced by low creatinine clearance characterizes both prerenal and acute renal failure. This results in retention of fluid causing edema, reduced urine volume, hypertension, uremia, and hyperkalemia in both prerenal and acute renal failure. The kidneys are not damaged in prerenal failure and, therefore, the microscopic examination is usually normal.

36. **A** In acute renal failure, reduced glomerular filtration coupled with decreased tubular secretion results in hyperkalemia. In chronic renal failure, scarring of the collecting tubules prevents salt and H_2O reabsorption. This results in normal or low serum potassium despite reduced glomerular filtration. The sediment in chronic renal failure is characterized by intermittent heavy hematuria and proteinuria.

37. **C** Decreased glomerular filtration in renal failure results in high serum creatinine, BUN, and uric acid concentrations. Failure of the tubules results in retention of hydrogen ions and phosphates, causing acidosis and an increased anion gap. The tubules fail to respond to parathyroid hormone, resulting in excessive loss of calcium in urine. Serum sodium level is usually normal or slightly increased, whereas hyperkalemia is a constant finding in acute renal failure.

38. **C** Although all four conditions are associated with proteinuria, it is greatest in the nephrotic syndrome. Urinary albumin loss is typically in excess of 4 g/day, causing dry reagent strip protein tests to give 3+ to 4+ reactions. In contrast to glomerulonephritis and pyelonephritis, the urinary sediment in nephrotic syndrome is not usually characterized by either hematuria or pyuria. Various casts, lipid-laden renal epithelial cells, and oval fat bodies are usually found.

39. Which of the following conditions is often a cause of glomerulonephritis?
  A. Hypertension
  B. CMV infection
  C. Systemic lupus erythematosus (SLE)
  D. Heavy metal poisoning

Body fluids/Apply knowledge of fundamental biological characteristics/Renal disease/2

40. Acute pyelonephritis is commonly caused by:
  A. Bacterial infection of medullary interstitium
  B. Circulatory failure
  C. Renal calculi
  D. Antigen-antibody reactions within the glomeruli

Body fluids/Apply knowledge of fundamental biological characteristics/Renal disease/2

41. All of the following are characteristics of the nephrotic syndrome *except*:
  A. Hyperlipidemia
  B. Hypoalbuminemia
  C. Hematuria and pyuria
  D. Severe edema

Body fluids/Correlate clinical and laboratory data/Renal disease/2

Answers to Questions 39–41

39. **C** Autoimmune diseases, diabetes mellitus, and nephrotoxic drugs are common causes of acute glomerulonephritis. Autoimmune damage may result from the deposition of antigen-antibody complexes and complement-mediated damage such as occurs in post– streptococcal glomerulonephritis or from the production of autoantibodies that attack the basement membrane, as in Goodpasture's syndrome. Acute glomerulonephritis is often classified by the pattern of injury rather than the cause. For example, insulin deficiency produces sclerotic vascular damage to the glomeruli, often resulting in crescentic glomerulonephritis. Group A streptococci and SLE result in immunologically mediated damage to the glomeruli, usually causing membranous or membranoproliferative glomerulonephritis, but different causes can result in the same pattern, and any one cause can result in different histological patterns in different persons. CMV infections and heavy metal poisoning cause damage to the tubules, resulting in nephrosis.

40. **A** Acute pyelonephritis is caused by infection of the medullary interstitium, usually by coliforms that enter from the lower urinary tract. *Escherichia coli* is the most commonly implicated bacterium. Since it is focused in the medulla, the disease involves mainly the tubules. As opposed to acute glomerulonephritis, pyelonephritis is not associated with reduced creatinine clearance, azotemia, or oliguria. Reabsorption of salt and water are blocked, resulting in hyperkalemia, acidosis, and polyuria.

41. **C** Although casts may be present, the urinary sediment in nephrotic syndrome is not characterized by RBCs and WBCs or by RBC, blood, and WBC casts. In nephrotic syndrome, unlike renal failure, the creatinine clearance and serum potassium are usually normal. Nephrotic syndrome often follows the anuric phase of acute glomerulonephritis, indicating a reversal of the inflammatory process.

42. Which of the following conditions is a characteristic finding in patients with obstructive renal disease?
   A. Polyuria
   B. Azotemia
   C. Dehydration
   D. Alkalosis

Body fluids/Correlate laboratory data with physiological processes/Renal disease/2

43. Whewellite and weddellite kidney stones are composed of:
   A. Magnesium ammonium phosphate
   B. Calcium oxalate
   C. Calcium phosphate
   D. Calcium carbonate

Body fluids/Apply knowledge of fundamental biological characteristics/Renal calculi/1

44. Which of the following abnormal crystals is often associated with formation of renal calculi?
   A. Cystine
   B. Ampicillin
   C. Tyrosine
   D. Leucine

Body fluids/Correlate clinical and laboratory data/Renal calculi/2

45. Which statement about renal calculi is true?
   A. Calcium oxalate and calcium phosphate account for about three quarters of all stones
   B. Uric acid stones can be seen by x-ray film
   C. Triple phosphate stones are found principally in the ureters
   D. Stones are usually made up of single salts

Body fluids/Apply knowledge of fundamental biological characteristics/Renal calculi/2

Answers to Questions 42–45

42. **B** Obstructive renal disease may result from renal or urinary tract calculi, benign prostatic hypertrophy, chronic urinary tract infection, or urogenital malignancy. Obstruction causes the hydrostatic pressure in Bowman's space to increase. This pressure opposes glomerular filtration. If the hydrostatic pressure in Bowman's space equals the hydrostatic pressure in the glomeruli, then filtrate will not be produced, resulting in anuria. Postrenal failure produces many of the same serum abnormalities as acute renal failure, including hyperkalemia, acidosis, edema, and azotemia. The urinary sediment is often abnormal as well. Bacteriuria and pyuria are common, and hematuria may result from rupture of the vasa recta or other blood vessels.

43. **B** Over three fourths of urinary tract stones are composed of calcium salts, and hyperparathyroidism is commonly associated with calcium stones. Stones composed of magnesium ammonium phosphate are called struvite and lodge in the renal pelvis, causing a characteristic "staghorn" appearance on radiographic examination. Stones mainly composed of calcium phosphate are called hydroxyapatite or bushite, depending upon the calcium composition. Stones of $CaCO_3$ are called carbonate apatite.

44. **A** Cystinuria is caused by an autosomal recessive defect in the tubular reabsorption of dibasic amino acids (a renal type aminoaciduria). Cystine crystals are highly insoluble and form kidney stones. Tyrosine crystals form fine dark sheaves or needles and may result from liver disease or tyrosinosis, an overflow aminoaciduria. Leucine crystals form yellow spheres with concentric rings and are seen in chronic liver disease. Ampicillin (rarely) forms long colorless prisms in sheaves in some patients being treated with high doses.

45. **A** Three fourths of all stones contain calcium and three fourths of these contain calcium oxalate. Stones are usually composed of several inorganic salts, but calcium oxalate is the most common component of urinary stones. Oxalates are hard, dark, and coarse stones. Uric acid stones are always pigmented yellow to reddish brown. They are small translucent stones not apparent on x-ray films. Stones made of primarily calcium phosphate (as hydroxyapatite) are light and crumble easily. Stones made of struvite (ammonium magnesium phosphate) are radiodense and lodge in the renal pelvis, forming an outline of the structures resembling the antlers of a deer (staghorn calculi).

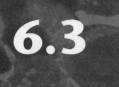

CEREBROSPINAL, SEROUS, AND SYNOVIAL FLUIDS

1. Cerebrospinal fluid (CSF) is formed by ultrafiltration of plasma through the:
   A. Choroid plexus
   B. Sagittal sinus
   C. Anterior cerebral lymphatics
   D. Arachnoid membrane

   Body fluids/Apply knowledge of fundamental biological characteristics/CSF/1

2. Which statement below regarding the CSF is true?
   A. Normal values for mononuclear cells are higher for infants than adults
   B. Absolute neutrophilia is not significant if the total WBC count is less than 25/μL
   C. The first aliquot of CSF should be sent to the microbiology laboratory
   D. Neutrophils constitute the majority of WBCs in normal CSF

   Body fluids/Apply principles of basic laboratory procedures/CSF/2

3. When collecting CSF, a difference between opening and closing fluid pressure greater than 100 mm H₂O indicates:
   A. Low CSF volume
   B. Subarachnoid hemorrhage
   C. Meningitis
   D. Hydrocephalus

   Body fluids/Correlate laboratory data with physiological processes/Cerebrospinal fluid/2

Answers to Questions 1–3

1. **A** CSF is formed by ultrafiltration of plasma though the choroid plexus, a tuft of capillaries in the pia mater located in the third and fourth ventricles. Endothelium of the choroid plexus vessels and ependymal cells lining the ventricles act as a barrier to the passage of proteins, drugs, and metabolites. Glucose in CSF is about 60% of the plasma glucose. Total protein in CSF is only 15–45 mg/dL, while chloride levels are 10%–15% higher than plasma. Approximately 500 mL of ultrafiltrate are produced per day, the bulk of which is returned to the circulation via the sagittal sinus. The normal volume of CSF in adults is 100–160 mL (10–60 mL for small children).

2. **A** Lymphocytes account for 40%–80% of WBCs in adults; monocytes and macrophages for 20%–50%. Neutrophils should be less than 10% of the WBCs. The reference range for WBCs in adults is 0–5/μL. Disease may be present when the WBC count is normal if the majority of WBCs are PMNs. In infants, monocytes account for 50%–90% of WBCs, and the upper limit for WBCs is 30/μL. The first aliquot is sent to the chemistry department because it may be contaminated with blood or skin flora.

3. **A** Normal CSF volume in adults is 100–160 mL. When volume is low, an abnormally high difference is observed between the opening and closing pressures. The difference is normally 10–30 mm H₂O, after removal of 15–20 mL. Low opening pressure is caused by reduced volume or block above the puncture site. High opening pressure may result from high CSF volume, CNS hemorrhage, or malignancy.

	WBCs	Lymphocytes	Monocytes	Eosinophils	Neutrophils	Neuroectodermal Cells
A	50/μL	44%	55%	0%	0%	1%
B	300/μL	75%	21%	3%	0%	1%
C	2000/μL	5%	15%	0%	80%	0%
D	2500/μL	40%	50%	0%	10%	0%

4. Which of the following findings is consistent with a subarachnoid hemorrhage rather than a traumatic tap?
   A. Clearing of the fluid as it is aspirated
   B. A clear supernatant after centrifugation
   C. Xanthochromia
   D. Presence of a clot in the sample

   Body fluids/Evaluate laboratory data to recognize health and disease states/CSF/2

5. The term used to denote a high WBC count in the CSF is:
   A. Empyema
   B. Neutrophilia
   C. Pleocytosis
   D. Hyperglycorrhachia

   Body fluids/Apply knowledge of fundamental biological characteristics/CSF/1

6. Which of the adult CSF values in the table above are consistent with bacterial meningitis?

   Body fluids/Evaluate laboratory data to recognize health and disease states/CSF/2

7. Given the following data, determine the corrected CSF WBC count.

	CSF Values	Peripheral Blood Values
RBCs	6000/μL	$4.0 \times 10^6/\mu L$
WBCs	150/μL	$5.0 \times 10^3/\mu L$

   A. 8 WBCs/μL
   B. 142 WBCs/μL
   C. 120 WBCs/μL
   D. 145 WBCs/μL

   Body fluids/Calculate/CSF hematology/2

Answers to Questions 4–7

4. **C** Xanthochromia is pigmentation of CSF caused by subarachnoid hemorrhage, high CSF protein, free hemoglobin, or bilirubin. The bilirubin may be caused by hepatic disease, CNS hemorrhage, or prior traumatic tap. In subarachnoid hemorrhage the fluid is pink if the RBC count is greater than 500/μL. It will turn orange as RBCs lyse in the first few hours and turn yellow after about 12 hours. Granulocyte infiltration occurs immediately after a subarachnoid hemorrhage and disappears after 24 hours. It is followed by an increase in macrophages showing evidence of erythrophagocytosis that remains for up to 2 weeks. After subarachnoid hemorrhage, D-dimer is present in CSF and can be used to distinguish between a traumatic tap and subarachnoid hemorrhage.

5. **C** Pleocytosis refers to an increase in WBCs within the CSF. Bacterial meningitis causes a neutrophilic pleocytosis, viral meningitis a lymphocytic pleocytosis, and tuberculous and fungal meningitis a mixed cell pleocytosis. Other causes of pleocytosis include multiple sclerosis, cerebral hemorrhage or infarction, and leukemia.

6. **C** Normal WBC counts for CSF are 0–5/μL for adults and 0–30/μL for children. Neutrophils predominate the differential count in bacterial meningitis, whereas lymphocytes predominate in viral meningitis. Hemorrhage and traumatic tap also cause increased PMNs, and WBC counts should be corrected using the CSF RBC count.

7. **B** Corrected WBC count = WBCs in CSF – [(Blood WBCs × CSF RBCs) ÷ Blood RBCs]

   Corrected WBC count = 150/μL– [(5000/μL WBCs × 6000/μL RBCs) ÷ 4,000,000/μL RBCs]

   Corrected WBC count = 150/μL–7.5/μL

   Corrected WBC count = 142/μL

8. **SITUATION:** What is the most likely cause of the following CSF results?

   > CSF glucose 20 mg/dL; CSF protein 100 mg/dL; CSF lactate 50 mg/dL

   A. Viral meningitis
   B. Viral encephalitis
   C. Cryptococcal meningitis
   D. Acute bacterial meningitis

   Body fluids/Evaluate laboratory data to recognize health and disease states/CSF/2

9. Which of the following conditions is most often associated with normal CSF glucose and protein?
   A. Multiple sclerosis
   B. Malignancy
   C. Subarachnoid hemorrhage
   D. Viral meningitis

   Body fluids/Correlate clinical and laboratory data/ Cerebrospinal fluid/2

10. The diagnosis of multiple sclerosis is often based upon which finding?
    A. The presence of elevated protein and low glucose
    B. An decreased IgG index
    C. The presence of oligoclonal bands by electrophoresis
    D. An increased level of CSF β-microglobulin

    Body Fluids/Correlate clinical and laboratory data/ CSF/2

11. Which of the following results is consistent with fungal meningitis?
    A. Normal CSF glucose
    B. Pleocytosis of mixed cellularity
    C. Normal CSF protein
    D. High CSF lactate

    Body fluids/Correlate clinical and laboratory data/CSF/2

8. **D** Acute bacterial meningitis causes increased production of immunoglobulins in CSF. Glucose levels are below normal (<40 mg/dL) because of consumption by PMNs and bacteria. Lactate levels rise due to increased pressure and hypoxia (>35 mg/dL being correlated with bacterial meningitis). When associated with increased PMNs and LD, these findings point to bacterial meningitis.

9. **D** In viral (aseptic) meningitis, the CSF glucose is usually above 40 mg/dL and the total protein is normal or slightly increased. Some types of viral meningitis can cause a low glucose level, which makes the differentiation of bacterial and viral meningitis difficult. Low CSF glucose and elevated total protein are also seen in malignancy, subarachnoid hemorrhage, and some persons with multiple sclerosis. Low glucose levels in malignancy and multiple sclerosis result from increased utilization. Glucose is reduced in subarachnoid hemorrhage as a result of release of glycolytic enzymes from RBCs. All three conditions result in high CSF protein, but multiple sclerosis (MS) is associated with an increased IgG index owing to local production of IgG.

10. **C** The total CSF protein is increased in less than half of persons with MS. The IgG index is increased in 80% or more of MS cases. Although the IgG index is sensitive, it is increased in many other disorders. The presence of oligoclonal banding (two or more discrete bands in the gamma zone following electrophoresis) is seen in 90% of persons with MS and in few other diseases. Although not entirely definitive, it is the single most effective laboratory test for the diagnosis of MS. When performing CSF electrophoresis, the serum pattern must be compared to the CSF pattern. At least some of the oligoclonal bands must *not* be found in the serum pattern for the test to be considered positive. β-2 Microglobulins are increased in CSF in inflammatory diseases (especially malignant diseases).

11. **B** In fungal meningitis the glucose and the total protein are elevated; however, unlike in bacterial meningitis, the lactate is usually below 35 mg/dL. Fungal meningitis usually produces a pleocytosis of mixed cellularity consisting of lymphocytes, PMNs, monocytes, and eosinophils. In some cases lymphocytes predominate, whereas in others PMNs make up the majority of WBCs.

12. In what suspected condition should a wet preparation using a warm slide be examined?
   A. Cryptococcal meningitis
   B. Amoebic meningoencephalitis
   C. *Mycobacterium tuberculosis* infection
   D. Neurosyphilis

   Body fluids/Select course of action/CSF/3

13. Which of the following CSF test results is most commonly increased in patients with multiple sclerosis?
   A. Glutamine
   B. Lactate
   C. IgG index
   D. Ammonia

   Body fluids/Correlate clinical and laboratory data/CSF/2

14. Which of the following is an inappropriate procedure for performing routine CSF analysis?
   A. A differential is done only if the total WBC count is higher than 10/μL
   B. A differential should be done on a stained CSF concentrate
   C. A minimum of 30 WBCs should be differentiated
   D. A Wright-stained slide should be examined rather than a chamber differential

   Body fluids/Apply principles of standard operating procedures/CSF/2

15. Which cell is present in the CSF in greater numbers in newborns than in older children or adults?
   A. Eosinophils
   B. Lymphocytes
   C. Monocytes
   D. Neutrophils

   Body fluids/Correlate clinical and laboratory data/CSF/2

16. Neutrophilic pleocytosis is usually associated with all of the following *except:*
   A. Cerebral infarction
   B. Malignancy
   C. Myelography
   D. Neurosyphilis

   Body fluids/Correlate clinical and laboratory data/CSF/2

Answers to Questions 12–16

12. **B** Amoeba in CSF appear very similar to monocytes in stained films but can be differentiated by their characteristic pseudopod mobility in a wet preparation on a prewarmed slide. *Naegleria fowleri* and *Acanthamoeba* spp. are causative agents of primary amoebic meningoencephalitis.

13. **C** IgG Index $= \dfrac{(\text{CSF IgG} \div \text{serum IgG})}{(\text{CSF albumin} \div \text{serum albumin})}$

   An IgG-albumin index is the ratio of CSF IgG: serum IgG divided by the CSF albumin:serum albumin. Values greater than 0.85 indicate CSF IgG production as seen in multiple sclerosis, or increased CSF production combined with increased permeability as seen in infection. Multiple sclerosis is characterized by the presence of oligoclonal banding in the CSF in more than 90% of patients with active disease. The total protein and myelin basic protein are often increased, and the glucose is decreased. Reye's syndrome results in hepatic failure, causing high CSF levels of ammonia and glutamine. CSF lactate is usually normal in patients with multiple sclerosis.

14. **A** A relative (percentage) increase in PMNs may be significant even when the WBC count does not exceed the upper limit of normal. For this reason a WBC differential using a concentrated CSF sample is always performed. Cytocentrifugation should be used to concentrate the cells followed by staining with Wright's stain.

15. **C** In newborns the upper reference limit (URL) for WBCs is 30/μL (URL for adults is 5/μL), with the majority of WBCs being monocytes or macrophages. In normal neonates, monocytes (including macrophages and histiocytes) account for about 75% of the WBCs, lymphocytes for about 20%, and PMNs for about 3%. In normal adults, lymphocytes account for about 60% of the WBCs, monocytes for about 35%, and PMNs for about 2%.

16. **D** Neutrophils may appear in CSF from many causes, making it necessary to correlate results of chemical assays with hematological findings. Low glucose and high protein levels occur in both malignancy and bacterial meningitis. LD isoenzymes and lactate may be helpful in distinguishing malignancy from bacterial meningitis. In neurosyphilis, there is usually an absolute lymphocytosis, increased total protein, and IgG index.

17. Which statement about CSF protein is true?
- **A.** An abnormal serum protein electrophoretic pattern does not affect the CSF pattern
- **B.** The upper reference limit for CSF total protein in newborns is one-half that of adult levels
- **C.** CSF IgG is increased in panencephalitis, malignancy, and neurosyphilis
- **D.** Antibodies to *Treponema pallidum* disappear after successful antibiotic therapy

Body fluids/Correlate clinical and laboratory data/CSF/2

18. Which of the following statements regarding routine microbiological examination of CSF is true?
- **A.** A Gram's stain is performed on the CSF prior to concentration
- **B.** The Gram stain is positive in fewer than 40% of cases of acute bacterial meningitis
- **C.** India ink and acid fast stains are indicated if neutrophilic pleocytosis is present
- **D.** All CSF specimens should be cultured using sheep blood agar, chocolate agar, and supplemented broth

Body fluids/Apply knowledge of standard operating procedures/CSF/2

19. Which organism is the most frequent cause of bacterial meningitis in neonates?
- **A.** *Neisseria meningitidis*
- **B.** Group B streptococci
- **C.** *Streptococcus pneumoniae*
- **D.** *Klebsiella pneumoniae*

Body fluids/Correlate clinical and laboratory data/CSF/2

20. Following a head injury, which protein will identify the presence of CSF leakage through the nose?
- **A.** Transthyretin
- **B.** Myelin basic protein
- **C.** Transferrin
- **D.** C-reactive protein

Body Fluids/Select test/CSF/2

17. **C** Although the blood-brain barrier excludes most plasma proteins, abnormal serum proteins can cause parallel CSF electrophoretic patterns. Therefore, an abnormal CSF pattern indicates CNS disease only if not duplicated by the serum pattern. Normal CSF total protein in newborns may be up to two times higher than those of adult levels. Antibodies to *T. pallidum* remain in CSF after treatment, but nontreponemal antibodies disappear. While the FTA-ABS test for specific antibodies is more sensitive, the VDRL test is often performed concurrently. A positive result for both tests is diagnostic of active tertiary syphilis.

18. **D** A culture should be performed on the sediment of the second aliquot of the CSF after it is centrifuged. Blood and chocolate agar and anaerobic broth should always be used, and if sterile held a minimum of 3 days. Blood cultures should be done because septicemia occurs in about one-half of bacterial meningitis cases. A Gram's stain is always performed using sediment of the CSF because it is positive in more than 70% of acute bacterial meningitis cases. India ink, acid-fast, and wet preparations may be ordered if an absolute monocytosis is present.

19. **B** Group B streptococci and *Escherichia coli* are the two most common isolates in neonates. *Haemophilus influenzae*, *S. pneumoniae*, and *N. meningitidis* are the most common isolates in children. *S. pneumoniae* is the most frequent isolate in the elderly.

20. **C** In cases of trauma, it may be necessary to differentiate rhinorrhea from CSF leakage, and this can be done by immunofixation electrophoresis to identify tau protein found in CSF but not serum. Tau protein is an enzymatically modified form of transferrin that migrates in the slow β-zone just behind unmodified transferrin. Transthyretin or prealbumin is present in far greater concentrations in CSF than blood but may not be seen if CSF is diluted with nasal fluid. Myelin basic protein is a component of nerve sheaths and is present in CSF in about 60% of persons with MS. It is also found in persons with other demyelinating diseases, SLE, stroke, and brain injury. C-reactive protein is elevated in the CSF of approximately two-thirds of persons with bacterial meningitis.

21. Which of the following statements regarding serous fluids is true?
  A. The normal volume of pleural fluid is 30–50 mL
  B. Mesothelial cells, PMNs, lymphocytes, and macrophages may be present in normal fluids
  C. X-ray films can detect a 10% increase in the volume of a serous fluid
  D. Normal serous fluids are colorless

Body fluids/Correlate clinical and laboratory data/Serous fluid/2

22. The term effusion refers to:
  A. A chest fluid that is purulent
  B. A serous fluid that is chylous
  C. An increased volume of serous fluid
  D. An inflammatory process affecting the appearance of a serous fluid

Body fluids/Apply knowledge of fundamental biological characteristics/Pleural fluid/1

23. Which of the following laboratory results is characteristic of a transudative fluid?
  A. SG = 1.018
  B. Total protein = 3.2 g/dL
  C. LD fluid/serum ratio = 0.25
  D. Total protein fluid/serum ratio = 0.65

Body fluids/Evaluate laboratory data to recognize health and disease states/Exudates/2

24. Which observation is *LEAST* useful in distinguishing a hemorrhagic serous fluid from a traumatic tap?
  A. Clearing of fluid as it is aspirated
  B. Presence of xanthochromia
  C. The formation of a clot
  D. Diminished RBC count in successive aliquots

Body fluids/Correlate laboratory data with physiological processes/Serous fluids/2

25. Which of the following laboratory results on serous fluid is most likely to be caused by a traumatic tap?
  A. An RBC count of 8000/μL
  B. A WBC count of 6000/μL
  C. An Hct of 35%
  D. A neutrophil count of 45%

Body fluids/Correlate laboratory data with physiological processes/Serous fluid/2

Answers to Questions 21–25

21. **B** The serous fluids include pleural, pericardial, and peritoneal fluid. They form from ultrafiltration of plasma through serous membranes. These are lined with specialized epithelium called mesothelium. They make up about 5% of the cells in serous fluid and may be difficult to differentiate from malignant cells. Pleural fluid volume is normally less than 10 mL. The volume of pericardial fluid is normally 10–50 mL and peritoneal fluid 30–50 mL. X-rays can detect an increase in serous fluids of 300 mL or more. Normal serous fluids are clear and range in color from straw to light yellow.

22. **C** Effusions are classified as either transudates, exudates, or chylous. Transudates result from abnormal hemodynamics (e.g., congestive heart failure, liver disease), and exudates and chylous fluids from local disease. A pleural fluid that is purulent is called an empyemic fluid. Such a fluid has a WBC count of 10,000/μL or greater.

23. **C** Transudative fluids are distinguished from exudative fluids by the physical appearance, SG, total protein, LD, cholesterol, and bilirubin. Exudative fluids have a fluid:serum LD ratio greater than 0.6 caused by release of the enzyme from inflammatory or malignant cells. Exudative fluids have a total protein greater than 3.0 g/dL, SG greater than 1.015, fluid:serum total protein ratio greater than 0.6, cholesterol greater than 60 mg/dL (fluid:serum ratio >0.3) and fluid:serum bilirubin ratio greater than 0.6. Exudates are caused by infection, infarction, malignancy, rheumatoid diseases, and trauma.

24. **C** Xanthochromia indicates either an exudative process or prior traumatic tap. Hemorrhagic pleural fluids usually have RBC counts greater than 100,000/μL and are usually caused by lung neoplasms. Clearing of fluid or diminished RBC counts in successive tubes favor a diagnosis of a traumatic tap. A clot may form in a hemorrhagic fluid or following a traumatic tap. However, a transudative fluid will not clot.

25. **A** Normal fluids have a WBC count less than 1000/μL, but counts between 1000 and 2500/μL may be seen in both exudates and transudates. All WBC types are present, but no type should account for more than 50% of the leukocyte count. An RBC count below 10,000/μL is usually caused by a traumatic tap. A fluid Hct similar to blood is caused by a hemothorax. Pleural fluids containing >100,000/μL RBCs are associated most often with malignancies but are also seen in trauma and pulmonary infarction.

26. Which of the following conditions is commonly associated with an exudative effusion?
    A. Congestive heart failure
    B. Malignancy
    C. Nephrotic syndrome
    D. Cirrhosis

    Body fluids/Correlate clinical and laboratory data/
    Transudate/2

27. Which of the following conditions is associated with a chylous effusion?
    A. Necrosis
    B. Pulmonary infarction or infection
    C. SLE or rheumatoid arthritis (RA)
    D. Lymphatic obstruction

    Body fluids/Correlate clinical and laboratory data/
    Exudates/2

28. Which of the following conditions is most often associated with a pleural fluid glucose below 30 mg/dL?
    A. Diabetes mellitus
    B. Pancreatitis
    C. Rheumatoid arthritis
    D. Bacterial pneumonia

    Body fluids/Correlate clinical and laboratory data/
    Pleural fluid/2

29. In which condition is the pleural fluid pH likely to be above 7.3?
    A. Bacterial pneumonia with parapneumonic exudate
    B. Rheumatoid pleuritis
    C. Esophageal rupture
    D. Pneumothorax

    Body fluids/Correlate clinical and laboratory data/
    Pleural fluid/2

Answers to Questions 26–29

26. **B** Transudative fluids are caused by circulatory problems, usually decreased oncotic pressure or increased hydrostatic pressure. In contrast, exudative effusions are caused by inflammatory processes and cellular infiltration as seen in malignancy. In addition to a RBC count $>100,000/\mu L$, malignancies often involve the lung, colon, breast, and pancreas and often produce carcinoembryonic antigen.

27. **D** Malignancy, pulmonary infarction, SLE, and RA are characterized by inflammation with increases in protein, WBCs, and LD. Exudates can also be caused by tuberculosis, pancreatitis, and lymphoma. Lymphatic obstruction is often associated with lymphoma and other malignancies that block the flow of lymph into the azygous vein. This causes a chylous effusion. Chylous effusions are also caused by traumatic injury to the thoracic duct. Necrosis causes a pseudochylous effusion. This resembles a chylous effusion in appearance but has a foul odor. Chylous fluids contain chylomicrons, stain positive for fat globules, show lymphocytosis, and have a triglyceride concentration over twofold higher than plasma (or >110 mg/dL). Pseudochylous effusions are characterized by mixed cellularity and an elevated cholesterol level.

28. **C** Normal pleural fluid has the same glucose concentration as plasma. Hyperglycemia is the only condition that is associated with a high pleural fluid glucose concentration. Low glucose levels (<60 mg/dL) may be seen in infection, malignancy, and rheumatic diseases. However, glucose levels are lowest (often below 30 mg/dL) and are a constant finding when rheumatoid disease affects the lungs. Pancreatitis causes an exudative peritoneal and pleural effusion with an elevated peritoneal fluid amylase (without a low glucose level).

29. **D** The pH of pleural fluid is approximately 7.64, and values below 7.30 are usually associated with a poorer prognosis and often require drainage. Esophageal rupture produces the lowest pH with values in the range of 6.0–6.3. In addition, pleural fluid pH is low in rheumatoid disease involving the lungs and pleura, some malignancies, and SLE. Low pH and glucose in pleural fluid are seen in lung abscess and exudative bacterial pneumonia (termed parapneumonic effusion). Pneumothorax results from air entering the pleural space and does not produce a low pH.

30. Which of the following hematological values best frames the upper reference limits for peritoneal fluid?

	WBC Count	Percentage of PMNs	RBC Count
A.	300/μL	25%	100,000/μL
B.	10,000/μL	50%	500,000/μL
C.	50,000/μL	50%	500,000/μL
D.	100,000/μL	75%	1,000,000/μL

Body fluids/Apply knowledge of fundamental biological characteristics/Serous fluids/2

31. Which of the following characteristics is higher for synovial fluid than for the serous fluids?
A. SG
B. Glucose
C. Total protein
D. Viscosity

Body fluids/Apply knowledge of fundamental biological characteristics/Synovial fluid/1

32. In which type of arthritis is the synovial WBC count likely to be greater than 50,000/μL?
A. Septic arthritis
B. Osteoarthritis
C. Rheumatoid arthritis
D. Hemorrhagic arthritis

Body fluids/Correlate clinical and laboratory data/Synovial fluid/2

33. What type of cell is a "ragocyte"?
A. Cartilage cell seen in inflammatory arthritis
B. A PMN with inclusions formed by immune complexes
C. A plasma cell seen in RA
D. A macrophage containing large inclusions

Body fluids/Apply knowledge of fundamental biological characteristics/Morphology/1

34. Which of the following crystals is the cause of gout?
A. Uric acid or monosodium urate
B. Calcium pyrophosphate or apatite
C. Calcium oxalate
D. Cholesterol

Body fluids/Apply knowledge of fundamental biological characteristics/Synovial fluid/1

30. **A** Peritoneal fluid normally has a WBC count of less than 300/μL. Neutrophils should account for no more than 25% of the WBCs. A majority of PMNs indicates bacterial infection of the peritoneum. Lymphocytosis suggests malignancy, tuberculosis, cirrhosis, and lymphatic leakage. Peritoneal fluid amylase is elevated in most cases of acute pancreatitis. Peritonitis is suspected when the fluid LD is greater than 40% of the serum level. Normal pleural fluid usually has a WBC count below 1000/μL. Exudative fluids usually have a WBC count above 10,000/μL, but values tend to overlap noninflammatory fluids. The PMNs should constitute 50% of the WBCs or less, and the RBC count should be less than 100,000/μL.

31. **D** Synovial fluid has approximately the same SG and glucose as plasma and the serous fluids but is far more viscous owing to a high content of mucoprotein (hyaluronate) secreted by the synovium. Viscosity is estimated by pulling the fluid from the tip of a syringe or pipette. Normal fluid gives a string longer than 4 cm. Low viscosity indicates inflammation. The total protein of synovial fluid is usually lower than that of serous fluids, the upper reference limit being 2.0 g/dL.

32. **A** The WBC count is elevated in all types of arthritis, but is greatest (50,000–100,000/μL) in septic arthritis. Neutrophils constitute less than 25% of WBCs in normal and noninflammatory arthritis but are above 50% in inflammatory and septic arthritis. Fluids are diluted in saline because acetic acid causes a mucin clot to form. . WBC counts should be performed within 1 hour of collection because the WBC count will diminish over time.

33. **B** Ragocytes are PMNs containing dark granules composed of immunoglobulins, but they may be seen in gout and septic arthritis as well as in RA. LE cells may be seen in fluid from patients with SLE, and Reiter's cells, macrophages with ingested globular inclusions, are seen in Reiter's syndrome and other inflammatory diseases.

34. **A** Although all of the crystals mentioned can cause crystal-induced arthritis, uric acid and sodium urate crystals cause gout and are seen in about 90% of gout patients.

35. Which crystal causes "pseudogout"?
- **A.** Oxalic acid
- **B.** Calcium pyrophosphate
- **C.** Calcium oxalate
- **D.** Cholesterol

Body fluids/Apply knowledge of fundamental biological characteristics/Synovial fluid/1

36. A synovial fluid sample is examined using a polarizing microscope with a red compensating filter. Crystals are seen that are yellow when the long axis of the crystal is parallel to the slow vibrating light. When the long axis of the crystal is perpendicular to the slow vibrating light, the crystals appear blue. What type of crystal is present?
- **A.** Calcium oxalate
- **B.** Calcium pyrophosphate
- **C.** Uric acid
- **D.** Cholesterol

Body fluids/Apply principles of special procedures/ Synovial fluid/2

37. In which condition is the synovial fluid glucose most likely to be within normal limits?
- **A.** Septic arthritis
- **B.** Inflammatory arthritis
- **C.** Hemorrhagic arthritis
- **D.** Gout

Body fluids/Correlate clinical and laboratory data/ Synovial fluid/2

38. Which statement about synovial fluid in RA is true?
- **A.** Synovial/serum IgG is usually 1:2 or higher
- **B.** Total hemolytic complement is elevated
- **C.** Ninety percent of RA cases test positive for rheumatoid factor in synovial fluid
- **D.** Demonstration of rheumatoid factor in joint fluid is diagnostic for RA

Body fluids/Correlate clinical and laboratory data/ Synovial fluid/2

39. Which of the following organisms accounts for the majority of septic arthritis cases in young and middle age adults?
- **A.** *H. influenzae*
- **B.** *N. gonorrhoeae*
- **C.** *Staphylococcus aureus*
- **D.** *Borrelia burgdorferi*

Body fluids/Apply knowledge of fundamental biological characteristics/Synovial fluid/2

Answers to Questions 35–39

35. **B** Calcium pyrophosphate crystals occur as needles or small rhombic plates and can be confused with uric acid. They rotate plane polarized light but not as strongly as uric acid. Synovial fluid should never be collected in tubes containing powdered EDTA because it may form crystals that can be mistaken for in vivo crystals. The recommended anticoagulant is sodium heparin, although liquid EDTA may be used.

36. **C** Polarized microscopy with a red compensating filter differentiates uric acid and pseudogout crystals. When the long axis of uric acid needles is parallel to the slow vibrating light, the crystals appear yellow. When the long axis is perpendicular to the slow vibrating light, the crystals appear blue. Calcium pyrophosphate gives the reverse effect.

37. **C** Synovial fluid glucose is normally less than 10 mg/dL below the serum glucose level and should be collected after an 8-hour fast to ensure that the fluid and plasma are equilibrated. In septic arthritis, the glucose level is often more than 40 mg/dL below the serum level and about 25–40 mg/dL lower in inflammatory arthritis, which includes gout. Osteoarthritis and hemorrhagic arthritis are not usually associated with low joint fluid glucose.

38. **A** Rheumatoid factor can be present in both serum and synovial fluids from patients with RA, SLE, and other inflammatory diseases. Rheumatoid factor is present in the synovial fluid of approximately 60% of patients with RA. Normally, IgG in synovial fluid is about 10% of the serum IgG level. CH_{50} levels in serum and synovium are more differential. Both are increased in Reiter's syndrome but are often low in SLE; synovial CH_{50} is decreased and serum CH_{50} is normal (or increased) in RA.

39. **B** Synovial fluid is normally sterile, and all of the organisms listed may cause septic arthritis. *N. gonorrhoeae* is responsible for about 75% of septic arthritis cases occurring in young and middle-aged adults. *Staphylococcus* spp. is responsible for the majority of cases involving the elderly. *Haemophilus* spp., *Staphylococcus* spp., and *Streptococcus* spp. are the most common causes of arthritis in children.

40. Which of the following hematology values best frames the upper reference limits for synovial fluid?

	WBC Count	Percentage of PMNs	RBC Count
A.	200/μL	25%	2000/μL
B.	5000/μL	50%	10,000/μL
C.	10,000/μL	50%	50,000/μL
D.	20,000/μL	5%	500,000/μL

Body fluids/Apply knowledge of fundamental biological characteristics/Synovial fluid/2

40. A The WBC count of normal joint fluid is 200/μL or less. Values above 5000/μL cause the fluid to be purulent and occur in septic arthritis, RA, and gout. WBC counts higher than 50,000 μL indicate septic arthritis. The majority of WBCs in normal fluid are monocytes, which usually account for 50%–65%. Neutrophils and lymphocytes should account for no more than 25% each. An increase in RBCs occurs in cases of infectious and hemorrhagic arthritis or results from a traumatic tap. Hemorrhagic fluid appears turbid, red to brown, and often clotted. Inflammatory arthritis can allow fibrinogen to enter the fluid and thus clot. Fluid from a hemophiliac will not clot in spite of its bloody appearance.

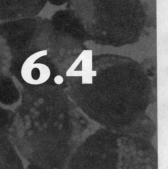

1. Which of the following statements about amniotic fluid bilirubin measured by scanning spectrophotometry is true?
   A. The 410-nm peak is due to hemoglobin and the 450-nm peak to bilirubin
   B. Baseline correction is not required if a scanning spectrophotometer is used
   C. Chloroform extraction is necessary only when meconium is present
   D. In normal amniotic fluid, bilirubin increases with gestational age

   Body fluids/Apply principles of special procedures/Amniotic fluid/2

2. Which test best correlates with the severity of hemolytic disease of the newborn (HDN)?
   A. Rh antibody titer of the mother
   B. Lecithin/sphingomyelin (L/S) ratio
   C. Amniotic fluid bilirubin
   D. Urinary estradiol

   Body Fluids/Correlate clinical and laboratory data/Amniotic fluid/2

Answers to Questions 1–2

1. **A** Amniotic fluid bilirubin reflects the extent of fetal RBC destruction in cases of HDN. It is measured by scanning the fluid from 350 to 600 nm, then drawing a baseline using the points at 365 nm and 550 nm. The delta absorbance (ΔA) of hemoglobin at 410 nm and bilirubin at 450 nm are determined by subtracting the absorbance of the baseline from the respective peaks. Samples that are not grossly hemolyzed can be corrected for oxyhemoglobin by subtracting 5% of the ΔA at 410 nm from the ΔA at 450 nm. When hemolysis is severe or meconium is present, the bilirubin must be extracted in chloroform before measuring absorbance. Bilirubin normally decreases with increasing gestational age because fetal urine contributes more to amniotic fluid volume as the fetus matures. The bilirubin concentration must be correlated with gestational age in order to correctly evaluate the severity of HDN.

2. **C** Amniotic fluid bilirubin is the best index of the severity of HDN and is measured by scanning spectrophotometry from 550–365 nm. When hemoglobin produces a positive slope at 410 nm, the bilirubin should be extracted with chloroform prior to scanning. Extraction methods give the best correlation with RBC destruction.

3. Which is the reference method for determining fetal lung maturity?

  A. Human placental lactogen
  B. L/S ratio
  C. Amniotic fluid bilirubin
  D. Urinary estriol

Body Fluids/Correlate laboratory data with physiological processes/L/S ratio/2

4. Which of the following statements regarding the L/S ratio is true?

  A. A ratio of 2:1 or greater usually indicates adequate pulmonary surfactant to prevent respiratory distress syndrome (RDS)
  B. A ratio of 1.5:1 indicates fetal lung maturity in pregnancies associated with diabetes mellitus
  C. Sphingomyelin levels increase during the third trimester, causing the L/S ratio to fall slightly during the last 2 weeks of gestation
  D. A phosphatidylglycerol (PG) spot indicates the presence of meconium in the amniotic fluid

Body fluids/Correlate clinical and laboratory data/L/S ratio/2

3. **B** Respiratory distress syndrome develops when surfactants are insufficient to prevent collapse of the infant's alveoli during expiration. Tests measuring pulmonary phospholipid surfactants are the most specific and sensitive indicators of respiratory distress syndrome. An L/S ratio greater than 2:1 (in some laboratories 2.5:1) is the most widely accepted measure of fetal lung maturity. An alternative to the L/S ratio used by many laboratories is the measurement of lecithin in amniotic fluid by fluorescence polarization immunoassay. This test measures the ratio of lecithin to albumin. Fluorescent dye is added to the sample, and the dye partitions between the albumin and lecithin. Dye bound to albumin produces plane polarized fluorescence, but dye bound to lecithin does not. Therefore, the intensity of plane polarized fluorescence is inversely related to lecithin concentration. Most of the surfactants in the amniotic fluid are present in the form of lamellar bodies. These can be counted using an electronic cell counter at the settings for enumerating platelets.

4. **A** Pulmonary surfactants are mainly disaturated lecithins produced by type II granular pneumocytes. The L/S ratio increases toward the end of the third trimester due to increased production of lecithin. The concentration of sphingomyelin remains constant throughout gestation and serves as an internal reference. Meconium contains less lecithin than amniotic fluid and usually decreases the L/S ratio; however, meconium produces a spot that can be misinterpreted as lecithin, leading to a falsely increased L/S ratio. Sufficient PG to produce a spot is seen only when the L/S ratio is 2:1 or higher. PG is not present in either blood or meconium and, therefore, its presence indicates fetal lung maturity. In diabetes the fetal lungs may mature more slowly than normal, and infants may develop RDS when the L/S ratio is 2:1 or slightly higher. For this reason, an L/S of 3:1 more closely correlates with fetal lung maturity when testing amniotic fluid from diabetic mothers. As in all other cases, when the amniotic fluid from a diabetic mother is positive for PG, fetal lung maturity is established.

5. Which of the following conditions is most likely to cause a falsely low L/S ratio?
   A. The presence of PG in amniotic fluid
   B. Freezing the specimen for one month at −20°C
   C. Centrifugation at 1000 × g for 10 min
   D. Maternal diabetes mellitus

Body fluids/Apply knowledge to recognize sources of error/Amniotic fluid/2

6. Which of the following statements accurately describes hCG levels in pregnancy?
   A. Levels of hCG rise throughout pregnancy
   B. In ectopic pregnancy serum hCG doubling time is below expected levels
   C. Molar pregnancies are associated with lower levels than expected for the time of gestation
   D. hCG returns to nonpregnant levels within 2 days following delivery, stillbirth, or abortion

Body fluids/Correlate clinical and laboratory data/Chorionic gonadotropin/2

7. Which of the following statements regarding pregnancy testing is true?
   A. β-Subunits of hCG, thyroid-stimulating hormone (TSH), and follicle-stimulating hormone (FSH) are very similar
   B. Antibodies against the β-subunit of hCG cross-react with luteinizing hormone (LH)
   C. A false-positive result may occur in patients with heterophile antibodies
   D. Serum should not be used for pregnancy tests because proteins interfere

Body fluids/Apply principles of basic laboratory procedures/Pregnancy test/2

Answers to Questions 5–7

5. **C** Pulmonary surfactants are largely present in the form of lamellar bodies and can be lost by centrifuging the amniotic fluid at high g force. Centrifuge speed should be the minimum required to spin down cells (450 g for 10 minutes at 4°C). Samples that cannot be measured immediately should be refrigerated or frozen. Samples are stable for up to 3 days at 2°C–8°C and for months when frozen at −20°C or lower. Meconium and blood may also introduce errors when measuring the L/S ratio. Blood has an L/S ratio of approximately 2:1 and falsely raises the L/S ratio when fetal lungs are immature and depresses the L/S ratio when fetal lungs are mature.

6. **B** In normal pregnancy hCG levels rise exponentially following implantation and peak at weeks 9–12, reaching in excess of 100,000 mIU/mL. Levels fall after the first trimester to about 20,000 mIU/mL and then remain at about that level through term. The hCG doubling time averages 2.2 days. In ectopic pregnancy the expected increase between consecutive days is below normal. Hydatiform moles are associated with greatly elevated levels of hCG. Serum hCG can take up to 4 weeks to return to nonpregnant (<25 mIU/mL) or baseline (<5 mIU/mL) levels following delivery, stillbirth, or abortion.

7. **C** The α-subunit of hCG is very similar to the α-subunit of TSH and FSH and identical to that of LH. Although the β-subunits of hCG and LH are very similar, antibodies can be made to the β-subunit of hCG that do not cross-react with LH or other pituitary hormones. Most enzyme immunoassay (EIA) methods utilize two monoclonal antibodies against different sites of the hCG molecule. One antibody is specific for the carboxy terminal end of the β-chain, and the other reacts with the α-chain, resulting in a positive test only when intact hCG is present. Because monoclonal antibodies are derived from mouse hybridomas, rare false-positive reactions may occur in patients who have antimouse Ig antibodies. Although the test can detect lower levels of hCG, 25 mIU/mL is the positive cutoff point for pregnancy. Serum is preferred over urine because serum levels are more consistently above the cutoff point than random urine in early pregnancy.

8. **SITUATION:** A pregnant female was seen by her physician, who suspects a molar pregnancy. An hCG test is ordered and found to be low. The sample was diluted tenfold and the assay was repeated. The result was found to be grossly elevated. What best explains this situation?
   A. The wrong specimen was diluted
   B. A pipetting error was made in the first analysis
   C. Antigen excess caused a falsely low result in the undiluted sample
   D. A inhibitor of the antigen–antibody reaction was present in the sample

   Body fluids/Apply knowledge to recognize sources of error/hCG/2

9. Most cases of Down's syndrome are the result of:
   A. Nondisjunction of an E chromosome (E trisomy)
   B. Nondisjunction of chromosome 21 (G trisomy)
   C. A 14–21 chromosome translocation
   D. Deletion of the long arm of G21

   Body fluids/Apply knowledge of fundamental biological characteristics/Cytogenetics/1

10. Which assay result is often approximately 25% below the expected level in pregnancies associated with Down's syndrome?
    A. Serum unconjugated estriol
    B. L/S ratio
    C. Amniotic fluid bilirubin
    D. Urinary chorionic gonadotropin

    Body Fluids/Correlate laboratory data with physiological processes/Cytogenetics/2

11. Which of the following statements about α-fetoprotein (AFP) is correct?
    A. Maternal serum may be used to screen for open neural tube defects
    B. Levels above 4 ng/mL are considered positive
    C. Elevated levels in amniotic fluid are specific for spina bifida
    D. AFP levels increase in pregnancies associated with Down's syndrome

    Body Fluids/Apply principles of special procedures/AFP/2

Answers to Questions 8–11

8. **C** Assays of intact hCG are double antibody sandwich immunoassays. One antibody reacts with the α-subunit and the other with the β-subunit. In assays in which both antibodies are added together, a process called the "hook effect" is known to occur. In extreme antigen excess, the hCG saturates both antibodies, preventing sandwich formation. This results in a falsely low measurements of hCG.

9. **B** Down's syndrome results from the presence of an extra chromosome 21. Although it can be caused by 14–21 translocation or isochromosome formation, most cases arise from nondisjunction. A quad marker screen consisting of maternal serum AFP, hCG, dimeric inhibin A, and unconjugated estriol is used to screen for Down's syndrome during the second trimester. If the test is positive, amniocentesis is performed, and 21 trisomy is investigated by chromosome karyotyping or FISH.

10. **A** Estriol is produced by the placenta as well as the fetal and maternal adrenal glands and liver. Free estriol produced by the placenta is rapidly conjugated by the maternal liver. Maternal serum unconjugated (free) estriol is almost all derived from the fetus and is a direct reflection of current fetal placental function. Serum unconjugated estriol (uE_3) measured during the second trimester is used along with serum AFP, hCG, and dimeric inhibin A as part of the quad marker screening test for Down's syndrome. AFP and uE_3 are decreased by approximately 25%, inhibin A is increased by a factor of approximately 1.8, and hCG is increased by a factor of approximately 2.5 in Down's syndrome pregnancies. When all four assays are combined with adjustments for maternal age, gestational age, race, maternal weight, and diabetes, the detection rate can be as high as 80% with a false-positive rate of 7%.

11. **A** Maternal serum AFP increases and amniotic fluid AFP decreases with gestational age. Because serum levels are dependent on gestational age, upper reference limits depend upon the last menstrual period dating. AFP is measured between 14 and 18 weeks' gestation, and levels are reported as multiples of the median in order to permit interlaboratory comparison. When serum levels are high, ultrasound is used to determine fetal age and rule out twins. Increased fetal AFP levels (>2.5 MoM) may result from many diseases in addition to open neural tube defects such as spina bifida. These include anencephaly, ventral wall defects, congenital hypothyroidism, and Turner's syndrome. Decreased levels (<0.75 MoM) may be seen in approximately 25% of Down's syndrome pregnancies.

12. First trimester screening for Down's syndrome can be performed using which markers?
  A. AFP and unconjugated estriol
  B. Free β-hCG and pregnancy-associated plasma protein A
  C. Intact hCG and dimeric inhibin A
  D. Dimeric inhibin B and AFP

  Body fluids/Apply knowledge of special procedures/Trisomy screening/2

13. When performing marker screening tests for Down's syndrome, why are results expressed in multiples of the median (MoM) rather than concentration?
  A. Concentration is not normally distributed
  B. MoM normalizes for gestational age
  C. Some tests cannot be reported in mass units
  D. Mean cannot be determined accurately for these analytes

  Body fluids/Apply knowledge of special procedures/ Trisomy screening/1

12. **B** Maternal serum AFP levels are too low to measure accurately during the first trimester and intact hCG and estriol do not discriminate well between 21 trisomy and normal pregnancy before the second trimester. First trimester screening for Down's syndrome (and trisomy 18) can be performed between weeks 10 and 13 using free β-hCG (almost twofold higher in Down's syndrome) and pregnancy-associated plasma protein A (PAPP-A), which has a median in Down's syndrome of less than half of that seen in normal pregnancy. These two markers, used together with high-resolution ultrasonography to determine nuchal fold thickness (NT) (swelling at the base of the neck), have a sensitivity as high as 85%–90%. NT in Down's syndrome averages 1.5 MoM compared to 1.0 MoM for normal pregnancy.

13. **B** Reporting of screening markers as multiples of the median has two advantages. It eliminates interlaboratory variation in reference ranges seen when concentration units are reported. Laboratories using different methods (antibodies or calibrators) may have significantly different mass unit results for the same sample, necessitating different reference ranges. The reference range in concentration units is also dependent on the gestational age at the time of sample collection; however, the average result for normals is always 1.0 MoM regardless of the gestational age of the cohort. Use of MoM obviates the need to report specific reference ranges based on method or gestational age and makes calculation of risk less complicated.

14. Which statement regarding the fetal fibronectin test is true?
    A. A positive test is correlated with a low probability of delivery within 14 days
    B. The test should not be performed before week 24 or after the end of week 34
    C. The test is performed on amniotic fluid
    D. The test is used to identify amniotic fluid after rupture of the fetal membranes

    Body Fluids/Apply principles of special laboratory procedures/Fetal fibronectin/1

15. What is the term for sperm when the anterior portion of the headpiece is smaller than normal?
    A. Azoospermia
    B. Microcephaly
    C. Acrosomal deficiency
    D. Necrozoospermia

    Body fluids/Apply knowledge of fundamental biological characteristics/Seminal fluid/1

16. What is the most common cause of male infertility?
    A. Mumps
    B. Klinefelter's syndrome
    C. Varicocele
    D. Malignancy

    Body fluids/Correlate clinical and laboratory data/ Seminal fluid/2

14. **B** The fetal fibronectin test is used to predict the possibility of preterm delivery in high risk pregnancies or in women with signs of preterm labor. Fetal fibronectin is a basement membrane protein produced by the amnion and chorion. It is present in cervical secretions in early pregnancy but disappears by about week 20. When there is inflammation in the membranes preceding delivery, fibronectin is released and can be found in cervicovaginal secretions. Fetal fibronectin is measured on a vaginal fluid sample by enzyme immunoassay after extracting it from a cervical swab. A positive test (>50 ng/mL) has a sensitivity of about 60% in predicting preterm birth. However, a negative test has a 92% negative predictive value for the likelihood of preterm delivery and effectively rules out preterm delivery within the next 2 weeks. Amniotic fluid that has escaped from ruptured membranes is identified by testing a vaginal swab for pH. Vaginal fluid is normally acidic, with a pH between 5.0 and 6.0. After rupture of the membranes, the pH of the fluid changes to 6.5–7.5. This change can be detected using nitrazine paper or a swab containing nitrazine yellow.

15. **C** Spermatozoa have a well-defined headpiece consisting of the acrosome and nucleus. The acrosome comprises the anterior portion of the head and contains nutrients and enzymes needed for penetration of the ovum. A thin filament, the neckpiece, connects the head and tail. The tail is divided into the midpiece, mainpiece, and endpiece. The midpiece is the thick anterior end of approximately 6 μ containing a 9 + 2 longitudinal arrangement of microtubules (two central microtubules surrounded by nine doublets so that a cross section appears like a pinwheel). This is called the axoneme and is surrounded by nine radial fibers. The longest portion of the tail (40–45 μ) is the mainpiece. It is thinner than the midpiece and lacks the outer radial fibers. The distal portion, called the endpiece, is approximately 5 μ. It contains the axoneme but is unsheathed.

16. **C** Varicocele is the hardening of veins that drain the testes. This causes blood from the adrenal vein to flow into the spermatic vein. Adrenal corticosteroids retard the development of spermatozoa. Mumps, Klinefelter's syndrome, and malignancy cause testicular failure, accounting for about 10% of infertility cases in men.

17. Which of the following values is the lower limit of normal for sperm concentration?
  A. 20 million/mL
  B. 40 million/mL
  C. 60 million/mL
  D. 100 million/mL

Body fluids/Evaluate laboratory data to recognize health and disease states/Seminal fluid/2

18. Which morphological abnormality of sperm is most often associated with varicocele?
  A. Tapering of the head
  B. Cytoplasmic droplet below the neckpiece
  C. Lengthened neckpiece
  D. Acrosomal deficiency

Body fluids/Correlate clinical and laboratory data/ Seminal fluid/2

19. Which of the following stains is used to determine sperm viability?
  A. Eosin Y
  B. Hematoxylin
  C. Papanicolaou
  D. Methylene blue

Body fluids/Apply principles of special procedures/ Seminal fluid/1

20. Which of the following semen analysis results is abnormal?
  A. Volume 1.0 mL
  B. Liquefaction 40 minutes
  C. pH 7.6
  D. Motility 50% rapid progressive movement

Body Fluids/Evaluate data to recognize abnormal results/Seminal fluid/2

Answers to Questions 17–20

17. **A** The broadest reference range for spermatozoa is 20–150×10^6/mL. Concentrations below 20×10^6/mL are considered abnormal. The sperm concentration is multiplied by the seminal fluid volume to determine the sperm count. The lower limit of normal for the sperm count is 40×10^6 per ejaculate. Lower sperm counts often result from obstruction of the ejaculatory duct or testicular failure.

18. **A** Acrosomal deficiency, nuclear abnormalities, and lengthened neckpiece are the most common morphological abnormalities of spermatozoa. Tapering of the head is a nuclear abnormality. Sperm morphology should be evaluated by classifying 200 mature sperm by strict criteria. The most commonly used strict criteria define the normal sperm head as having a length of 4.0–5.0 μ, a width of 2.5–3.5 μ, a L:W ratio of 1.5–1.75, and an acrosomal area of 40%–70%. Using strict criteria, there is a high likelihood of infertility when the number of normal forms is below 15%. However, when nonstrict criteria are used, ≥60% of sperm should be normal.

19. **A** Eosin Y is excluded by living sperm and is used to determine the percentage of living cells. Papanicolaou, Giemsa, and hematoxylin stains are used to evaluate sperm morphology, but Wright's stain is not recommended. The viability test should be performed whenever the results of the motility test are subnormal.

20. **A** The normal volume of seminal fluid is 2.0–5.0 mL. A lower volume than 2.0 mL causes a low sperm count (sperm/mL × volume) and can be caused by the absence of the seminal vesicles or prostate, ductal obstruction, or retrograde ejaculation of seminal fluid into the urinary bladder. The seminal fluid should coagulate within 5 min after ejaculation as a result of secretions of the seminal vesicles. Proteases such as PSA hydrolyze semenogelin and fibronectin, causing liquefaction to occur within 1 hour at room temperature. The seminal fluid pH should be between 7.2 and 8.0. Motility is evaluated by grading 100 sperm in 4–6 high power fields. It is normal when ≥25% show rapid progressive movement or when ≥50% show rapid progressive or slow progressive movement.

21. Which of the following sample collection and processing conditions leads to inaccurate seminal fluid analysis results?

- **A.** Sample stored at room temperature for 1 hour before testing
- **B.** Sample collected following coitus
- **C.** Sample collected without an anticoagulant
- **D.** Sample collected without use of a condom

Body fluids/Apply knowledge to recognize sources of error/Seminal fluid/2

22. When performing a seminal fluid analysis, what is the upper limit of normal for WBCs?

- **A.** 1×10^6/mL
- **B.** 5×10^6/mL
- **C.** 10×10^6/mL
- **D.** 20×10^6/mL

Body fluids/Evaluate laboratory data to recognize health and disease states/Seminal fluid/2

23. Which carbohydrate measurement is clinically useful when performing a seminal fluid analysis?

- **A.** Glucose
- **B.** Galactose
- **C.** Fructose
- **D.** Maltose

Body Fluids/Apply knowledge of special procedures/Seminal fluid/1

24. Which condition is most often associated with gastric ulcers?

- **A.** Cancer of the stomach
- **B.** *Helicobacter pylori* infection
- **C.** Zollinger-Ellison syndrome
- **D.** Pernicious anemia

Body Fluids/Gastric/Correlate clinical and laboratory data/2

Answers to Questions 21–24

21. **B** A seminal fluid sample should not be collected following coitus. The patient should abstain from ejaculation for 3 days prior to submitting the sample. A condom should not be used because it may contain spermicides. The sample should be collected at the testing site in a sterile jar with a wide opening and stored at room temperature. The specimen should be analyzed as soon as possible. The time between collection and delivery to the laboratory must be documented. Motility should be determined as soon as the fluid has liquefied (maximum storage time is 4 hours). Anticoagulants are not used; if the sample fails to liquefy it can be treated with chymotrypsin before analysis.

22. **A** When evaluating sperm morphology, the number of immature spermatozoons and white blood cells (round cells) should also be determined. The number of each is counted along with 200 mature sperm, then divided by 2 to determine their percentage. This is multiplied by the sperm concentration to give the absolute count per mL. An increased number of WBCs is an indicator of infection and is usually associated with prostatitis. Round cells are also estimated by noting their number per high power field. Each round cell per field counted with the 40 × objective corresponds to one million per mL. The upper limit of normal for WBCs is 1×10^6/mL, and for immature sperm 5×10^6/mL.

23. **C** Fructose is the primary nutrient in the seminal fluid and is needed for motility. It is supplied by the seminal vesicles and is low when the vas deferens or seminal vesicles are absent. The lower limit of normal is 150 mg/dL or 13 μmol per ejaculate.

24. **B** Peptic ulcer disease may be caused by either gastric or duodenal ulcers, which are associated with discomfort, hyperacidity, and bleeding. Hyperacidity is most often caused by *H. pylori* infection, which can cause both gastric and duodenal ulcers. In the absence of a positive test for *H. pylori* (e.g., endoscopic biopsy, breath test, ELISA, PCR) and no history of drug-induced ulcers, Zollinger-Ellison syndrome (gastrinoma) should be suspected and can usually be identified by a plasma gastrin assay. Cancer of the stomach is associated with increased gastric fluid volume but not hyperacidity. Pernicious anemia is associated with gastric hypoacidity and not ulcers.

25. In which condition is the highest level of serum gastrin usually seen?
 A. Atrophic gastritis
 B. Pernicious anemia
 C. Zollinger-Ellison syndrome
 D. Cancer of the stomach

Body fluids/Correlate clinical and laboratory data/
Gastric function/2

26. In determining free HCl, the gastric fluid is titrated to pH ___?
 A. 6.5
 B. 4.5
 C. 3.5
 D. 2.0

Body fluids/Apply principles of special procedures/
Gastric pH/1

25. **C** Gastrin is produced by specialized epithelium of the stomach and stimulates secretion of HCl by parietal cells. Secretion is controlled by negative feedback causing levels to be high in conditions associated with achlorhydria such as atrophic gastritis. Zollinger-Ellison syndrome results from a gastrin-secreting tumor, gastrinoma, usually originating in the pancreas. It is characterized by very high levels of plasma gastrin and excessive gastric acidity. In duodenal ulcers, increased gastric acidity occurs, but fasting plasma gastrin levels are normal. However, postprandial gastrin levels may be elevated in these patients because they do not respond to the negative feedback signal caused by HCl release. In stomach cancer, gastric volume is increased but acidity is not, and plasma gastrin levels are variable.

26. **C** Gastric analysis is performed rarely because endoscopic procedures usually are sufficient to diagnose hypo- and hyperacidity states. In difficult cases analysis of gastric fluid can be used to make a definitive diagnosis. Free HCl in gastric residue from a 12-hour fasting sample obtained by nasogastric suction is measured by titrating with 0.1 N NaOH to a pH 3.5. Total acidity is titrated to pH 7.0 and includes contributions of other acids, including proteins and salts of chloride. Basal acid output (BAO) and peak acid output (PAO) are determined using timed collection of gastric sample aliquots before and after stimulation of HCl release by pentagastrin. In achlorhydria the fasting gastric pH is often greater than 6.0, and this is considered diagnostic. The BAO:PAO ratio is normally less than 0.2. Patients with gastric ulcers may also have a ratio less than 0.2 or between 0.2 and 0.4. In duodenal ulcers the ratio is usually between 0.2 and 0.6. The ratio is greater than 0.6 only in Zollinger-Ellison syndrome.

27. Which test can identify persons with gastrin-secreting tumors who do not demonstrate a definitively increased plasma gastrin concentration?
   A. Secretin stimulation
   B. Pentagastrin
   C. Cholecystokinin pancreozymin
   D. Trypsinogen

Body Fluids/Select tests/Gastrointestinal function/2

28. Which of the following tests would be normal in pancreatic insufficiency?
   A. Secretin stimulation
   B. D-xylose absorption
   C. 24-hour fecal fat
   D. β-Carotene absorption

Body fluids/Correlate clinical and laboratory data/Pancreatic function/2

29. Which of the following is commonly associated with occult blood?
   A. Colon cancer
   B. Atrophic gastritis
   C. Pernicious anemia
   D. Pancreatitis

Body fluids/Correlate clinical and laboratory data/Occult blood/2

30. Which statement regarding fecal trypsin screening is true?
   A. Deficiency of trypsin causes clearing of an x-ray film
   B. It is useful in screening adults for steatorrhea
   C. Fecal trypsin deficiency in newborns is associated with cystic fibrosis
   D. Stool is diluted in phosphate buffer at pH 7.0

Body fluids/Correlate clinical and laboratory data/Fecal trypsin/2

27. A Plasma gastrin levels higher than 1000 pg/mL are usually diagnostic of Zollinger-Ellison syndrome. Smaller elevations can occur in other types of hyperacidity, including gastric ulcers, in renal disease, and after vagotomy. Zollinger-Ellison syndrome can be differentiated from the others by the secretin stimulation test. Secretin is administered intravenously, and timed plasma samples are collected and measured for gastrin. In Zollinger-Ellison syndrome at least one specimen should show an increase of 200 pg/mL above the baseline for gastrin. CCK-PZ is a hormone produced by the small intestine that simulates HCl production by the stomach and pancreatic release of bicarbonate and intestinal motility. It may be measured to diagnose intestinal malabsorption or used along with secretin to evaluate pancreatic secretion. Trypsinogen is a precursor of trypsin and is produced by the pancreas. Urinary trypsinogen is increased in acute pancreatitis, whereas fecal trypsin and chymotrypsin are decreased in cystic fibrosis because of pancreatic duct obstruction.

28. B The xylose absorption test differentiates pancreatic insufficiency from malabsorption syndrome (both cause deficient fat absorption). Xylose is absorbed by the small intestine without the aid of pancreatic enzymes. It is not metabolized and is excreted into urine. Low levels indicate gastrointestinal malabsorption.

29. A Blood in feces is a very sensitive indicator of gastrointestinal bleeding and is an excellent screening test to detect asymptomatic ulcers and malignancy of the gastrointestinal tract. However, the test is nonspecific and contamination with vaginal blood is a frequent source of error.

30. C In cystic fibrosis obstruction of pancreatic ducts causes deficient delivery of trypsin into the small intestine. This can be detected by the inability of feces to hydrolyze the gelatin of an x-ray film. However, this test is not useful in screening adults because trypsin inhibitors are present in the stool. Fecal trypsin activity should be measured at a pH of 8.0. A more sensitive measure of pancreatic function is the quantitative measurement of fecal chymotrypsin. A synthetic substrate coupled to *p*-nitroanilide at the amino terminal end is used. When the peptide is hydrolyzed by chymotrypsin, *p*-nitroaniline is liberated, which causes an increase in light absorption at 450 nm.

1. Given the following dry reagent strip urinalysis results, select the most appropriate course of action:

> pH = 8.0; protein = 1+; glucose = Neg; ketone = Neg; blood = Neg; nitrite = Neg; bilirubin = Neg

A. Report the results assuming acceptable quality control

B. Check pH with a pH meter before reporting

C. Perform a turbidimetric protein test and report instead of the dipstick protein

D. Request a new specimen

Body fluids/Evaluate laboratory data to recognize problems/Urinalysis/3

2. Given the following urinalysis results, select the most appropriate course of action:

> pH = 8.0; protein = tr; glucose = Neg; ketone = sm; blood = Neg; nitrite = Neg; 0–2 RBCs/HPF; 20–50 WBCs/HPF; bacteria = Lg; CaCO₃ crystals = Sm

A. Call for a new specimen because urine was contaminated in vitro

B. Recheck pH because calcium carbonate (CaCO₃) does not occur at alkaline pH

C. No indication of error is present; results indicate a urinary tract infection

D. Report all results except bacteria because the nitrite test was negative

Body fluids/Evaluate laboratory data to recognize inconsistent results/Urinalysis/3

3. **SITUATION:** A 6-mL pediatric urine sample is processed for routine urinalysis in the usual manner. The sediment is prepared by centrifuging all of the urine remaining after performing the biochemical tests. The following results are obtained:

> SG = 1.015; protein = 2+; blood = Lg; 5–10 RBCs/HPF; 5–10 WBCs/HPF

Select the most appropriate course of action.

A. Report these results; blood and protein correlate with microscopic results

B. Report biochemical results only; request a new sample for the microscopic examination

C. Request a new sample and report as quantity not sufficient (QNS)

D. Recentrifuge the supernatant and repeat the microscopic examination

Body fluids/Apply knowledge to recognize sources of error/Urinalysis/3

Answers to Questions 1–3

1. **C** Highly buffered alkaline urine may cause a false-positive dry reagent strip protein test by titrating the acid buffer on the reagent pad. The turbidimetric test with SSA is not subject to positive interference by highly buffered alkaline urine.

2. **C** A positive nitrite test requires infection with a nitrate-reducing organism, dietary nitrate, and incubation of urine in the bladder. The test is positive in about 70% of urinary tract infection cases. Alkaline pH, bacteriuria, and leukocytes point to a urinary tract infection.

3. **B** This discrepancy between the blood reaction and RBC count resulted from spinning less than 12 mL of urine. When volume is below 12 mL, the sample should be diluted with saline to 12 mL before concentrating. Results are multiplied by the dilution (12 mL/mL urine) to give the correct range.

4. Given the urinalysis results below, select the most appropriate course of action:

> pH = 6.5; protein = Neg; glucose = Neg; ketone = tr; blood = Neg; bilirubin = Neg; mucus = Sm; ammonium biurate crystals = Lg

A. Recheck urine pH

B. Report these results, assuming acceptable quality control

C. Repeat the dry reagent strip tests to confirm the ketone result

D. Request a new sample and repeat the urinalysis

Body fluids/Evaluate laboratory data to recognize problems/Urinalysis/3

5. Given the following urinalysis results, select the most appropriate course of action:

> Color = amber; transparency = clear; pH = 6.0; protein = Neg; glucose = Neg; ketone = Neg; blood = Neg; bilirubin = Neg; bilirubin granules = Sm

A. Perform a tablet test for bilirubin before reporting

B. Request a new sample

C. Recheck the pH

D. Perform a test for urinary urobilinogen

Body fluids/Evaluate laboratory data to determine possible inconsistent results/Urinalysis/3

6. A biochemical profile gives the following results:

> Creatinine = 1.4 mg/dL; BUN = 35 mg/dL; K = 5.5 mmol/L

All other results are normal and all tests are in control. Urine from the patient has an osmolality of 975 mOsm/kg. Select the most appropriate course of action:

A. Check for hemolysis

B. Repeat the BUN and report only if normal

C. Repeat the serum creatinine and report only if elevated

D. Report these results

Body fluids/Evaluate laboratory data to recognize problems/Renal function/3

7. A 2 p.m. urinalysis has a trace glucose by the dry reagent strip test. A fasting blood glucose sample drawn 8 hours earlier is 100 mg/dL. No other results are abnormal. Select the most appropriate course of action.

A. Repeat the urine glucose and report if positive

B. Perform a test for reducing sugars and report the result

C. Perform a quantitative urine glucose; report as trace if greater than 100 mg/dL

D. Request a new urine specimen

Body fluids/Evaluate laboratory data to determine possible inconsistent results/Glucose/3

8. Following a transfusion reaction, urine from a patient gives positive tests for blood and protein. The SG is 1.015. No RBCs or WBCs are seen in the microscopic examination. These results:

A. Indicate renal injury induced by transfusion reaction

B. Support the finding of an extravascular transfusion reaction

C. Support the finding of an intravascular transfusion reaction

D. Rule out a transfusion reaction caused by RBC incompatibility

Body fluids/Correlate clinical and laboratory data/Urinalysis/3

Answers to Questions 4–8

4. **A** Ammonium biurate crystals occur at alkaline pH only. The pH should be checked, and if below 7.0, the crystals should be reviewed in order to identify correctly. The trace ketone does not require confirmation provided that the quality control of the reagent strips is acceptable.

5. **A** Bilirubin crystals cannot occur in urine without bilirubin. The tablet test is more sensitive than the dry reagent test and will confirm the presence of bilirubin. If negative, the crystals should be reviewed before reporting. Abnormal crystals occur only in acid or neutral urine.

6. **D** Patients with prerenal failure usually have a BUN:creatinine ratio greater than 20:1. Reduced renal blood flow causes increased urea reabsorption and high urine osmolality. Patients are usually hypertensive and show fluid retention and hyperkalemia.

7. **A** The urine glucose is determined by the blood glucose at the time the urine is formed. The postprandial glucose (2 p.m.) level exceeded the renal threshold, resulting in trace glycosuria. Tests for reducing sugars are not used to confirm a positive urine glucose test.

8. **C** RBCs usually remain intact at a SG of 1.015. The absence of RBCs, WBCs, and casts points to hemoglobinuria caused by intravascular hemolysis rather than glomerular injury. A positive protein reaction occurs if sufficient hemoglobin is present.

9. A urine sample taken after a suspected transfusion reaction has a positive test for blood, but intact RBCs are not seen on microscopic examination. Which one test result would rule out an intravascular hemolytic transfusion reaction?
A. Negative urine urobilinogen
B. Serum unconjugated bilirubin below 1.0 mg/dL
C. Serum potassium below 6.0 mmol/L
D. Normal plasma haptoglobin

Body Fluids/Select routine laboratory procedures to verify test results/Transfusion reaction/3

10. Given the following urinalysis results, select the most appropriate course of action:

pH = 5.0; protein = Neg;
glucose = 1000 mg/dL; ketone = Mod;
blood = Neg;
bilirubin = Neg; SSA protein = 1+

A. Report the SSA protein result instead of the dry reagent strip result
B. Call for a list of medications administered to the patient
C. Perform a quantitative urinary albumin
D. Perform a test for microalbuminuria

Body fluids/Evaluate laboratory data to determine possible inconsistent results/Urinalysis/3

11. Urinalysis results from a 35-year-old woman are:

SG = 1.015; pH = 7.5; protein = Tr;
glucose = Sm; ketone = Neg; blood = Neg;
leukocyte esterase = Mod; 5–10 RBCs/HPF;
25–50 WBCs/HPF

Select the most appropriate course of action:
A. Recheck the blood reaction; if negative look for budding yeasts
B. Repeat the WBC count
C. Report all results except blood
D. Request a list of medications

Body fluids/Evaluate laboratory data to recognize sources of error/Urinalysis/3

12. A routine urinalysis gives the following results:

pH = 6.5; protein = Neg; glucose = Tr;
ketone = Neg; blood = Neg;
5–10 blood casts/LPF;
mucus = Sm; amorphous crystals = Lg

These results are most likely explained by:
A. False-negative blood reaction
B. False-negative protein reaction
C. Pseudocasts of urate mistaken for true casts
D. Mucus mistaken for casts

Body fluids/Evaluate laboratory data to determine possible inconsistent results/Urinalysis/3

13. SITUATION: When examining a urinary sediment under 40× magnification, the technologist noted many red blood cells as having cytoplasmic blebs and an irregular distribution of the hemoglobin. This phenomenon is most often caused by:
A. Intravascular hemolytic anemia
B. Glomerular disease
C. Hypotonic or alkaline urine
D. Severe dehydration

Body Fluids/Correlate clinical and laboratory data/Hematuria/2

Answers to Questions 9–13

9. D The plasma free hemoglobin will be increased immediately after a hemolytic transfusion reaction, and the haptoglobin will be decreased. The hemoglobin will be eliminated by the kidneys, but the haptoglobin will remain low or undetectable for 2–3 days. Normal urine urobilinogen and serum unconjugated bilirubin help in ruling out extravascular hemolysis. Pretransfusion potassium is needed to evaluate the contribution of hemolysis to the post-transfusion result.

10. B The combination of glucose- and ketone-positive urine points to a patient with insulin-dependent diabetes. A false-positive SSA test is likely if tolbutamide (Orinase) has been administered.

11. A A nonhemolyzed trace may have been overlooked and the blood test should be repeated. A false-negative (e.g., megadoses of vitamin C) rarely occurs. Yeast cells often accompany pyuria and glycosuria and are easily mistaken for RBCs.

12. C At pH 6.5 amorphous crystals are most often urate. These form yellow- or reddish-brown refractile deposits sometimes resembling blood or granular casts. The number of blood casts reported could not have occurred with negative protein and blood tests.

13. B When RBCs pass through the damaged endothelial wall of the glomerulus they become distorted, and such cells are described as dysmorphic in appearance. They are characterized by uneven distribution of hemoglobin, cytoplasmic blebs, or extruded cytoplasm, and an asymmetrical membrane distinct from crenation. The cytoplasm may be extruded from the cell and may aggregate at the membrane, giving the cell a wavy appearance. A predominance of dysmorphic RBCs in the microscopic examination points to glomerular bleeding as opposed to hematuria from other causes. Intravascular hemolytic anemia causes hemoglobinuria rather than hematuria. RBCs lyse in hypotonic and alkaline urine. Severe dehydration is not a cause of hematuria.

14. **SITUATION:** Urine is dark orange and turns brown after storage in the refrigerator overnight. The technologist requests a new specimen. The second specimen is bright orange and is tested immediately. Which test result would differ between the two specimens?
  A. Ketone
  B. Leukocyte esterase
  C. Urobilinogen
  D. Nitrite

Body Fluids/Apply knowledge to recognize sources of error/Urobilinogen/3

15. A toluidine blue chamber count on CSF gives the following values:

CSF Counts	Peripheral Blood Counts
WBCs 10×10^6/L	WBCs 5×10^9/L
RBCs 1000×10^6/L	RBCs 5×10^{12}/L

After correcting the WBC count in CSF, one should next:
  A. Report the WBC count as 9×10^6/L without additional testing
  B. Report the WBC count and number of PMNs identified by the chamber count
  C. Perform a differential on a direct smear of the CSF
  D. Concentrate CSF using a cytocentrifuge and perform a differential count

Body fluids/Apply knowledge of standard operating procedures/CSF/3

16. A blood-tainted pleural fluid is submitted for culture. Which test result would be most conclusive in classifying the fluid as an exudate?

	Test	Result
A.	LD fluid/serum	0.65
B.	Total protein	3.2 g/dL
C.	RBC count	10,000/μL
D.	WBC count	1500/μL

Body fluids/Correlate clinical and laboratory data/ Pleural fluid/3

17. A pleural fluid submitted to the laboratory is milky in appearance. Which test would be most useful in differentiating between a chylous and pseudochylous effusion?
  A. Fluid to serum triglyceride ratio
  B. Fluid WBC count
  C. Fluid total protein
  D. Fluid to serum LD ratio

Body fluids/Select test/Pleural fluid/2

14. **C** Urinary urobilinogen is increased in persons with extravascular hemolysis or hepatocellular liver disease. A freshly voided specimen is needed to detect urobilinogen because it is rapidly photo-oxidized to urobilin. This is accompanied by a color change from orange to brown. Urobilin does not react with 2,4 dimethylaminobenzaldehyde or 4-methoxybenzene diazonium tetrafluoroborate, which is used to detect urobilinogen. Consequently, the urobilinogen test in the first sample will be normal but increased in the second sample if tested immediately after collection. The best sample for detecting urobilinogen is a 2-hour timed urine sample collected in the mid-afternoon when urobilinogen excretion is highest. Ketones and nitrites do not alter the pigment of the urine sample. Leukocytes cause the urine to be turbid but do not cause abnormal color. These three tests are stable for 24 hours when urine is refrigerated within 30 minutes of collection.

15. **D** A differential is performed using CSF concentrate regardless of the WBC count. A toluidine blue chamber count of PMNs is not sufficiently sensitive to detect neutrophilic pleocytosis.

16. **A** A traumatic tap makes classification of fluids difficult on the basis of cell counts and protein. The values reported for protein, RBCs, and WBCs can occur in either an exudate or bloody transudate, but the LD ratio is significant.

17. **A** Chylous effusions are caused by extravasation of lymphatic fluid into the pleural cavity. Pseudochylous effusions are caused by necrosis. Both fluids often appear white and opalescent but both effusions can also be bloody, green, or yellow in addition to being turbid. However, chylous effusions are odorless and have a twofold higher triglyceride level than the plasma. They also usually show a lymphocytosis. Pseudochylous effusions are foul-smelling, usually have a mixed cellularity, and show an elevated cholesterol. They may have an increased triglyceride concentration, but it is usually below 50 mg/dL. Chylous effusions are most often caused by lymphoma or other malignancy or trauma, and like pseudochylous effusions may have an increased LD fluid:serum ratio, total protein, and WBC count.

18. A CSF sample from an 8-year-old child with a fever of unknown origin was tested for glucose, total protein, lactate, and IgG index. The glucose level was 180 mg/dL but all other results were within the reference range. The CSF WBC count was 9×10^6/L, and the RBC count was 10×10^6/L. The differential showed 50% lymphocytes, 35% monocytes, 10% macrophages, 3% neutrophils, and 2% neuroectodermal cells. What is the most likely cause of these results?
A. Aseptic meningitis
B. Traumatic tap
C. Subarachnoid hemorrhage
D. Hyperglycemia

Body Fluids/Apply knowledge to recognize inconsistent results/CSF/2

19. A WBC count and differential performed on ascites fluid gave a WBC count of 20,000 µL with 90% macrophages. The gross appearance of the fluid was described by the technologist as "thick and bloody." It was noted on the report that several clusters of these cells were observed and that the majority of the cells contained many vacuoles resembling paper-punch holes. What do the observations above suggest?
A. Malignant mesothelial cells were counted as macrophages
B. Adenocarcinoma from a metastatic site
C. Lymphoma infiltrating the peritoneal cavity
D. Nodular sclerosing Hodgkin's disease

Body Fluids/Apply knowledge to recognize inconsistent results/Serous fluids/3

20. Given the data for creatinine clearance below, select the most appropriate course of action:

Volume = 2.8 L/day; surface area = 1.73 m²;
urine creatinine = 100 mg/dL;
serum creatinine = 1.2 mg/dL

A. Report a creatinine clearance of 162 mL/min
B. Repeat the urine creatinine; results point to a dilution error
C. Request a new 24-hour urine sample
D. Request the patient's age and sex

Body fluids/Evaluate laboratory data to recognize problems/Creatinine clearance/3

21. An elevated amylase level is obtained on a *stat* serum collected at 8 p.m.. A delta-check flag for amylase occurs because of a normal result from 8 a.m. Amylase is also ordered on a 6 p.m. urine sample. Select the most appropriate course of action:
A. Repeat the *stat* amylase; report only if the delta-check limit is not exceeded

B. Repeat both the a.m. and p.m. amylase tests and report only if they agree
C. Request a new specimen; do not report results of the stat sample
D. Review amylase on the 6 p.m. urine sample; if elevated, report the *stat* amylase result

Body fluids/Apply knowledge to recognize inconsistent results/Amylase/3

Answers to Questions 18–21

18. D CSF glucose is approximately 60% of the plasma glucose but may be somewhat lower in a diabetic person. The reference range is approximately 40–70 mg/dL. A CSF glucose above 70 mg/dL is caused by a high plasma glucose that equilibrated with the CSF. Therefore hyperglycorrhachia is caused by hyperglycemia. The WBC count in a child between 5–12 years is $0–10 \times 10^6$/L (0–10/µL). The normal RBC count and protein rule out subarachnoid hemorrhage and traumatic tap. Although aseptic meningitis cannot be ruled out conclusively, it is unlikely given a normal WBC count and IgG index.

19. A Bloody, exudative fluids with a preponderance of a singular cell type are suggestive of malignancy. The cellularity in malignancy is variable, but lymphocytosis occurs in about half of cases. Mesothelial cells normally make up less than 10% of the cells in serous fluid. They may be resting cells, reactive, degenerate, or phagocytic in nonmalignant conditions. In inflammatory conditions, they are often increased and resemble macrophages. However, clusters or balls of such cells and paper-punch vacuoles throughout the cytoplasm and over the nucleus are characteristics of malignant mesothelial cells. Such cells secrete hyaluronic acid, making the fluid highly viscous. The gross appearance of this fluid suggests malignancy. The description of these cells points to mesothelioma, and this specimen should be referred for cytological examination in order to confirm the diagnosis.

20. C A calculated clearance in excess of 140 mL/min is greater than the upper physiological limit. The high volume per day suggests addition of H_2O to the sample. The result should be considered invalid.

21. D Serum amylase often peaks 2–10 hours after an episode of acute pancreatitis and may cause a delta-check flag in the absence of laboratory error. Urinary amylase parallels serum amylase; a positive urine test at 6 p.m. makes sample collection error unlikely.

22. Results of a fetal lung maturity (FLM) study from a patient with diabetes mellitus are:

L/S = 2.0; PG = pos; creatinine = 2.5 mg/dL

Given these results one should:

A. Report the result and recommend repeating the L/S ratio in 24 hours

B. Perform scanning spectrophotometry on the fluid to determine if blood is present

C. Repeat the L/S ratio after 4 hours and report those results

D. Report results as invalid

Body fluids/Correlate laboratory data to verify test results/L/S ratio/3

23. A 24-hour urine sample from an adult submitted for catecholamines gives a result of 140 μg/day (upper reference limit 150 μg/day). The 24-hour urine creatinine level is 0.6 g/day. Select the best course of action:

A. Check the urine pH to verify that it is less than 2.0

B. Report the result in μg catecholamines per mg creatinine

C. Request a new 24-hour urine sample

D. Measure the VMA and report the catecholamine result only if elevated

Body fluids/Evaluate to recognize problems/ Catecholamines/3

24. A 5-hour urinary D-xylose test on a 7-year-old boy who was given 0.5 g of D-xylose per pound is 15%. The 2-hour timed blood D-xylose is 15 mg/dL (lower reference limit 30 mg/dL). Select the most appropriate action:

A. Request that a β-carotene absorption test be performed

B. Repeat the urinary result because it is borderline

C. Request a retest using a 25-g dose of D-xylose

D. Request a retest using only a 1-hour timed blood sample

Body fluids/Apply principles of special procedures/ D-xylose absorption/3

25. A quantitative serum hCG is ordered on a male patient. One should:

A. Perform the test and report the result

B. Request that the order be cancelled

C. Perform the test and report the result if negative

D. Perform the test and report the result only if higher than 25 IU/L

Body fluids/Apply knowledge of standard operating procedures/hCG/3

Answers to Questions 22–25

22. **A** In patients with diabetes, lung maturity may be delayed and an L/S ratio of 2:1 may be associated with respiratory distress syndrome. A positive PG spot correlates with an L/S ratio of 2:1 or higher and rules out a falsely increased result caused by blood contamination. The best course of action is to wait an additional 24 hours and perform another L/S ratio on a fresh sample of amniotic fluid because an L/S ratio of 3:1 would indicate a high probability of fetal lung maturity.

23. **C** Urine creatinine of less than 0.8 g/day indicates incomplete sample collection. The patient's daily catecholamine excretion would be misinterpreted from this result.

24. **D** Urinary xylose excretion is less reliable in children under the age of 10, and peak blood levels occur sooner than in adults. A 60-minute blood sample should have been used. A serum D-xylose level greater than 30 mg/dL at 1 hour is considered normal.

25. **A** hCG may be produced in men by tumors of trophoblastic origin, such as teratoma and seminoma, and is an important marker for nontrophoblastic tumors as well.

BIBLIOGRAPHY

1. Brunzel, N.A.: Fundamentals of Urine and Body Fluid Analysis. W.B. Saunders, Philadelphia, 1994.
2. Burtis, C.A., Ashwood, E.R., and Bruns, D.E.: Tietz Textbook of Clinical Chemistry and Molecular Diagnostics. ed 4. Elsevier Saunders, St. Louis, 2006.
3. Haber, M.H.: Urinary Sediment: A Textbook Atlas. ASCP, Chicago, 1981.
4. Henry, J.B. (ed.): Clinical Diagnosis and Management by Laboratory Methods. ed 20. W.B. Saunders, Philadelphia, 2001..
5. Kaplan, L.A., and Pesce, A.J. (eds.): Clinical Chemistry Theory Analysis and Correlation. ed 4. Mosby, St. Louis. 2003.
6. Kjeldsberg, C.R., and Knight, J.A.: Body Fluids. ed 3. ASCP Press, Chicago, 1993.
7. Strasinger, S.K., and DiLorenzo, M.S.: Urinalysis and Body Fluids. ed 4,. FA Davis, Philadelphia, 2001.

CHAPTER **7**

Microbiology

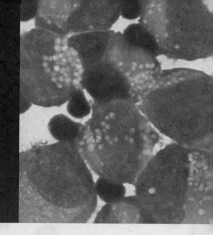

7.1   SPECIMEN COLLECTION, MEDIA, AND METHODS

7.2   ENTEROBACTERIACEAE

7.3   NONFERMENTATIVE BACILLI

7.4   MISCELLANEOUS AND FASTIDIOUS GRAM-NEGATIVE RODS

7.5   GRAM-POSITIVE AND GRAM-NEGATIVE COCCI

7.6   AEROBIC GRAM-POSITIVE RODS, SPIROCHETES, MYCOPLASMAS AND UREAPLASMAS, AND CHLAMYDIA

7.7   ANAEROBIC BACTERIA

7.8   MYCOBACTERIA

7.9   MYCOLOGY

7.10 VIROLOGY

7.11 PARASITOLOGY

7.12 PROBLEM SOLVING IN MICROBIOLOGY AND PARASITOLOGY

357

1. The aseptic collection of blood cultures requires that the skin be cleansed with:

A. 2% iodine and then 70% alcohol solution

B. 70% alcohol and then 2% iodine or an iodophor

C. 70% alcohol and then 95% alcohol

D. 95% alcohol only

Microbiology/Apply knowledge of standard operating procedures/Specimen collection/1

2. When cleansing the skin with alcohol and then iodine for the collection of a blood culture, the iodine (or iodophor) should remain intact on the skin for at least:

A. 10 sec

B. 30 sec

C. 60 sec

D. 5 min

Microbiology/Apply knowledge of standard operating procedures/Specimen collection and handling/1

3. What is the purpose of adding 0.025%–0.050% sodium polyanethol sulfonate (SPS) to nutrient broth media for the collection of blood cultures?

A. It inhibits phagocytosis and complement

B. It promotes formation of a blood clot

C. It enhances growth of anaerobes

D. It functions as a preservative

Microbiology/Apply knowledge of standard operating procedures/Media/1

4. A flexible calcium alginate nasopharyngeal swab is the collection device of choice for recovery of which organism from the nasopharynx?

A. *Staphylococcus aureus*

B. *Streptococcus pneumoniae*

C. *Corynebacterium diphtheriae*

D. *Bacteroides fragilis*

Microbiology/Apply knowledge of standard operating procedure/Specimen collection and handling/1

5. Semisolid transport media such as Amies, Stuart, or Cary-Blair are suitable for the transport of swabs for culture of most pathogens *except:*

A. *Neisseria gonorrhoeae*

B. Enterobacteriaceae

C. *Campylobacter fetus*

D. *Streptococcus pneumoniae*

Microbiology/Select methods/Reagents/Media/Specimen collection and handling/2

Answers to Questions 1–5

1. **B** In order to attain asepsis of the skin, 70% alcohol followed by 2% iodine is used for obtaining blood cultures.

2. **C** The iodine should remain on the skin for 1 min because instant antisepsis does not occur when cleansing the skin for a blood culture.

3. **A** SPS is used in most commercial blood culture products because it functions as an anticoagulant and prevents phagocytosis and complement activation. In addition, SPS neutralizes aminoglycoside antibiotics. Addition of SPS may inhibit some *Neisseria* and *Peptostreptococcus*, but this can be reversed with 1.2% gelatin.

4. **C** *C. diphtheriae* must be recovered from the deep layers of the pseudomembrane that forms in the nasopharyngeal area. A flexible calcium alginate nasopharyngeal swab is the best choice for collecting a specimen from the posterior nares and pharynx.

5. **A** Specimens for culture of *N. gonorrhoeae* are best if plated immediately or transported in a medium containing activated charcoal to absorb inhibitory substances that hinder their recovery.

6. Select the method of choice for recovery of anaerobic bacteria from a deep abscess.
   A. Cotton fiber swab of the abscess area
   B. Skin snip of the surface tissue
   C. Needle aspirate after surface decontamination
   D. Swab of the scalpel used for débridement

Microbiology/Apply knowledge of standard operating procedure/Specimen collection and handling/2

7. Select the primary and differential media of choice for recovery of most fecal pathogens.
   A. MacConkey, blood, birdseed, and *Campylobacter* (Campy) agars
   B. Hektoen, MacConkey, Campy, colistin-nalidixic acid (CNA) agars
   C. CNA and Christensen urea agars and thioglycollate media
   D. Blood, Campy, Mueller-Hinton agars, and thioglycollate media

Microbiology/Select methods/Reagents/Media/Stool culture/2

8. Select the media of choice for recovery of *Vibrio cholerae* from a stool specimen.
   A. MacConkey agar and thioglycollate media
   B. Thiosulfate-citrate-bile-sucrose (TCBS) agar and alkaline peptone water (APW) broth
   C. Blood agar and selenite-F (SEL) broth
   D. CNA agar

Microbiology/Select methods/Reagents/Media/Stool culture/2

9. Colistin-nalidixic acid agar (CNA) is used primarily for the recovery of:
   A. *Neisseria* species
   B. Enterobacteriaceae
   C. *Pseudomonas aeruginosa*
   D. *Staphylococcus aureus*

Microbiology/Select methods/Reagents/Media/Gram-positive cocci/2

10. In the United States, most blood agar plates are prepared with 5% or 10% red blood cells (RBCs) obtained from:
   A. Sheep
   B. Horses
   C. Humans
   D. Dogs

Microbiology/Select methods/Reagents/Media/Culture/1

11. All of the following are appropriate when attempting to isolate *N. gonorrhoeae* from a genital specimen *except:*
   A. Transport the genital swab in charcoal transport medium
   B. Plate the specimen on Modified Thayer-Martin (MTM) medium
   C. Plate the specimen on New York City or Martin-Lewis agar
   D. Culture specimens in ambient oxygen at 37°C

Microbiology/Select methods/Reagents/Media/Culture/1

Answers to Questions 6–11

6. **C** Anaerobic specimens are easily contaminated with organisms present on the skin or mucosal surfaces when a swab is used. Needle aspiration of an abscess following surface decontamination provides the least exposure to ambient oxygen.

7. **B** Hektoen agar selectively isolates pathogenic coliforms, especially *Salmonella* and *Shigella*. MacConkey agar differentiates lactose fermenters from nonfermenters. CNA agar contains antibiotics that prohibit growth of gram-negative coliforms but not gram-positive cocci. Campy agar contains the antibiotics cephalothin, trimethoprim, vancomycin, polymyxin B, and amphotericin B to prevent growth of Enterobacteriaceae, *Pseudomonas* spp, and fungi.

8. **B** TCBS agar is used to grow *Vibrio cholerae*, which appear as yellow colonies as a result of the use of both citrate and sucrose. APW is used as an enrichment broth and should be subcultured to TCBS agar for further evaluation of *Vibrio* colonies.

9. **D** CNA agar inhibits the growth of gram-negative bacteria and is used to isolate gram-positive cocci from specimens. This medium is especially useful for stool and wound cultures because these may contain large numbers of gram-negative rods.

10. **A** Sheep RBCs are used in blood agar plates because they are readily available and less inhibitory than cells of other species. The type of hemolysis is determined by the source of RBCs. Sheep RBCs are chosen because of the characteristically clear hemolysis produced by β-hemolytic streptococci, *Staphylococcus*, and other pathogens producing β-hemolysins. Sheep blood does not support the growth of *Haemophilus haemolyticus*, eliminating the possibility of confusing it with β-hemolytic streptococci in throat cultures.

11. **D** MTM, New York City, and Martin-Lewis agars contain blood factors needed to support the growth of *N. gonorrhoeae* as well as antibiotics that prevent growth of normal genital flora. Cultures must be incubated in 3%–7% CO_2 at 35°C. Cultures should be held a minimum of 48 hours before being considered negative.

12. Chocolate agar and modified Thayer-Martin agar are used for the recovery of:
- **A.** *Haemophilus* spp and *Neisseria* spp, respectively
- **B.** *Haemophilus* spp and *N. gonorrhoeae*, respectively
- **C.** *Neisseria* spp and *Streptococcus* spp, respectively
- **D.** *Streptococcus* spp and *Staphylococcus* spp, respectively

Microbiology/Select methods/Reagents/Media/Stool culture/2

13. Cycloserine-cefoxitin-fructose agar (CCFA) is used for the recovery of:
- **A.** *Yersinia enterocolitica*
- **B.** *Yersinia intermedia*
- **C.** *Clostridium perfringens*
- **D.** *Clostridium difficile*

Microbiology/Select methods/Reagents/Media/Stool culture/1

14. Deoxycholate agar (DCA) is useful for the isolation of:
- **A.** Enterobacteriaceae
- **B.** *Enterococcus* spp
- **C.** *Staphylococcus* spp
- **D.** *Neisseria* spp

Microbiology/Select methods/Reagents/Media/Stool culture/1

15. Xylose lysine deoxycholate (XLD) agar is a highly selective medium used for the recovery of which bacteria?
- **A.** *Staphylococcus* spp from normal flora
- **B.** *Yersinia* spp that do not grow on Hektoen agar
- **C.** Enterobacteriaceae from gastrointestinal specimens
- **D.** *Streptococcus* spp from stool cultures

Microbiology/Select methods/Reagents/Media/Stool culture/1

16. A sheep blood agar plate is used as a primary isolation medium when all of the following organisms are to be recovered from a wound specimen *except*:
- **A.** β-Hemolytic streptococci and coagulase-positive staphylococci
- **B.** *Haemophilus influenzae* and *Haemophilus parainfluenzae*
- **C.** *Proteus* spp and *Escherichia coli*
- **D.** *Pseudomonas* spp and *Acinetobacter* spp

Microbiology/Select methods/Reagents/Media/Wound culture/2

17. Prereduced and vitamin K_1-supplemented blood agar plates are recommended isolation media for:
- **A.** *Mycobacterium marinum* and *Mycobacterium avium-intracellulare*
- **B.** *Bacteroides*, *Peptostreptococcus*, and *Clostridium* spp
- **C.** *Proteus* spp
- **D.** *Enterococcus* spp

Microbiology/Select methods/Reagents/Media/Anaerobes/2

Answers to Questions 12–17

12. **B** Chocolate agar provides X factor (hemin) and V factor (NAD) required for the growth of *Haemophilus* spp. MTM is a chocolate agar containing the antibiotics vancomycin, colistin, nystatin, and trimethoprim. These permit isolation of *N. gonorrhoeae* in specimens containing large numbers of gram-negative bacteria, including commensal *Neisseria* species.

13. **D** CCFA is used for recovery of *C. difficile* from stool cultures. Cycloserine and cefoxitin inhibit growth of gram-negative coliforms in the stool specimen. *C. difficile* ferments fructose, forming acid that, in the presence of neutral red, causes the colonies to become yellow.

14. **A** DCA inhibits gram-positive organisms. *N. gonorrhoeae* and *Neisseria meningitidis* are too fastidious to grow on DCA. Citrate and deoxycholate salts inhibit growth of gram-positive bacteria. The media contain lactose and neutral red, allowing differentiation of lactose fermenters (pink colonies) from nonfermenters (colorless).

15. **C** XLD agar is selective for gram-negative coliforms because of a high concentration (0.25%) of deoxycholate, which inhibits gram-positive bacteria. In addition, XLD is differential for *Shigella* and *Salmonella* spp. The medium contains xylose, lactose, and sucrose, which are fermented by most normal intestinal coliforms producing yellow colonies. *Shigella* does not ferment the sugars and produces red (or clear) colonies. *Salmonella* spp ferment xylose; however, they also decarboxylate lysine in the medium, causing production of ammonia. Therefore, *Salmonella* first appear yellow but become red. Some *Salmonella* produce hydrogen sulfide (H_2S) from sodium thiosulfate and therefore appear as red colonies with black centers.

16. **B** Both gram-positive cocci and gram-negative bacilli will grow on blood agar plates, but the medium is used in conjunction with a selective medium such as CNA agar for gram-positive cocci and MacConkey agar for gram-negative bacilli. *H. influenzae* requires X and V factors, and *H. parainfluenzae* requires V factor; the primary isolation medium for *Haemophilus* is chocolate agar.

17. **B** Anaerobic culture media can be prereduced before sterilization by boiling, saturation with oxygen-free gas, and addition of cysteine or other thiol compounds. The final oxidation reduction potential (Eh) of the medium should be approximately –150 mV to minimize the effects of exposure of organisms to oxygen during inoculation.

18. Which procedure is appropriate for culture of genital specimens in order to recover *Chlamydia* spp?
  A. Inoculate cycloheximide-treated McCoy cells
  B. Plate onto blood and chocolate agar
  C. Inoculate into thioglycollate (THIO) broth
  D. Plate onto modified Thayer-Martin agar within 24 hours

Microbiology/Select methods/Reagents/Media/Virus culture/1

19. Specimens for virus culture should be transported in media containing:
  A. Antibiotics and 5% sheep blood
  B. Saline and 5% sheep blood
  C. 22% bovine albumin
  D. Antibiotics and nutrient

Microbiology/Select methods/Reagents/Media/Virus culture/1

20. Cerebrospinal fluid (CSF) should be cultured immediately, but if delayed the specimen should be:
  A. Refrigerated at 4° to 6°C
  B. Frozen at –20°C
  C. Stored at room temperature for not longer than 24 hours
  D. Incubated at 37°C and cultured as soon as possible

Microbiology/Apply knowledge of standard operating procedure/Specimen collection and transport/1

21. The most sensitive method for the detection of β-lactamase in bacteria is by the use of:
  A. Chromogenic cephalosporin
  B. Penicillin
  C. Oxidase
  D. Chloramphenicol acetyltransferase

Microbiology/Select methods/Reagents/Media/Sensitivity testing/2

22. The breakpoint of an antimicrobial drug refers to:
  A. The amount needed to cause bacteriostasis
  B. A minimum inhibitory concentration (MIC) of 16 μg/mL or greater
  C. A MIC of 64 μg/mL or greater
  D. The level of drug that is achievable in serum

Microbiology/Apply principle of theory and practice related to laboratory operations/Sensitivity testing/2

23. Which of the following variables may change the results of an MIC?
  A. Inoculum size
  B. Incubation time
  C. Growth rate of the bacteria
  D. All of the above

Microbiology/Apply knowledge to identify sources of error/Sensitivity testing/2

18. **A** *Chlamydia* are strict intracellular organisms and must be cultured using living cells. Direct smears can also be made at the time of culture. Staining cells with iodine may reveal the characteristic reddish-brown inclusions sometimes seen in *Chlamydia* infections. Fluorescein-conjugated monoclonal antibodies may be used to identify the organisms in infected cells.

19. **D** Media for transporting specimens for virus culture include Hanks balanced salt solution with bovine albumin, Stuart transport media, and Leibovitz-Emory media. Media used for transporting specimens for viral culture are similar to those for bacteria with the addition of a nutrient such as fetal calf serum or albumin and antibiotics. Specimens should be refrigerated after being placed in the transport media until the culture media can be inoculated.

20. **D** Fastidious organisms such as *Neisseria* and *Haemophilus* frequently isolated from the CSF of patients with bacterial meningitis are preserved by placing the fluid in 3%–7% CO_2 at 35°–37°C (or at room temperature for no longer than 30 min), if the specimen cannot be cultured immediately.

21. **A** β-Lactamase production by bacteria that are resistant to penicillin and cephalosporin is detected using one of these drugs as a substrate. Penicillin is hydrolyzed by β-lactamase into acidic products that can be detected as a color change by a pH indicator. In the iodometric method, a disk containing a penicillin-starch substrate turns blue when a drop of iodine is added. A loop of β-lactamase–positive organisms applied to the center of the blue spot will reduce the iodine to iodide, causing the area to clear. The most sensitive method of detection is based upon the ability of the organism to hydrolyze the β-lactam ring of a chromogenic cephalosporin.

22. **D** The breakpoint refers to an antimicrobial concentration in the serum associated with optimal therapy using the customary dosing schedule. An organism is susceptible if the MIC is at or below the breakpoint.

23. **D** In vitro testing of drugs is reliable if the method is standardized. In addition to the first three variables, the type of media and the stability of antibiotics affect the results of MIC testing and must be carefully controlled.

24. According to the Kirby-Bauer standard antimicrobial susceptibility testing method, what should be done when interpreting the zone size of a motile, swarming organism such as a *Proteus* species?
   A. The swarming area should be ignored
   B. The results of the disk diffusion method are invalid
   C. The swarming area should be measured as the growth boundary
   D. The isolate should be retested after diluting to a 0.05 McFarland standard

Microbiology/Apply knowledge of standard operating procedures/Sensitivity testing/2

25. Which class of antibiotics is used for the treatment of serious gram-negative infections as well as infections with *Mycobacterium tuberculosis*?
   A. Cephalosporins
   B. Penicillins
   C. Tetracyclines
   D. Aminoglycosides

Microbiology/Apply knowledge of fundamental biological characteristics/Antibiotics/1

24. A A thin film of growth appearing in the zone area of inhibition around the susceptibility disk should be ignored when swarming *Proteus* or other organisms are encountered. Discontinuous, poor growth or tiny colonies near the end of the zone should also be ignored.

25. D The aminoglycoside antibiotics are bactericidal agents that act by inhibiting protein synthesis. They show a low incidence of bacterial resistance but must be monitored carefully because at high doses they can cause ototoxicity and nephrotoxicity. The group includes amikacin, gentamicin, tobramycin, kanamycin, streptomycin, and spectinomycin. These drugs are usually administered intravenously or intramuscularly because they are poorly absorbed from the gastrointestinal tract.

1. **Biochemically, the Enterobacteriaceae are gram-negative rods that:**
   A. Ferment glucose, reduce nitrate to nitrite, and are oxidase-negative
   B. Ferment glucose, produce indophenol oxidase, and form gas
   C. Ferment lactose and reduce nitrite to nitrogen gas
   D. Ferment lactose and produce indophenol oxidase

   Microbiology/Apply knowledge of fundamental biological characteristics/Biochemical/Gram-negative bacilli/1

2. **The ortho-nitrophenyl-β-galactopyranoside (ONPG) test is most useful when differentiating:**
   A. *Salmonella* spp from *Pseudomonas* spp
   B. *Shigella* spp from some strains of *Escherichia coli*
   C. *Klebsiella* spp from *Enterobacter* spp
   D. *Proteus vulgaris* from *Salmonella* spp

   Microbiology/Apply principles of basic laboratory procedures/Biochemical/2

3. **The Voges-Proskauer (VP) test detects which end product of glucose fermentation?**
   A. Acetoin
   B. Nitrite
   C. Acetic acid
   D. Hydrogen sulfide

   Microbiology/Apply principles of basic laboratory procedures/Biochemical/1

4. **At which pH does the methyl red (MR) test become positive?**
   A. 7.0
   B. 6.5
   C. 6.0
   D. 4.5

   Microbiology/Apply principles of basic laboratory procedures/Biochemical/1

5. **A positive Simmons citrate test is seen as a:**
   A. Blue color in the medium after 24 hours incubation at 35°C
   B. Red color in the medium after 18 hours incubation at 35°C
   C. Yellow color in the medium after 24 hours' incubation at 35°C
   D. Green color in the medium after 18 hours incubation at 35°C

   Microbiology/Apply principles of basic laboratory procedures/Biochemical/1

Answers to Questions 1–5

1. **A** The family Enterobacteriaceae consists of more than 100 species and represents the most commonly encountered isolates in clinical specimens. All Enterobacteriaceae ferment glucose and are oxidase-negative and nonsporulating. Most Enterobacteriaceae are motile, but the genera *Shigella* and *Klebsiella* are not.

2. **B** The ONPG test detects β-galactosidase activity and is most useful in distinguishing late lactose fermenters from lactose nonfermenters. Some strains of *E. coli* are slow lactose fermenters and may be confused with *Shigella* spp, which do not ferment lactose. *E. coli* are ONPG-positive while *Shigella* spp are ONPG-negative.

3. **A** Acetoin or carbinol, an end product of glucose fermentation, is converted to diacetyl after the addition of the VP reagents (α-naphthol and 40% potassium hydroxide [KOH]). Diacetyl is seen as a red- to pink-colored complex.

4. **D** Both MR and VP tests detect acid production from the fermentation of glucose. However, a positive MR test denotes a more complete catabolism of glucose to highly acidic end products such as formate and acetate than occurs with organisms that are VP-positive only (e.g., *Klebsiella pneumoniae*).

5. **A** The Simmons citrate test determines if an organism can utilize citrate as the sole source of carbon. The medium turns blue, indicating the presence of alkaline products such as carbonate. Tubes are incubated a minimum of 24 hours at 35°C with a loose cap before reading.

6. In the test for urease production, ammonia reacts to form which product?
   A. Ammonium citrate
   B. Ammonium carbonate
   C. Ammonium oxalate
   D. Ammonium nitrate

   Microbiology/Apply principles of basic laboratory procedures/Biochemical/1

7. Which of the following reagents is added to detect the production of indole?
   A. *p*-Dimethylaminobenzaldehyde
   B. Bromcresol purple
   C. Methyl red
   D. Cytochrome oxidase

   Microbiology/Apply principles of basic laboratory procedures/Biochemical/1

8. Decarboxylation of the amino acids lysine, ornithine, and arginine results in the formation of:
   A. Ammonia
   B. Urea
   C. CO_2
   D. Amines

   Microbiology/Apply principles of basic laboratory procedures/Biochemical/1

9. Lysine iron agar (LIA) showing a purple slant and a blackened butt indicates:
   A. *E. coli*
   B. *Citrobacter* spp
   C. *Salmonella* spp
   D. *Proteus* spp

   Microbiology/Evaluate laboratory data to make identifications/Gram-negative bacilli/2

10. Putrescine is an alkaline amine product of which bacterial enzyme?
    A. Arginine decarboxylase
    B. Phenylalanine deaminase
    C. Ornithine decarboxylase
    D. Lysine decarboxylase

    Microbiology/Apply principles of basic laboratory procedures/Biochemical/1

11. Which genera are positive for phenylalanine deaminase?
    A. *Enterobacter, Escherichia,* and *Salmonella*
    B. *Morganella, Providencia,* and *Proteus*

C. *Klebsiella* and *Enterobacter*
D. *Proteus, Escherichia,* and *Shigella*

Microbiology/Evaluate laboratory data to make identifications/Gram-negative bacilli/2

Answers to Questions 6–11

6. **B** The test for urease production is based on the ability of the colonies to hydrolyze urea in Stuart broth or Christensen agar to form CO_2 and ammonia. These products form ammonium carbonate, resulting in alkalinization. This turns the pH indicator (phenol red) pink at pH 8.0.

7. **A** The indole test detects the conversion of tryptophan (present in the media) to indole by the enzyme tryptophanase. Indole is detected by the reaction with the aldehyde group of *p*-dimethylaminobenzaldehyde (the active reagent in Kovac's and Ehrlich's reagents) in acid, forming a red complex.

8. **D** Specific decarboxylases split dibasic amino acids (lysine, arginine, and ornithine), forming alkaline amines. These products turn the pH indicators in the medium (cresol red and bromcresol purple) from yellow to purple.

9. **C** LIA is used as an aid for the identification of *Salmonella* species. It contains phenylalanine, lysine, glucose, thiosulfate, ferric ammonium citrate, and bromcresol purple. *Salmonella* produce H_2S from thiosulfate. This reduces ferric ammonium citrate, forming ferrous sulfate and causing the butt to blacken. *Salmonella* also decarboxylate lysine to produce alkaline amines, giving the slant its purple color and differentiating it from *Citrobacter* spp, which are lysine decarboxylase–negative.

10. **C** Putrescine is the amine product of the decarboxylation of ornithine.

11. **B** Phenylalanine deaminase oxidatively deaminates phenylalanine, forming phenylpyruvic acid. When a solution of ferric chloride is added the iron reacts with phenylpyruvic acid, forming a green-colored complex. Phenylalanine deaminase is found in the genera *Morganella, Providencia,* and *Proteus* and is an excellent test to determine if an organism belongs to this group. Rarely, isolates of *Enterobacter* may be phenylalanine deaminase–positive as well.

12. Kligler iron agar (KIA) differs from triple sugar iron agar (TSI) in the:
   A. Ratio of lactose to glucose
   B. Ability to detect H_2S production
   C. Use of sucrose in the medium
   D. Color reaction denoting production of acid

Microbiology/Apply principles of basic laboratory procedures/Methods/Reagents/Media/Gram-negative bacilli/2

13. The malonate test is most useful in differentiating which members of the Enterobacteriaceae?
   A. *Shigella*
   B. *Proteus*
   C. *Salmonella* subgroups 2, 3 (the former *Arizona*)
   D. *Serratia*

Microbiology/Evaluate laboratory data to make identifications/Gram-negative bacilli/2

14. Which genera of the Enterobacteriaceae are known to cause diarrhea and are considered enteric pathogens?
   A. *Enterobacter, Klebsiella, Providencia,* and *Proteus*
   B. *Escherichia, Salmonella, Shigella,* and *Yersinia*
   C. *Pseudomonas, Moraxella, Acinetobacter,* and *Aeromonas*
   D. *Enterobacter, Citrobacter,* and *Morganella*

Microbiology/Apply knowledge of fundamental biological characteristics/Gram-negative bacilli/1

15. An isolate of *E. coli* recovered from the stool of a patient with severe bloody diarrhea should be tested for which sugar before sending it to a reference laboratory for serotyping?
   A. Sorbitol (fermentation)
   B. Mannitol (oxidation)
   C. Raffinose (fermentation)
   D. Sucrose (fermentation)

Microbiology/Evaluate laboratory data to recognize health and disease states/Gram-negative bacilli/3

16. Care must be taken when identifying biochemical isolates of *Shigella* because serological cross-reactions occur with:
   A. *E. coli*
   B. *Salmonella* spp
   C. *Pseudomonas* spp
   D. *Proteus* spp

Microbiology/Apply knowledge of fundamental biological characteristics/Gram-negative bacilli/2

17. Which species of *Shigella* is most commonly associated with diarrheal disease in the United States?
   A. *S. dysenteriae*
   B. *S. flexneri*
   C. *S. boydii*
   D. *S. sonnei*

Microbiology/Apply knowledge of fundamental biological characteristics/Gram-negative bacilli/2

Answers to Questions 12–17

12. **C** Both KIA and TSI contain tenfold more lactose than glucose, peptone, and phenol red to detect acid production (turns yellow) and sodium thiosulfate and ferrous ammonium sulfate to detect H_2S production. However, TSI contains sucrose and KIA does not. Organisms fermenting either sucrose or lactose will turn the slant of the agar tube yellow. Therefore, some organisms, (e.g., many species of *Cedecea, Citrobacter, Edwardsiella,* and *Serratia*) will produce a yellow slant on TSI but a red slant on KIA.

13. **C** The malonate test determines whether an organism can utilize sodium malonate as the sole source of carbon. Malonate is broken down, forming alkaline metabolites that raise the pH of the broth above 7.6. This causes bromthymol blue to turn from green to deep blue (Prussian blue). *E. coli, Shigella,* and most *Salmonella* are malonate-negative, whereas *Enterobacter* and *Salmonella* (formerly *Arizona*) subgroups 2, 3a, and 3b are positive. *Proteus* and *Providencia* and *Serratia* and *Yersinia* are also malonate-negative.

14. **B** *Escherichia, Salmonella, Shigella,* and *Yersinia* are responsible for the majority of enteric diarrhea cases attributable to the Enterobacteriaceae family.

15. **A** An isolate of *E. coli* recovered from a stool culture in hemorrhagic colitis can be definitely identified only by serotyping. The isolate is identified as *E. coli* by the usual biochemical reactions. The strain of *E. coli* responsible for hemorrhagic colitis is O157:H7 and is usually negative for sorbitol fermentation. Colonies of this strain of *E. coli* appear colorless on MacConkey agar with sorbitol added.

16. **A** Serological confirmation of *Shigella* isolates is based upon O antigen typing. If a suspected *Shigella* spp is serologically typed with polyvalent sera before it has been correctly identified biochemically, a false-positive confirmation may occur with an isolate that is *E. coli* (i.e., anaerogenic nongas-producing, lactose-negative or delayed, and non-motile strains). These strains were formerly known as the Alkalescens-Dispar serotype.

17. **D** The *Shigella* spp are lactose nonfermenters that for the most part are biochemically inert and are classified into serogroups A, B, C, and D as a result of their biochemical similarity. *S. sonnei* is the species most often isolated from diarrhea cases in the United States. It is more active biochemically than the other species owing to ornithine decarboxylase and β-galactosidase activity. These enzymes, found in most strains of *S. sonnei*, distinguish it from other *Shigella* species.

18. Which of the following tests best differentiates *Shigella* species from *E. coli*?
- **A.** Hydrogen sulfide, VP, citrate, and urease
- **B.** Lactose, indole, ONPG, and motility
- **C.** Hydrogen sulfide, MR, citrate, and urease
- **D.** Gas, citrate, and VP

Microbiology/Evaluate laboratory data to make identifications/Gram-negative bacilli/2

19. Which genera of Enterobacteriaceae are usually nonmotile at 36°C?
- **A.** *Shigella*, *Klebsiella*, and *Yersinia*
- **B.** *Escherichia*, *Edwardsiella*, and *Enterobacter*
- **C.** *Proteus*, *Providencia*, and *Salmonella*
- **D.** *Serratia*, *Morganella*, and *Hafnia*

Microbiology/Apply knowledge of fundamental biological characteristics/Gram-negative bacilli/2

20. Fever, abdominal cramping, watery stools, and fluid and electrolyte loss preceded by bloody stools 2–3 days before is characteristic of shigellosis but may also result from infection with:
- **A.** *Campylobacter* spp
- **B.** *Salmonella* spp
- **C.** *Proteus* spp
- **D.** *Yersinia* spp

Microbiology/Apply knowledge of fundamental biological characteristics/Gram-negative bacilli/2

21. Cold enrichment of feces (incubation at 4°C) in phosphate-buffered saline prior to subculture onto enteric media enhances the recovery of:
- **A.** Enterotoxigenic *E. coli*
- **B.** *Salmonella paratyphi*
- **C.** *Hafnia alvei*
- **D.** *Y. enterocolitica*

Microbiology/Apply principles of special procedures/Gram-negative bacilli/2

22. Which group of tests, along with colonial morphology on primary media, aids most in the rapid identification of the Enterobacteriaceae?
- **A.** MR and VP, urease and blood agar plate
- **B.** Phenylanine deaminase, urease, and CDC agar plate
- **C.** Bacitracin, β-lactamase, and MacConkey agar plate
- **D.** Indole, oxidase, MacConkey, and blood agar plates

Microbiology/Select methods/Reagents/Media/Gram-negative bacilli/2

Answers to Questions 18–22

18. **B** *E. coli*, positive for lactose, indole, and ONPG, are usually motile. *Shigella* species do not ferment lactose or produce indole, lack β-galactosidase, and are nonmotile.

19. **A** *Shigella* spp and *Klebsiella* spp are for the most part nonmotile. *Yersinia* can be motile at 22°C but is nonmotile at 36°C. Other members of the Enterobacteriaceae that have been isolated from human specimens and are usually nonmotile include *Leminorella*, *Rahnella*, and *Tatumella*.

20. **A** *Shigella* spp and *Campylobacter* spp are both causes of diarrhea, abdominal pain, fever, and sometimes vomiting. Blood is present in the stools of patients infected with *Shigella* as a result of invasion and penetration of the bowel. Young children may also exhibit bloody stools when infected with *Campylobacter*.

21. **D** Cold enrichment is especially useful when specimens contain large numbers of normal flora that are sensitive to prolonged exposure to near-freezing temperature. In addition to *Yersinia*, the technique has been used to enhance recovery of *Listeria monocytogenes* from specimens containing other bacteria.

22. **D** The Enterobacteriaceae are all oxidase-negative. Because *E. coli* and *Proteus* spp comprise a majority of the organisms recovered from clinical specimens, they can be initially identified through rapid testing without additional overnight testing. *E. coli* display a positive indole test, and the colonial morphology on MacConkey agar is distinctive, showing flat, pink (lactose-positive) colonies with a ring of bile precipitation. *Proteus* spp swarm on blood agar and are indole-negative.

23. A routine, complete stool culture procedure should include media for the isolation of *E. coli* O157:H7 as well as:

A. *Salmonella, Shigella, Yersinia, Campylobacter*, and *Staphylococcus aureus*

B. *Vibrio cholerae, Brucella*, and *Yersinia* spp

C. *S. aureus*, group B streptococci, and group D streptococci

D. *Clostridium difficile, Clostridium perfringens*, and *Yersinia* spp

Microbiology/Select methods/Reagents/Media/Gram-negative bacilli/2

24. Which group of tests best identifies the *Morganella* and *Proteus* genera?

A. Motility, urease, and phenylalanine deaminase

B. Malonate, glucose fermentation, and deoxyribonuclease (DNase)

C. Indole, oxidase, MR, and VP

D. Indole, citrate, and urease

Microbiology/Evaluate laboratory data to make identifications/Gram-negative bacilli/2

25. Which group of tests best differentiates *Enterobacter aerogenes* from *Edwardsiella tarda*?

A. Motility, citrate, and urease

B. Hydrogen sulfide (H₂S) production, sucrose fermentation, indole, and VP

C. Lysine decarboxylase, urease, and arginine dihydrolase

D. Motility, H₂S production, and DNase

Microbiology/Evaluate laboratory data to make identifications/Gram-negative bacilli/2

26. *Enterobacter sakazakii* can best be differentiated from *Enterobacter cloacae* by its:

A. Yellow pigmentation and negative sorbitol fermentation

B. Pink pigmentation and positive arginine dihydrolase

C. Yellow pigmentation and positive urease

D. H₂S production on TSI

Microbiology/Evaluate laboratory data to make identifications/Gram-negative bacilli/2

27. Members of the genus *Cedecea* are best differentiated from *Serratia* spp by which test result?

A. Positive motility

B. Positive urease

C. Positive phenylalanine deaminase

D. Negative DNase

Microbiology/Evaluate laboratory data to make identifications/Gram-negative bacilli/2

Answers to Questions 23–27

23. **A** *V. cholerae* and *C. difficile* are usually not included in a routine stool culture. If *Vibrio* spp are suspected, a special request should be included. Although MacConkey agar will support the growth of *Vibrio* spp, normal enteric flora overgrow and occlude these organisms. *C. difficile* culture requires special media (CCFA) that inhibit other anaerobic flora and facultative anaerobic flora and should be requested specifically if symptoms warrant. MacConkey agar with sorbitol will allow the *E. coli* O157:H7 to be recovered. *Yersinia* spp can be detected on a regular MacConkey agar plate.

24. **A** *Morganella* and *Proteus* spp are motile, produce urease, and deaminate phenylalanine.

25. **B**

Test	*E. aerogenes* (% positive)	*E. tarda* (% positive)
H₂S	0	100
Sucrose	>90	0
Indole	<20	100
VP	100	0
Citrate	95	0

26. **A** *E. sakazakii* is called a yellow-pigmented *E. cloacae* and is best differentiated from *E. cloacae* by sorbitol fermentation (95% positive for *E. cloacae* and 0% for *E. sakazakii*). In addition, *E. cloacae* is usually positive for urease and malonate (65% and 75%, respectively) and *E. sakazakii* is usually negative (1% and <20%, respectively). Both species are usually motile and arginine dihydrolase–positive.

27. **D** DNase is not produced by *Cedecea* spp but is produced (along with proteinases) by *Serratia* spp. Other key differential tests include lipase (positive for *Cedecea*, negative for *Serratia*) and gelatin hydrolysis (negative for *Cedecea*, positive for *Serratia*).

28. Which of the following organisms is often confused with the *Salmonella* species biochemically and on plated media?
  A. *E. coli*
  B. *Citrobacter freundii*
  C. *Enterobacter cloacae*
  D. *Shigella dysenteriae*

Microbiology/Apply knowledge of fundamental biological characteristics/Gram-negative bacilli/2

29. A gram-negative rod is recovered from a catheterized urine sample from a nursing home patient. The lactose-negative isolate tested positive for indole, urease, ornithine decarboxylase, and phenylalanine deaminase and negative for H_2S. The most probable identification is:
  A. *Ewardsiella* spp
  B. *Morganella* spp
  C. *Ewingella* spp
  D. *Shigella* spp

Microbiology/Evaluate laboratory data to make identifications/Gram-negative bacilli/3

30. Which single test best separates *Klebsiella oxytoca* from *K. pneumoniae*?
  A. Urease
  B. Sucrose
  C. Citrate
  D. Indole

Microbiology/Evaluate laboratory data to make identifications/Gram-negative bacilli/2

31. Which of the following organisms, found in normal fecal flora, may be mistaken biochemically for the genus *Yersinia*?
  A. *Klebsiella* spp
  B. *Proteus* spp
  C. *E. coli*
  D. *Enterobacter* spp

Microbiology/Apply knowledge of fundamental biological characteristics/Gram-negative bacilli/2

32. Why might it be necessary for both pink (lactose-positive) and colorless (lactose-negative) colonies from an initial stool culture on MacConkey agar to be subcultured and tested further for possible pathogens?
  A. Most *Shigella* strains are lactose-positive
  B. Most *Salmonella* strains are maltose-negative
  C. Most *Proteus* spp are lactose-negative
  D. Pathogenic *E. coli* can be lactose-positive or lactose-negative

Microbiology/Evaluate laboratory data to make identifications/Gram-negative bacilli/2

Answers to Questions 28–32

28. **B** Biochemical differentiation is essential because *Citrobacter* isolates may give a false-positive agglutination test with *Salmonella* grouping sera. *C. freundii* strains, like *Salmonella* spp, are usually H_2S producers and may be confused with *Salmonella* spp unless the proper biochemical tests are utilized. *C. freundii* and *Salmonella* spp are adonitol-, indole-, and malonate-negative. However, *C. freundii* is KCN-positive, whereas *Salmonella* spp are KCN-negative.

29. **B** *Morganella* are biochemically similar to *Proteus* spp, both being lactose-negative, motile, and positive for phenylalanine deaminase and urease. However, *Morganella* can be differentiated from *Proteus* spp based upon H_2S, indole, ornithine decarboxylase, and xylose fermentation. *Ewingella* spp are usually positive (70%) for lactose fermentation, whereas the other three genera are lactose-negative.

30. **D** *K. oxytoca* and *K. pneumoniae* are almost identical biochemically except for the ability to produce indole. Both organisms are usually positive for urease, sucrose, and citrate. However, *K. oxytoca* is indole-positive and *K. pneumoniae* is indole-negative.

31. **B** *Proteus* spp are urease-positive as are approximately 70% of *Y. enterocolitica* isolates. Both organisms are lactose-negative and motile. However, *Yersinia* is motile at 22°C and not at 35°C (demonstrated using motility media).

32. **D** Possible pathogenic strains of *E. coli* should be picked from MacConkey agar and subcultured onto MacConkey agar with sorbitol. After subculture, these strains can be serotyped or sent to a reference laboratory. Most *E. coli* normal flora ferment D-sorbitol and appear pink to red on MacConkey-sorbitol agar. The *E. coli* strain O157:H7 causes the enteric disease hemorrhagic colitis. It ferments D-sorbitol slowly or not at all and appears as colorless colonies on MacConkey-sorbitol agar.

33. Which agar that is used for routine stool cultures is the medium of choice for the isolation of *Yersinia* strains from stool specimens?
A. *Salmonella-Shigella* agar
B. Hektoen enteric agar
C. MacConkey agar
D. CNA agar

Microbiology/Select methods/Reagents/Media/Gram-negative bacilli/2

34. Which organism is sometimes mistaken for *Salmonella* and will agglutinate in *Salmonella* polyvalent antiserum?
A. *C. freundii* strains
B. *Proteus mirabilis* strains
C. *S. sonnei* strains
D. *E. coli*

Microbiology/Apply knowledge of fundamental biological characteristics/Gram-negative bacilli/2

35. A bloody stool from a 26-year-old woman with 3 days of severe diarrhea showed the following results at 48 hours after being plated on the following media:

> MacConkey agar: little normal flora with many nonlactose-fermenting colonies
>
> Hektoen enteric agar: many blue-green colonies
>
> *Campylobacter* blood agar and *C. difficile* agar: no growth
>
> Clear colonies (from MacConkey agar) tested negative for oxidase, indole, urease, motility, and H$_2$S

The most likely identification is:
A. *Shigella* spp
B. *Salmonella* spp
C. *Proteus* spp
D. *E. coli*

Microbiology/Evaluate laboratory data to make identifications/Gram-negative bacilli/2

36. Which of the following organisms are generally positive for β-galactosidase?
A. *Salmonella* spp
B. *Shigella* spp
C. *Proteus* spp
D. *E. coli*

Microbiology/Evaluate laboratory data to make identifications/Gram-negative bacilli/2

33. **C** Cefsulodin-irgasan-novobiocin (CIN) medium is the best agar for the isolation of *Yersinia* strains because it inhibits growth of other coliforms, but it is not used routinely in clinical laboratories. *Yersinia* spp grow well on MacConkey agar incubated at 37°C, but the colonies are much smaller than the other Enterobacteriaceae; therefore, 25°C is the temperature recommended for isolation. Some serotypes of *Yersinia* may be inhibited on more selective media, such as *Salmonella-Shigella* or Hektoen. CNA agar inhibits the growth of gram-negative bacteria.

34. **A** *C. freundii* and *Salmonella* spp are H$_2$S-positive and indole, VP, and phenylalanine deaminase–negative. Biochemical characteristics that help to differentiate *C. freundii* from *Salmonella* include lactose fermentation (50% of *C. freundii* are lactose-positive, whereas 100% of *Salmonella* are lactose-negative) and urease production (70% of *Citrobacter* are positive and >99% of *Salmonella* are negative).

35. **A** *Shigella* is the most likely organism biochemically. *E. coli* are usually indole- and motility-positive, and *Proteus* are motility and urease-positive. Most *Salmonella* are H$_2$S-positive. *Shigella* and *Campylobacter* cause bloody diarrhea because they invade the epithelial cells of the large bowel; however, *Campylobacter* spp do not grow on MacConkey agar, and they are oxidase-positive.

36. **D** Enterobacteriaceae are grouped according to their ability to ferment lactose, a β-galactoside. *Salmonella*, *Shigella*, *Proteus*, *Providencia*, and *Morganella* are usually lactose nonfermenters. Others, including certain strains of *E. coli*, *S. sonnei*, *Hafnia alvei*, *Serratia marcescens*, and some *Yersinia*, appear to be lactose nonfermenters because they lack the permease enzyme that actively transports lactose across the cell membrane. However, true lactose nonfermenters do not possess β-galactosidase. The test for β-galactosidase uses the substrate *o*-nitrophenyl-β-galactopyranoside. At an alkaline pH, β-galactosidase hydrolyses the substrate, forming *o*-nitrophenol, which turns the medium yellow.

37. In the Kauffmann-White schema, the combined antigens used for serological identification of the *Salmonella* spp are:
- **A.** O antigens
- **B.** H antigens
- **C.** Vi and H antigens
- **D.** O, Vi, and H antigens

Microbiology/Apply knowledge of fundamental biological characteristics/Gram-negative bacilli/1

38. The drugs of choice for treatment of infections with Enterobacteriaceae are:
- **A.** Aminoglycosides, trimethoprim-sulfamethoxazole, third-generation cephalosporins
- **B.** Ampicillin and nalidixic acid
- **C.** Streptomycin and isoniazid
- **D.** Chloramphenicol, ampicillin, and colistin

Microbiology/Apply knowledge of fundamental biological characteristics/Gram-negative bacilli/2

39. The Shiga-like toxin (verotoxin) is produced mainly by which Enterobacteriaceae?
- **A.** *Klebsiella pneumoniae*
- **B.** *E. coli*
- **C.** *Salmonella typhimurium*
- **D.** *Enterobacter cloacae*

Microbiology/Apply knowledge of fundamental biological characteristics/Gram-negative bacilli/2

40. Infections caused by *Yersinia pestis* are rare in the United States. Those cases that do occur are most frequently located in which region?
- **A.** New Mexico, Arizona, and California
- **B.** Alaska, Oregon, and Utah
- **C.** North and South Carolina and Virginia
- **D.** Ohio, Michigan, and Indiana

Microbiology/Apply knowledge of fundamental biological characteristics/Gram-negative bacilli/2

41. A leg culture from a nursing home patient grew gram-negative rods on MacConkey agar as pink to dark pink oxidase-negative colonies. Given the following results, which is the most likely organism?

TSI = A/A	Indole = Neg
MR = Neg	VP = +
Citrate = +	H₂S = Neg
Urease = +	Motility = Neg

Antibiotic susceptibility: resistant to carbenicillin and ampicillin
- **A.** *Serratia marcescens*
- **B.** *Proteus vulgaris*

- **C.** *Enterobacter cloacae*
- **D.** *Klebsiella pneumoniae*

Microbiology/Evaluate laboratory data to make identifications/Gram-negative bacilli/3

Answers to Questions 37–41

37. **D** The Kaufmann-White schema groups the salmonellae on the basis of the somatic O (heat-stable) antigens and subdivides them into serotypes based on their flagellar H (heat-labile) antigens. The Vi (or K) antigen is a capsular polysaccharide that may be removed by heating. There are over 2200 serotypes of *Salmonella*.

38. **A** The drugs of choice for the Enterobacteriaceae vary, and several genera display patterns of resistance that aid in their identification. *K. pneumoniae* and *Citrobacter diversus* are resistant to ampicillin and carbenicillin; most *Enterobacter* spp and *Hafnia* are resistant to ampicillin and cephalothin. *Proteus*, *Morganella*, and *Serratia* are resistant to colistin. *Providencia* and *Serratia* are resistant to multiple drugs. Several genera are resistant to chloramphenicol and most are resistant to penicillin.

39. **B** Strains of *E. coli* that produce one or both of the shiga-like toxins (SLT I and SLT II) can cause bloody diarrhea (hemorrhagic colitis). In the United States, *E. coli* strain O157:H7 is the serotype most often associated with hemorrhagic colitis.

40. **A** Approximately 15 cases of *Y. pestis* infection are confirmed in the United States annually. Most originate in the Southwest. It is necessary to be aware of this regional occurrence because untreated cases are associated with a mortality rate of approximately 60%. *Y. pestis* is not fastidious and grows well on blood agar. It is inactive biochemically, which helps to differentiate it from other Enterobacteriaceae.

41. **D** *K. pneumoniae* and *E. cloacae* display similar IMViC (indole, MR, VP, and citrate) reactions (00++) and TSI results. However, approximately 65% of *E. cloacae* strains are urease-positive compared with 98% of those of *K. pneumoniae*. *Enterobacter* spp are motile and *Klebsiella* are nonmotile. The antibiotic pattern of resistance to carbenicillin and ampicillin is characteristic for *Klebsiella*.

42. Four blood cultures were taken over a 24-hour period from a 20-year-old woman with severe diarrhea. The cultures grew motile (room temperature), gram-negative rods. A urine specimen obtained by catheterization also showed gram-negative rods, 100,000 col/mL. Given the following results, which is the most likely organism?

TSI = A/A gas   Indole = +
VP = Neg   MR = +
H_2S = Neg   Citrate = Neg
Urease = Neg   Lysine decarboxylase = +
Phenylalanine deaminase = Neg

A. Proteus vulgaris
B. Salmonella typhi
C. Yersinia enterocolitica
D. E. coli

Microbiology/Evaluate laboratory data to make identifications/Gram-negative bacilli/3

43. A stool culture from a 30-year-old man suffering from bloody mucoid diarrhea gave the following results on differential enteric media:

MacConkey agar = clear colonies;
XLD agar = clear colonies;
Hektoen agar = green colonies;
Salmonella-Shigella agar = small, clear colonies

Which tests are most appropriate for identification of this enteric pathogen?
A. TSI, motility, indole, urease, *Shigella* typing with polyvalent sera
B. TSI, motility, indole, lysine, *Salmonella* typing with polyvalent sera
C. TSI, indole, MR, VP, citrate
D. TSI, indole, MR, and urease

Microbiology/Evaluate laboratory data to make identifications/Gram-negative bacilli/3

44. A leg-wound culture from a hospitalized 70-year-old diabetic man grew motile, lactose-negative colonies on MacConkey agar. Given the following biochemical reactions at 24 hours, what is the most probable organism?

H_2S (TSI) = Neg   Indole = Neg
MR = Neg   VP = +
Phenylalanine deaminase = Neg   DNase = +
Citrate = +   Urease = Neg
Ornithine and lysine decarboxylase = +
Arginine decarboxylase = Neg
Gelatin hydrolysis = +

A. Proteus vulgaris
B. Serratia marcescens
C. Proteus mirabilis
D. Enterobacter cloacae

Microbiology/Evaluate laboratory data to make identifications/Gram-negative bacilli/3

45. Three blood cultures taken from a 30-year-old cancer patient receiving chemotherapy and admitted with a urinary tract infection grew lactose-negative, motile, gram-negative rods prior to antibiotic therapy. Given the following biochemical reactions, which is the most likely organism?

H_2S (TSI) = +   Indole = +
MR = +   VP = Neg
Phenylalanine deaminase = +   DNase = +
Citrate = Neg   Urease = +
Gelatin hydrolysis = +   Ornithine decarboxylase = Neg

A. Proteus vulgaris
B. Proteus mirabilis
C. Serratia marcescens
D. Klebsiella pneumoniae

Microbiology/Evaluate laboratory data to make identifications/Gram-negative bacilli/3

Answers to Questions 42–45

42. D Typically, the IMViC reactions for the organisms listed are:

E. coli	(++00)
S. typhi	(0+00)
Y. enterocolitica	(V+00)
P. vulgaris	(++00)

Note: Indole reaction is variable (V) for *Y. enterocolitica*.

43. A The most likely organism is a species of *Shigella*. Typically, *Salmonella* spp produce H_2S-positive colonies that display black centers on the differential media (except on MacConkey agar). The biochemical tests above are necessary to differentiate *Shigella* from *E. coli* because some *E. coli* strains cross-react with *Shigella* typing sera. *Shigella* spp are one of the most common causes of bacterial diarrhea; group D (*S. sonnei*) and group B (*S. flexneri*) are the species most often isolated.

44. B *S. marcescens* has been implicated in numerous nosocomial infections and is recognized as an important pathogen with invasive properties. Gelatin hydrolysis and DNase are positive for both the *Proteus* spp and *Serratia*, but the negative urease and phenylalanine deaminase are differential. *E. cloacae* does not produce DNase, gelatinase, or lysine decarboxylase.

45. A Although *P. mirabilis* is more frequently recovered from patients with urinary tract infections, *P. vulgaris* is commonly recovered from immunosuppressed patients. *P. mirabilis* is indole-negative and ornithine decarboxylase-positive but otherwise is very similar to *P. vulgaris*.

46. Three consecutive stool cultures from a 25-year-old male patient produced scant normal fecal flora on MacConkey and Hektoen agars. However, colonies on CIN agar (cefsoludin-irgasan-novobiocin) displayed "bulls-eye" colonies after 48 hours incubation. The patient had been suffering from enterocolitis with fever, diarrhea, and abdominal pain for 2 days. What is the most likely identification of this gram-negative rod?
    A. *E. coli*
    B. *Proteus mirabilis*
    C. *Yersinia enterocolitica*
    D. *Klebsiella pneumoniae*

Microbiology/Evaluate laboratory data to make identifications/Gram-negative bacilli/3

47. A 6-year-old female patient was admitted to the hospital following two days of severe diarrhea. Cultures from three consecutive stool samples contained blood and mucus.

    Patient history revealed a hamburger lunch at a fast-food restaurant 3 days earlier. Which pathogen is most likely responsible for the following results?

    Growth on:
    XLD agar = yellow colonies
    HE agar = yellow colonies
    Mac agar = light pink and dark pink colonies
    Mac with sorbitol agar = few dark pink and many colorless colonies
    A. *Salmonella* spp
    B. *Shigella* spp
    C. *E. coli* O157:H7
    D. *Yersinia enterocolitica*

Microbiology/Evaluate laboratory data to make identifications/Gram-negative bacilli/3

48. Following a 2-week camping trip to the Southwest (US), a 65-year-old male patient was hospitalized with a high fever and an inflammatory swelling of the axilla and groin lymph nodes. Several blood cultures were obtained, resulting in growth of gram-negative rods resembling "closed-safety pins." The organism grew on MacConkey's agar showing non-lactose–fermenting colonies. Testing demonstrated a nonmotile rod that was biochemically inert. The most likely identification is?

A. *Yersinia pestis*
B. *Klebsiella pneumoniae*
C. *Proteus vulgaris*
D. *Morganella morganii*

Microbiology/Evaluate laboratory data to make identifications/Gram-negative bacilli/3

Answers to Questions 46–48

46. **C** Most members of the Enterobacteriaceae family produce detectable growth on MacConkey agar within 24 hours. *Yersinia enterocolita* produces non-lactose–fermenting colonies on MacConkey agar, salmon-colored colonies on Hektoen agar, and yellow or colorless colonies on XLD agar. If *Yersinia enterocolitica* is suspected, specialized agar (CIN) is employed. The typical bulls-eye colonies, dark red with a translucent border, can be confused with *Aeromonas* spp that appear similarly on CIN agar. To differentiate, an oxidase test must be performed, since *Yersinia* spp are oxidase-negative and *Aeromonas* spp are oxidase-positive.

47. **C** Inflammation with bleeding of the mucosa of the large intestine (hemorrhagic colitits) is a result of an enterohemorrhagic *E. coli* (EHEC) infection associated with certain serotypes, such as *E. coli* O157:H7. The source of the *E. coli* infection is from ingestion of undercooked ground beef contaminated with fecal matter or drinking raw milk.

48. **A** *Yersinia pestis* is the cause of bubonic and pneumonic plague. Bubonic plague causes swelling of the groin lymph nodes (bubos). whereas pneumonic plague involves the lungs. The infection caused by bubonic plague may result in fulminant bacteremia that is usually fatal. The transmission is from rodents (rats, ground squirrels, or prairie dogs) to humans by the bite of fleas (vectors) or by ingestion of contaminated animal tissues. Pneumonic plague is acquired via the airborne route when there is close contact with other pneumonic plague victims.

49. The majority of clinical laboratories with a microbiology department should have the capability of serotyping which pathogenic Enterobacteriaceae?

  A. *Yersinia enterocolitica, Shigella* spp

  B. *E. coli* O157:H7, *Salmonella* spp, *Shigella* spp

  C. *Yersinia pestis, Salmonella* spp

  D. *Edwardiella* spp, *Salmonella* spp

Microbiology/Apply knowledge of standard operating procedures/Identification/2

50. Direct spread of pneumonic plague disease occurs by which route?

  A. Fecal-oral route

  B. Rat bite

  C. Ingestion of contaminated tissue

  D. Inhalation of contaminated airborne droplets

Microbiology/Apply knowledge of epidemiology of transmission/2

Answers to Questions 49–50

49. **B** Preliminary serological grouping of the *Salmonella* spp *and Shigella* spp should be performed, since reliable commercial polyvalent antisera are available. Sorbitol-negative (MacConkey agar with sorbitol) colonies of *E. coli* should be tested using commercially available antisera for somatic "O" antigen 157 and flagellar "H" antigen 7. However, *Yersinia pestis* isolates should be sent to a public health laboratory for testing, since clinical laboratories generally do not have the typing sera available.

50. **D** Bubonic plague involves an inflammatory swelling of the lymph nodes of the axilla and groin, whereas pneumonic plague is associated with an airborne route involving the lungs. Both infections are caused by the same member of the Enterobacteriaceae family, *Yersinia pestis*.

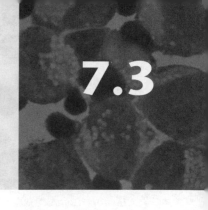

1. What are the most appropriate screening tests to presumptively differentiate and identify the nonfermentative gram-negative bacilli (NFB) from the Enterobacteriaceae?
   A. Catalase, decarboxylation of arginine, growth on blood agar
   B. Motility, urease, morphology on blood agar
   C. Oxidase, TSI, nitrate reduction, growth on MacConkey agar
   D. Oxidase, indole, and growth on blood agar

   Microbiology/Evaluate laboratory data to make identifications/NFB/2

2. Presumptive tests used for identification of the *Pseudomonas* spp are:
   A. Oxidase, oxidation-fermentation (OF) glucose (open), OF glucose (sealed), motility, pigment production
   B. Growth on blood agar plate (BAP) and eosin-methylene blue (EMB) agars, lysine decarboxylation, catalase
   C. Growth on MacConkey, EMB, and XLD agars and motility
   D. Growth on mannitol salt agar and flagellar stain

   Microbiology/Evaluate laboratory data to make identifications/NFB/2

3. Which tests are most appropriate to differentiate between *Pseudomonas aeruginosa* and *Pseudomonas putida*?
   A. Oxidase, motility, pyoverdin
   B. Oxidase, motility, lactose
   C. Oxidase, ONPG, DNase
   D. Mannitol, nitrate reduction, growth at 42°C

   Microbiology/Evaluate laboratory data to make identifications/NFB/2

4. Which test group best differentiates *Acinetobacter baumannii* from *P. aeruginosa*?
   A. Oxidase, motility, NO$_3$ reduction
   B. MacConkey growth, 37°C growth, catalase
   C. Blood agar growth, oxidase, catalase
   D. Oxidase, TSI, MacConkey growth

   Microbiology/Evaluate laboratory data to make identifications/NFB/2

Answers to Questions 1–4

1. **C** NFB will grow on the slant of TSI or KIA but they do not acidify the butt (glucose fermentation), as do the Enterobacteriaceae. NFB can be cytochrome oxidase–positive or –negative, but all the Enterobacteriaceae are oxidase-negative. The Enterobacteriaceae grow well on MacConkey agar and reduce nitrate to nitrite, but the NFB grow poorly or not at all and most do not reduce nitrate. Nearly 70% of the NFB recovered from clinical specimens are:

   Strains of *P. aeruginosa*

   Acinetobacter baumannii (*A. anitratus*)

   Stenotrophomonas (*Xanthomonas*) *maltophilia*

2. **A** The use of OF tubes helps to determine the presumption of a nonfermentative bacillus (glucose oxidation–positive and glucose fermentation–negative). The positive cytochrome oxidase test and pigment production indicate a possible *Pseudomonas* species. Several NFB produce pigments that aid in species identification: *P. aeruginosa* produces yellow pyoverdins (fluorescein) and/or pyocyanin (blue aqua pigment). The characteristic grapelike odor of aminoacetophenone as well as growth at 42°C are characteristics of *P. aeruginosa*.

3. **D** Both organsims are oxidase-positive, motile, and produce pyoverdin. Both are negative for ONPG and DNase. The differentiating tests are:

Test	P. aeruginosa	P. putida
Mannitol	+	Neg
Reduce NO$_3$ to NO$_2$	+	Neg
42°C growth	+	Neg

4. **A** *Acinetobacter* are nonmotile rods that appear as coccobacillary forms from clinical specimens. All are oxidase-negative and catalase-positive. *P. aeruginosa* reduces NO$_3$ to NO$_2$ while *A. baumannii* does not.

5. In addition to motility, which test best differentiates *Acinetobacter* spp and *Alcaligenes* spp?
  A. TSI
  B. Oxidase
  C. Catalase
  D. Flagellar stain

Microbiology/Select methods/Reagents/Media/NFB/ Identification/2

6. The most noted differences between *P. aeruginosa* and *S. (X.) maltophilia* are:
  A. Oxidase, catalase, and TSI
  B. Oxidase, catalase, and ONPG
  C. Oxidase, 42°C growth, and polar tuft of flagella
  D. Catalase, TSI, and pigment

Microbiology/Evaluate laboratory data to make identifications/NFB/2

7. Which *Pseudomonas* is usually associated with a lung infection related to cystic fibrosis?
  A. *P. fluorescens*
  B. *P. aeruginosa*
  C. *P. putida*
  D. *Burkholderia (P.) pseudomallei*

Microbiology/Apply knowledge of fundamental biological characteristics/NFB/2

8. A nonfermenter recovered from an eye wound is oxidase-positive, motile with polar monotrichous flagella, and grows at 42°C. Colonies are dry, wrinkled or smooth, buff to light brown in color, and are difficult to remove from the agar. In which DNA homology group should this organism be placed?
  A. *Pseudomonas stutzeri*
  B. *Pseudomonas fluorescens*
  C. *Pseudomonas alcaligenes*
  D. *Pseudomonas diminuta*

Microbiology/Apply knowledge of fundamental biological characteristics/NFB/2

9. Which organism is associated with immunodeficiency syndromes and melioidosis (a glanders-like disease in Southeast Asia and northern Australia)?
  A. *Pseudomonas aeruginosa*
  B. *Pseudomonas stutzeri*
  C. *Pseudomonas putida*
  D. *Burkholderia (P.) pseudomallei*

Microbiology/Apply knowledge of fundamental biological characteristics/NFB/2

10. Which biochemical tests are needed to differentiate *Burkholderia (P.) cepacia* from *S. (X.) maltophilia*?
  A. Pigment on blood agar, oxidase, DNase
  B. Pigment on MacConkey agar, flagellar stain, motility
  C. Glucose, maltose, lysine decarboxylase
  D. TSI, motility, oxidase

Microbiology/Evaluate laboratory data to make identifications/NFB/2

Answers to Questions 5–10

5. **B** The two genera, *Acinetobacter* and *Alcaligenes*, are very similar. Both use oxidation for the metabolism of carbohydrate, with some strains being nonsaccharolytic. Both grow well on MacConkey agar. However, *Acinetobacter* is nonmotile and oxidase-negative. *Alcaligenes* is motile by peritrichous flagella and oxidase-positive.

6. **C** The two genera, *Pseudomonas* and *Stenotrophomonas* (*Xanthomonas*), are motile and grow well on MacConkey agar. However, *P. aeruginosa* is oxidase-positive and grows at 42°C but is motile only by polar monotrichous flagella. *S. (X.) maltophilia* is oxidase-negative, does not grow at 42°C, and is motile by a polar tuft of flagella.

7. **B** *P. aeruginosa* is often recovered from the respiratory secretions of cystic fibrosis patients. If the patient is chronically infected with the mucoid strain of *P. aeruginosa*, the biochemical identification is very difficult. The mucoid strain results from production of large amounts of alginate, a polysaccharide that surrounds the cell.

8. **A** *P. stutzeri* produces dry, wrinkled colonies that are tough and adhere to the media as well as smooth colonies. *B. (P.) pseudomallei* produces similar colony types but is distinguished by biochemical tests and susceptibility to the polymixins. The colonies of *P. stutzeri* are buff to light brown because of the relatively high concentration of cytochromes.

9. **D** *B. (P.) pseudomallei* produces wrinkled colonies resembling *P. stutzeri*. Infections are usually asymptomatic and can be diagnosed only by serological methods. The organism exists in soil and water in an area of latitude 20° north and south of the equator (mainly in Thailand and Vietnam). Thousands of U.S. military personnel were infected with these bacteria during the 1960s and 1970s. The disease may reactivate many years after exposure and has been called the "Vietnamese time bomb."

10. **A** Both organisms produce yellowish pigment and have polar tuft flagella, but the oxidase and DNase tests are differential.

Test	B. (P.) cepacia	S. (X.) maltophilia
Pigment on BAP	Green-yellow	Lavender-green
Oxidase	+	Neg
DNase	Neg	+
Motility	+	+
Glucose OF (open)	+	+
Maltose OF (open)	+	+
Lysine decarboxylase	+	+

11. The following results were obtained from a pure culture of gram-negative rods recovered from the pulmonary secretions of a 10-year-old cystic fibrosis patient with pneumonia:

Oxidase = +	Motility = +
Glucose OF (open) = +	Gelatin hydrolysis = +
Pigment = Red (nonfluorescent)	Arginine dihydrolase = +
Growth at 42°C = +	Flagella = + (polar monotrichous)

Which is the most likely organism?
A. *Burkholderia (P.) pseudomallei*
B. *Pseudomonas stutzeri*
C. *Burkholderia (P.) cepacia*
D. *Pseudomonas aeruginosa*

Microbiology/Evaluate laboratory data to make identifications/NFB/3

12. *Alcaligenes faecalis* (formerly *A. odorans*) is distinguished from *Bordetella bronchiseptica* with which test?
A. Urease (rapid)
B. Oxidase
C. Growth on MacConkey agar
D. Motility

Microbiology/Evaluate laboratory data to make identifications/NFB/2

13. *Flavobacterium* spp are easily distinguished from *Acinetobacter* spp by which of the following two tests?
A. Oxidase, growth on MacConkey agar
B. Oxidase and OF (glucose)
C. TSI and urea hydrolysis
D. TSI and VP

Microbiology/Evaluate laboratory data to make identifications/NFB/2

14. A gram-negative coccobacillus was recovered on chocolate agar from the CSF of an immunosuppressed patient. The organism was nonmotile and positive for indophenol oxidase but failed to grow on MacConkey agar. The organism was highly susceptible to penicillin. The most probable identification is:
A. *Acinetobacter* spp
B. *Pseudomonas aeruginosa*
C. *Pseudomonas stutzeri*
D. *Moraxella lacunata*

Microbiology/Evaluate laboratory data to make identifications/NFB/2

15. Cetrimide agar is used as a selective isolation agar for which organism?
A. *Acinetobacter* spp
B. *Pseudomonas aeruginosa*
C. *Moraxella* spp
D. *Stenotrophomonas (X.) maltophilia*

Microbiology/Select methods/Reagents/Media/NFB/Identification/2

Answers to Questions 11–15

11. D The oxidase test and red pigment (pyorubin), as well as growth at 42°C, distinguish *P. aeruginosa* from the other pseudomonads listed, particularly *B. cepacia*, which is also associated with cystic fibrosis.

12. A *Alcaligenes* and *Bordetella* are genera belonging to the Alcaligenaceae family. The two organisms are very similar biochemically, but *B. bronchiseptica* is urease-positive. Both organisms are oxidase-positive, grow on MacConkey agar, and are motile by peritrichous flagella. *B. bronchiseptica* grows well on MacConkey agar but other species of *Bordetella* are fastidious gram-negative rods.

13. A *Flavobacterium* spp and *Acinetobacter* spp often produce a yellow pigment on blood or chocolate agar and are nonmotile. *Acinetobacter* spp are oxidase-negative, grow on MacConkey agar, and are coccobacillary on the Gram stain smear. In contrast, *Flavobacterium* spp are oxidase-positive, do not grow on MacConkey agar, and are typically rod-shaped. *Flavobacterium meningosepticum* is highly pathogenic for premature infants.

14. D *Moraxella* spp are oxidase-positive and nonmotile, which distinguishes them from *Acinetobacter* spp and most *Pseudomonas* spp. *Moraxella* spp are highly sensitive to penicillin, but *Acinetobacter* spp and *Pseudomonas* spp are penicillin-resistant. *M. lacunata* is implicated in infections involving immunosuppressed patients.

15. B Cetrimide (acetyl trimethyl ammonium bromide) agar is used for the isolation and identification of *P. aeruginosa*. With the exception of *P. fluorescens*, the other pseudomonads are inhibited along with related nonfermentative bacteria.

16. A specimen from a 15-year-old female burn patient was cultured after débridement, and the following results were obtained:

Oxidase = +   Lysine decarboxylase = Neg

Catalase = +   Motility = +

Ornithine decarboxylase   Glucose = + for oxidation
= Neg   (open tube)

Arginine dihydrolase = +   Maltose = Neg for oxidation
                                 (open tube)

Penicillin = Resistant   Aminoglycosides = Susceptible

Colistin (Polymixin B) = Susceptible

These results indicate which of the following organisms?

A. *Acinetobacter (calcoaceticus) baumannii*

B. *Moraxella lacunata*

C. *Pseudomonas aeruginosa*

D. *Acinetobacter lwoffii*

Microbiology/Evaluate laboratory data to make identifications/NFB/3

17. A yellow pigment–producing organism that is oxidase-positive, nonmotile, and does not grow on MacConkey agar is:

A. *Acinetobacter (calcoaceticus) baumannii*

B. *Acinetobacter lwoffii*

C. *Burkholderia (P.) cepacia*

D. *Flavobacterium meningosepticum*

Microbiology/Evaluate laboratory data to make identifications/NFB/2

18. Which reagent(s) is(are) used to develop the red color indicative of a positive reaction in the nitrate reduction test?

A. Sulfanilic acid and α-naphthylamine

B. Ehrlich's and Kovac's reagents

C. *o*-Nitrophenyl-β-D-galactopyranoside

D. Kovac's reagent

Microbiology/Apply knowledge of biochemical reactions/bacteria/1

19. A culture from an intra-abdominal abscess produced orange-tan colonies on blood agar that gave the following results:

Oxidase = +   Nitrate reduction = +

KIA = Alk/Alk (H_2S)+   Motility = + (single polar flagellum)

DNase = +   Ornithine decarboxylase = +

Growth at 42°C = Neg

The most likely identification is:

A. *Shewanella (Pseudomonas) putrefaciens*

B. *Acinetobacter* spp

C. *Pseudomonas aeruginosa*

D. *Flavobacterium* spp

Microbiology/Evaluate laboratory data to make identifications/NFB/3

20. *Flavobacterium* spp and *B. (P.) cepacia* are easily differentiated by which test?

A. Motility

B. OF glucose

C. Oxidase

D. Cetrimide agar

Microbiology/Evaluate laboratory data to make identifications/NFB/2

Answers to Questions 16–20

16.   C *P. aeruginosa* is a cause of a significant number of burn wound infections; these organisms can exist in distilled water and underchlorinated water. *Acinetobacter* spp are oxidase-negative and *Moraxella* spp are highly susceptible to penicillin, ruling them out as possible causes.

17.   D All species of *Acinetobacter* are oxidase-negative and grow on MacConkey agar. *Flavobacterium* spp produce yellow pigment (like *Acinetobacter*) but are oxidase-positive and do not grow on MacConkey agar. *B. (P.) cepacia* also produces a yellow pigment but is motile.

18.   A In the nitrate test, nitrites formed by bacterial reduction of nitrates will diazotize sulfanilic acid. The diazonium compound complexes with α-naphthylamine, forming a red product. Media containing nitrates are used for the identification of nonfermenters. When testing nonfermenters, it is wise to confirm a negative reaction using zinc dust. The diazonium compound detects nitrite only, and the organism may have reduced the nitrates to nitrogen, ammonia, nitrous oxide, or hydroxylamine. Zinc ions reduce residual nitrates in the media to nitrites. A red color produced after addition of zinc indicates the presence of residual nitrates, confirming a true negative reaction. If a red or pink color does not occur after adding zinc, then the organism reduced the nitrate to a product other than nitrite, and the test is considered positive.

19.   A *S. putrefaciens* produces abundant H_2S on KIA or TSI (the alkaline butt distinguishes it from other dextrose-negative nonfermentative bacilli).

20.   A *B. (P.) cepacia* (93%) are weakly oxidase-positive and motile. *Flavobacterium* spp are oxidase-positive but are nonmotile.

21. A 15-year-old female complained of a severe eye irritation after removing her soft-contact lenses. A swab of the infected right eye was obtained by an ophthalmologist, who ordered a culture and sensitivity test. The culture was plated on blood agar and MacConkey agar. At 24 hours, growth of a gram-negative rod that tested cytochrome oxidase–positive was noted . The Mueller-Hinton sensitivity plate showed a bluish-green "lawn" of growth that proved highly resistant to most of the antibiotics tested except amikacin, tobramycin, and ciprofloxacin. The most likely identification is?

A. *Burkholderia cepacia*
B. *Pseudomonas aeruginosa*
C. *Stenotrophomonas maltophilia*
D. *Acinetobacter baumannii*

Microbiology/Apply knowledge of laboratory data to make identifications/GNNFB/3

22. Which of the *Pseudomonas* spp. below is associated with the following virulence factors: exotoxin A, endotoxins, proteolytic enzymes, antimicrobial resistance, and production of alginate?

A. *P. fluorescens*
B. *P. putida*
C. *P. stutzeri*
D. *P. aeruginosa*

Microbiology/Apply knowledge of virulence/Identification/GNNFB/2

23. A 20 year-old horse groomer exhibited a "glanders-like" infection. His history indicated he had suffered several open wounds on his hands 2 weeks before the swelling of his lymph nodes. A gram-negative rod was recovered from a blood culture that grew well on blood and MacConkey agars. Most of the biochemical tests were negative, including the cytochrome oxidase test. What is the most likely identification?

A. *Burkholderia mallei*
B. *Pseudomonas aeruginosa*
C. *Pseudomonas stutzeri*
D. *Burkholderia pseudomallei*

Microbiology/Apply epidemiology for ID/GNNFB/3

24. A Vietnam War veteran presented with a "glanders-like" infection (melioidosis). Several blood cultures produced gram-negative rods that were cytochrome oxidase–positive, oxidized glucose and xylose, and grew at 42° C. The most likely organism is?

A. *Stenotrophomonas maltophilia*
B. *Burkholderia pseudomallei*
C. *Pseudomonas aeruginosa*
D. *Acinetobacter* spp

Microbiology/Apply knowledge for identification/GNNFB/2

25. Cytochrome oxidase-positive, nonfermentative gram-negative bacilli were recovered from the stool of a cystic fibrosis (CF) patient. The isolates produced wet (mucoidy) colonies on blood agar. Which identification is most likely?

A. *Acinetobacter* spp.
B. *Pseudomonas alcaligenes*
C. *Pseudomonas stutzeri*
D. *Pseudomonas aeruginosa*

Microbiology/Apply knowledge for identification/NFGNB/2

Answers to Questions 21–25

21. **B** *P. aeruginosa* is an opportunistic organism that is not part of the human normal flora. Contact lens solution contamination, eye injury, or contact lens eye trauma are factors that contribute to *P. aeruginosa* eye infections. The characteristic blue-green pigment on Mueller-Hinton agar (pyocyanin pigment) produced by *P. aeruginosa* and the highly resistant nature to antibiotics aid in its identification.

22. **D** *P. aeruginosa* is highly resistant to many antimicrobial drugs as well as being one of the most often cultured opportunistic organisms. This virulence factor allows for many nosocomial infections such as those of the urinary tract, wounds (burn patients), bacteremia, respiratory tract, and CNS.

23. **A** *Burkholderia mallei* is rarely transmitted to humans. It is the causative agent of glanders in mules, donkeys, and horses. It is not part of the human skin flora and the most likely transmission to humans is through broken skin.

24. **B** *Burkholderia pseudomallei* infections often produce abscesses in organs (liver, spleen, lungs) as well as on the skin, in soft tissue, and in joints and bones. Vietnam War veterans especially may harbor these organisms, which are limited to tropical and subtropical environments (Southeast Asia and Australia). The organism may surface years later after surviving in a latent state within phagocytes. The surfaces of rice paddies in Northern Thailand have a high prevalence of this organism.

25. **D** Infected CF patients usually do not escape *P. aeruginosa* infections completely. *P. aeruginosa* produces alginate that accounts for the "wet, mucoidy" appearance of colonies. This overproduction of alginate is thought to cause the inhibition of phagocytosis. The result is chronic infections in CF patients with the "wet" form of *P. aeruginosa*.

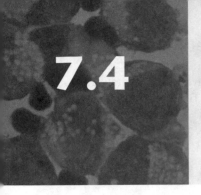

1. A visitor to South America who returned with diarrhea is suspected of being infected with *V. cholerae*. Select the best medium for recovery and identification of this organism.
   A. MacConkey agar
   B. Blood agar
   C. TCBS agar
   D. XLD agar

   Microbiology/Select methods/Reagents/Media/Bacteria/ Identification/2

2. A curved gram-negative rod producing oxidase-positive colonies on blood agar was recovered from a stool culture. Given the following results, what is the most likely identification?

Lysine decarboxylase = +	Arginine decarboxylase = Neg	Indole = + Lactose = Neg
KIA = Alk/Acid	VP = Neg	TCBS agar =
Urease = ±	String test = Neg	Green colonies

   A. *Vibrio cholerae*
   B. *Vibrio parahaemolyticus*
   C. *Shigella* spp
   D. *Salmonella* spp

   Microbiology/Evaluate laboratory data to make identifications/Bacteria/3

3. A gram-negative S-shaped rod recovered from selective media for *Campylobacter* species gave the following results:

Catalase = +	Oxidase = +
Motility = +	Hippurate hydrolysis = +
Growth at 42°C = +	Nalidixic acid = Susceptible
Pigment = Neg	Grape odor = Neg
Cephalothin = Resistant	

   The most likely identification is:
   A. *Pseudomonas aeruginosa*
   B. *Campylobacter jejuni*
   C. *Campylobacter fetus*
   D. *Pseudomonas putida*

   Microbiology/Evaluate laboratory data to make identifications/Bacteria/3

4. Which atmospheric condition is needed to recover *Campylobacter* spp from specimens inoculated onto a Campy-selective agar at 35°–37°C and 42°C?
   A. 5% O_2, 10% CO_2, and 85% N_2
   B. 20% O_2, 10% CO_2, and 70% N_2
   C. 20% O_2, 20% CO_2, and 60% N_2
   D. 20% O_2, 5% CO_2, and 75% N_2

   Microbiology/Apply knowledge of fundamental biological characteristics/Bacteria/2

Answers to Questions 1–4

1. **C** The growth of yellow colonies on TCBS agar (citrate utilization and acid from sucrose) is diagnostic for *V. cholerae*. On blood agar, *V. cholerae* of the El Tor biotype appear as large, translucent, β-hemolytic colonies and will agglutinate chicken erythrocytes.

2. **B** *V. parahaemolyticus* appear as green colonies on TCBS agar, whereas *V. cholerae* appear as yellow colonies on TCBS. *V. cholerae* is the only *Vibrio* species that causes a positive string test. In the test, a loopful of bacterial colonies is suspended in sodium deoxycholate, 0.5%, on a glass slide. After 60 sec, the inoculating loop is lifted out of the suspension. *V. cholerae* forms a long string resembling a string of pearls. *Salmonella* spp and *Shigella* spp are oxidase-negative.

3. **B** The only *Campylobacter* spp that hydrolyze hippurate are *C. jejuni* and subsp *doylei*. However, some strains of *P. aeruginosa* grow on agar selective for *Campylobacter* at 42°C. *C. fetus* will not grow at 42°C but will grow at 25°C and 37°C.

4. **A** *Campylobacter* spp. are best recovered in a microaerophilic atmosphere (reduced O_2). The use of a CO_2 incubator or candle jar is not recommended because the amount of O_2 and CO_2 do not permit any but the most aerotolerant *Campylobacter* to survive. Cultures for *Campylobacter* should be incubated for 48–72 hours before reporting no growth.

5. Which group of tests best differentiates *Helicobacter pylori* from *C. jejuni*?
   A. Catalase, oxidase, and Gram stain
   B. Catalase, oxidase, and nalidixic acid sensitivity
   C. Catalase, oxidase, and cephalothin sensitivity
   D. Urease, nitrate, and hippurate hydrolysis

Microbiology/Select methods/Reagents/Media/Bacteria/ Identification/2

6. Which of the following tests should be done first in order to differentiate *Aeromonas* spp from the Enterobacteriaceae?
   A. Urease
   B. OF glucose
   C. Oxidase
   D. Catalase

Microbiology/Select methods/Reagents/Media/Bacteria/ Identification/2

7. Which is the best rapid test to differentiate *Plesiomonas shigelloides* from a *Shigella* species on selective enteric agar?
   A. Oxidase
   B. Indole
   C. TSI
   D. Urease

Microbiology/Select methods/Reagents/Media/Bacteria/ Identification/2

8. Which are the best two tests to differentiate *A. hydrophilia* from *P. shigelloides*?
   A. Oxidase and motility
   B. DNase and VP
   C. Indole and lysine decarboxylase
   D. Growth on MacConkey and blood agar

Microbiology/Select methods/Reagents/Media/Bacteria/ Identification/2

Answers to Questions 5–8

5. D *Helicobacter pylori* is found in specimens from gastric secretions and biopsies and has been implicated as a cause of gastric ulcers. It is found only in the mucus-secreting epithelial cells of the stomach. Both *H. pylori* and *C. jejuni* are catalase- and oxidase-positive. However, *Helicobacter* spp are urease-positive, which differentiates them from *Campylobacter* spp.

Test	H. pylori	C. jejuni
Nitrate reduction	Neg	+
Hippurate hydrolysis	Neg	+
Urease	+	Neg
Cephalothin sensitivity	Sensitive	Resistant
Nalidixic acid sensitivity	Resistant	Sensitive

6. C *Aeromonas hydrophilia* and other *Aeromonas* spp have been implicated in acute diarrheal disease as well as cellulitis and wound infections. Infections usually follow exposure to contaminated soil, water, or food. *Aeromonas* growing on enteric media are differentiated from the Enterobacteriaceae by demonstrating that colonies are oxidase-positive. The *Aeromonas* are sometimes overlooked as pathogens because most strains grow on selective enteric agar as lactose fermenters.

7. A *P. shigelloides* is a lactose nonfermenter that will resemble *Shigella* spp on MacConkey agar. Both are TSI Alk/Acid and urease-negative. *Plesiomonas* produces indole and *Shigella* usually causes delayed production of indole. However, *Plesiomonas* is oxidase-positive, whereas *Shigella* spp are oxidase-negative.

8. B Both of these bacteria cause diarrhea, grow well on enteric agar, and may be confused with Enterobacteriaceae. Both organisms are positive for oxidase, motility, indole, and lysine decarboxylase. The following reactions are differential:

Test	A. hydrophilia	P. shigelloides
β-Hemolysis on sheep blood agar	+	Neg
DNase	+	Neg
VP	+	Neg

9. Which genus (in which most species are oxidase- and catalase-positive) of small gram-negative coccobacilli is associated mainly with animals but may cause endocarditis, bacteremia, and wound and dental infections in humans?
   A. *Actinobacillus*
   B. *Pseudomonas*
   C. *Campylobacter*
   D. *Vibrio*

   Microbiology/Apply fundamental biological characteristics/Bacteria/2

10. Which of the following tests may be used to differentiate *Cardiobacterium hominis* from *Actinobacillus* spp?
    A. Gram stain
    B. Indole
    C. Anaerobic incubation
    D. Oxidase

    Microbiology/Select methods/Reagents/Media/Bacteria/ Identification/2

11. A mixture of slender gram-negative rods and coccobacilli with rounded ends was recovered from blood cultures following a patient's root canal surgery. Given the following results after 48 hours, what is the most likely organism?

Catalase = Neg	Ornithine decarboxylase = +
Urease = Neg	Lysine decarboxylase = +
Oxidase = +	X and V requirement = Neg
Indole = Neg	Growth on blood and chocolate
Carbohydrates = Neg	agar = + (with pitting of agar)
(no acid produced)	Growth on MacConkey agar = Neg

    A. *Eikenella corrodens*
    B. *Actinobacillus* spp
    C. *Cardiobacterium hominis*
    D. *Proteus* spp

    Microbiology/Evaluate laboratory data to make identifications/Bacteria/3

12. *Kingella kingae* can best be differentiated from *Eikenella corrodens* using which medium?
    A. Sheep blood agar
    B. Chocolate agar
    C. MacConkey agar
    D. XLD agar

    Microbiology/Select methods/Reagents/Media/Bacteria/ Identification/2

13. *Kingella kingae* is usually associated with which type of infection?
    A. Middle ear
    B. Endocarditis
    C. Meningitis
    D. Urogenital

Microbiology/Apply fundamental biological characteristics/Bacteria/1

Answers to Questions 9–13

9. **A** *Actinobacillus* spp (formerly CDC groups HB-3 and HB-4) share many biochemical characteristics of the *Haemophilus* spp. Infections most often associated with this gram-negative coccobacillus are subacute bacterial endocarditis and periodontal disease (its main habitat is the mouth). The most common human isolate is *Actinobacillus actinomycetemcomitans*, which grows slowly on chocolate agar. It is positive for catalase, nitrate reduction, and glucose fermentation. It does not grow on MacConkey agar and is negative for oxidase, urease, indole, X, and V requirements.

10. **B** *C. hominis* is a gram-negative coccobacillus biochemically similar to *Actinobacillus* spp. Like *Actinobacillus*, it is a cause of endocarditis. However, *Cardiobacterium* spp are positive for cytochrome oxidase and negative for nitrate reduction, while most *Actinobacillus* are negative for oxidase and positive for nitrate reduction. *C. hominis* will grow on blood agar after 48–72 hours in 5% CO_2 at 35°C, but *Actinobacillus* requires chocolate agar.

11. **A** *E. corrodens* is a part of the normal flora of the upper respiratory tract and the mouth. It is often seen after trauma to the head and neck, dental infections, and human bite wounds. It requires blood for growth. The organism causes a pitting of the agar where colonies are located. The smell of bleach may be apparent when the plates are uncovered for examination. *Actinobacillus* spp and *C. hominis* both utilize several carbohydrates, and *Proteus* spp are oxidase-negative.

12. **A** Both *Kingella kingae* and *E. corrodens* are gram-negative rods that are oxidase-positive and catalase-negative. Both grow well on blood and chocolate agars and cause pitting of the media, and neither grows on MacConkey or XLD agar. However, *K. kingae* strains produce a narrow zone of β-hemolysis on blood agar (sheep) similar to that of group B streptococci.

13. **B** *Kingella* spp are gram-negative coccobacilli or plump-looking rods. They are part of the normal flora of the upper respiratory and urogenital tracts of humans. Infection is seen primarily in patients having underlying heart disease, poor oral hygiene, or iatrogenic mucosal ulcerations (e.g., radiation therapy), in whom the organism is recovered from blood cultures.

14. Cultures obtained from a dog bite wound produced yellow, tan, and slightly pink colonies on blood and chocolate agar with a margin of fingerlike projections appearing as a film around the colonies. Given the following results at 24 hours, which is the most likely organism?

> Oxidase = +   Catalase = +
> Growth on MacConkey agar =
> Neg Motility = Neg

   A. *Actinobacillus* spp
   B. *Eikenella* spp
   C. *Capnocytophaga* spp
   D. *Pseudomonas* spp

Microbiology/Evaluate laboratory data to make identifications/Bacteria/3

15. Smooth gray colonies showing no hemolysis are recovered from an infected cat scratch on blood and chocolate agar but fail to grow on MacConkey agar. The organisms are gram-negative pleomorphic rods that are both catalase- and oxidase-positive and strongly indole-positive. The most likely organism is:
   A. *Capnocytophaga* spp
   B. *Pasteurella* spp
   C. *Proteus* spp
   D. *Pseudomonas* spp

Microbiology/Evaluate laboratory data to make identifications/Bacteria/3

16. Which media should be used to recover *Bordetella pertussis* from a nasopharyngeal specimen?
   A. Chocolate agar
   B. Blood agar
   C. MacConkey agar
   D. Bordet-Gengou agar

Microbiology/Select methods/Reagents/Media/Bacteria/ Identification/2

17. Which medium is recommended for the recovery of *Brucella* spp from blood and bone marrow specimens?
   A. Biphasic Castenada bottles with *Brucella* broth
   B. Blood culture bottles with *Brucella* broth
   C. Bordet-Gengou agar plates and THIO broth
   D. Blood culture bottles with THIO broth

Microbiology/Select methods/Reagents/Media/Bacteria/ Identification/2

18. In addition to CO_2 requirements and biochemical characteristics, *Brucella melitensis* and *Brucella abortus* are differentiated by growth on media containing which two dyes?
   A. Basic fuchsin and thionin
   B. Methylene blue and crystal violet
   C. Carbol fuchsin and iodine
   D. Safranin and methylene blue

Microbiology/Select methods/Reagents/Media/Bacteria/ Identification/2

14. C *Capnocytophaga gingivalis*, *C. sputigena*, and *C. ochracea* are part of the normal oropharyngeal flora of humans; however, *C. canimorsus* and *C. cynodegmi* (formerly CDC groups DF-2 and DF-2-like bacteria) are associated with infections resulting from dog bite wounds.

15. B *Pasteurella multocida* (*P. canis*) is part of the normal mouth flora of cats and dogs and is frequently recovered from wounds inflicted by them. It produces large amounts of indole and therefore an odor resembling colonies of *E. coli*. *Pseudomonas* spp are also catalase- and oxidase-positive but can be ruled out because they grow on MacConkey agar and do not produce indole.

16. D *B. pertussis* is an oxidase-positive, nonmotile gram-negative coccobacillus and appears as small, round colonies resembling droplets of mercury. It is fastidious and does not grow on chocolate or MacConkey agar. However, *B. pertussis* adapts to blood agar, growing within 3–6 days. This organism is the cause of whooping cough, which has declined with the policy of mandatory diphtheria, tetanus, pertussis (DPT) immunization of infants in the United States. The DPT vaccine contains diphtheria and tetanus toxoids and killed whole-cell *B. pertussis*.

17. A Although blood agar will support the growth of *Brucella* spp, Castenada bottles are the medium of choice. Castenada bottles contain a slant of enriched agar medium that is partially submerged and surrounded by an enriched broth medium. As the specimen is injected into the bottles and mixed, the agar slant is simultaneously coated with the blood (or bone marrow). *Brucella* is the cause of undulant fever and is responsible for many cases of fever of unknown origin. *Brucella* spp are facultative intracellular organisms and grow very slowly, usually requiring 4–6 weeks for recovery. *Brucella melitensis* is the most frquently recovered species.

18. A *B. abortus* can be differentiated from *B. melitensis* by the reactions shown at the bottom of the page:

	H$_2$S	Urease	CO_2 Requirement	Basic Fuchsin	Thionin (20 mg)
B. melitensis	Neg	V	Neg	+	+
B. abortus	+	+	+/V	+	Neg

19. Which of the following amino acids are required for growth of *Francisella tularensis*?
- **A.** Leucine and ornithine
- **B.** Arginine and lysine
- **C.** Cysteine and cystine
- **D.** Histidine and tryptophan

Microbiology/Apply fundamental biological characteristics/Bacteria/1

20. Which medium is best for recovery of *Legionella pneumophila* from clinical specimens?
- **A.** Chocolate agar
- **B.** Bordet-Gengou agar
- **C.** New yeast extract agar
- **D.** Buffered charcoal-yeast extract (CYE) agar

Microbiology/Select methods/Reagents/Media/Bacteria/Identification/1

21. *Haemophilus influenzae*, which requires X and V factors for growth, can be differentiated from subspecies *Haemophilus aegyptius* by which two tests?
- **A.** Indole and xylose
- **B.** Glucose and urease
- **C.** Oxidase and catalase
- **D.** Indole and oxidase

Microbiology/Select methods/Reagents/Media/Bacteria/Identification/2

22. *Haemophilus* species that require the V factor (NAD) are easily recovered on which agar plate?
- **A.** Blood agar made with sheep red cells
- **B.** Blood agar made with horse red cells
- **C.** Chocolate agar
- **D.** Xylose agar

Microbiology/Select methods/Reagents/Media/Bacteria/Identification/2

23. Which of the following products is responsible for satellite growth of *Haemophilus* spp around colonies of *Staphylococcus* and *Neisseria* spp on sheep blood agar?
- **A.** NAD
- **B.** Hemin
- **C.** Indole
- **D.** Oxidase

Microbiology/Apply fundamental biological characteristics/Bacteria/1

Answers to Questions 19–23

19. **C** *F. tularensis* is a fastidious gram-negative rod that is best recovered from lymph node aspirates and tissue biopsies. It is oxidase-negative, nonmotile, and inert biochemically. Cysteine blood agar is the medium of choice, but *F. tularensis* will grow on commercially prepared chocolate agar because it contains X factor and is supplemented with a growth enrichment (IsoVitaleX) that contains cysteine. *F. tularensis* may not grow well on MacConkey agar.

20. **D** *L. pneumophila* should be recovered on buffered CYE agar. This agar is nonselective but can be made more selective for *Legionella* spp by addition of the antibiotics cefamandole, polymyxin B, and anisomycin. Any small, glistening, convex colonies on buffered CYE agar after 2–3 days of incubation that do not grow on L-cysteine–deficient buffered CYE agar or routine nonselective media should be further tested by the direct fluorescent antibody test (DFA) for confirmation of *L. pneumophila*.

21. **A** *H. influenzae* and subspecies *H. aegyptius* are both glucose, urease, oxidase, and catalase-positive. *H. influenzae* (biotype II) is positive for both indole and xylose, whereas *H. aegyptius* is negative for both tests. Biotype II encompasses 40%–70% of *H. influenzae* strains recovered from clinical specimens. *H. influenzae* subspecies *aegyptius* is responsible for epidemics of conjunctivitis in children.

22. **C** The V factor, NAD, must first be released from RBCs before it can be assimilated by *Haemophilus* spp. Chocolate agar is made by heating blood agar in order to lyse RBCs. The released NAD is directly available to those *Haemophilus* species requiring it. Chocolate agar also contains the X factor (hemin). All *Haemophilus* except *H. ducreyi* and *H. aphrophilus* require V factor, while X factor is required by *H. influenzae*, *H. haemolyticus*, and *H. ducreyi*.

23. **A** Colonies growing on sheep blood agar secreting NAD (V factor) or producing β-hemolysins (which lyse the sheep RBCs releasing NAD) allow pinpoint-size colonies of *Haemophilus* spp to grow around them. Sheep blood agar alone does not support the growth of *Haemophilus* spp, which require V factor because of the presence of V factor–inactivating enzymes that are present in the agar.

	H. influenzae	H. parainfluenzae	H. haemolyticus	H. parahaemolyticus	H. aphrophilus	H. aegyptius	H. ducreyi
X factor	+	Neg	+	Neg	Neg	+	+
V factor	+	+	+	+	Neg	+	Neg
Hemolysis	Neg	Neg	+	+	Neg	Neg	Neg

24. Which of the following plates should be used in order to identify *Haemophilus haemolyticus* and *Haemophilus parahaemolyticus*?
 A. Sheep blood agar and chocolate agar
 B. Horse blood agar and Mueller-Hinton agar with X and V strips
 C. Brain-heart infusion agar with sheep red cells added
 D. Chocolate agar and Mueller-Hinton agar with X factor added

Microbiology/Select methods/Reagents/Media/Bacteria/ Identification/2

25. The majority of *Haemophilus influenzae* infections are caused by which of the following capsular serotypes?
 A. a
 B. b
 C. c
 D. d

Microbiology/Correlate clinical and laboratory data/ Bacteria/Haemophilus/2

26. Which *Haemophilus* species is generally associated with endocarditis?
 A. *H. influenzae*
 B. *H. ducreyi*
 C. *H. aphrophilus*
 D. *H. haemolyticus*

Microbiology/Correlate clinical and laboratory data/ Bacteria/Haemophilus/2

27. Which *Haemophilus* species is difficult to isolate and recover from genital ulcers and swollen lymph nodes?
 A. *H. aphrophilus*
 B. *H. ducreyi*
 C. *H. haemolyticus*
 D. *H. parahaemolyticus*

Microbiology/Correlate clinical and laboratory data/ Bacteria/Haemophilus/2

28. Which of the following is a characteristic of strains of *Haemophilus influenzae* that are resistant to ampicillin?
 A. Production of β-lactamase enzymes
 B. Hydrolysis of chloramphenicol
 C. Hydrolysis of urea
 D. All of the above

Microbiology/Apply fundamental biological characteristics/Bacteria/1

Answers to Questions 24–28

24. **B** Production of β-hemolysis is used to distinguish these two species from other *Haemophilus* with the same X and V requirements. Horse blood agar furnishes X factor and, when supplemented with yeast extract, supports the growth of *Haemophilus* spp. Sheep blood agar is not used because it contains growth inhibitors for some *Haemophilus* spp. The chart at the top of this page summarizes the characteristics of the *Haemophilus* spp.

25. **B** The majority of *H. influenzae* infections occur in children under 5 years old and are caused by capsular serotype b, one of six serotypes designated a through f. This strain appears to contain a virulence factor making it resistant to phagocytosis and intracellular killing by neutrophils. Serotyping of *Haemophilus* is performed by mixing colonies with agglutinating antibodies available as commercial agglutination kits.

26. **C** *H. aphrophilus* does not require either X or V factor for growth and is differentiated from the other *Haemophilus* species by its ability to produce acid from lactose and a positive δ-aminolevulinic acid (ALA) test. *H. influenzae* and *H. haemolyticus* are incapable of synthesizing protoporphyrin from δ-ALA and are negative for this test.

27. **B** *H. ducreyi* requires exogenous X factor and causes genital lesions referred to as "soft chancres." The medium used for recovery is commercial chocolate agar or gonococcus base medium containing 1%–2% hemoglobin, 5% fetal calf serum, and 1% IsoVitaleX enrichment. The plates must be incubated in a 3%–5% CO_2 environment for 2–3 days. Most specimens are recovered from heterosexuals, and outbreaks in the United States are traced to female prostitutes.

28. **A** Roughly 20% of *H. influenzae* strains produce β-lactamase, which hydrolyses and inactivates the β-lactam ring of ampicillin (and penicillin).

29. A small, gram-negative coccobacillus recovered from the CSF of a 2-year-old gave the following results:

Indole = +   Glucose = + (acid)
X requirement = +   V requirement = +
Urease = +   Lactose = Neg
Sucrose = Neg   Hemolysis = Neg

Which is the most likely identification?
A. *Haemophilus parainfluenzae*
B. *Haemophilus influenzae*
C. *Haemophilus ducreyi*
D. *Haemophilus aphrophilus*

Microbiology/Evaluate laboratory data to make identifications/Bacteria/3

30. The δ-ALA test (for porphyrins) is a confirmatory procedure for which test used for identification of *Haemophilus* species?
A. X factor requirement
B. V factor requirement
C. Urease production
D. Indole production

Microbiology/Apply knowledge to recognize sources of error/Bacteria/Identification/3

29. **B** Although several biotypes of *H. parainfluenzae* produce indole and urease, *H. parainfluenzae* does not require X factor for growth. *H. ducreyi* requires X factor but not V factor. *H. aphrophilus* does not require either X factor or V factor for growth.

30. **A** The X factor requirement for growth is the cause of many inaccuracies when identifying *Haemophilus* spp requiring this factor. False-negative results have been attributed to the presence of small amounts of hemin in the basal media, or X factor carryover from colonies transferred from primary media containing blood. The δ-ALA test determines the ability of an organism to synthesize protoporphyrin intermediates in the biosynthetic pathway to hemin from the precursor compound δ-aminolevulinic acid. *Haemophilus* species that need exogenous X factor to grow are unable to synthesize protoporphyrin from δ-ALA and are negative for the δ-ALA test. These include *H. influenzae*, *H. haemolyticus*, *H. aegyptius*, and *H. ducreyi*.

1. The test used most often to separate the Micrococ-caceae family from the Streptococcaceae family is:
   A. Bacitracin
   B. Catalase
   C. Hemolysis pattern
   D. All of the above

   Microbiology/Select methods/Reagents/Media/Bacteria/Identification/1

2. *Micrococcus* and *Staphylococcus* species are differentiated by which test(s)?
   A. Fermentation of glucose (OF tube)
   B. Catalase test
   C. Gram stain
   D. All of the above

   Microbiology/Select methods/Reagents/Media/Bacteria/Identification/1

3. Lysostaphin is used to differentiate *Staphylococcus* from which other genus?
   A. *Streptococcus*
   B. *Stomatococcus*
   C. *Micrococcus*
   D. *Planococcus*

   Microbiology/Select methods/Reagents/Media/Bacteria/Identification/2

Answers to Questions 1–3

1. **B** The catalase test (utilizing a 3% hydrogen peroxide [H_2O_2] solution stored in a brown bottle under refrigeration) is positive for the four genera belonging to the Micrococcaceae family: *Planococcus*, *Micrococcus*, *Stomatococcus*, and *Staphylococcus*. Members of the Streptococcaceae family are negative. *Planococcus* spp are associated with marine life and not human infections. *Stomatococcus* spp are implicated in endocarditis following cardiac catheterization; they are weakly catalase-positive and produce white or transparent sticky colonies on agar, which help to differentiate them from *Staphylococcus*.

2. **A** Both micrococci and staphylococci are catalase-positive and gram-positive cocci. On direct smears they both appear as pairs, short chains (resembling *Streptococcus* spp), or clusters. However, the micrococci fail to produce acid from glucose under anaerobic conditions. The OF tube reactions are:

	Staphylococcus spp	*Micrococcus* spp
Open tube (oxidation)	+	+
Closed tube (fermentation)	+	Neg

3. **C** Lysostaphin is an endopeptidase that cleaves the glycine-rich pentapeptide crossbridges in the staphylococcal cell wall peptidoglycan. The susceptibility of the staphylococci to lysostaphin is used to differentiate them from the micrococci. Staphylococci are susceptible and show a 10–16 mm zone of inhibition, while micrococci are not inhibited.

4. Which of the following tests is used routinely to identify *Staphylococcus aureus*?

   A. Slide coagulase test

   B. Tube coagulase test

   C. Latex agglutination

   D. All of the above

   Microbiology/Select methods/Reagents/Media/Bacteria/ Identification/2

5. Which of the following enzymes contribute to the virulence of *S. aureus*?

   A. Urease and lecithinase

   B. Hyaluronidase and β-lactamase

   C. Lecithinase and catalase

   D. Cytochrome oxidase

   Microbiology/Apply knowledge of fundamental biological characteristics/Bacteria/1

6. Toxic shock syndrome is attributed to infection with:

   A. *Staphylococcus epidermidis*

   B. *Staphylococcus hominis*

   C. *Staphylococcus aureus*

   D. *Staphylococcus saprophyticus*

   Microbiology/Correlate clinical and laboratory data/Bacteria/Staphylococcus/2

7. Which *Staphylococcus* species, in addition to *S. aureus*, also produces coagulase?

   A. *S. intermedius*

   B. *S. saprophyticus*

   C. *S. hominis*

   D. All of the above

   Microbiology/Correlate clinical and laboratory data/Bacteria/Staphylococcus/2

8. *Staphylococcus epidermidis* (coagulase-negative) is recovered from which of the following sources?

   A. Prosthetic heart valves

   B. Intravenous catheters

   C. Urinary tract

   D. All of the above

   Microbiology/Correlate clinical and laboratory data/Bacteria/Staphylococcus/2

9. Slime production is associated with which *Staphylococcus* species?

   A. *S. aureus*

   B. *S. epidermidis*

   C. *S. intermedius*

   D. *S. saprophyticus*

   Microbiology/Apply knowledge of fundamental biological characteristics/Bacteria/1

4. **D** The slide coagulase test using rabbit plasma with ethylenediaminetetraacetic acid (EDTA) detects bound coagulase or "clumping factor" on the surface of the cell wall, which reacts with the fibrinogen in the plasma. This test is not positive for all strains of *S. aureus*, and a negative result must be confirmed by the tube method for detecting "free coagulase" or extracellular coagulase. The tube test is usually positive within 4 hours at 35°C; however, a negative result must then be incubated at room temperature for the remainder of 18–24 hours. Some strains produce coagulase slowly or produce fibrinolysin, which dissolves the clot at 35°C. Latex agglutination procedures utilize fibrinogen and IgG-coated latex beads that detect protein A on the staphylococcal cell wall.

5. **B** In addition to coagulase, the virulence of *S. aureus* is attributed to hyaluronidase, which damages the intercellular matrix (basement membrane) of tissues. β-Lactamase–producing strains are able to inactivate penicillin and ampicillin, making the organism resistant to these antibiotics. Lecithinase is not produced by *S. aureus*, and urease is not a virulence factor.

6. **C** *S. aureus* is the organism most often recovered from female patients. These strains produce toxic shock syndrome toxin 1 (TSST-1). Toxic shock syndrome is attributed to the use of certain highly absorbent tampons by menstruating females. The toxin is also recovered from sites other than the genital area and produces fever and life-threatening systemic damage as well as shock.

7. **A** *S. intermedius* infects mammals and certain birds but not usually humans. Cases involving humans result from animal bites and are most often seen in persons who work closely with animals.

8. **D** *S. epidermidis* represents 50%–80% of all coagulase-negative *Staphylococcus* spp recovered from numerous clinical specimens. It is of special concern in nosocomial infections because of its high resistance to antibiotics.

9. **B** *S. epidermidis* produces an extracellular slime that enhances the adhesion of these organisms to indwelling plastic catheters. The slime production is considered a virulence factor and is associated with infections from prostheses.

10. Strains of *Staphylococcus* species resistant to the β-lactam antibiotics by standardized disk diffusion and broth microdilution susceptibility methods are called:

A. Heteroresistant

B. Bacteriophage group 52A

C. Cross-resistant

D. Plasmid altered

Microbiology/Apply knowledge of fundamental biological characteristics/Bacteria/1

11. *Staphylococcus saprophyticus* is best differentiated from *Staphylococcus epidermidis* by resistance to:

A. 5 μg of lysostaphin

B. 5 μg of novobiocin

C. 10 units of penicillin

D. 0.04 unit of bacitracin

Microbiology/Correlate clinical and laboratory data/Bacteria/Staphylococcus/2

12. The following results were observed by using a tube coagulase test:

Coagulase at 4 hours = +   Coagulase at 18 hours = Neg
Novobiocin = Sensitive   Hemolysis on blood agar = β
(16-mm zone)   Mannitol salt plate = + (acid
DNase = +   production)

What is the most probable identification?

A. *Staphylococcus saprophyticus*

B. *Staphylococcus epidermidis*

C. *Staphylococcus aureus*

D. *Staphylococcus hominis*

Microbiology/Evaluate laboratory data to make identifications/Bacteria/3

13. *Staphylococcus aureus* recovered from a wound culture gave the following antibiotic sensitivity pattern by the standardized Kirby-Bauer method (S = sensitive; R = resistant):

Penicillin = R   Ampicillin = S (moderate)
Cephalothin = R   Cefoxitin = R
Vancomycin = S   Methicillin = R
(moderate)

Which is the drug of choice for treating this infection?

A. Penicillin

B. Ampicillin

C. Cephalothin

D. Vancomycin

Microbiology/Correlate clinical and laboratory data/Bacteria/Staphylococcus/2

14. Which of the following tests should be used to differentiate *Staphylococcus aureus* from *Staphylococcus intermedius*?

A. Acetoin

B. Catalase

C. Slide coagulase test

D. Urease

Microbiology/Select methods/Reagents/Media/Bacteria/Identification/2

Answers to Questions 10–14

10. **A** Methicillin-resistant *S. aureus* (MRSA) and methicillin-resistant *S. epidermidis* (MRSE) are termed heteroresistant. This refers to two subpopulations in a culture, one that is susceptible and the other that is resistant to antibiotic(s). The resistant population grows more slowly than the susceptible one and can be overlooked. Therefore, the more resistant subpopulation should be promoted growthwise by using a neutral pH (7.0–7.4), cooler incubation temperatures (30°–35°C), the addition of 2%–4% NaCl, and incubation up to 48 hours.

11. **B** *S. saprophyticus* is coagulase-negative and resistant to 5 μg of novobiocin. Using the standardized Kirby-Bauer sensitivity procedure, a 6–12 mm zone of growth inhibition is considered resistant. Susceptible strains measure 16–27 mm (inhibition) zones.

12. **C** *S. aureus* can produce fibrinolysins that dissolve the clot formed by the coagulase enzyme. The tube method calls for an incubation of 4 hours at 35°–37°C and 18–24 hours at room temperature. Both must be negative to interpret the result as coagulase-negative. This organism is coagulase-positive and, therefore, identified as *S. aureus*.

13. **D** Vanomycin, along with rifampin, is used for strains of *S. aureus* that are resistant to the β-lactams. MRSA strains pose problems when reading the zone sizes for these strains. Their heteroresistance results in a film of growth consisting of very small colonies formed within the defined inhibition zone surrounding the antibiotic disk. Initially, this appears as a mixed culture or contaminant.

14. **A** The production of acetoin by *S. aureus* from glucose or pyruvate differentiates it from *S. intermedius*, which is also coagulase-positive. This test is also called the VP test. Acetoin production is detected by addition of 40% KOH and 1% α-napthol to the VP test broth after 48 hours of incubation. A distinct pink color within 10 minutes denotes a positive test.

15. A gram-positive coccus recovered from a wound ulcer from a 31-year-old diabetic patient showed pale yellow, creamy, β-hemolytic colonies on blood agar. Given the following test results, what is the most likely identification?

> Catalase = +
>
> Glucose OF: positive open tube, negative sealed tube
>
> Mannitol salt = Neg
>
> Slide coagulase = Neg

A. *Staphylococcus aureus*
B. *Staphylococcus epidermidis*
C. *Micrococcus* spp
D. *Streptococcus* spp

Microbiology/Evaluate laboratory data to make identifications/Bacteria/3

16. Urine cultured from the catheter of an 18-year-old female patient produced more than 100,000 col/mL on a CNA plate. Colonies were catalase-positive, coagulase-negative by the latex agglutination slide method as well as the tube coagulase test. The best single test for identification is:

A. Lactose fermentation
B. Urease
C. Catalase
D. Novobiocin susceptibility

Microbiology/Select methods/Reagents/Media/Bacteria/Identification/3

17. A *Staphylococcus* spp recovered from a wound (cellulitis) was negative for the slide coagulase test (clumping factor) and negative for novobiocin resistance. The next test(s) needed for identification is (are):

A. Tube coagulase test
B. β-Hemolysis on blood agar
C. Mannitol salt agar plate
D. All of the above

Microbiology/Select methods/Reagents/Media/Bacteria/Identification/3

18. Furazolidone (furoxone) susceptibility is a test used to differentiate:

A. *Staphylococcus* spp from *Micrococcus* spp
B. *Streptococcus* spp from *Staphylococcus* spp
C. *Staphylococcus* spp from *Pseudomonas* spp
D. *Streptococcus* spp from *Micrococcus* spp

Microbiology/Select methods/Reagents/Media/Bacteria/Identification/2

19. Bacitracin resistance (0.04 unit) is used to differentiate:

A. *Micrococcus* spp from *Staphylococcus* spp
B. *Staphylococcus* spp from *Neisseria* spp
C. *Planococcus* spp from *Micrococcus* spp
D. *Staphylococcus* spp from *Streptococcus* spp

Microbiology/Select methods/Reagents/Media/Bacteria/Identification/2

20. Which of the following tests will rapidly differentiate micrococci from staphylococci?

A. Catalase
B. Coagulase
C. Modified oxidase
D. Novobiocin susceptibility

Microbiology/Select methods/Reagents/Media/Bacteria/Identification/2

Answers to Questions 15–20

15. **C** *Micrococcus* spp utilize glucose oxidatively but not under anaerobic conditions (sealed tube). *Staphylococcus* spp utilize glucose oxidatively and anaerobically. The catalase differentiates the Micrococcaceae family (positive) from the Streptococcaceae family (negative).

16. **D** *S. epidermidis* and *S. saprophyticus* are the two possibilities because they are both catalase-positive, coagulase-negative, urease-positive, and ferment lactose. Novobiocin susceptibility is the test of choice for differentiating these two species. *S. epidermidis* is sensitive but *S. saprophyticus* is resistant to 5 μg of novobiocin.

17. **D** *S. aureus* is novobiocin-sensitive and cannot be ruled out by a negative clumping factor test. Most *S. aureus* produce β-hemolysis on sheep blood agar plates and are mannitol salt–positive (produce acid and are not inhibited by the high salt concentration). The tube test should be performed because the slide test was negative.

18. **A** Staphylococci are susceptible to furazolidone, giving zones of inhibition that are 15 mm or greater. *Micrococcus* spp are resistant to furazolidone, giving zones of 6–9 mm. The test is performed as a disk susceptibility procedure using a blood agar plate.

19. **A** A bacitracin disk (0.04 unit) is used to identify group A β-hemolytic streptococci, but it will also differentiate catalase-positive organisms. A zone of 10 mm or greater is considered susceptible. The *Staphylococcus* species are resistant and grow up to the disk, while *Micrococcus* species are sensitive.

20. **C** The modified oxidase test is used to rapidly identify catalase-positive gram-positive cocci as *Micrococcus* spp (positive) or *Staphylococcus* spp (negative). Filter paper disks that are saturated with oxidase reagent (tetramethyl-*p*-phenylenediamine in dimethylsulfoxide) are used. A colony of the isolate is rubbed onto the paper. Oxidase-positive organisms produce a purple color within 30 sec.

21. *Streptococcus* species exhibit which of the following properties?

A. Aerobic, oxidase-positive, and catalase-positive

B. Facultative anaerobe, oxidase-negative, catalase-negative

C. Facultative anaerobe, β-hemolytic, catalase-positive

D. May be α-, β-, or γ-hemolytic, catalase-positive

Microbiology/Apply knowledge of fundamental biological characteristics/Streptococci/1

22. Which group of streptococci is associated with erythrogenic toxin production?

A. Group A

B. Group B

C. Group C

D. Group G

Microbiology/Apply knowledge of fundamental biological characteristics/Bacteria/1

23. A fourfold rise in titer of which antibodies is the best indicator of a recent infection with group A β-hemolytic streptococci?

A. Anti-streptolysin O

B. Anti-streptolysin S

C. Anti-A

D. Anti-B

Microbiology/Select methods/Reagents/Media/Bacteria/Identification/1

24. Bacitracin A disks (0.04 unit) are used for the presumptive identification of which group of β-hemolytic streptococci?

A. Group A

B. Group B

C. Group C

D. Group F

Microbiology/Select methods/Reagents/Media/Bacteria/Identification/1

25. Trimethoprim-sulfamethoxazole (SXT) disks are used along with bacitracin disks to differentiate which streptococci?

A. α-Hemolytic streptococci

B. β-Hemolytic streptococci

C. *Streptococcus pneumoniae*

D. *Enterococcus faecalis*

Microbiology/Select methods/Reagents/Media/Bacteria/Identification/1

26. β-Hemolytic streptococci, not of group A or B, usually exhibit which of the following reactions?

	Bacitracin	Trimethoprim–sulfamethoxazole
A.	Susceptible	Resistant
B.	Resistant	Resistant
C.	Resistant	Susceptible
D.	Susceptible	Indeterminate

Microbiology/Correlate clinical and laboratory data/Bacteria/Streptococci/2

Answers to Questions 21–26

21. B *Streptococcus* species are facultative anaerobes that grow aerobically as well, and are oxidase- and catalase-negative. In order to demonstrate streptolysin O on blood agar, it is best to stab the agar to create anaerobiosis because streptolysin O is oxygen-labile.

22. A Group A β-hemolytic streptococci are the cause of scarlet fever, and some strains produce toxins (pyrogenic exotoxins A, B, and C) that cause a scarlatiniform rash.

23. A The antistreptolysin O (ASO) titer is used to indicate a recent infection with group A β-hemolytic streptococci. Streptolysin O may also be produced by some strains of groups C and G streptococci.

24. A The bacitracin disk test is used in conjunction with other confirmatory tests for the β-hemolytic streptococci. In addition to group A, groups C, F, and G are also β-hemolytic and give a positive test for bacitracin (a zone of inhibition of any size). Therefore, a positive test does not confirm the presence of group A β-hemolytic streptococci.

25. B β-Hemolytic streptococci are the only streptococci that should be tested. *S. pneumoniae*, which is α-hemolytic, is susceptible to small concentrations of bacitracin, as are other α-hemolytic streptococci. SXT is inhibitory to most streptococci except *Streptococcus pyogenes* and *Streptococcus agalactiae*. For this reason, SXT is used in a commercially available streptococcal selective agar (SSA) as a primary plating agar for the detection of group A streptococci.

26. C Streptococci that are not group A or B may be either resistant or susceptible to bacitracin but are usually susceptible to SXT.

β Hemolytic Streptococci	Bacitracin	Trimethoprim-sulfamethoxazole
Group A	Sensitive	Resistant
Group B	Resistant	Resistant
Non-A, non-B groups	Sensitive or Resistant	Sensitive

27. A false-positive CAMP test for the presumptive identification of group B streptococci may occur if the plate is incubated in a(n):
   A. Candle jar or CO_2 incubator
   B. Ambient air incubator
   C. 35°C incubator
   D. 37°C incubator

Microbiology/Apply knowledge to identify sources of error/Identification/Streptococci/3

28. Which test is used to differentiate the viridans streptococci from the group D streptococci and enterococci?
   A. Bacitracin disk test
   B. CAMP test
   C. Hippurate hydrolysis test
   D. Bile esculin test

Microbiology/Select methods/Reagents/Media/Bacteria/ Identification/2

29. The bile solubility test causes the lysis of:
   A. *Streptococcus bovis* colonies on a blood agar plate
   B. *Streptococcus pneumoniae* colonies on a blood agar plate
   C. Group A streptococci in broth culture
   D. Group B streptococci in broth culture

Microbiology/Apply knowledge to identify sources of error/Identification/Streptococci/1

30. *S. pneumoniae* and the viridans streptococci can be differentiated by which test?
   A. Optochin disk test, 5 μg/mL or less
   B. Bacitracin disk test, 0.04 unit
   C. CAMP test
   D. Bile esculin test

Microbiology/Select methods/Reagents/Media/Bacteria/ Identification/2

31. The salt tolerance test (6.5% salt broth) is used to presumptively identify:
   A. *Streptococcus pneumoniae*
   B. *Streptococcus bovis*
   C. *Streptococcus equinus*
   D. *Enterococcus faecalis*

Microbiology/Select methods/Reagents/Media/Bacteria/ Identification/2

32. In addition to *Enterococcus faecalis*, which other streptococci will grow in 6.5% salt broth?
   A. Group A streptococci
   B. Group B streptococci
   C. *Streptococcus pneumoniae*
   D. Group D streptococci (nonenterococci)

Microbiology/Correlate clinical and laboratory data/ Bacteria/Streptococci/2

Answers to Questions 27–32

27. **A** The CAMP (hemolytic phenomenon first described by Christie, Atkins, and Munch-Petersen in 1944) test refers to a hemolytic interaction that is seen on a blood agar plate between the β-hemolysins produced by most strains of *S. aureus* and an extracellular protein produced by both hemolytic and nonhemolytic isolates of group B streptococci. When performing a CAMP test, the plate must be placed in an ambient air incubator at 35°–37°C. Group A streptococci may be CAMP-positive if the plate is incubated in a candle jar, high CO_2 atmosphere, or anaerobically.

28. **D** The bile esculin test differentiates those bacteria that can hydrolyze esculin and also grow in the presence of 4% bile salts or 40% bile. The bile esculin slant is inoculated on the surface and incubated for 24–48 hours in a non-CO_2 incubator. Group D streptococci (enterococci and nonenterococci) are positive, causing blackening of half or more of the slant within 48 hours. Viridans streptococci are negative (do not grow or hydrolyze esculin).

29. **B** The bile solubility test can be performed directly by dropping 2% sodium deoxycholate onto a few well-isolated colonies of *S. pneumoniae*. The bile salts speed up the autolysis observed in pneumococcal cultures. The colonies lyse and disappear when incubated at 35°C for 30 min, leaving a partially hemolyzed area on the plate. The same phenomenon can be seen using a broth culture; addition of 10% deoxycholate to broth containing *S. pneumoniae* results in visible clearing of the suspension after incubation at 35°C for 3 hours.

30. **A** Optochin at a concentration of 5 μg/mL or less inhibits the growth of *S. pneumoniae* but not viridans streptococci. However, optochin at a concentration in excess of 5 μg/mL inhibits viridans streptococci as well. A zone of inhibition of 14 mm or more around the 6-mm disk is considered a presumptive identification of *S. pneumoniae*. A questionable zone size should be confirmed by performing a bile solubility test.

31. **D** *Enterococcus faecalis* will grow in 6.5% salt and the nonenterococci (*S. bovis* and *S. equinus*) will not. This test distinguishes the enterococci group from *S. bovis* and *S. equinus* (nonenterococci group). Both groups grow on bile esculin agar.

32. **B** Approximately 80% of group B streptococci are capable of growing in 6.5% salt broth; however, they do not hydrolyze esculin or grow in media containing 4% bile salts.

33. The quellung test is used to identify which *Streptococcus* species?
   A. *S. pyogenes*
   B. *S. agalactiae*
   C. *S. sanguis*
   D. *S. pneumoniae*

Microbiology/Apply knowledge of fundamental biological characteristics/Streptococci/1

34. The L-pyrrolidonyl-β-napthylamide (PYR) hydrolysis test is a presumptive test for which streptococci?
   A. Group A and D (enterococcus) streptococci
   B. Group A and B β-hemolytic streptococci
   C. Nongroup A or B β-hemolytic streptococci
   D. *Streptococcus pneumoniae* and group D streptococci (nonenterococcus)

Microbiology/Apply knowledge of fundamental biological characteristics/Streptococci/1

35. A pure culture of β-hemolytic streptococci recovered from a leg wound ulcer gave the following reactions:

CAMP test = Neg	Hippurate hydrolysis = Neg
Bile esculin = Neg	6.5% salt = Neg
PYR = Neg	Bacitracin = Resistant
Optochin = Resistant	SXT = Sensitive

The most likely identification is:
   A. Group A streptococci
   B. Group B streptococci
   C. *Enterococcus faecalis*
   D. Nongroup A, nongroup B, nongroup D streptococci

Microbiology/Evaluate laboratory data to make identifications/Bacteria/3

36. β-Hemolytic streptococci, more than 50,000 col/mL, were isolated from a urinary tract catheter. Given the following reactions, what is the most likely identification?

CAMP test = Neg	Hippurate hydrolysis = ±
Bile solubility = Neg	6.5% salt = +
PYR = +	Bile esculin = +
SXT = Resistant	Bacitracin = Resistant
Optochin = Resistant	

   A. Group A streptococci
   B. Group B streptococci
   C. *Enterococcus faecalis*
   D. Nongroup A, nongroup B, nongroup D streptococci

Microbiology/Evaluate laboratory data to make identifications/Bacteria/3

37. Nutritionally variant streptococci (NVS) require specific thiol compounds, cysteine, or the active form of vitamin B_6. Which of the following tests supplies these requirements?
   A. CAMP test
   B. Bacitracin susceptibility test
   C. Bile solubility test
   D. Staphylococcal cross-streak test

Microbiology/Apply knowledge of fundamental biological characteristics/Streptococci/1

Answers to Questions 33–37

33.   D A precipitin reaction seen microscopically with methylene blue stain (microprecipitin reaction) occurs between the carbohydrate of the capsule of *S. pneumoniae* and anticapsular antibody. The antibody may be type-specific or polyvalent. Binding of antibodies to the bacteria causes the capsule to swell, identifying the organisms as *S. pneumoniae*.

34.   A The PYR hydrolysis test is highly specific for group A streptococci and group D enterococci. The test detects the pyrrolidonylarylamidase enzyme, which hydrolyzes PYR.

35.   D The β-hemolytic streptococci, not of groups A, B, or D, are sensitive to SXT and may be either sensitive or resistant to bacitracin. Groups A and B are both resistant to SXT. Group A and *Enterococcus faecalis* are PYR-positive. *Enterococcus faecalis* is also positive for bile esculin and 6.5 % salt broth.

36.   C Group A streptococci are sensitive to bacitracin and negative for bile esculin and 6.5% salt broth. Group B streptococci will grow in 6.5% salt broth but are negative for bile esculin and PYR. The nongroup A, B, or D streptococci will not grow in 6.5% salt broth and are sensitive to SXT. Some group D streptococci will hydrolyze hippurate. *Enterococcus faecalis* is positive for bile esculin, 6.5% salt broth, and PYR.

37.   D The staphylococcal streak, across the NVS inoculum, provides the nutrients needed. Very small colonies of NVS can be seen growing adjacent to the staphylococcal streak on the blood agar plate in a manner similar to the satellite phenomenon of *Haemophilus* spp around *S. aureus*.

38. Many α-hemolytic streptococci recovered from a wound were found to be penicillin-resistant. Given the following results, what is the most likely identification?

Bile esculin = +   PYR = +   6.5% salt = +

Hippurate hydrolysis = +   Bile solubility = Neg   SXT = Resistant

A. *Enterococcus faecalis*
B. *Streptococcus pneumoniae*
C. *Streptococcus bovis*
D. Group B streptococci

Microbiology/Evaluate laboratory data to make identifications/Bacteria/3

39. Which two tests best differentiate *S. bovis* (group D streptococcus, nonenterococcus) from *Streptococcus salivarius*?

A. Bile esculin and 6.5% salt broth
B. Starch hydrolysis and acid production from mannitol
C. Bacitracin and PYR
D. Trimethoprim-sulfamethoxazole susceptibility and PYR

Microbiology/Select methods/Reagents/Media/Bacteria/Identification/2

40. Two blood cultures on a newborn grew β-hemolytic streptococci with the following reactions:

CAMP test = +	Hippurate hydrolysis = +
Bile solubility = Neg	6.5% salt = +
Bacitracin = Resistant	Bile esculin = Neg
PYR = Neg	Trimethoprim-sulfamethoxazole = Resistant

Which is the most likely identification?

A. Group A streptococci
B. Group B streptococci
C. Group D streptococci
D. Nongroup A, nongroup B, nongroup D streptococci

Microbiology/Evaluate laboratory data to make identifications/Bacteria/3

41. MTM medium is used primarily for the selective recovery of which organism from genital specimens?

A. *Neisseria gonorrhoeae*
B. *Neisseria lactamica*
C. *Neisseria sicca*
D. *Neisseria flavescens*

Microbiology/Select methods/Reagents/Media/Bacteria/Identification/1

42. Variation in colony types seen with fresh isolates of *Neisseria gonorrhoeae* and sometimes with *Neisseria meningitidis* are the result of:

A. Multiple nutritional requirements
B. Pili on the cell surface
C. Use of a transparent medium
D. All of the above

Microbiology/Apply knowledge of fundamental biological characteristics/Neisseria/2

Answers to Questions 38–42

38. **A** *E. faecalis* is highly resistant to penicillin and ampicillin as well as some of the aminoglycoside antibiotics. Pneumococci, group B streptococci, and *S. bovis* are PYR-negative.

39. **B** *S. bovis* and *S. salivarius* are physiologically and biochemically similar. They are both PYR and 6.5% salt broth–negative and bile esculin–positive, but only *S. bovis* is positive for mannitol and starch reactions. See chart below.

	Bacitracin	PYR	Bile Esculin	6.5% Salt	Mannitol	Starch
S. bovis	R	Neg	+	Neg	+	+
S. salivarius	R	Neg	+	Neg	Neg	Neg

40. **B** Group B streptococci (*S. agalactiae*) are resistant to both bacitracin and SXT. Unlike group A and group D streptococci, the group B streptococci are negative for PYR. With some exceptions, group B streptococci will grow in 6.5% salt broth.

41. **A** Both *N. gonorrhoeae* and *N. meningitidis* grow selectively on MTM owing to the addition of vancomycin and colistin, which inhibit gram-positive and gram-negative bacteria, respectively. Trimethoprim is added to inhibit swarming of *Proteus* spp because a rectal swab may be used for culture. Nystatin and amphotericin B are used to prevent growth of yeasts and molds from vaginal specimens.

42. **D** Upon subculture from a primary plate, various sizes and appearances of gonococci are the result of multiple nutritional requirements, such as arginine-hypoxanthine-uracil (AHU)-requiring strains. Colony size and coloration (or light reflection) are the basis of Kellogg's scheme (types T1 through T5). Types T1 and T2 have pili on the surface and T3, T4, and T5 do not. Transparent media are not used routinely, but opaque and transparent colonial differences of the gonococci can be seen when using it.

43. Gram-negative diplococci recovered from an MTM plate and giving a positive oxidase test can be presumptively identified as:

A. *Neisseria gonorrhoeae*

B. *Neisseria meningitidis*

C. *Neisseria lactamica*

D. All of the above

Microbiology/Evaluate laboratory data to make identifications/Bacteria/2

44. The Superoxol test is used as a rapid presumptive test for:

A. *Neisseria gonorrhoeae*

B. *Neisseria meningitidis*

C. *Neisseria lactamica*

D. *Moraxella (Branhamella) catarrhalis*

Microbiology/Apply knowledge of fundamental biological characteristics/Neisseria/1

45. Nonpathogenic *Moraxella* spp capable of growing on selective media for *Neisseria* can be differentiated from *Neisseria* spp by which test?

A. Catalase test

B. 10-unit penicillin disk

C. Oxidase test

D. Superoxol test

Microbiology/Select methods/Reagents/Media/Bacteria/ Identification/2

46. A Gram stain of a urethral discharge from a man showing extracellular and intracellular gram-negative diplococci within segmented neutrophils is a presumptive identification for:

A. *Neisseria gonorrhoeae*

B. *Neisseria meningitidis*

C. *Moraxella (Branhamella) catarrhalis*

D. *Neisseria lactamica*

Microbiology/Evaluate laboratory data to make identifications/Bacteria/3

47. The β-galactosidase test aids in the identification of which *Neisseria* species?

A. *N. lactamica*

B. *N. meningitidis*

C. *N. gonorrhoeae*

D. *N. flavescens*

Microbiology/Apply knowledge of fundamental biological characteristics/Neisseria/1

48. Cystine tryptic digest (CTA) media used for identification of *Neisseria* spp should be inoculated and cultured in:

A. A CO_2 incubator at 35°C for 24 hours

B. A CO_2 incubator at 42°C for up to 72 hours

C. A non-CO_2 incubator at 35°C for up to 72 hours

D. An anaerobic incubator at 35°C for up to 72 hours

Microbiology/Apply knowledge of basic laboratory procedures/Gram-negative cocci/1

Answers to Questions 43–48

43. **D** All of the listed *Neisseria* spp grow on MTM and are oxidase-positive. *N. lactamica* is a nonpathogenic component of normal throat flora resembling *N. meningitidis* but it grows well on selective MTM agar. Presumptive identification of *N. meningitidis* or *N. gonorrhoeae* is stated only if the source of the specimen (i.e., urogenital or CSF) is given. The identification must be confirmed by further testing such as carbohydrate utilization tests, DNA tests, or rapid latex slide agglutination tests.

44. **A** *N. gonorrhoeae* colonies recovered from selective MTM media give an immediate positive reaction (bubbling) when 30% H_2O_2 is added. The catalase test uses 3% H_2O_2. This is a presumptive test for *N. gonorrhoeae*; *N. meningitidis* and *N. lactamica* give a weak or delayed bubbling reaction. *M. (B.) catarrhalis* is catalase-positive, superoxol-negative, and has a variable growth pattern on MTM.

45. **B** *Moraxella* spp are oxidase- and catalase-positive, as are the gonococci. *Neisseria* spp and *M. (B.) catarrhalis* will keep their typical coccal morphology after overnight incubation on blood agar with a 10-unit penicillin disk (CO_2 incubation). Other *Moraxella* species form long filaments or long spindle-shaped cells when grown near a 10-unit penicillin disk.

46. **A** A Gram stain of urethral discharge (in men only) showing typical gonococcal cells in PMNs should be reported "presumptive *N. gonorrhoeae*, confirmation to follow." With female patients, the normal vaginal flora contain gram-negative cocci and diplococci resembling gonococci and, therefore, no presumptive identification should be reported for *N. gonorrhoeae* from the vaginal Gram stain smear.

47. **A** *N. lactamica* utilizes lactose by producing the enzyme β-galactosidase. All other *Neisseria* spp that grow on MTM media are lactose-negative.

48. **C** CTA agar with 1% carbohydrate and phenol red pH indicator added is used for the identification of *Neisseria* species. CTA carbohydrates must be placed in an ambient air incubator because a high CO_2 concentration may reduce the pH, causing a false-positive (acid) result. The utilization of carbohydrates by some fastidious gonococcal strains may take up to 72 hours in order to produce a color change in the pH indicator.

49. Culture on MTM media of a vaginal swab produced several colonies of gram-negative diplococci that were catalase- and oxidase-positive and Superoxol-negative. Given the following carbohydrate reactions, select the most likely identification.

Glucose = +   Sucrose = Neg   Lactose = +

Maltose = +   Fructose = Neg

A. Neisseria gonorrhoeae
B. Neisseria sicca
C. Neisseria flavescens
D. Neisseria lactamica

Microbiology/Evaluate laboratory data to make identifications/Bacteria/3

50. Sputum from a patient with pneumonia produced many colonies of gram-negative diplococci on a chocolate plate that were also present in fewer numbers on MTM after 48 hours. Given the results below, what is the most likely identification?

Catalase = +   Oxidase = +
DNase = +   Tributyrin hydrolysis = +
Glucose = Neg   Sucrose = Neg
Lactose = Neg   Maltose = Neg
Fructose = Neg

A. Moraxella (Branhamella) catarrhalis
B. Neisseria flavescens
C. Neisseria sicca
D. Neisseria elongata

Microbiology/Apply knowledge of fundamental biological characteristics/Gram-negative cocci/1

Answers to Questions 49–50

49. **D** N. lactamica is part of the normal vaginal and throat flora and is the only Neisseria species that grows on MTM that utilizes lactose. Other saprophytic Neisseria spp may utilize lactose but do not grow on MTM media.

50. **A** M. (B.) catarrhalis is part of the normal upper respiratory flora but is implicated in lower respiratory infections, including pneumonia. It produces stunted growth on MTM and is DNase-positive, characteristics differentiating it from the other saprophytic Neisseria species.

1. A large gram-positive spore-forming rod growing on blood agar as large, raised, β-hemolytic colonies that spread and appear as frosted green-gray glass is most likely a:
   A. *Pseudomonas* spp
   B. *Bacillus* spp
   C. *Corynebacterium* spp
   D. *Listeria* spp

   Microbiology/Apply knowledge of fundamental biological characteristics/Bacteria/2

2. *Bacillus anthracis* and *Bacillus cereus* can best be differentiated by which tests?
   A. Motility and β-hemolysis on a blood agar plate
   B. Oxidase and β-hemolysis on a blood agar plate
   C. Lecithinase and glucose
   D. Lecithinase and catalase

   Microbiology/Select methods/Reagents/Media/Bacteria/ Identification/2

3. Which is the specimen of choice for proof of food poisoning by *Bacillus cereus*?
   A. Sputum
   B. Blood
   C. Stool
   D. Food

   Microbiology/Apply knowledge of fundamental biological characteristics/GPB/2

4. A suspected *Bacillus anthracis* culture obtained from a wound specimen produced colonies that had many outgrowths (Medusa-head appearance), but were not β-hemolytic on sheep blood agar. Which test should be performed next?
   A. Penicillin (10-unit) susceptibility test
   B. Lecithinase test
   C. Glucose test
   D. Motility test

   Microbiology/Select course of action/GPB/3

Answers to Questions 1–4

1. **B** The only spore former listed is the *Bacillus* spp, which grow as large, spreading colonies on blood agar plates. *Pseudomonas* spp are gram-negative rods; *Corynebacterium* spp appear as small, very dry colonies on BAP; *Listeria* spp appear as very small β-hemolytic colonies on BAP resembling *Streptococcus* species.

2. **A** Both species of *Bacillus* are catalase- and lecithinase-positive and produce acid from glucose. *B. cereus* is β-hemolytic and motile, but *B. anthracis* is neither. See chart below.

3. **D** The best specimen is the suspected food itself. Stool cultures are not useful because *B. cereus* is part of the normal fecal flora. The suspected food can be the source of food poisoning by *B. cereus* if 100,000 or greater organisms per gram of infected food are demonstrated.

4. **A** The best differentiating test to perform on a suspected *B. anthracis* culture is the 10-unit penicillin disk test. *B. anthracis* is susceptible but other *Bacillus* spp are not. Organisms suspected to be *B. anthracis* should be sent to a reference laboratory for final confirmation. All tests should be performed in a biological safety hood, and personnel should wear protective clothing to reduce risk from possible production of aerosols.

	β Hemolysis	Motility	Oxidase	Catalase	Lecithinase	Glucose
B. cereus	+	+	Neg	+	+	+
B. anthracis	Neg	Neg	Neg	+	+	+

5. Which of the following tests should be performed for initial differentiation of *Listeria monocytogenes* from group B streptococci?
   A. Gram stain, motility at room temperature, catalase
   B. Gram stain, CAMP test, H₂S/TSI
   C. Oxidase, CAMP test, glucose
   D. Oxidase, bacitracin

   Microbiology/Select methods/Reagents/Media/Bacteria/2

6. Culture of a finger wound specimen from a meat packer produced short gram-positive bacilli on a blood agar plate with no hemolysis. Given the following test results at 48 hours, what is the most likely identification?

   Catalase = Neg   H₂S/TSI = +
       Motility (wet prep) = Neg
       Motility (media) = Neg (bottle brush growth
       in stab culture)

   A. *Bacillus cereus*
   B. *Listeria monocytogenes*
   C. *Erysipelothrix rhusiopathiae*
   D. *Bacillus subtilis*

   Microbiology/Evaluate laboratory data to make identifications/Bacteria/3

7. A nonspore-forming, slender gram-positive rod forming palisades and chains was recovered from a vaginal culture and grew well on tomato juice agar. The most likely identification is:
   A. *Lactobacillus* spp
   B. *Bacillus* spp
   C. *Neisseria* spp
   D. *Streptococcus* spp

   Microbiology/Evaluate laboratory data to make identifications/Bacteria/2

8. A *Corynebacterium* species recovered from a throat culture is considered a pathogen when it produces:
   A. A pseudomembrane of the oropharynx
   B. An exotoxin
   C. Gray-black colonies with a brown halo on Tinsdale's agar
   D. All of the above

   Microbiology/Apply knowledge of fundamental biological characteristics/GPB/2

9. A presumptive diagnosis of *Gardnerella vaginalis* can be made using which of the following findings?
   A. Oxidase and catalase tests
   B. Pleomorphic bacilli heavily colonized on vaginal epithelium
   C. Hippurate hydrolysis test
   D. All of the above

   Microbiology/Select methods/Reagents/Media/Gardnerella/2

Answers to Questions 5–9

5. **A** *Streptococcus* spp are catalase-negative and *L. monocytogenes* is catalase-positive. *L. monocytogenes* appears on the Gram stain smear as gram-positive short, thin, diphtheroidal shapes, whereas streptococci usually appear as short, gram-positive chains. The reactions shown in the chart below differentiate *L. monocytogenes* from the group B streptococci.

	Catalase	Motility	CAMP	H₂S	Bile Esculin
L. monocytogenes	+	+	+	Neg	+
Group B streptococci	Neg	Neg	+	Neg	Neg

6. **C** *E. rhusiopathiae* is catalase-negative, whereas the other three organisms are catalase-positive. *E. rhusiopathiae* are seen primarily as skin infections on the fingers of meat and poultry workers. Colonies growing on blood agar are small and transparent, may be either smooth or rough, and are often surrounded by a green tinge. *E. rhusiopathiae* is characterized by H₂S production in the butt of a TSI slant, which differentiates it from other catalase-negative, gram-positive rods.

7. **A** *Lactobacillus* spp produce both long, slender rods or short coccobacilli that form chains. It is part of the normal flora of the vagina (is not considered a pathogen) and is sometimes confused with the streptococci.

8. **D** *Corynebacterium* species recovered from a throat culture are usually considered part of the normal throat flora. *C. diphtheriae* is an exception and should be suspected when one of the conditions described occurs. In this event, direct inoculation on Loeffler serum medium or tellurite medium and the following biochemical tests should be performed to confirm the identification of *C. diphtheriae*.

   Gelatin hydrolysis = Neg   Catalase = +
   Motility = +   Urease = +
   Acid from glucose = +   Carbohydrate fermentation = +

9. **D** A Gram stain smear from vaginal secretion showing many squamous epithelial cells loaded with pleomorphic gram-variable (positive and negative) bacilli is considered presumptive for *G. vaginalis*. Other important findings are:

   β-Hemolysis on BAP = +   Catalase = Neg

   Oxidase = Neg   Hippurate hydrolysis = +

10. A gram-positive branching filamentous organism recovered from a sputum specimen was found to be positive with a modified acid-fast stain method. What is the most likely presumptive identification?
  A. *Bacillus* spp
  B. *Nocardia* spp
  C. *Corynebacterium* spp
  D. *Listeria* spp

Microbiology/Evaluate laboratory data to make identifications/Bacteria/2

11. Routine laboratory testing for *Treponema pallidum* involves:
  A. Culturing
  B. Serological analysis
  C. Acid-fast staining
  D. Gram's staining

Microbiology/Select methods/Reagents/Media/Spirochetes/1

12. Spirochetes often detected in the hematology laboratory, even before the physician suspects the infection, are:
  A. *Borrelia* spp
  B. *Treponema* spp
  C. *Campylobacter* spp
  D. *Leptospira* spp

Microbiology/Apply knowledge of fundamental biological characteristics/Spirochetes/1

13. Which of the following organisms is the cause of Lyme disease?
  A. *Treponema pallidum*
  B. *Neisseria meningitidis*
  C. *Babesia microti*
  D. *Borrelia burgdorferi*

Microbiology/Apply knowledge of fundamental biological characteristics/Spirochetes/1

14. The diagnostic method most commonly used for the identification of Lyme disease is:
  A. Serology
  B. Culture
  C. Gram stain
  D. Acid-fast stain

Microbiology/Select methods/Reagents/Media/Spirochetes/1

15. Primary atypical pneumonia is caused by:
  A. *Streptococcus pneumoniae*
  B. *Mycoplasma pneumoniae*
  C. *Klebsiella pneumoniae*
  D. *Mycobacterium tuberculosis*

Microbiology/Apply knowledge of fundamental biological characteristics/1

Answers to Questions 10–15

10. B *Nocardia* spp should be suspected if colonies that are partially acid-fast by the traditional method are positive with the modified acid-fast method using Kinyoun stain and 1% sulfuric acid as the decolorizing agent. The other organisms above are acid-fast-stain–negative.

11. B Serological tests of the patient's serum for evidence of syphilis is routinely performed but culturing is not because research animals must be used for inoculation of the suspected spirochete. *T. pallidum* does not stain by either the Gram or acid-fast technique. Darkfield microscopy for direct visualization or indirect immunofluorescence using fluorescein-conjugated antihuman globulin (the fluorescent treponemal antibody-absorption test, FTA-ABS) may be used to identify syphilis.

12. A *Borrelia* spp are often seen on Wright's-stained smears of peripheral blood as helical bacteria with 3–10 loose coils. They are gram-negative but stain well with Giemsa's stain.

13. D Lyme disease may result in acute arthritis and meningitis and is caused by *B. burgdorferi*. This spirochete is carried by the deer tick belonging to the *Ixodes* genus (*I. dammini* in the Eastern and North-central United States and *I. pacificus* in the Northwest United States). The life cycle of the tick involves small rodents such as the white-footed mouse and the white-tailed deer.

14. A Serological analysis using immunofluorescence or an enzyme immunoassay is the method of choice for diagnosis of Lyme disease. Titers of IgM remain high throughout the infection. *B. burgdorferi* can be cultured directly from lesions, and darkfield microscopy can be used for detection of spirochetes in blood cultures after 2–3 weeks of incubation at 34°–37°C.

15. B A common cause of respiratory tract illness, *M. pneumoniae*, generally causes a self-limited infection (3–10 days) and usually does not require antibiotic therapy. *M. pneumoniae* can be cultured from the upper and lower respiratory tracts onto specially enriched (diphasic) media but is most frequently diagnosed by the change in antibody titer from acute to convalescent serum using enzyme immunoassay or other serological methods.

16. Which organism typically produces "fried-egg" colonies on agar within 1–5 days of culture from a genital specimen?
    A. *Mycoplasma hominis*
    B. *Borrelia burgdorferi*
    C. *Leptospira interrogans*
    D. *Treponema pallidum*

    Microbiology/Apply knowledge of fundamental biological characteristics/1

17. The manganous chloride–urea test is used for the identification of which organism?
    A. *Mycoplasma pneumoniae*
    B. *Ureaplasma urealyticum*
    C. *Bacillus cereus*
    D. *Borrelia burgdorferi*

    Microbiology/Select methods/Reagents/Media/ Mycoplasma/1

18. A gram-positive (gram-variable), beaded organism with delicate branching was recovered from the sputum of a 20-year-old patient with leukemia. The specimen produced orange, glabrous, waxy colonies on Middlebrook's agar that showed partial acid-fast staining with the modified Kinyoun stain. What is the most likely identification?
    A. *Rhodococcus* spp
    B. *Actinomadura* spp
    C. *Streptomyces* spp
    D. *Nocardia* spp

    Microbiology/Evaluate laboratory data to make identifications/Bacteria/3

19. A direct smear from a nasopharyngeal swab stained with Loeffler methylene blue stain showed various letter shapes and deep blue, metachromatic granules. The most likely identification is:
    A. *Corynebacterium* spp
    B. *Nocardia* spp
    C. *Listeria* spp
    D. *Gardnerella* spp

    Microbiology/Evaluate laboratory data to make identifications/Bacteria/3

20. Which of the following is the best, rapid, noncultural test to perform when *Gardnerella vaginalis* is suspected in a patient with vaginosis?
    A. 10% KOH test
    B. 3% H_2O_2 test
    C. 30% H_2O_2 test
    D. All of the above

    Microbiology/Select methods/Reagents/Media/ Gardnerella/2

Answers to Questions 16–20

16. **A** Genital mycoplasmas (*M. hominis* and *Ureaplasma urealyticum*) are grown on specific agars. *M. hominis* is grown on "M" agar containing arginine and phenol red. Colonies of mycoplasma are 50–300 μm in diameter and display a "fried-egg" appearance with red holes. *U. urealyticum* is isolated from genital specimens on "U" agar (containing urea and phenol red), then subcultured to A7/A8 agar. Colonies of *Ureaplasma* are small and golden brown on A7/A8 agar.

17. **B** *U. urealyticum* is the only human mycoplasma that hydrolyzes urea. The manganous chloride-urea test utilizes manganous chloride ($MnCl_2$) in the presence of urea. Urease produced by the organism hydrolyzes the urea to ammonia. This reacts with $MnCl_2$ forming manganese oxide, which is insoluble and forms a dark brown precipitate around the colonies. The reaction is observed under a dissecting microscope and is a rapid test for the identification of *U. urealyticum*.

18. **D** All of the listed organisms produce mycelium (aerial or substrate), causing them to appear branched when Gram-stained, but only the *Nocardia* spp are modified acid-fast stain-positive. *Nocardia* is an opportunistic pathogen, and cultures typically have a musty basement odor.

19. **A** *Corynebacterium* spp are part of the normal upper respiratory tract flora. Organisms display typical pleomorphic shapes often resembling letters such as Y or L, and metachromatic granules. Identification of *C. diphtheriae*, however, requires selective culture media and biochemical testing.

20. **A** The "whiff" test is used for a presumptive diagnosis of an infection with *G. vaginalis*. A fishlike odor is noted after the addition of 1 drop of 10% KOH to the vaginal washings. This odor results from the high concentration of amines found in women with vaginosis caused by *G. vaginalis*.

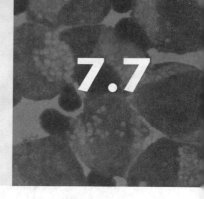

1. Obligate anaerobes, facultative anaerobes, and microaerophiles are terms referring to bacteria requiring:
   A. Increased nitrogen
   B. Decreased CO_2
   C. Increased O_2
   D. Decreased O_2

   Microbiology/Apply principles of fundamental biological characteristics/Anaerobes/1

2. Which of the following most affects the oxidation-reduction potential (Eh or redox potential) of media for anaerobic bacteria?
   A. O_2
   B. Nitrogen
   C. pH
   D. Glucose

   Microbiology/Apply principles of fundamental biological characteristics/Anaerobes/1

3. Which of the following is the medium of choice for the selective recovery of gram-negative anaerobes?
   A. Kanamycin-vancomycin (KV) agar
   B. Phenylethyl alcohol (PEA) agar
   C. Cycloserine-cefoxitin-fructose agar (CCFA)
   D. THIO broth

   Microbiology/Select methods/Reagents/Media/Anaerobes/2

4. Anaerobic bacteria are routinely isolated from all of the following types of infections *except*:
   A. Lung abscesses
   B. Brain abscesses
   C. Dental infections
   D. Urinary tract infections

   Microbiology/Apply principles of fundamental biological characteristics/Anaerobes/1

Answers to Questions 1–4

1. **D** The anaerobic bacteria are subdivided according to their requirement for O_2. Obligate anaerobes are killed by exposure to atmospheric O_2 for 10 min or longer. Facultative anaerobes grow under aerobic or anaerobic conditions. Microaerophilic organisms do not grow in an aerobic incubator on solid media and only minimally under anaerobic conditions. However, they will grow in minimal oxygen (5% O_2). Superoxide dismutase (SOD) is produced by many anaerobes, which catalyzes the conversion of superoxide radicals to less toxic H_2O_2 and molecular O_2.

2. **C** The Eh is most affected by pH and is expressed at pH 7.0. In cultivating anaerobic bacteria, reducing agents such as thioglycollate and L-cysteine are added to anaerobic transport and culture media in order to maintain a low Eh. Certain anaerobes do not grow in the media above a specific critical Eh level.

3. **A** KV allows the growth of *Bacteroides* spp, *Prevotella* spp, and *Fusobacterium* spp and inhibits most facultative anaerobic gram-negative rods and gram-positive bacteria (both aerobic and anaerobic). PEA inhibits facultative gram-negative bacteria but will support gram-positive aerobes and anaerobes and gram-negative obligate anaerobes. CCFA is selective for *C. difficile* from stool, while THIO broth supports gram-positive and gram-negative aerobes and anaerobes.

4. **D** The incidence of anaerobic bacteria recovered from the urine is approximately 1% of isolates. The other three types of infection are associated with a 60%–93% incidence of anaerobic recovery. Urine is not cultured routinely under anaerobic conditions unless obtained surgically (e.g., suprapubic aspiration).

5. Methods other than packaged microsystems used to identify anaerobes include:

A. Antimicrobial susceptibility testing

B. Gas-liquid chromatography (GLC)

C. Special staining

D. Enzyme immunoassay

Microbiology/Select methods/Reagents/Media/Anaerobes/1

6. Which broth is used for the cultivation of anaerobic bacteria in order to detect volatile fatty acids as an aid to identification?

A. Prereduced peptone-yeast extract-glucose (PYG)

B. THIO broth

C. Gram-negative (GN) broth

D. Selenite (SEL) broth

Microbiology/Select methods/Reagents/Media/Anaerobes/1

7. A gram-positive spore-forming bacillus growing on sheep-blood agar anaerobically produces a double zone of β-hemolysis and is positive for lecithinase. What is the presumptive identification?

A. *Bacteroides ureolyticus*

B. *Bacteroides fragilis*

C. *Clostridium perfringens*

D. *Clostridium difficile*

Microbiology/Evaluate laboratory data to make identifications/Bacteria/2

8. Egg yolk agar is used to detect which enzyme produced by *Clostridium* species?

A. Lecithinase

B. β-Lactamase

C. Catalase

D. Oxidase

Microbiology/Apply principles of fundamental biological characteristics/Anaerobes/1

9. Which of the following organisms will display lipase activity on egg yolk agar?

A. *Clostridium botulinum*

B. *Clostridium sporogenes*

C. *Clostridium novyi* (A)

D. All of the above

Microbiology/Evaluate laboratory data to make identifications/Bacteria/2

10. Which spore type and location is found on *Clostridium tetani*?

A. Round, terminal spores

B. Round, subterminal spores

C. Ovoid, subterminal spores

D. Ovoid, terminal spores

Microbiology/Apply principles of fundamental biological characteristics/Anaerobes/1

5. **B** Anaerobic bacteria can be identified by analysis of metabolic products using gas-liquid chromatography. Results are evaluated along with Gram staining characteristics, spore formation, and cellular morphology in order to make the identification.

6. **A** Peptone yeast and chopped meat with carbohydrates support the growth of anaerobic bacteria. The end products from the metabolism of the peptone and carbohydrates are volatile fatty acids that help to identify the bacteria. After incubation the broth is centrifuged. and the supernatant injected into a gas-liquid chromatograph. Peaks for acetic, butyric, or formic acid, for example, can be identified by comparison to the elution time of volatile organic acid standards.

7. **C** *C. perfringens* produces a double zone of β-hemolysis on blood agar, which makes identification relatively easy. The inner zone of complete hemolysis is caused by a θ-toxin and the outer zone of incomplete hemolysis is caused by an α-toxin (lecithinase activity). The *Bacteroides* spp are gram-negative bacilli, and *C. difficile* is lecithinase-negative and does not produce a double zone of β-hemolysis.

8. **A** Egg yolk agar (modified McClung's or neomycin egg yolk agar) is used to determine the presence of lecithinase activity, which causes an insoluble, opaque, whitish precipitate within the agar. Lipase activity is indicated by an iridescent sheen or pearly layer on the surface of the agar.

9. **D** Lipase is produced by some *Clostridium* spp and is seen as an iridescent pearly layer on the surface of the colonies that extends onto the surface of the egg yolk agar medium surrounding them. *C. perfringens*, the most frequently isolated *Clostridium* species, is negative for lipase production.

10. **A** Spore appearance and location, along with Gram stain morphology, aids in distinguishing the *Clostridium* spp. Round, terminal spores are demonstrated when *C. tetani* is grown in chopped meat with glucose broth. Recognition of spores is particularly important because *C. tetani* sometimes appears as gram-negative.

	Spores	Motility	Lecithinase	Double-Zone Hemolysis	GLC Products
C. tetani	Terminal*	+	Neg	Neg	A,B
C. perfringens	Subterminal	Neg	+	+	A,B
C. novyi (B)	Subterminal	+	+	Neg	A,B,P†
C. sporogenes	Subterminal	+	Neg	Neg	A,B

*Usually lacking
†Proprionic acid

11. Gram-positive bacilli recovered from two blood cultures from a 60-year-old diabetic patient gave the following results:

Spores seen = Neg   Hemolysis = + (double zone)

Motility = Neg   Lecithinase = +

Volatile acids by GLC (PYG) = acetic acid (A) and butyric acid (B)

What is the most likely identification?
A. *Clostridium tetani*
B. *Clostridium perfringens*
C. *Clostridium novyi* (B)
D. *Clostridium sporogenes*

Microbiology/Evaluate laboratory data to make identifications/Bacteria/3

12. Which mechanism is responsible for botulism in infants caused by *Clostridium botulinum*?
A. Ingestion of spores in food or liquid
B. Ingestion of preformed toxin in food
C. Virulence of the organism
D. Lipase activity of the organism

Microbiology/Apply principles of fundamental biological characteristics/Anaerobes/2

13. The classic form of foodborne botulism is characterized by the ingestion of:
A. Spores in food
B. Preformed toxin in food
C. Toxin H
D. All of the above

Microbiology/Apply principles of fundamental biological characteristics/Anaerobes/2

14. Which test is performed in order to confirm an infection with *Clostridium botulinum*?
A. Toxin neutralization
B. Spore-forming test

C. Lipase test
D. Gelatin hydrolysis test

Microbiology/Select methods/Reagents/Media/Anaerobes/2

Answers to Questions 11–14

11. **B** Spores are generally not demonstrated from clinical specimens containing *C. perfringens*, which is the only species above producing a double zone of hemolysis. The reactions in the chart above distinguish the four species listed.

12. **A** Infant botulism is the most frequent form occurring in the United States. Epidemiological studies have demonstrated that infant botulism results from the ingestion of spores via breast-feeding or exposure to honey. Preformed toxin has not been detected in food or liquids taken by the infants. *C. botulinum* multiplies in the gut of the infant and produces the neurotoxin in situ.

13. **B** Foodborne botulism in adults and children is caused by ingestion of the preformed toxin (botulinum toxins A, B, E, and F) in food. The neurotoxins of *C. botulinum* are protoplastic proteins made during the growing phase and released during lysis of the organisms. Confirmation of botulism is made by demonstration of the toxin in serum, gastric, or stool specimens.

14. **A** *C. botulinum* and *C. sporogenes* have similar characteristics biochemically (see chart below), and definitive identification of *C. botulinum* is made by the mouse neutralization test for its neurotoxins in serum or feces.

	Spore Type	Motility	Lipase	GLC Products
C. botulinum	Subterminal	+	+	A, (P)*, B, (IB)†, IV‡
C. sporogenes	Subterminal	+	+	A, (P), B, (IB), IV

*Variable
†Isobutyric acid
‡Isovaleric acid

15. Which *Clostridium* spp causes pseudomembranous colitis or antibiotic-associated colitis?
   A. *C. ramosum*
   B. *C. difficile*
   C. *C. perfringens*
   D. *C. sporogenes*

Microbiology/Apply principles of fundamental biological characteristics/Anaerobes/2

16. Identification of *Clostridium tetani* is based upon:
   A. Gram stain of the wound site
   B. Anaerobic culture of the wound site
   C. Blood culture results
   D. Clinical findings

Microbiology/Apply principles of fundamental biological characteristics/Anaerobes/2

17. Obligate anaerobic gram-negative bacilli that do not form spores grow well in 20% bile and are resistant to penicillin 2-unit disks are most likely:
   A. *Porphyromonas* spp
   B. *Bacteroides* spp
   C. *Fusobacterium* spp
   D. *Prevotella* spp

Microbiology/Evaluate laboratory data to make identifications/Bacteria/2

18. Which *Bacteroides* spp is noted for "pitting" of the agar and is sensitive to penicillin 2-unit disks?
   A. *B. vulgatus*
   B. *B. ovatus*
   C. *B. thetaiotaomicron*
   D. *B. ureolyticus*

Microbiology/Evaluate laboratory data to make identifications/Bacteria/2

19. Which gram-negative bacilli produce black pigment and brick red fluorescence when exposed to an ultraviolet light source?
   A. *Porphyromonas* spp and *Prevotella* spp
   B. *Fusobacterium* spp and *Actinomyces* spp
   C. *Bacteroides* spp and *Fusobacterium* spp
   D. All of the above

Microbiology/Evaluate laboratory data to make identifications/Bacteria/2

20. The following characteristics of an obligate anaerobic gram-negative bacilli best describe which of the genera below?

   Gram stain: long slender rods with pointed ends

   Colonial appearance: dry bread crumbs or "fried-egg" appearance

   Penicillin 2-unit disk test: Susceptible

   A. *Bacteriodes* spp
   B. *Fusobacterium* spp
   C. *Prevotella* spp
   D. *Porphyromonas* spp

Microbiology/Evaluate laboratory data to make identifications/Bacteria/3

Answers to Questions 15–20

15. **B** *C. difficile* is also implicated in hospital-acquired diarrhea and colitis. Clinical testing for *C. difficile* includes culture and cytotoxin testing. Because culture takes 3 days and will detect nontoxigenic strains that do not cause diarrheal disease, immunoassays using antibodies against either the A toxin or both the A and B toxins are most frequently employed. Assays detecting both toxins are only slightly more sensitive, since infections producing only B toxin are infrequent. The cytotoxin assay requires that specimens be shipped to a reference laboratory on dry ice or kept at 4°–6°C if done in-house.

16. **D** The culture and Gram stain of the puncture wound site usually does not produce any evidence of *C. tetani*. The diagnosis is usually based upon clinical findings, which are characterized by spastic muscle contractions, lockjaw, and backward arching of the back caused by muscle contraction.

17. **B** The *Bacteroides* group grows well in 20% bile and is resistant to penicillin 2-unit disks with the exception of *B. ureolyticus*. Most *Prevotella* are also resistant to penicillin 2-unit disks, but most *Fusobacterium* and *Porphyromonas* are sensitive.

18. **D** *B. ureolyticus* is the only species listed that is susceptible to penicillin and produces urease. The other organisms listed are resistant to penicillin.

19. **A** Pigmenting *Porphyromonas* spp and *Prevotella* spp also show hemolysis on sheep blood agar.

20. **B** *Fusobacterium* spp are usually spindle-shaped, slim rods, whereas the other genera are small rods (variable length for *Bacteroides* spp and tiny coccoid rods for *Prevotella* and *Porphyromonas* spp). *Fusobacterium* spp and *Porphyromonas* spp are susceptible to penicillin 2-unit disks, while most *Bacteroides* spp and *Prevotella* spp are resistant.

21. All of the following genera are anaerobic cocci that stain gram-positive *except*:
  A. *Peptococcus* spp
  B. *Peptostreptococcus* spp
  C. *Streptococcus* spp
  D. *Veillonella* spp

Microbiology/Apply principles of fundamental biological characteristics/Anaerobes/2

22. The gram-positive nonspore–forming anaerobic rods most frequently recovered from blood cultures as a contaminant are:
  A. *Proprionibacterium acnes*
  B. *Clostridium perfringens*
  C. *Staphylococcus intermedius*
  D. *Veillonella parvula*

Microbiology/Apply knowledge of fundamental biological characteristics/Anaerobes/2

23. Which *Clostridium* sp is most often recovered from a wound infection with gas gangrene?
  A. *C. sporogenes*
  B. *Clostridium sordellii*
  C. *C. novyi*
  D. *C. perfringens*

Microbiology/Apply knowledge of fundamental biological characteristics/Anaerobes/1

24. Gram stain of a smear taken from the periodontal pockets of a 30-year-old man with poor dental hygiene showed sulfur granules containing gram-positive rods (short diphtheroids and some unbranched filaments). Colonies on blood agar resembled "molar teeth" in formation. The most likely organism is:
  A. *Actinomyces israelii*
  B. *Propionibacterium acnes*
  C. *Staphylococcus intermedius*
  D. *Peptostreptococcus anaerobius*

Microbiology/Evaluate laboratory data to make identifications/Bacteria/3

25. Antimicrobial susceptibility testing of anaerobes is done by which of the following methods?
  A. Broth disk elution
  B. Disk agar diffusion
  C. Microtube broth dilution
  D. β-Lactamase testing

Microbiology/Apply knowledge of standard operating procedures/Anaerobes/1

Answers to Questions 21–25

21. **D** *Veillonella* spp are gram-negative cocci. All four genera are part of the normal human flora and are the anaerobic cocci most frequently isolated from blood cultures, abscesses, wounds, and body fluids. The *Streptococcus* spp are facultative anaerobes, but only *Streptococcus intermedius* is classified as an obligate anaerobe.

22. **A** *P. acnes* is a nonspore former and is described as a diphtheroid-shaped rod. It is part of the normal skin, nasopharynx, genitourinary, and gastrointestinal tract flora but is implicated as an occasional cause of endocarditis.

23. **D** Wounds infected with clostridia are characterized by invasion and liquefactive necrosis of muscle tissue with gas formation. The most frequent isolate is *C. perfringens* followed by *C. novyi* and *C. septicum*.

24. **A** *A. israelii* is part of the normal flora of the mouth and tonsils but may cause upper or lower respiratory tract infections. The sulfur granules are granular microcolonies with a purulent exudate. Like *Nocardia*, *Actinomyces* produces unbranched mycelia and is sometimes (erroneously) considered a fungus. It has also been implicated in pelvic infection associated with intrauterine contraceptive devices (IUDs).

25. **C** The anaerobes are not suited for the broth disk elution or disk agar diffusion tests because of their slow rate of growth. Kirby-Bauer method reference charts are not designed to be used as a reference of susceptibility for anaerobes.

7.8

MYCOBACTERIA

1. The best specimen for recovery of the mycobacteria from a sputum sample is:
   A. First morning specimen
   B. 10-hour evening specimen
   C. 12-hour pooled specimen
   D. 24-hour pooled specimen

   Microbiology/Apply knowledge of standard operating procedures/Mycobacteria/1

2. What concentration of sodium hydroxide (NaOH) is used to prepare a working decontamination solution for the processing of not normally sterile specimens for mycobacteria?
   A. 1% NaOH
   B. 4% NaOH
   C. 8% NaOH
   D. 12% NaOH

   Microbiology/Apply knowledge of standard operating procedures/Mycobacteria/1

3. Which is the most appropriate nonselective medium for recovery of mycobacteria from a heavily contaminated specimen?
   A. Löwenstein-Jensen agar
   B. Middlebrook 7H10 agar
   C. Petragnani's agar
   D. American Thoracic Society medium

   Microbiology/Select method/Reagents/Media/ Mycobacteria/2

4. Mycobacteria stained by the Ziehl-Neelsen or Kinyoun methods with methylene blue counterstain are seen microscopically as:
   A. Bright red rods against a blue background
   B. Bright yellow rods against a yellow background
   C. Orange-red rods against a black background
   D. Bright blue rods against a pink background

   Microbiology/Apply knowledge of fundamental biological characteristics/Mycobacteria/1

Answers to Questions 1–4

1. **A** Contamination by fungi and other bacteria contributes to lower yields of mycobacteria in a 24-hour sample. The first morning specimen collected by expectoration or nebulization produces the highest concentration of mycobacteria in sputum.

2. **B** A strong decontamination solution (6% NaOH or greater) may kill or severely damage the mycobacteria. A 4% NaOH solution is mixed with an equal volume of N-acetyl-L-cysteine (NALC), a digestant or mucolytic agent, to yield a final working concentration of 2% NaOH. The time of exposure of the specimen to the digestion/decontamination solution must be monitored because overtreatment may result in fewer positive cultures.

3. **C** All four media contain malachite green as an inhibitory agent of nonmycobacteria, but Petragnani's medium contains a higher concentration (0.052 g/dL) than Löwenstein-Jensen (0.025 g/dL), Middlebrook 7H10 (0.0025 g/dL), or American Thoracic Society medium (0.02 g/dL). The last is used for normally sterile specimens, such as from CSF and bone marrow.

4. **A** The carbolfuchsin (fuchsin with phenol) stains the mycobacteria red and does not decolorize after the acid-alcohol is added. The background and any other bacterial elements will decolorize and are counterstained blue by the methylene blue. A fluorescent staining procedure may be used as an alternative to acid-fast staining. Auramine fluorochrome produces bright yellow fluorescent mycobacteria and auramine-rhodamine causes an orange-red (gold) fluorescence against a dark background. A fluorescent microscope must be used, but with this method the smear can be scanned with a 25× objective instead of the 100× objective, permitting more rapid identification of mycobacteria.

5. Acid-fast staining of a smear prepared from a digested sputum showed slender, slightly curved, beaded, red mycobacterial rods. Growth on Middlebrook 7H10 slants produced buff-colored microcolonies with a serpentine pattern after 14 days at 37°C. Niacin and nitrate reduction tests were positive. What is the most probable presumptive identification?
- **A.** Mycobacterium tuberculosis
- **B.** Mycobacterium ulcerans
- **C.** Mycobacterium kansasii
- **D.** Mycobacterium avium-intracellulare complex

Microbiology/Evaluate laboratory data to make identifications/Mycobacteria/3

6. Which organism, associated with tuberculosis in cattle, causes tuberculosis in humans, especially in regions where dairy farming is prevalent?
- **A.** Mycobacterium avium-intracellulare complex
- **B.** Mycobacterium kansasii
- **C.** Mycobacterium marinum
- **D.** Mycobacterium bovis

Microbiology/Apply knowledge of fundamental biological characteristics/Mycobacteria/1

7. Which of the following organisms are used as controls for rapid-growers and slow-growers?
- **A.** Mycobacterium fortuitum and Mycobacterium tuberculosis
- **B.** Mycobacterium avium-intracellulare complex and Mycobacterium tuberculosis
- **C.** Mycobacterium chelonei and Mycobacterium fortuitum
- **D.** Mycobacterium kansasii and Mycobacterium tuberculosis

Microbiology/Apply knowledge of fundamental biological characteristics/Mycobacteria/2

8. Which of the following Mycobacterium spp produce pigmented colonies in the dark (is a scotochromogen)?
- **A.** M. szulgai
- **B.** M. kansasii
- **C.** M. tuberculosis
- **D.** All of the above

Microbiology/Apply knowledge of fundamental biological characteristics/Mycobacteria/2

9. All of the following mycobacteria are associated with skin infections *except*:
- **A.** Mycobacterium marinum
- **B.** Mycobacterium haemophilum
- **C.** Mycobacterium ulcerans
- **D.** Mycobacterium kansasii

Microbiology/Apply knowledge of fundamental biological characteristics/Mycobacteria/

Answers to Questions 5–9

5. A M. tuberculosis is niacin accumulation–positive, while the other three species are niacin–negative. M. ulcerans is associated with skin infections (in the tropics), does not grow at 37°C (optimal temperature is 33°C), and is not recovered from sputum. A serpentine pattern of growth indicates production of cording factor, a virulence factor for M. tuberculosis.

6. D M. bovis is also called the bovine tubercle bacillus. A nonvirulent strain, bacillus Calmette-Guérin (BCG), is used as a tuberculosis vaccine throughout the world. Infections with M. bovis resemble infections caused by M. tuberculosis and are seen in circumstances where there is close contact between humans and cattle.

7. A Growth rates of mycobacteria are used along with biochemical tests as an aid to identification. M. fortuitum grows within 3–5 days at 37°C and is used as the control for rapid growers. M. tuberculosis grows in 12–25 days at 37°C and is a control organism for slow growers. In addition to M. fortuitum, M. chelonei is a rapid grower (3–5 days at 28°–35°C). In addition to M. tuberculosis, M. avium and M. kansasii are slow growers (10–21 days at 37°C).

8. A M. tuberculosis does not produce pigmentation in the dark or after exposure to light (photochromogen). A common tapwater scotochromogen is Mycobacterium gordonae. The pathogenic scotochromogens are Mycobacterium szulgai, Mycobacterium scrofulaceum, and Mycobacterium xenopi. M. kansasii is a photochromogen producing a yellow pigment following exposure to light and red β-carotene crystals after long incubation periods.

9. D M. kansasii is a photochromogen that causes chronic pulmonary disease (classic tuberculosis). The other three species cause cutaneous or subcutaneous disease. It is important to culture skin lesions at the correct temperature to facilitate growth.

	Optimum temperature	Growth at 37°C
M. marinum	30°C–32°C	Poor
M. haemophilum	28°C–32°C	Poor or no
M. ulcerans	33°C	No

10. All of the following *Mycobacterium* spp produce the enzyme required to convert niacin to niacin ribonucleotide *except:*

A. *M. kansasii*

B. *M. tuberculosis*

C. *M. avium-intracellulare* complex

D. *M. szulgai*

Microbiology/Apply knowledge of fundamental biological characteristics/Mycobacteria/2

11. The catalase test for mycobacteria differs from that used for other types of bacteria by using:

A. 1% H_2O_2 and 10% Tween 80

B. 3% H_2O_2 and phosphate buffer, pH 6.8

C. 10% H_2O_2 and 0.85% saline

D. 30% H_2O_2 and 10% Tween 80

Microbiology/Select method/Reagents/Media/ Mycobacteria/2

12. Growth inhibition by thiophene-2-carboxylic hydrazide (T_2H) is used to differentiate *M. tuberculosis* from which other *Mycobacterium* sp?

A. *M. bovis*

B. *M. avium-intracellulare* complex

C. *M. kansasii*

D. *M. marinum*

Microbiology/Apply knowledge of fundamental biological characteristics/Mycobacteria/2

13. Which of the following *Mycobacterium* spp is best differentiated by the rapid hydrolysis of Tween 80?

A. *M. fortuitum*

B. *M. chelonae*

C. *M. kansasii*

D. *M. gordonae*

Microbiology/Apply knowledge of fundamental biological characteristics/Mycobacteria/2

14. Mycobacteria isolated from the hot water system of a hospital grew at 42°C. Colonies on Löwenstein-Jensen medium were not pigmented after exposure to light and were negative for niacin accumulation and nitrate reduction. The most likely identification is:

A. *Mycobacterium xenopi*

B. *Mycobacterium marinum*

C. *Mycobacterium ulcerans*

D. *Mycobacterium haemophilum*

Microbiology/Evaluate laboratory data to make identifications/Mycobacteria/3

Answers to Questions 10–14

10. **B** Niacin production is common to all mycobacteria. However, the niacin accumulates as a water-soluble metabolite in the culture medium when the organism cannot form niacin ribonucleotide. *M. tuberculosis*, *M. simiae*, and some strains of *M. marinum*, *M. chelonae*, and *M. bovis* lack the enzyme and therefore are termed niacin-positive because of the accumulation of niacin detected in the test medium.

11. **D** One milliliter of an equal mixture of 30% H_2O_2 (Superoxal) and Tween 80 (a strong detergent) is added to a 2-week-old subculture on Löwenstein-Jensen medium and placed upright for 5 minutes. Catalase activity is determined semiquantitatively by measuring the height of the column of bubbles produced above the culture surface.

12. **A** *M. bovis* and *M. tuberculosis* are very similar biochemically, and some strains of *M. bovis* also accumulate niacin. The T_2H test differentiates *M. tuberculosis* from *M. bovis*. *M. tuberculosis* is not inhibited by T_2H.

13. **C** The hydrolysis of Tween 80 is usually positive when testing the clinically insignificant mycobacteria. *M. fortuitum*, *M. chelonae*, and *M. gordonae* are saprophytic (and opportunistic) species, but *M. kansasii* is a pathogen. *M. kansasii* hydrolyses Tween 80 more rapidly than the other species (within 3–6 hours). A positive reaction is indicated by a change in the color of neutral red from yellow to pink.

14. **A** *M. xenopi* causes a pulmonary infection resembling *M. tuberculosis* and is frequently isolated from patients with an underlying disease such as alcoholism, AIDS, diabetes, or malignancy. It is often recovered from hot water taps and contaminated water systems and is a possible source of nosocomial infection. The other three species cause skin infections and grow on artificial media at a much lower temperature than *M. xenopi* (below 32°C).

15. A *Mycobacterium* species recovered from a patient with AIDS gave the following results:

Niacin = Neg	T$_2$H = +
Tween 80 hydrolysis = Neg	Nitrate reduction = Neg
Heat-stable catalase (68°C) = ±	Nonphotochromogen

What is the most likely identification?
A. *M. gordonae*
B. *M. bovis*
C. *M. avium-intracellulare* complex
D. *M. kansasii*

Microbiology/Evaluate laboratory data to make identifications/Mycobacteria/3

16. The urease test is needed to differentiate *Mycobacterium scrofulaceum* from which of the following mycobacteria?
A. *M. gordonae*
B. *M. kansasii*
C. *M. avium-intracellulare* complex
D. *M. bovis*

Microbiology/Apply knowledge of fundamental biological characteristics/Mycobacteria/2

17. A laboratory provides the following services for identification of mycobacteria:

> Acid-fast staining of clinical specimens
>
> Inoculation of cultures
>
> Shipment of positive cultures to a reference laboratory for identification

According to the American Thoracic Society's definition for levels of service this laboratory is:
A. Level I
B. Level II
C. Level III
D. Level IV

Microbiology/Apply knowledge of laboratory operations/Mycobacteria/2

18. According to the College of American Pathologists (CAP) guidelines, which services for mycobacteria would be performed by a level II laboratory?
A. No procedures performed
B. Acid-fast staining, inoculation, and referral to a reference laboratory
C. Isolation and identification of *Mycobacterium tuberculosis;* preliminary identification of other species

D. Definitive identification of all mycobacteria

Microbiology/Apply knowledge of laboratory operations/Mycobacteria/2

Answers to Questions 15–18

15. **C** With the exception of *M. tuberculosis, M. avium-intracellulare* (MAI) complex is the *Mycobacterium* species most often isolated from AIDS patients. It is biochemically inert, which is a distinguishing factor for identification. MAI complex is highly resistant to the antibiotics used to treat tuberculosis, including multidrug therapy. Treatment with streptomycin, rifampin, ethionamide, ethambutol with cycloserine, or kanamycin has shown little success.

16. **A** Both pathogenic and saprophytic mycobacteria may produce urease, and urease production is used to differentiate several mycobacteria species. Biochemically, *M. scrofulaceum* is identical to *M. gordonae*, except for the urease reaction for which *M. scroflaceum* is positive and *M. gordonae* is negative. Urease reactions for the other pathogenic mycobacteria are:

M. tuberculosis = +	M. kansasii = +
M. bovis = +	M. avium-intracellulare complex = Neg

17. **A** The American Thoracic Society recognizes three levels of laboratory services for mycobacteria testing. Level I laboratories are those that grow mycobacteria and perform acid-fast stains but do not identify *M. tuberculosis* (they may or may not perform drug susceptibility tests on *M. tuberculosis*). Level II laboratories perform all of the functions of level I laboratories and also identify *M. tuberculosis*. Level III laboratories identify all mycobacteria species from clinical specimens and perform drug susceptibility tests on all species.

18. **B** The CAP lists four options for laboratories to follow in order to correlate the services provided with guidelines for inspection and accreditation. A laboratory's performance on CAP proficiency tests is evaluated by interlaboratory comparison with laboratories within these levels of performance.

19. Culture of a skin (hand) wound from a manager of a tropical fish store grew on Löwenstein-Jensen agar slants at 30°C in 10 days but did not grow on the same media at 37°C in 20 days. Given the results below, what is the most likely identification?

Photochromogen = +	Niacin = Neg
Urease = +	Heat-stable catalase (68°C) = Neg
Nitrate reduction = Neg	Tween 80 hydrolysis = +

A. *Mycobacterium marinum*
B. *Mycobacterium kansasii*
C. *Mycobacterium avium-intracellulare* complex
D. *Mycobacterium tuberculosis*

Microbiology/Evaluate laboratory data to make identifications/Mycobacteria/3

20. Which nonpathogenic *Mycobacterium* sp is isolated most often from clinical specimens and is called the "tapwater bacillus"?
A. *M. kansasii*
B. *M. avium-intracellulare* complex
C. *M. leprae*
D. *M. gordonae*

Microbiology/Apply knowledge of laboratory operations/Mycobacteria/2

21. Which of the following drugs are first-line antibiotics used to treat classic tuberculosis for which susceptibility testing is performed by the disk diffusion method on 7H11 agar plates?
A. Ampicillin, penicillin, and carbenicillin
B. Ampicillin, penicillin, and methicillin
C. Vancomycin, methicillin, and carbenicillin
D. Isonicotinic acid hydrazide (INH), rifampin, ethambutol

Microbiology/Apply principles of special procedures/Mycobacteria/2

22. How long should *Mycobacterium tuberculosis*-positive cultures be kept by the laboratory after identification and antibiotic susceptibility testing have been performed?
A. 1–2 months
B. 2–4 months
C. 5–6 months
D. 6–12 months

Microbiology/Apply knowledge of standard operating procedures/Mycobacteria/2

23. According to the reporting standards of the American Lung Association (ALA), one or more acid-fast bacilli (AFB) per oil immersion field are reported as:
A. Numerous or 3+.
B. Few or 1+.
C. Rare or 2+.
D. Indeterminate; a new specimen should be requested.

Microbiology/Apply knowledge of standard operating procedures/Mycobacteria/1

Answers to Questions 19–23

19. **A** *M. marinum* is typically recovered from cutaneous wounds resulting from infection when the skin is traumatized and comes into contact with inadequately chlorinated fresh water or salt water, such as in swimming pools or fish aquariums. The other three species are slow-growers at 37°C. *M. tuberculosis* and *M. avium-intracellulare* complex are nonphotochromogens. *M. avium-intracellulare* complex is urease-negative, *M. tuberculosis* is positive for niacin and nitrate, and *M. kansasii* is positive for nitrate and catalase.

20. **D** *M. gordonae* is a nonpathogen, scotochromogen, and rapid-grower (7 days at 37°C). Rarely, it is implicated in opportunistic infections in patients with shunts, prosthetic heart values, or hepatoperitoneal disease. The other three species are pathogenic mycobacteria.

21. **D** Streptomycin and pyrazinamide are also included as first-line drugs. The first-line antibiotics, except for ethambutol, are bactericidal. Second-line antibiotics used to treat first-line drug-resistant tuberculosis include *p*-aminosalicylic acid, cycloserine, ethionamide, kanamycin, amikacin, viomycin, and capreomycin.

22. **D** Standard therapy using INH and rifampin for classic, uncomplicated pulmonary tuberculosis is 9 months. The patient may not respond to therapy, even when the organism is susceptible to the antibiotics in vitro; therefore, cultures must be kept for up to 1 year in order to facilitate testing of additional antibiotics should the infection become refractory to therapy.

23. **A** Acid-fast smears are standardized by the ALA for reporting the number of AFB seen. The following criteria should be used to uniformly report results:

1–2 AFB per smear: report negative and request another sample

3–9 AFB per smear: report as rare (1+)

10 or more per smear: report as few (2+)

1 or more per oil immersion field: report as numerous (3+)

24. Which of the following *Mycobacterium* spp would be most likely to grow on a MacConkey agar plate?
A. *M. chelonae-fortuitum* complex
B. *M. ulcerans*
C. *M. marinum*
D. *M. avium-intracellulare* complex

Microbiology/Apply knowledge of fundamental biological characteristics/Mycobacteria/1

25. Rapid methods for identifying classic infection with *M. tuberculosis* include:
A. Gas-liquid chromatography
B. Nucleic acid probes
C. Acid-fast smears
D. All of the above

Microbiology/Apply principles of special procedures/ Mycobacteria/2

24. A Mycobacteria growing on MacConkey agar are usually nonpathogens. *M. chelonae* and *M. fortuitum* are both nonpathogenic rapid-growers that will grow on MacConkey agar (with no crystal violet) within 5 days. MAI complex is variable on MacConkey agar but takes much longer to grow. *M. marinum* and *M. ulcerans* do not grow on MacConkey agar.

25. D *M. tuberculosis* is a slow-grower with a prolonged culture time of 12–25 days and requires 3–6 weeks for definitive identification and antibiotic susceptibility testing. The acid-fast smear remains the number one rapid test for the detection of mycobacterial infection. A positive smear has a predictive value of 96% when all laboratory and clinical findings are considered. GLC is used to evaluate cell wall lipid patterns for identification. DNA probes are available for rapid identification of *M. tuberculosis*, *M. bovis*, *M. avium-intracellulare* complex, and *M. gordonae*. PCR for mycobacterial detection involves amplification of a species-specific region of DNA with a labeled (biotinylated) oligonucleotide primer. The PCR product is detected by denaturation and hybridization to a capture probe. After washing to remove unbound DNA, strepavidin conjugated to an enzyme is added. After washing to remove unbound conjugate, substrate is added. The presence of product indicates a positive result.

1. All of the following are examples of appropriate specimens for the recovery of fungi *except:*
   A. Tissue biopsy
   B. CSF
   C. Aspirate of exudate
   D. Swab

   Microbiology/Apply knowledge to identify sources of error/Mycology/1

2. For which clinical specimens is the KOH direct mount technique for examination of fungal elements used?
   A. Skin
   B. CSF
   C. Blood
   D. Bone marrow

   Microbiology/Apply principles of basic laboratory procedures/Mycology/1

3. The India ink stain is used as a presumptive test for the presence of which organism?
   A. *Aspergillus niger* in blood
   B. *Cryptococcus neoformans* in CSF
   C. *Histoplasma capsulatum* in CSF
   D. *Candida albicans* in blood or body fluids

   Microbiology/Correlate clinical and laboratory data/Mycology/2

4. Cutaneous disease involving skin, hair, and nails usually indicates an infection with a:
   A. Dimorphic fungus
   B. Dermatophyte
   C. Zygomycetes
   D. *Candida* species

   Microbiology/Correlate clinical and laboratory data/Mycology/2

5. What is the first step to be performed in the identification of an unknown yeast isolate?
   A. Gram stain smear
   B. India ink stain
   C. Catalase test
   D. Germ tube test

   Microbiology/Select methods/Reagents/Media/ Mycology/2

1. **D** Specimens for fungal culture must be kept in a moist, sterile environment. Swabs that are dried out or submitted with insufficient material on them should be rejected. Generally, swabs are inadequate for the recovery of fungi because they are easily contaminated by surrounding skin flora.

2. **A** A solution of 10% KOH is used for contaminated specimens such as skin, nail scrapings, hair, and sputum to clear away background debris that may resemble fungal elements. Normally sterile specimens (CSF, blood, and bone marrow) do not require KOH for clearing.

3. **B** Meningitis caused by *C. neoformans* is diagnosed through culture, biochemical reactions, and rapid agglutination tests for cryptococcal antigen. The India ink test is not diagnostic for cryptococcal meningitis because positive staining results are demonstrated in less than 50% of confirmed cases. A positive India ink test shows yeast cells in CSF with a surrounding clear area (the capsule) because the capsule of *C. neoformans* is not penetrated by ink particles.

4. **B** Superficial dermatophytes rarely invade the deeper tissues and are the cause of most cutaneous fungal infections. Fungal infections of the skin are most often caused by *Microsporum* spp, *Trichophyton* spp, and *Epidermophyton* spp, although *Candida* spp are sometimes implicated as the cause of nail infections.

5. **D** The true germ tube (filamentous extension from a yeast cell) is approximately one half the width and three to four times the length of the cell with no true hyphae constriction at the point of origin. *C. albicans* produce germ tubes (95%), and a positive test is considered a presumptive identification.

6. An isolate produced a constriction that was interpreted as a positive germ tube, but *Candida albicans* was ruled out when confirmatory tests were performed. Which of the following fungi is the most likely identification?
   A. *Candida tropicalis*
   B. *Cryptococcus neoformans*
   C. *Candida glabrata*
   D. *Rhodotorula rubra*

   Microbiology/Apply knowledge of fundamental biological characteristics/Mycology/2

7. Cornmeal agar with Tween 80 is used to identify which characteristic of an unknown yeast isolate?
   A. Hyphae (true and pseudo)
   B. Blastospores and arthrospores
   C. Chlamydospores
   D. All of the above

   Microbiology/Apply knowledge of basic laboratory procedures/Mycology/1

8. Blastospores (blastoconidia) are the beginning of which structures?
   A. Arthrospores
   B. Germ tubes
   C. Pseudohyphae
   D. True hyphae

   Microbiology/Apply knowledge of fundamental biological characteristics/Mycology/1

9. An isolate from CSF growing on cornmeal agar produces the following structures:

   Blastospores = +   Pseudohyphae = Neg
   Chlamydospores = Neg   Arthrospores = Neg

   Which tests should be performed next?
   A. Birdseed agar and urease
   B. Germ tube and glucose
   C. India ink and germ tube
   D. All of the above

   Microbiology/Select methods/Reagents/Media/Mycology/2

10. Which of the following yeast enzymes is detected using birdseed (niger seed) agar?
    A. Phenol oxidase
    B. Catalase
    C. Urease
    D. Nitrate reductase

    Microbiology/Apply knowledge of fundamental biological characteristics/Mycology/2

11. Which of the following yeasts is characteristically positive for germ tube production?
    A. *Candida tropicalis*
    B. *Candida pseudotropicalis*
    C. *Cryptococcus neoformans*
    D. *Candida albicans*

    Microbiology/Apply knowledge of fundamental biological characteristics/Mycology/1

Answers to Questions 6–11

6. **A** *C. tropicalis* forms pseudohyphae that resemble true germ tubes by producing a constriction at the point of origin of the yeast cell. A germ tube represents a true hyphae without constriction, and therefore the test should have been repeated along with carbohydrate tests before making a presumptive identification. The other three species of yeast listed do not form hyphae.

7. **D** Cornmeal agar with Tween 80 (polysorbate) reduces the surface tension and allows for enhanced formation of hyphae, blastospores, and chlamydospores.

8. **C** Pseudohyphae are the result of a pinching-off process, blastoconidiation, with the growth of filaments with constrictions. Germ tubes are the beginning of true hyphae (no constrictions). Arthrospores are the result of a breaking-off process of true septate hyphae resulting in square conidia.

9. **A** A yeast isolated from the CSF producing blastospores is most likely to be *C. neoformans*, which is positive for urease and produces brown colonies on birdseed agar.

10. **A** Most isolates of *C. neoformans* produce phenol oxidase when grown on *Guizotia abyssinica* medium (birdseed medium), producing brown to black pigmented colonies. *C. neoformans* is the only *Cryptococcus* species that oxidizes *o*-diphenol to melanin, which is responsible for the color.

11. **D** *C. albicans* and *Candida stellatoidea*, a variant of *C. albicans*, are the only yeasts that produce germ tubes within 1–3 hours of incubation at 37°C. *C. tropicalis* produces pseudohyphae after incubation for 3 hours, which may be mistaken for germ tubes. A careful evaluation of the tube origin for constriction is required in order to avoid a false-positive interpretation.

12. Arthrospore (arthroconidia) production is used to differentiate which two yeast isolates?
    A. *Candida albicans* and *Candida. stellatoidea*
    B. *Trichosporon pullulans* and *Cryptococcus neoformans*
    C. *Candida albicans* and *Candida tropicalis*
    D. *Saccharomyces cerevisiae* and *Candida (Torulopsis) glabrata*

    Microbiology/Apply knowledge of fundamental biological characteristics/Mycology/2

13. The urease test, niger seed agar test, and the germ tube test are all used for the presumptive identification of:
    A. *Rhodotorula rubra*
    B. *Cryptococcus neoformans*
    C. *Trichosporon pullulans*
    D. *Candida albicans*

    Microbiology/Apply knowledge of fundamental biological characteristics/Mycology/2

14. Which of the following yeasts produces only blastospores on cornmeal Tween 80 agar?
    A. *Candida* spp
    B. *Trichosporon* spp
    C. *Geotrichum* spp
    D. *Cryptococcus* spp

    Microbiology/Apply knowledge of fundamental biological characteristics/Mycology/2

15. Ascospores are formed by which yeast isolate?
    A. *Saccharomyces cerevisiae*
    B. *Candida albicans*
    C. *Cryptococcus neoformans*
    D. All of the above

    Microbiology/Apply knowledge of fundamental biological characteristics/Mycology/2

16. A germ tube–negative, pink yeast isolate was recovered from the respiratory secretions and urine of a patient with AIDS. Given the following results, what is the most likely identification?

Cornmeal Tween 80 Agar	
Blastospores = +	Pseudohyphae = Neg
Arthrospores = Neg	Urease = +

    A. *Candida albicans*
    B. *Rhodotorula* spp
    C. *Cryptococcus* spp
    D. *Trichosporon* spp

    Microbiology/Evaluate laboratory data to make identifications/Mycology/3

Answers to Questions 12–16

12. **B** *T. pullulans* and *C. neoformans* are both urease-positive, but *T. pullulans* produces arthrospores and *C. neoformans* does not. In addition to *Trichosporon* spp, arthrospores are produced by *Geotrichum* spp.

13. **B** A germ tube negative isolate producing dark brown to black colonies on niger seed agar and a positive urease test are presumptive identifications of *C. neoformans*. A positive germ tube test is a presumptive identification for *C. albicans* as well as for *C. stellatoidea*. See the following chart.

	C. neoformans	R. rubra	T. pullulans	C. albicans
Urease	+	+	+	Neg
Germ tube	Neg	Neg	Neg	+
Brown and black colonies on niger seed agar	+	Neg	Neg	Neg

14. **D** *Cryptococcus* spp do not form either pseudohyphae or arthrospores. *Candida* spp produce blastospores or pseudohyphae. *Trichosporon* spp and *Geotrichum* spp produce pseudohyphae, blastospores, and arthrospores. See the following chart.

	Blastospores	Pseudohyphae	Arthrospores
Cryptococcus spp	+	Neg	Neg
Candida spp	+	+	Neg
Trichosporon spp	+	+	+
Geotrichum spp	+	+	+

15. **A** Sexual spore production is a characteristic of the *Ascomycotina*, which produce an ascus (saclike structure) after the union of two nuclei. The resulting spore is termed an ascospore. *S. cerevisiae* produces ascospores when grown on ascospore agar for 10 days at 25°C.

16. **B** *Rhodotorula* spp produce pink- to coral-colored colonies on Sabouraud's agar and cornmeal agar. It is usually considered a contaminant but is an opportunistic pathogen and must be identified when found in specimens from immunosuppressed patients.

17. Chlamydospore production is demonstrated by which *Candida* species?
A. *C. glabrata*
B. *C. krusei*
C. *C. albicans*
D. *C. tropicalis*

Microbiology/Apply knowledge of fundamental biological characteristics/Mycology/1

18. Carbohydrate assimilation tests are used for the identification of yeast isolates by inoculating media:
A. Free of carbohydrates
B. Free of niger seed
C. Containing carbohydrates
D. Containing yeast extract

Microbiology/Apply principles of basic laboratory procedures/Mycology/1

19. Yeast recovered from the urine of a catheterized patient receiving chemotherapy for cancer gave the following results:

Cornmeal Tween 80 Agar		
Germ tube = +	Blastospores = +	
Pseudohyphae = +	Arthrospores = Neg	Chlamydospores = +

What further testing is necessary?
A. Carbohydrate assimilation and urease
B. Urease and niger seed
C. Nitrate reductase and carbohydrate fermentation
D. No further testing is needed for identification

Microbiology/Select course of action/Mycology/3

20. A blood agar plate inoculated with sputum from a patient with diabetes mellitus grew very few bacterial flora and a predominance of yeast. Given the following results, what is the most likely identification of the yeast isolate?

Cornmeal Tween 80 Agar	
Germ tube = Neg	Pseudohyphae = +
Arthrospores = Neg	Blastoconidia = + (arranged
Chlamydospores = Neg	along pseudohyphae)

A. *Candida tropicalis*
B. *Candida pseudotropicalis*
C. *Trichosporon beigelii*
D. *Geotrichum candidum*

Microbiology/Evaluate laboratory data to make identifications/Mycology/3

21. Dimorphic molds are found in infected tissue in which form?
A. Mold phase
B. Yeast phase
C. Encapsulated
D. Latent

Microbiology/Apply knowledge of fundamental biological characteristics/Mycology/1

Answers to Questions 17–21

17. **C** Cornmeal Tween 80 agar supports the growth of *C. albicans* and the formation of its distinctive thick-walled, terminal (at the tip of the pseudohyphae) chlamydospores. *C. stellatoidea* may also produce chlamydospores, but it is considered a variant of *C. albicans* and is not usually differentiated.

18. **A** The yeast isolate is inoculated directly into the molten agar base free of carbohydrates or is poured as a suspension onto a yeast nitrogen agar base plate. Carbohydrate disks are then added to the surface of the agar, and the plates are incubated for 24–48 hours at 30°C. Growth around the disk indicates the ability of the yeast to utilize the carbohydrate(s) as a sole source of carbon.

19. **D** This isolate is *C. albicans*, which also produces some true hyphae along with pseudohyphae. A positive germ tube is a presumptive identification; no further testing is needed because no other yeast produces blastospores and chlamydospores along with pseudohyphae.

20. **A** *C. tropicalis* and *C. pseudotropicalis* differ in their arrangement of blastoconidia along the pseudohyphae. *C. pseudotropicalis* forms elongated blastoconidia arranged in parallel clusters that simulate logs in a stream. *Trichosporon* spp and *Geotrichum* spp form arthrospores.

21. **B** Dimorphic molds are in the yeast form in infected tissues because they are in the yeast form at 37°C. Specimens are cultured and incubated at both room temperature and 35°–37°C. To prove that a mold growing at room temperature (or 30°C) is a dimorphic fungus, conversion to the yeast form must be demonstrated via subculture and incubation at 37°C.

22. The mycelial form of which dimorphic mold produces thick-walled, rectangular, or barrel-shaped alternate arthroconidia?
    A. *Coccidioides immitis*
    B. *Sporothrix schenckii*
    C. *Histoplasma capsulatum*
    D. *Blastomyces dermatitidis*

    Microbiology/Apply knowledge of fundamental biological characteristics/Mycology/2

23. The yeast form of which dimorphic fungus appears as oval or elongated cigar shapes?
    A. *Coccidioides immitis*
    B. *Sporothrix schenckii*
    C. *Histoplasma capsulatum*
    D. *Blastomyces dermatitidis*

    Microbiology/Apply knowledge of fundamental biological characteristics/Mycology/2

24. The mycelial form of *Histoplasma capsulatum* seen on agar resembles:
    A. *Sepedonium* spp
    B. *Penicillium* spp
    C. *Sporothrix* spp
    D. *Coccidioides* spp

    Microbiology/Apply knowledge of fundamental biological characteristics/Mycology/2

25. The yeast form of which dimorphic mold shows a large parent yeast cell surrounded by smaller budding yeast cells?
    A. *Paracoccidioides brasiliensis*
    B. *Sporothrix schenckii*
    C. *Coccidioides immitis*
    D. *Histoplasma capsulatum*

    Microbiology/Apply knowledge of fundamental biological characteristics/Mycology/2

26. Which group of molds can be ruled out when septate hyphae are observed in a culture?
    A. Dematiaceous
    B. Zygomycetes
    C. Dermatophytes
    D. Dimorphic molds

    Microbiology/Apply knowledge of fundamental biological characteristics/Mycology/1

27. Tinea versicolor is a skin infection caused by:
    A. *Malassezia furfur*
    B. *Trichophyton rubrum*
    C. *Trichophyton schoenleinii*
    D. *Microsporum gypseum*

    Microbiology/Apply knowledge of fundamental biological characteristics/Mycology/1

Answers to Questions 22–27

22. **A** The mold form of *C. immitis* shows barrel-shaped arthroconidia separated by empty cells (ghost cells) that cause an uneven staining effect when they are examined under a microscope. *S. schenckii*, *H. capsulatum*, and *B. dermatitidis* produce conidia that are round or oval in shape in the mold phase.

23. **B** *S. schenckii* is usually acquired by humans through thorns or splinters because it is commonly found on living or dead vegetation. It is called "rose gardener's disease" because gardeners, florists, and farmers are most often infected. *S. schenckii* is often recovered from exudates of unopened subcutaneous nodules or open draining lesions.

24. **A** *Sepedonium* spp are saprophytic molds that do not have a yeast phase and produce large spherical tuberculate macroconidia like *H. capsulatum*. Histoplasmosis is a chronic granulomatous infection primarily found in the lungs that invades the reticuloendothelial system. Infection occurs via spores released from decaying bird or chicken droppings that are inhaled when disturbed.

25. **A** *P. brasiliensis* yeast forms are sometimes seen as a "mariner's wheel" because multiple budding cells completely surround the periphery of the parent cell.

26. **B** Zygomycetes commonly recovered from clinical specimens are *Rhizopus* spp and *Mucor* spp. Both display aseptate hyphae, while the other groups above display septate hyphae. Zygomycetes usually not encountered in clinical specimens are also aseptate and include *Absidia* spp, *Rhizomucor* spp, *Cincinella* spp, *Cunninghamella* spp, and *Syncephalastrum* spp.

27. **A** *M. furfur* has a worldwide distribution and causes a superficial, brownish, dry, scaly patch on the skin of light-skinned persons and lighter patches on persons with dark skin. *M. furfur* is not cultured because diagnosis can be made from microscopic examination of the skin scales. Skin scrapings prepared in KOH show oval or bottle-shaped cells that exhibit monopolar budding in the presence of a cell wall and also produce small hyphae.

28. Which of the following structures is invaded by the genus *Trichophyton*?
A. Hair
B. Nails
C. Skin
D. All of the above

Microbiology/Apply knowledge of fundamental biological characteristics/Mycology/1

29. An organism cultured from the skin produces colonies displaying a cherry red color on Sabouraud dextrose agar after 3–4 weeks and teardrop-shaped microconidia along the sides of the hyphae. The most likely identification is:
A. *Trichophyton rubrum*
B. *Trichophyton tonsurans*
C. *Trichophyton schoenleinii*
D. *Trichophyton violacium*

Microbiology/Apply knowledge of fundamental biological characteristics/Mycology/1

30. Which *Microsporum* species causes an epidemic form of tinea capitis in children?
A. *Microsporum canis*
B. *Microsporum audouinii*
C. *Microsporum gypseum*
D. All of the above

Microbiology/Correlate clinical and laboratory data/Mycology/2

31. Microscopic examination of a fungus cultured from a patient with athlete's foot showed large, smooth-walled, club-shaped macroconidia appearing singly or in clusters of two to three from the tips of short conidiophores. The colonies did not produce microconidia. What is the most likely identification?
A. *Trichophyton* spp
B. *Alternaria* spp
C. *Epidermophyton* spp
D. *Microsporum* spp

Microbiology/Evaluate laboratory data to make identifications/Mycology/2

32. Which *Trichophyton* species causes the favus type of tinea capitis seen in the Scandinavian countries and in the Appalachian region of the United States?
A. *T. verrucosum*
B. *T. violaceum*
C. *T. tonsurans*
D. *T. schoenleinii*

Microbiology/Correlate clinical and laboratory data/Mycology/2

Answers to Questions 28–32

28. **D** *Trichophyton* spp, *Microsporum* spp, and *Epidermophyton* spp are the organisms causing human dermatomycoses or cutaneous infections. *Trichophyton* spp infect hair and nails as well as skin. Infections with members of the genus *Microsporum* are confined to the hair and skin, while infections caused by the genus *Epidermophyton* are seen only on the skin and nails.

29. **A** Members of the genus *Microsporum* produce club-shaped microconidia and are usually pigmented white, buff, yellow, or brown. *Epidermophyton* does not display microconidia and produces yellow-green or yellow-tan colonies. *T. rubrum* can be differentiated from the other members of the genus by its distinctive cherry red color. *Trichophyton mentagrophytes* may also produce a red pigment, but it is usually rose-colored or orange, or deep red. *T. tonsurans* produces white-tan to yellow suedelike colonies. *T. schoenleinii* produces white to cream-colored colonies, and *T. violaceum* produces port wine to deep violet colonies.

30. **B** *M. audouinii* and *T. tonsurans* may both cause epidemic tinea capitis in children. *M. audouinii* causes a chronic infection transmitted directly via infected hairs on caps, hats, combs, upholstery, and hair clippers. Infected hair shafts fluoresce yellow-green under a Wood's lamp. *M. audouinii* does not usually sporulate in culture and forms atypical vegetative forms such as antler and racquet hyphae and terminal chlamydospores. In contrast, *M. canis* produces spindle-shaped, thick-walled multicelled macroconidia, and *M. gypseum* produces ellipsoidal, multicellular macroconidia.

31. **C** *Epidermophyton* spp do not produce microconidia; this differentiates them from *Trichophyton* spp and *Microsporum* spp. *Alternaria* is not a dermatophyte. *Epidermophyton floccosum* is the most frequently isolated member of the genus and infects the skin but not the hair.

32. **D** *T. schoenleinii* is identified microscopically by its characteristic antler-shaped hyphae and chlamydospores in the absence of conidia.

33. The Hair Baiting Test is used to differentiate which two species of *Trichophyton* that produce red colonies on Sabouraud agar plates?
  A. *T. mentagrophytes* and *T. rubrum*
  B. *T. tonsurans* and *T. schoenleinii*
  C. *T. tonsurans* and *T. violaceum*
  D. *T. verrucosum* and *T. rubrum*

  Microbiology/Correlate clinical and laboratory data/Mycology/2

34. A mold that produces colonies with a dark brown, green-black, or black appearance of both the surface and reverse side is classified as a:
  A. Dematiaceous mold
  B. Dermatophyte
  C. Hyaline mold
  D. Dimorphic fungus

  Microbiology/Apply knowledge of fundamental biological characteristics/Mycology/1

35. A rapidly growing hyaline mold began as a white colony but soon developed a black "pepper" effect on the agar surface. The older colony produced a black matte, making it resemble a dematiaceous mold. What is the most likely identification?
  A. *Penicillium notatum*
  B. *Aspergillus niger*
  C. *Paecilomyces* spp
  D. *Scopulariopsis* spp

  Microbiology/Apply knowledge of fundamental biological characteristics/Mycology/1

36. Which dematiaceous mold forms flask-shaped phialides, each with a flask-shaped collarette?
  A. *Phialophora* spp
  B. *Exophila* spp
  C. *Wangiella* spp
  D. All of the above

  Microbiology/Apply knowledge of fundamental biological characteristics/Mycology/1

37. Which *Aspergillus* species, recovered from sputum or bronchial mucus, is the most common cause of pulmonary aspergillosis?
  A. *A. niger*
  B. *A. flavus*
  C. *A. fumigatus*
  D. All of the above

  Microbiology/Correlate clinical and laboratory data/ Mycology/2

38. A hyaline mold recovered from a patient with AIDS produced rose-colored colonies with lavender centers on Sabouraud dextrose agar. Microscopic examination showed multiseptate macroconidia appearing as sickles or canoes. What is the most likely identification?
  A. *Fusarium* spp
  B. *Wangiella* spp
  C. *Exophiala* spp
  D. *Phialophora* spp

  Microbiology/Evaluate laboratory data to make identifications/Mycology/3

Answers to Questions 33–38

33. **A** *T. mentagrophytes* may produce a deep red pigment seen through the reverse side of the agar plate that resembles the cherry red pigment produced by *T. rubrum*. However, *T. mentagrophytes* can be differentiated by its ability to invade the hair shaft. *T. rubrum* grows on the surface of the hair but does not penetrate the shaft.

34. **A** The dematiaceous molds are easily recognized and confirmed by observing dark yellow or brown septate hyphae upon microscopic examination.

35. **B** *A. niger* is the only species listed producing black conidia, which causes a "pepper" effect as the colony grows. The reverse side of the agar plate remains buff- or cream-colored, which differentiates it from the dematiaceous (dark) molds.

36. **A** *Phialophora*, *Exophila*, and *Wangiella* all produce phialides, but the last two genera form elongated, tubelike phialides without a collarette, as opposed to the flask-shaped phialides of *Phialophora*, which contain clusters of conidia at the tips.

37. **C** *A. fumigatus* is most often associated with compost piles and is found in the soil of potted plants. *A. niger* is the cause of cavitary fungus ball lesions of the lungs and nasal passages.

38. **A** *Fusarium* spp are usually a contaminant but are sometimes seen as a cause of mycotic eye, nail, or skin infection in debilitated patients. *Fusarium* spp is a hyaline Hyphomycetes and grows on Sabouraud agar plates at 30°C within 4 days. The other three organisms are members of the Dematiaceae family (dark molds).

39. Material from a fungus-ball infection produced colonies with a green surface on Sabouraud agar in 5 days at 30°C. Microscopic examination showed club-shaped vesicles with sporulation only from the top half of the vesicle. This hyaline mold is most probably which *Aspergillus* spp?
   A. *A. niger*
   B. *A. fumigatus*
   C. *A. flavus*
   D. *A. terreus*

Microbiology/Evaluate laboratory data to make identifications/Mycology/3

40. A rapidly growing nonseptate mold produced colonies with a gray surface resembling cotton candy that covered the entire plate. Microscopic examination revealed sporangiophores arising between, not opposite, the rhizoids and producing pear-shaped sporangia. What is the most likely identification?
   A. *Absidia* spp
   B. *Penicillium* spp
   C. *Rhizopus* spp
   D. *Aspergillus* spp

Microbiology/Evaluate laboratory data to make identifications/Mycology/3

41. An India ink test was performed on CSF from an HIV-infected male patient. Many encapsulated yeast cells were seen in the centrifuged sample.

Further testing revealed a positive urease test and growth of brown colonies on niger-seed agar. The diagnosis of meningitis was caused by which yeast?
   A. *Candida albicans*
   B. *Cryptococcus neoformans*
   C. *Cryptococcus laurentii*
   D. *Candida tropicalis*

Microbiology/Apply knowledge for identification/Mycology/3

42. A bone marrow sample obtained from an immunocompromised patient revealed small intracellular cells using a Wright's stain preparation. Growth on Sabouraud-dextrose agar plates of a mold phase at 25°C and a yeast phase at 37°C designates the organism as dimorphic. The mold phase produced thick, spherical tuberculated macroconidia. What is the most likely identification?
   A. *Histoplasma capsulatum*
   B. *Sepedonium* spp
   C. *Sporothrix schenckii*
   D. *Coccidioides immitis*

Microbiology/Apply knowledge for identification/Mycology/3

43. A lung biopsy obtained from an immunocompromised patient showed many "cup-shaped" cysts (gray to black) in a foamy exudate (green background) with

Gomori methenamine silver (GMS) stain. The organism cannot be cultured because it does not grow on routine culture media for molds. The patient was diagnosed with pneumonia that resisted antibiotic treatment. The most likely identification is?
   A. *Pneumocystis carinii*
   B. *Histoplasma capsulatum*
   C. *Sporothrix schenckii*
   D. *Scopulariopsis* spp

Microbiology/Apply knowledge for identification/Mycology/3

Answers to Questions 39–43

39. B *A. fumigatus* is the most common cause of aspergillosis. It is characterized by sporulation only from the upper half or two-thirds of the vesicle. Colonies of *A. niger* are white with black pepper growth and produce phialides over the entire vesicle, forming the classic "radiate" head. *A. flavus* colonies are yellow to yellow-green and produce phialides that cover the entire vesicle and point out in all directions. *A. terreus* produces brown colonies and phialides that also cover the entire vesicle.

40. A *Absidia* spp are similar to *Rhizopus* spp except for the location of rhizoids (rootlike hyphae). The rhizoids of *Rhizopus* spp are located at the point where the stolons and sporangiophores meet, whereas those of *Absidia* spp arise at a point on the stolon between the rhizoids. *Penicillium* spp and *Aspergillus* spp do not form rhizoids.

41. B Immunocompromised patients are at risk for invasion of *Cryptococcus neoformans*. The polysaccharide capsule of *C. neoformans* is not recognized by phagocytes that allow patients with impaired cell-mediated immunity to become readily infected with *C. neoformans*.

42. A Thermally dimorphic *Histoplasma capsulatum* produce microconidia and hyphal fragments at 37°C (yeast phase), whereas at 25°C (mold phase) the organism displays large, thick-walled, round macroconidia with knobby or knob-like projections. The yeast form is able to survive within circulating monocytes or tissue macrophages that can be demonstrated with Giemsa's or Wright's stain.

43. A *Pneumocystis carinii*, most recently classified as a fungus but formerly as a parasite, is best recovered by bronchoalveolar lavage in immunocompromised patients. Open lung biopsy sample was the specimen of choice before the AIDS epidemic. Gomori methenamine silver stain is used to identify the organism; it stains the cyst form but not the trophozoites.

44. Upon direct examination of a sputum specimen, several spherules were noted that contained endospores. Growth on Sabouraud-dextrose agar showed aerial mycelial elements. The septate hyphae produced barrel-shaped arthroconidia. What is the most likely identification?

A. *Penicillium marneffei*
B. *Scopulariopsis* spp
C. *Cryptococcus neoformans*
D. *Coccidioides immitis*

Microbiology/Evaluate laboratory data to make identifications/Mycology/3

45. A bone marrow specimen was obtained from an immunocompromised patient who tested positive for HIV. The organism grew rapidly at 3 days showing a mold form (at 25°C), displaying conidiophores with four to five terminal metulae with each having four to six phialides. The conidia at the end of the phialides were oval and in short chains. They appear as a fan or broom when viewing under 10× and 40×. At 37°C, the yeast form grew more slowly, showing conidia that formed hyphal elements breaking at the septa to produce oval arthroconidia. This thermo-dimorphic mold is most likely?

A. *Paecilomyces* spp
B. *Penicillium marneffei*

C. *Rhizomucor* spp
D. *Aspergillus fumigatus*

Microbiology/Evaluate laboratory data to make identifications/Mycology/3

Answers to Questions 44–45

44. **D** *Coccidioides immitis* endospores are often confused with yeast cells but they do not bud. *C. immitis* is endemic in the southwestern US. Since the arthroconidia are highly infectious, an open plate should not be used, and a slide culture test should **not** be performed. Rather, tubed media is used for testing, and all work should be performed in a biological safety cabinet.

45. **B** Other *Penicillium* spp are differentiated from *P. marneffei* (thermally dimorphic) through conversion from the mold to yeast phase. *P. marneffei* are seen as yeast at 35–37°C on 5% sheep blood agar or in BHI broth. Other *Penicillium* spp do not display a yeast phase. *P. marneffei* are recovered from blood, skin, lymph nodes, bone marrow, and internal organs of immunocompromised patients.

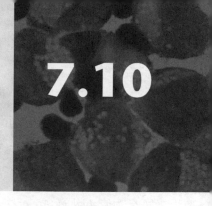

1. Classification of viruses is made by:
   A. Complement fixation serology
   B. Electron microscopy
   C. Nucleic acid composition
   D. Cellular inclusion bodies

   Microbiology/Apply knowledge of fundamental biological characteristics/Viruses/1

2. Which virus is the most common etiological agent of viral respiratory diseases in infants and children?
   A. Respiratory syncytial virus (RSV)
   B. Measles virus
   C. Coxsackie A virus
   D. Coxsackie B virus

   Microbiology/Apply knowledge of fundamental biological characteristics/Viruses/1

3. The most common viral syndrome of pericarditis, myocarditis, and pleurodynia (pain upon breathing) is caused by:
   A. Herpes simplex virus
   B. Respiratory syncytial virus
   C. Epstein-Barr virus
   D. Coxsackie B virus

   Microbiology/Apply knowledge of fundamental biological characteristics/Viruses/1

4. Which of the following viruses is implicated along with Epstein-Barr virus as a cause of infectious mononucleosis?
   A. Cytomegalovirus (CMV)
   B. Coxsackie A virus
   C. Coxsackie B virus
   D. Hepatitis B virus

   Microbiology/Apply knowledge of fundamental biological characteristics/Viruses/1

5. The most common causes of viral pneumonia in adults are:
   A. Influenza and adenovirus
   B. Hepatitis A and B viruses
   C. Coxsackie A and B viruses
   D. Herpes simplex and CMV

   Microbiology/Apply knowledge of fundamental biological characteristics/Viruses/1

Answers to Questions 1–5

1. **C** True viruses have nucleic acid that is either RNA or DNA, and this serves as the basis for initial classification. Members of these classes are further divided into groups that cause human disease based upon the mode of transmission, tissues invaded, diseases produced, and antigenic characteristics.

2. **A** RSV is the cause of croup, bronchitis, bronchiolitis, and interstitial pneumonia. Children under 1 year old who are hospitalized are the most susceptible group.

3. **D** Coxsackie A virus, coxsackie B virus, and the echoviruses are most commonly implicated in myocarditis and other syndromes, including acute cerebellar ataxia and hepatitis. Like poliovirus, infections are more common in the summer and fall and gain entry through the gastrointestinal tract.

4. **A** CMV infection in a previously healthy individual causes a self-limited mononucleosis syndrome. CMV is an opportunistic pathogen that may produce lifelong infections and can cause a variety of diseases, including congenital and neonatal infection, hepatitis, pneumonia, and disseminated infection in immunocompromised patients.

5. **A** Influenza and adenoviruses are the main causes of respiratory infections, including the common cold, tracheobronchitis, and pneumonia. Adenoviruses also cause conjunctivitis, keratitis, cystitis, and gastroenteritis.

6. Which virus belonging to the Reoviridae group causes gastroenteritis in infants and young children but an asymptomatic infection in adults?
   A. Coxsackie B virus
   B. Rotavirus
   C. Respiratory syncytial virus
   D. Rhabdovirus

Microbiology/Apply knowledge of fundamental biological characteristics/Viruses/1

7. A very small, single-stranded DNA virus that causes a febrile illness with a rash and is called the fifth childhood disease after rubeola, rubella, varicella, and roseola is:
   A. Rotavirus
   B. Adenovirus type 40
   C. Coxsackie A virus
   D. Parvovirus B19

Microbiology/Apply knowledge of fundamental biological characteristics/Viruses/1

8. Hepatitis B virus can be transmitted by:
   A. Acupuncture
   B. Tattoos
   C. Sexual contact
   D. All of the above

Microbiology/Apply knowledge of fundamental biological characteristics/Viruses/1

9. Which virus has been implicated in adult gastroenteritis resulting from ingestion of contaminated food (especially shellfish) and water?
   A. Norwalk-like viruses
   B. Rotavirus
   C. Hepatitis C virus
   D. Coronavirus

Microbiology/Apply knowledge of fundamental biological characteristics/Viruses/1

10. Which virus is associated with venereal and respiratory tract warts and produces lesions of skin and mucous membranes?
   A. Polyomavirus
   B. Poxvirus
   C. Adenovirus
   D. Papillomavirus

Microbiology/Apply knowledge of fundamental biological characteristics/Viruses/1

11. A clinical test used for the detection and identification of viral infections other than culture is:
   A. Hemagglutination
   B. Hemadsorption
   C. Viral antigen detection
   D. All of the above

Microbiology/Apply principles of basic laboratory procedures/Viruses/1

Answers to Questions 6–11

6. **B** Rotaviruses have been implicated in both nosocomial infections and epidemic gastroenteritis. Children 3–24 months old are most commonly affected. Diarrhea begins after an incubation period of 3 days, lasts for 2–10 days, and is associated with vomiting and dehydration. In immunosuppressed children, rotavirus causes a chronic infection.

7. **D** Parvovirus causes a fever and characteristic "slapped cheek" rash in young children. Adults are usually immune, but immunocompromised persons may exhibit an arthritis or anemia (the virus infects immature RBCs in the bone marrow).

8. **D** Although the most common mode of transmission of hepatitis B is via needle puncture, it may also be transmitted by other parenteral means, including sexual transmission and contact with contaminated blood through broken skin or mucous membranes.

9. **A** Norwalk-like viruses are small RNA viruses that have been implicated in epidemics of community gastroenteritis as well as sporadic infections. Unlike rotaviruses, which cause gastroenteritis in infants and young children, Norwalk-like viruses produce infections in all age groups.

10. **D** The human papillomaviruses (HPVs) cause genital warts. Several strains, including HPV-6, HPV-11, HPV-16, and HPV-18, are associated with cervical and vaginal neoplasia. Because the virus cannot be cultured in vitro, diagnosis is usually made using DNA probes. A diagnostic characteristic of infected cells is koilocytosis, a perinuclear clearing in the squamous epithelium accompanied by nuclear atypia.

11. **D** In addition to serological tests for antibodies against the virus and DNA probes that identify viral DNA or RNA, the methods above aid in the rapid diagnosis of several viruses. Various species of animal RBCs are used for identification of viruses that contain receptors that agglutinate the RBCs. Some influenza A and parainfluenza viruses may be detected only by hemagglutination or hemadsorption. Testing for viral antigen in culture is used for detection of RSV, CMV, and varicella-zoster.

12. Which technique is most widely used for the confirmation of infection with human immunodeficiency virus (HIV-1)?
   A. Western blot (immunoblot) assay
   B. Enzyme-linked immunosorbent assay (ELISA)
   C. Complement fixation
   D. Polymerase chain reaction

   Microbiology/Select methods/Reagents/Media/Viruses/2

13. A 13-year-old boy was admitted to the hospital with a diagnosis of viral encephalitis. History revealed that the boy harbored wild racoons from a nearby woods. What is the best method to determine if the boy has contracted rabies?
   A. Remove the brain stems from all of the racoons and examine for cytopathic effects
   B. Request immunofluorescent test for antibody on the saliva from all of the racoons
   C. Request immunofluorescent test for antigen in cutaneous nerves obtained by nuchal biopsy of the patient
   D. Isolate the virus from the saliva of both the animals and the patient

   Microbiology/Select methods/Reagents/Media/Viruses/3

14. A 65-year-old woman was admitted to the hospital with acute respiratory distress, fever, myalgia, and headache. Influenza A or B was suspected after ruling out bacterial pneumonia. Which of the following methods could be used to confirm influenza infection?
   A. Influenza virus culture in Madin-Darby canine kidney
   B. Hemagglutination-inhibition test for antibodies in the patient's serum
   C. Direct examination of nasal epithelium for virus using fluorescent antibody stain
   D. All of the above

   Microbiology/Select methods/Reagents/Media/Viruses/3

15. The most rapid definitive diagnosis of a genital herpes simplex (HSV-2) infection in a 20-year-old man is made by which method?
   A. Direct immunofluorescence test for viral antigen in vesicle fluid
   B. Titer of serum and seminal fluid for antibodies to herpes simplex
   C. Detection of antiherpes simplex in seminal fluid
   D. Cell culture of vesicle fluid

   Microbiology/Select methods/Reagents/Media/Viruses/2

Answers to Questions 12–15

12. **A** The Western blot assay is most often used to confirm a positive serological test of antibodies to HIV. A sample is confirmed positive if antibodies are demonstrated against two of the three major regions (env, pol, and gag).

13. **C** Using direct immunofluorescence, rabies antigen can be detected in the cutaneous nerves surrounding the hair follicles of the posterior region of the neck (nuchal biopsy) and in epithelial cells obtained by a corneal impression. Antibodies to rabies can be detected in the serum and CSF of infected persons within 8–10 days of illness; however, infection usually occurs several months before the onset of symptoms. Isolation of virus from the saliva of the patient may be accomplished by mouse inoculation or by inoculation of susceptible cell culture lines with subsequent detection by immunofluorescent antibodies.

14. **D** Influenza virus types A, B, and C may be grown and isolated in embryonated hen eggs or cell cultures using Madin-Darby canine kidney (MDCK), rhesus monkey, or cynomolgus monkey kidney cells. Cell culture using MDCK cells is the most rapid technique, permitting identification within 1–3 days. The hemagglutination inhibition test can be used to titer antibody to influenza virus and to distinguish virus subtypes, if specific antisera is available. Direct fluorescent and enzyme immunoassays using monoclonal antibodies to nucleoprotein antigens in infected nasal epithelium are used for rapid diagnosis of both influenza A and influenza B infections.

15. **A** Direct immunofluorescence testing of vesicle (lesion) fluid for virus using fluorescein-conjugated antibodies is the most rapid method for diagnosis of genital herpes infection. Immunofluorescence and immunoperoxidase methods are also used to distinguish HSV-1 and HSV-2. However, the most sensitive method is viral cell culture, which may yield a positive result within 24 hours when fluid contains a high concentration of virus. Vero cells or primary human embryonic cells are inoculated with vesicle fluid and examined for cytopathic effects (CPE), the most common of which are large "balloon" cells and multinucleated giant cells.

16. A 20-year-old female college student complained of a sore throat and extreme fatigue. The physician noted lymphadenopathy and ordered a rapid test for infectious mononucleosis antibodies that was negative. Bacterial cultures were negative, as were serological tests for influenza A and B, HIV-1, CMV, hepatitis B, and antistreptolysin O. What would be the next line of viral testing to establish a diagnosis?
A. Herpes simplex
B. Rubella
C. Epstein-Barr
D. West Nile

Microbiology/Select testing for identification/Virology/3

17. A 60-year-old male gardener from New York state was hospitalized with flu-like symptoms and eventually diagnosed with encephalitis. While working in his garden, he noticed several dead birds around his bird feeder. The region was known to be heavily infested with mosquitoes. What is the most likely cause of his illness?
A. West Nile virus
B. Epstein-Barr virus
C. Parvovirus
D. Hantavirus

Microbiology/Select diagnosis/Virology/2

18. A 30-year-old male patient who was a contractor and building inspector in the southwestern U.S. complained of difficulty breathing and was admitted to the hospital with severe respiratory disease. The physician noted a high fever and cough. Two days before, the patient had inspected an old warehouse, abandoned and infested with rodents. The patient was given intravenous antibiotics, but two days into therapy the pneumonia worsened and he developed pulmonary edema. Which organism should be suspected of causing his illness?
A. Hantavirus
B. Rotavirus
C. West Nile virus
D. Norwalk-like virus

Microbiology/Select diagnosis/Virology/2

19. A 3-year-old female was admitted to the hospital following a two-day visit with relatives over the Christmas holidays. Vomiting and diarrhea left the child severely dehydrated. No other members of the family were affected. All bacterial cultures proved negative. A stool sample should be tested for which virus?

A. CMV
B. EBV
C. Hepatitis D
D. Rotavirus

Microbiology/Select testing for identification/Virology/2

Answers to Questions 16–19

16. **C** Epstein-Barr virus serological testing for IgM-VCA (viral capsid antigen) during the acute phase would be indicated because testing for infectious mononucleosis antibodies may or may not be positive. Patients who present with an infectious mononucleosis-like syndrome should be tested for both EBV and CMV. Both viruses cause the same symptoms during the acute phase of the illness.

17. **A** West Nile virus causes neurological diseases with meningitis and encephalitis at the top of the list. The animal reservoirs are birds with humans being accidental hosts. Transmission of West Nile virus is from mosquito to bird. The primary site of infection for Norwalk and rotavirus is the gastrointestinal area and for hantavirus the pulmonary sector.

18. **A** Hantavirus is transmitted by a rodent host, the deer mouse, and is endemic in the southwestern U.S. The name of the hantavirus responsible for outbreaks in this region is the Sin Nombre virus. Breathing in excrement from the mouse is the most common route of infection, and the lung is the site of initial infection. Diagnosis is usually made using an IgM ELISA assay.

19. **D** Rotavirus is one of the most common causes of gastroenteritis in infants and young children (6 months to 2 years old). Vomiting and diarrhea are also common symptoms of Norwalk virus infections, but the prevalence of rotavirus during the winter months and the lack of illness in other family members make rotavirus a more likely cause. Commercial availability of immunoassays for rotavirus makes its diagnosis easier to establish and rule out than infection with Norwalk-like viruses.

20. A 25-year-old male patient was diagnosed with HIV-1 by enzyme immunoassay, testing positive twice, and the diagnosis was confirmed by Western blot testing. Which laboratory testing should be performed prior to initiating antiviral therapy?
   A. Quantitative plasma virus concentration (viral load testing)
   B. Quantitation of CD4 lymphocytes
   C. Phenotype/genotype resistance testing
   D. All of the above

Microbiology/Select tests/Virology/3

21. A 6-month-old male infant was hospitalized with a respiratory infection. He was diagnosed with apnea and bronchiolitis. Further testing revealed congenital heart disease. Bacterial cultures were negative for *Streptococcus pneumoniae* and *Haemophilus influenzae*. What further testing should be done?
   A. Respiratory syncytial virus (RSV)
   B. Rotavirus
   C. Norwalk virus
   D. HIV

Microbiology/Select testing for identification/Viruses/2

22. A young male hunter encountered a fox in his path during a walk in the woods. The fox was staggering but appeared nonthreatening. The man tried to avoid contact but was attacked and bitten on the leg. The bite broke the skin but was not deep. Wildlife officials were unable to locate the fox for testing. What procedure should take place next for the hunter?
   A. Spinal tap with CSF testing for rabies virus
   B. Administration of hyperimmune antirabies globulin and rabies vaccine
   C. Biopsy of the wound site
   D. Throat culture and blood culture

Microbiology/Evaluate information for testing and identification/Virology/2

23. A 40-year-old female experienced a respiratory infection after returning home from a visit to her homeland of China. A rapid onset of pneumonia in the lower respiratory area prompted the physician to place her in isolation. She was diagnosed presumptively with severe acute respiratory syndrome (SARS) and placed on a respirator. What type of testing should be done next to diagnose this disease?
   A. Molecular technique and cell culture
   B. Latex agglutination test
   C. Blood culture
   D. Complement fixation

Microbiology/Select tests for identification/Virology/2

Answers to Questions 20–23

20. **D** The decision to initiate antiviral therapy is based upon the presence or absence of symptoms, CD4 lymphocyte count, and the viral load. For example, treatment is usually withheld from patients with CD4 counts >350/μL and viral load <55,000/mL and is instituted in asymptomatic patients if the CD4 count is <200/μL regardless of viral load. Treatment failure within the first year with three-drug regimens is 35%-45%, and drug resistance testing (genotype and/or phenotype testing) is recommended to identify drug-resistant strains prior to initiating treatment.

21. **A** Respiratory syncytial virus (RSV) is spread by large particle droplets such as dust and is one of the most common causes of hospitalization for respiratory illness of infants less than 1 year old. RSV causes bronchiolitis, pneumonia, and croup in infants and upper respiratory illness in children. It has also been found to cause nosocomial infection in nursing homes. Diagnosis is made by EIA, fluorescent antibody (FA) staining, and cell culture.

22. **B** Rabies virus can be detected by FA staining and PCR testing. The virus replicates at the site of the bite and penetrates the surrounding tissue, finding its way to the central nervous system. Since the source cannot be tested, the best course of action is to initate postexposure prophylaxis with antirabies globulin and to immunize the patient with rabies vaccine.

23. **A** SARS virus was discovered in China in 2003. The virus belongs to the common cold group of coronaviruses, and is easily transmitted to health care workers having close contact with infected patients. It is the cause of a severe lower respiratory infection that can be fatal. Laboratory confirmation may be done by PCR testing that is available commercially, cell culture, EIA, or IFA. Typically, PCR is used on two different specimen types or the same specimen type submitted at least two days apart. If both tests are positive, the infection is confirmed.

24. A pregnant 25-year-old female with genital lesions delivered a premature newborn with complications. The baby tested negative for bacterial infection (cultures of blood and urine). Antigen testing of the baby's urine proved negative for group B streptococci and *Streptococcus pneumoniae*. The mother tested negative for bacterial sexually transmitted diseases and for group B streptococci. The baby was treated with acyclovir and failed to survive. What was the most likely cause of death?

A. CMV
B. Human deficiency virus
C. Respiratory syncial virus
D. Herpes simplex virus

Microbiology/Select diagnosis/Viruses/2

25. A young father of two small children complained of a rash on the torso of his body. The children had been diagnosed with chickenpox and confined to their home. The father had experienced chickenpox as a child and knew he did not have the same rash as his children. What is the most likely cause of the father's rash?

A. Herpes simplex 1 virus
B. Varicella-zoster virus

C. Herpes simplex 2 virus
D. Epstein-Barr virus

Microbiology/Select diagnosis/Viruses/2

Answers to Questions 24–25

24. D Herpes simplex virus type 2 infections produce genital lesions. Infants born prematurely with disseminated infection of HSV type 2 from HSV-positive mothers have a mortality rate of 50%-60%. Testing of pregnant women for antibody and Cesarean section delivery can prevent most neonatal HSV infections because the virus enters the fetus during the delivery process.

25. B Varicella-zoster virus is the cause of an infection with chickenpox. As an adult, the father is experiencing shingles, a reactivation of the virus. The virus lies dormant in the sensory (dorsal root) ganglia of the spinal nerves, and its reactivation produces a nonweeping blister-like rash on an inflamed skin base that follows the path of the underlying nerves.

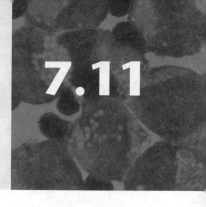

1. The *incorrect* match between organism and the appropriate diagnostic procedure is:
   A. *Onchocerca volvulus*—examination of skin snips
   B. *Cryptosporidium*—modified acid-fast stain
   C. *Echinococcus granulosus*—routine ova and parasite examination
   D. *Schistosoma haematobium*—examination of urine sediment

   Microbiology/Apply knowledge of diagnostic techniques/Parasitology/2

2. In a patient with diarrhea, occasionally *Entamoeba histolytica/E. dispar* (four nucleated cysts, no chromatoidal bars) are identified as being present; however, these cells, which are misdiagnosed as protozoa, are really:
   A. Macrophages
   B. Polymorphonuclear leukocytes
   C. Epithelial cells
   D. Eosinophils

   Microbiology/Apply knowledge of the morphology of artifacts/Parasitology/3

3. Charcot-Leyden crystals in stool may be associated with an immune response and are thought to be the breakdown products of:
   A. Neutrophils
   B. Eosinophils
   C. Monocytes
   D. Lymphocytes

   Microbiology/Apply knowledge of the morphology of artifacts/Parasitology/1

4. Parasitic organisms that are most often transmitted sexually include:
   A. *Entamoeba gingivalis*
   B. *Dientamoeba fragilis*
   C. *Trichomonas vaginalis*
   D. *Diphyllobothrium latum*

   Microbiology/Apply knowledge of life cycles and epidemiology/Parasitology/1

Answers to Questions 1–4

1. **C** The appropriate procedure for the diagnosis of *E. granulosus* (hydatid disease) would involve the microscopic examination of hydatid fluid aspirated from a cyst. Immature scolices and/or hooklets would be found in the centrifuged fluid sediment and could be identified under the microscope.

2. **B** As polymorphonuclear leukocytes (PMNs) in stool begin to fragment and appear to have four nuclei, they will resemble *E. histolytica/E. dispar* cysts. However, *E. histolytica/E. dispar* cysts are rarely seen in cases of diarrhea. The species name *E. histolytica* is reserved for the true pathogen, whereas *E. dispar* is used for the nonpathogenic species. Unfortunately, morphologically they look identical. The only time *E. histolytica* could be identified morphologically would be from trophozoites containing ingested red blood cells (RBCs). Nonpathogenic *E. dispar* would not contain ingested RBCs. The correct way to report these organisms is *E. histolytica/E. dispar* (no trophozoites containing ingested RBCs) or *E. histolytica* (trophozoites seen that contain ingested RBCs). Physicians may treat based on patient symptoms.

3. **B** When eosinophils disintegrate, the granules reform into Charcot-Leyden crystals.

4. **C** *T. vaginalis* has been well documented to be a sexually transmitted flagellate.

5. The *incorrect* match between the organism and one method of acquiring the infection is:
   A. *Trypanosoma brucei rhodesiense*—bite of sand fleas
   B. *Giardia lamblia*—ingestion of water contaminated with cysts
   C. Hookworm—skin penetration of larvae from soil
   D. *Toxoplasma gondii*—ingestion of raw or rare meats

Microbiology/Apply knowledge of fundamental life cycles/Parasitology/1

6. Upon examination of stool material for *Isospora belli*, one would expect to see:
   A. Cysts containing sporozoites
   B. Precysts containing chromatoidal bars
   C. Oocysts that are acid-fast
   D. Sporozoites that are hematoxylin-positive

Microbiology/Apply knowledge of life cycles and organism morphology/Parasitology/1

7. Which specimen is the *LEAST* likely to provide recovery of *Trichomonas vaginalis*?
   A. Urine
   B. Urethral discharge
   C. Vaginal discharge
   D. Feces

Microbiology/Apply knowledge of pathogenesis and diagnostic procedures/Parasitology/2

8. Which of the following is the best technique to identify *Dientamoeba fragilis* in stool?
   A. Formalin concentrate
   B. Trichrome-stained smear
   C. Modified acid fast–stained smear
   D. Giemsa's stain

Microbiology/Apply knowledge of diagnostic procedures/Parasitology/2

9. One of the following protozoan organisms has been implicated in waterborne and foodborne outbreaks within the United States. The suspect organism is:
   A. *Trichomonas hominis*
   B. *Dientamoeba fragilis*
   C. *Giardia lamblia*
   D. *Balantidium coli*

Microbiology/Apply knowledge of life cycles and epidemiology/Parasitology/1

10. A Gram stain from a gum lesion showed what appeared to be amoebae. A trichrome smear showed amoebae with a single nucleus and partially digested PMNs. The correct identification is:
   A. *Trichomonas tenax*
   B. *Entamoeba histolytica/E. dispar*
   C. *Entamoeba gingivalis*
   D. *Entamoeba polecki*

Microbiology/Apply knowledge of organism morphology and body site/Parasitology/3

11. An *Entamoeba histolytica* trophozoite has the following characteristics:
   A. Central karyosome in the nucleus, ingested RBCs, and clear pseudopodia
   B. Ingested RBCs, clear pseudopodia, and uneven chromatin on the nuclear membrane
   C. Ingested RBCs, clear pseudopodia, and large glycogen vacuoles in cytoplasm
   D. Large, blotlike karyosome, ingested white blood cells (WBCs), and granular pseudopods

Answers to Questions 5–11

5. A East and West African trypanosomiasis (*T. b. rhodesiense* and *T. b. gambiense*) are caused when infective forms are introduced into the human body through the bite of the tsetse fly, not sand fleas.

6. C *I. belli* oocysts in various stages of maturity would be seen in the concentrate sediment or possibly the direct, wet preparation; these oocysts would stain positive with modified acid-fast stains.

7. D *T. vaginalis* is site-specific. The organisms are found in the urogenital tract; thus, the intestinal tract is not the normal site for these organisms.

8. B Because there is no known cyst form, the best technique to recover and identify *D. fragilis* trophozoites would be the trichrome-stained smear.

9. C For a number of years, *G. lamblia* has been implicated in both waterborne and foodborne outbreaks from the ingestion of infective cysts within contaminated water and food.

10. C *E. gingivalis* is known to be an inhabitant of the mouth and is characterized by morphology that resembles *E. histolytica/E. dispar*. However, *E. gingivalis* tends to ingest PMNs, whereas *E. histolytica/E. dispar* do not.

11. A The trophozoite of *E. histolytica* has evenly arranged chromatin on the nuclear membrane; a central, compact karyosome in the nucleus; clear pseudopodia; and ingested RBCs in the cytoplasm.

12. A 12-year-old girl is brought to the emergency room with meningitis and a history of swimming in a warm-water spring. Motile amoebae that measure 10 μ in size are seen in the CSF and are most likely:
   A. *Iodamoeba bütschlii* trophozoites
   B. *Endolimax nana* trophozoites
   C. *Dientamoeba fragilis* trophozoites
   D. *Naegleria fowleri* trophozoites

Microbiology/Apply knowledge of life cycle and epidemiology/Parasitology/3

13. Characteristics of the rhabditiform (noninfective) larvae of *Strongyloides stercoralis* include a:
   A. Short buccal capsule and large genital primordium
   B. Long buccal capsule and pointed tail
   C. Short buccal capsule and small genital primordium
   D. Small genital primordium and notch in tail

Microbiology/Apply knowledge of organism morphology and life cycle/Parasitology/2

14. Visceral larva migrans is associated with which of the following organisms?
   A. *Toxocara*—serology
   B. *Onchocerca*—skin snips
   C. *Dracunculus*—skin biopsy
   D. *Angiostrongylus*—CSF examination

Microbiology/Apply knowledge of life cycle and diagnostic procedures/Parasitology/2

15. The following organisms are linked with specific, relevant information. The incorrect combination is:
   A. *Strongyloides stercoralis*—internal autoinfection
   B. *Echinococcus granulosus*—hydatid examination
   C. *Pneumocystis carinii*—more than 50% of population antibody-positive by age 4
   D. *Balantidium coli*—common within the United States

Microbiology/Apply knowledge of life cycle and epidemiology/Parasitology/2

16. Examination of 24-hour unpreserved urine specimen is sometimes helpful in the recovery of:
   A. *Trichomonas vaginalis* trophozoites
   B. *Schistosoma haematobium* eggs
   C. *Enterobius vermicularis* eggs
   D. *Strongyloides stercoralis* larvae

Microbiology/Apply knowledge of life cycle and diagnostic methods/Parasitology/1

17. The examination of sputum may be necessary to diagnose infection with:
   A. *Paragonimus westermani*
   B. *Trichinella spiralis*
   C. *Wuchereria bancrofti*
   D. *Fasciola hepatica*

Microbiology/Apply knowledge of life cycle and diagnostic methods/Parasitology/1

18. Two helminth eggs that may resemble one another are:
   A. *Diphyllobothrium latum* and *Paragonimus westermani*
   B. *Opisthorchis sinensis* and *Fasciolopsis buski*
   C. *Taenia saginata* and *Hymenolepis nana*
   D. *Ascaris lumbricoides* and *Trichostrongylus*

Microbiology/Apply knowledge of organism morphology/Parasitology/2

Answers to Questions 12–18

12. **D** *N. fowleri* are free-living soil and water amoebae that cause primary amoebic meningoencephalitis, or PAM. The number of cases reported is few; however, the infection is very acute and almost always fatal.

13. **A** The rhabditiform larvae of *S. stercoralis* are characterized by the short buccal capsule (mouth) and large genital primordium, whereas hookworm larvae have a long buccal capsule and very small genital primordium.

14. **A** *Toxocara* spp are the cause of visceral larva migrans and occur when humans accidentally ingest the infective eggs of the dog or cat ascarid. The larvae migrate through the deep tissues, including the eye. The test of choice is the serology.

15. **D** *B. coli* is a ciliate that can cause watery diarrhea in humans; however, it is not commonly found within the United States. It is the largest of the intestinal protozoa and can be found in proficiency testing specimens. Therefore although it is not common, laboratories must still be able to identify these organisms.

16. **B** *S. haematobium* blood flukes reside in the veins over the bladder. When the eggs are passed from the body, they are often found in urine; egg viability can also be determined in unpreserved urine.

17. **A** *P. westermani* adult worms are found in the lung, and eggs may be coughed up in the sputum. Consequently, both sputum and stool (if the sputum containing the eggs is swallowed) are the recommended specimens for examination for the eggs.

18. **A** Both *D. latum* and *P. westermani* eggs are operculated and approximately the same size. The morphology is similar, although *D. latum* has a knob at the abopercular end and *P. westermani* has a thickened abopercular end and shoulders into which the operculum fits.

19. Eating poorly cooked pork can lead to an infection with:
  A. *Taenia solium* and *Trichinella spiralis*
  B. *Taenia saginata* and *Hymenolepis nana*
  C. *Trichuris trichiura* and *Hymenolepis diminuta*
  D. *Diphyllobothrium latum* and *Ascaris lumbricoides*

  Microbiology/Apply knowledge of organism life cycle/Parasitology/1

20. An operculated cestode egg that can be recovered from human feces is:
  A. *Clonorchis sinensis*
  B. *Diphyllobothrium latum*
  C. *Paragonimus westermani*
  D. *Dipylidium caninum*

  Microbiology/Apply knowledge of organism morphology/Parasitology/1

21. The adult tapeworm of *Echinococcus granulosus* is found in the intestine of:
  A. Dogs
  B. Sheep
  C. Humans
  D. Cattle

  Microbiology/Apply knowledge of life cycle/Parasitology/1

22. In infections with *Taenia solium*, humans can serve as the:
  A. Definitive host
  B. Intermediate host
  C. Either the definitive or the intermediate host
  D. None of the above

  Microbiology/Apply knowledge of life cycle/Parasitology/2

23. Humans acquire infections with *Diphyllobothrium latum* adult worms by:
  A. Ingestion of freshwater crabs
  B. Skin penetration of cercariae
  C. Ingestion of water chestnuts
  D. Ingestion of raw freshwater fish

  Microbiology/Apply knowledge of life cycle/Parasitology/1

24. Humans can serve as both the intermediate and definitive host in infections caused by:
  A. *Enterobius vermicularis*
  B. *Hymenolepis nana*
  C. *Schistosoma japonicum*
  D. *Ascaris lumbricoides*

  Microbiology/Apply knowledge of life cycle/Parasitology/1

25. *Babesia* is an organism that has been implicated in disease from both splenectomized and nonsplenectomized patients. Morphologically, the parasites resemble:
  A. *Plasmodium falciparum* rings
  B. *Leishmania donovani* amastigotes
  C. *Trypanosoma cruzi* trypomastigotes
  D. *Pneumocystis carinii* cysts

  Microbiology/Apply knowledge of parasite morphology/Parasitology/2

Answers to Questions 19–25

19. **A** Both *T. solium* (pork tapeworm) and *T. spiralis* can be acquired from the ingestion of raw or poorly cooked pork.

20. **B** *D. latum* is the only operculated cestode egg that is found in humans; the infection is acquired from the ingestion of raw freshwater fish.

21. **A** Although the hydatid cysts are found in sheep or in humans (accidental intermediate host), the adult tapeworms of *E. granulosus* are found in the intestine of the dog.

22. **C** If humans ingest *T. solium* cysticerci in uncooked or rare pork, the adult tapeworm will mature within the intestine (human will serve as definitive host); if eggs from the adult tapeworm are ingested, then the cysticerci will develop in human tissues (accidental intermediate host), causing cysticercosis.

23. **D** The ingestion of raw freshwater fish containing the encysted larvae of *D. latum* will result in the development of an adult tapeworm within the human intestine.

24. **B** In infections with *H. nana*, humans serve as both intermediate and definitive hosts. When ingested, the oncosphere penetrates the intestinal mucosa, develops into the mature cysticercoid (human is intermediate host), and returns to the gut, where the adult tapeworm matures (human is definitive host).

25. **A** *Babesia* is an intracellular parasite that closely resembles the ring forms (early trophozoites) of *P. falciparum*. Often in babesiosis there are more rings per cell and the ring form is the only stage seen.

26. Organisms (and infections) that under normal conditions cannot be transmitted in the laboratory are:
A. *Cryptosporidium*—cryptosporidiosis
B. *Taenia solium*—cysticercosis
C. *Ascaris lumbricoides*—ascariasis
D. *Enterobius vermicularis*—pinworm infections

Microbiology/Apply knowledge of life cycles/ Parasitology/2

27. *Toxoplasma gondii* is characterized by:
A. Possible congenital infection and ingestion of oocysts
B. Cosmopolitan distribution and possible difficulties with interpretation of serological results
C. None of the above
D. Both A and B

Microbiology/Apply knowledge of all areas of parasite biology, diagnostic procedures/Parasitology/3

28. Oocysts of *Cryptosporidium* spp can be detected in stool specimens using:
A. Modified Ziehl-Neelsen acid-fast stain
B. Gram's stain
C. Methenamine silver stain
D. Trichrome stain

Microbiology/Apply knowledge of diagnostic procedures, staining characteristics/Parasitology/1

29. Which microfilariae are usually *not* found circulating in the peripheral blood?
A. *Brugia malayi*
B. *Wuchereria bancrofti*
C. *Onchocerca volvulus*
D. *Loa loa*

Microbiology/Apply knowledge of diagnostic procedures, staining characteristics/Parasitology/1

30. Massive hemolysis, blackwater fever, and central nervous system involvement are most common with:
A. *Plasmodium vivax*
B. *Plasmodium falciparum*
C. *Plasmodium ovale*
D. *Plasmodium malariae*

Microbiology/Apply knowledge of disease pathogenesis/ Parasitology/2

31. Organisms that should be considered in a nursery school outbreak of diarrhea include:
A. *Endolimax nana*, *Giardia lamblia*, and *Entamoeba coli*
B. *Giardia lamblia*, *Dientamoeba fragilis*, and *Cryptosporidium parvum*
C. *Cryptosporidium parvum*, *Trichomonas vaginalis*, and *Entamoeba coli*
D. *Trichomonas hominis*, *Dientamoeba fragilis*, and *Endolimax nana*

Microbiology/Apply knowledge of epidemiology/ Parasitology/2

32. The *incorrect* match between disease and symptoms is:
A. Paragonimiasis—hemoptysis
B. Cryptosporidiosis—watery diarrhea
C. Toxoplasmosis in compromised host—central nervous system symptoms
D. Enterobiasis—dysentery

Microbiology/Apply knowledge of life cycles/ Parasitology/2

Answers to Questions 26–32

26. **C** *A. lumbricoides* eggs require a period of development in the soil before they are infective for humans. The other organisms listed can be transmitted within the laboratory or in the hospital setting.

27. **D** Infection with *T. gondii* is acquired through the ingestion of rare or raw meats, infective oocysts from cat feces, or as a congenital transmission. The organism has a cosmopolitan distribution and although serological testing is generally the test of choice, the results may be very difficult to interpret in certain situations (e.g., congenital infection and immunocompromised patients).

28. **A** The oocysts of *C. parvum* can be found and identified using microscopic examination of fecal smears stained with modified acid-fast stains. They appear as purple-red-pink round objects, measuring approximately 4–6 μ. Often the four sporozoites and residual body can be seen within the oocyst wall.

29. **C** The microfilariae of *O. volvulus* are normally found in the fluid right under the outer layer of skin. Therefore, the skin snip is the proper specimen to examine.

30. **B** The pathogenic sequelae of malarial infections with *P. falciparum* are the most severe of the four species. They can include massive hemolysis, blackwater fever, and multiple organ involvement, including the central nervous system (cerebral malaria).

31. **B** *G. lamblia*, *D. fragilis*, and *C. parvum* have been implicated in nursery school outbreaks. Among the many protozoa and coccidia found in the human, these three organisms have become the most likely parasites in this type of setting.

32. **D** Infections with *E. vermicularis* (the pinworm) may cause anal itching, sleeplessness, and possibly some vaginal irritation or discharge; however, dysentery (bloody diarrhea) has not been associated with this infection.

33. The formalin-ether (ethyl acetate) concentration procedure for feces is used to demonstrate:
  A. Motility of helminth larvae
  B. Protozoan cysts and helminth eggs
  C. Formation of amoebic pseudopods
  D. Trophozoites

Microbiology/Apply knowledge of diagnostic procedures/Parasitology/2

34. Cysts of *Iodamoeba bütschlii* typically have:
  A. Chromatoidal bars with rounded ends
  B. A heavily vacuolated cytoplasm
  C. A large glycogen vacuole
  D. Many ingested bacteria and yeast cells

Microbiology/Apply knowledge of morphology/Parasitology/1

35. The miracidial hatching test helps to demonstrate the viability of eggs of:
  A. *Taenia* species
  B. *Schistosoma* species
  C. Hookworm species
  D. *Opisthorchis* species

Microbiology/Apply knowledge of diagnostic procedures/Parasitology/1

36. Organisms that should be considered in a waterborne outbreak of diarrheal disease include:
  A. *Giardia lamblia* and *Cryptosporidium parvum*
  B. *Endolimax nana* and *Entamoeba histolytica*
  C. *Blastocystis hominis* and *Trichomonas vaginalis*
  D. *Toxoplasma gondii* and *Schistosoma mansoni*

Microbiology/Apply knowledge of epidemiology/Parasitology/2

37. The bronchoalveolar lavage (BAL) specimen has become much more widely used in:
  A. Any suspect patient with both toxoplasmosis and cryptosporidiosis
  B. Pediatric patients with pulmonary paragonimiasis
  C. AIDS patients with suspected *Pneumocystis* pneumonia
  D. Immunocompromised patients with disseminated strongyloidiasis

Microbiology/Apply knowledge of pathogenesis and diagnostic procedures/Parasitology/3

38. Primary infections with the microsporidia may originate in:
  A. The lung
  B. The nervous system
  C. The gastrointestinal tract
  D. Mucocutaneous lesions

Microbiology/Apply knowledge of life cycles/Parasitology/2

Answers to Questions 33–38

33. B The ova and parasite examination contains three components: the direct wet film (demonstrates protozoan trophozoite motility), the formalin-ethyl acetate concentration (demonstrates protozoan cysts, coccidian oocysts, and helminth eggs), and the trichrome or iron hematoxylin–stained smear (confirms protozoan cysts and trophozoites).

34. C The cyst of *I. bütschlii* is characterized by a large glycogen vacuole that is seen on the wet smear (stains brown with iodine) and on the permanent stained smear (vacuole will appear clear). Occasionally the vacuole will be so large that the organism will collapse on itself.

35. B The determination of egg viability is important in schistosomiasis; therefore, the miracidial hatching test is helpful in demonstrating the egg viability of *Schistosoma* species. Once the eggs are hatched, the living miracidium larvae will be visible in the water.

36. A Both *G. lamblia* and *C. parvum* have been implicated in waterborne outbreaks or diarrheal disease. These infections would result from the ingestion of *G. lamblia* cysts and/or *C. parvum* oocysts.

37. C With the advent of AIDS, the use of less invasive procedures for the diagnosis of *Pneumocystis* pneumonia, including the BAL method, has become much more common. These patients are often not able to tolerate an "open" procedure like the lung biopsy (more commonly used in non-AIDS patients).

38. C With the possible exception of direct inoculation infection in the eye, the microsporidia are thought to initially infect the gastrointestinal (GI) tract through ingestion of the infective spores; infections in other body sites are thought to disseminate from the GI tract.

39. Eye infections with *Acanthamoeba* spp have most commonly been traced to:
   A. Use of soft contact lenses
   B. Use of hard contact lenses
   C. Use of contaminated lens care solutions
   D. Failure to remove lenses while swimming

Microbiology/Apply knowledge of epidemiology/ Parasitology/2

40. Select the most sensitive recovery method for *Acanthamoeba* spp from lens care solutions or corneal biopsies.
   A. The trichrome staining method
   B. The use of monoclonal reagents for the detection of antibody
   C. The use of non-nutrient agar cultures seeded with *Escherichia coli*
   D. The Giemsa stain method

Microbiology/Apply knowledge of diagnostic procedures/Parasitology/2

41. The microsporidia are protozoans that have been implicated in human disease primarily in:
   A. Immunocompromised patients
   B. Pediatric patients under the age of 5
   C. Adult patients with congenital immunodeficiencies
   D. Patients who have been traveling in the tropics

Microbiology/Apply knowledge of pathogenesis and epidemiology/Parasitology/2

42. When staining *Isospora belli* oocysts with modified acid-fast stains, the important difference between these methods and the acid-fast stains used for acid-fast bacilli (AFB) is:
   A. The staining time is much longer with regular AFB acid-fast stains.
   B. The decolorizer is weaker than acid alcohol used for AFB decolorizing.
   C. A counterstain must be used for the modified methods.
   D. The stain is more concentrated when staining for AFB.

Microbiology/Apply knowledge of diagnostic procedures/Parasitology/2

43. The *incorrect* match between symptoms and disease is:
   A. Dysentery and amebiasis
   B. Malabsorption syndrome and giardiasis
   C. Cardiac involvement and chronic Chagas' disease
   D. Myalgias and trichuriasis

Microbiology/Apply knowledge of life cycle and pathogenesis/Parasitology/2

44. The *incorrect* match between organism and characteristic is:
   A. *Chilomastix mesnili* and Shepherd's crook and lemon shape
   B. *Plasmodium malariae* and "band troph"
   C. *Hymenolepis nana* and striated shell
   D. *Wuchereria bancrofti* and sheathed microfilariae

Microbiology/Apply knowledge of morphology/ Parasitology/2

Answers to Questions 39–44

39. C The majority of eye infections with *Acanthamoeba* spp have resulted from the use of contaminated eye care solutions, primarily the use of homemade saline. It is recommended that all solutions be discarded at the expiration date. Continued use may increase the risk of environmental contamination of the fluids.

40. C Currently, the most sensitive method for the recovery of *Acanthamoeba* spp from clinical specimens is the non-nutrient agar culture seeded with *E. coli*. The amoebae feed on the bacteria; both trophozoites and cysts can be recovered from the agar surface.

41. A Although the microsporidia have been known as pathogens in many groups of animals, their involvement in humans has primarily been in immunocompromised patients, especially those with AIDS. Microsporidia can be found in different tissues, and currently there are eight genera implicated in human disease.

42. B The decolorizer in modified acid-fast stains (Kinyoun's cold method, modified hot method) is usually 1%–3% sulfuric acid rather than the stronger acid alcohol used in the routine AFB stains.

43. D *T. trichiura* (whipworm) may cause diarrhea and occasionally dysentery in very heavy infections; however, the worms are confined to the intestine, and myalgias are not seen in this helminth infection.

44. C *H. nana* has a thin eggshell containing a six-hooked embryo (oncosphere) and polar filaments that lie between the eggshell and the embryo. The striated eggshell is generally associated with *Taenia* spp eggs.

45. The *incorrect* match between method and method objective is:
   A. Direct wet examination and detection of organism motility
   B. Knott's concentration and the recovery of operculated helminth eggs
   C. Baermann's concentration and the recovery of *Strongyloides*
   D. Permanent stained fecal smear and confirmation of protozoa

Microbiology/Apply knowledge of diagnostic procedures/Parasitology/2

46. The *incorrect* match between organism and characteristic is:
   A. *Dientamoeba fragilis* and tetrad karyosome in the nucleus
   B. *Toxoplasma gondii* and diagnostic serology
   C. *Echinococcus granulosus* and daughter cysts
   D. *Schistosoma mansoni* and egg with terminal spine

Microbiology/Apply knowledge of morphology/Parasitology/2

47. There are few procedures considered *stat* in parasitology. The most obvious situation would be:
   A. Ova and parasite examination for giardiasis
   B. Baermann's concentration for strongyloidiasis
   C. Blood films for malaria
   D. Culture of amoebic keratitis

Microbiology/Apply knowledge of pathogenesis and diagnostic procedures/Parasitology/3

48. An immunosuppressed man has several episodes of pneumonia, intestinal pain, sepsis with gram-negative rods, and a history of military service in Southeast Asia 20 years earlier. The most likely cause is infection with:
   A. *Trypanosoma cruzi*
   B. *Strongyloides stercoralis*
   C. *Naegleria fowleri*
   D. *Paragonimus westermani*

Microbiology/Apply knowledge of pathogenesis and life cycles/Parasitology/3

49. In a non-AIDS patient, the recommended clinical specimen for recovery of *Pneumocystis carinii* is the:
   A. Tracheobronchial aspirate
   B. Bronchoalveolar lavage (BAL)
   C. Bronchial brushings
   D. Open-lung biopsy

Microbiology/Apply knowledge of pathogenesis and life cycle/Parasitology/2

50. Eosinophilic meningoencephalitis is a form of larva migrans, causing fever, headache, stiff neck, and increased cells in the spinal fluid. It is generally a mild and self-limited infection and is caused by:
   A. *Necator americanus*
   B. *Angiostrongylus cantonensis*
   C. *Ancylostoma braziliense*
   D. *Strongyloides stercoralis*

Microbiology/Apply knowledge of pathogenesis and life cycle/Parasitology/2

Answers to Questions 45–50

45. **B** The Knott concentration is designed to allow the recovery of microfilariae from a blood specimen. Dilute formalin (2%) is used; blood is introduced into the formalin, the red cells lyse, and the sediment can be examined as a wet preparation or permanent stained smear (Giemsa or hematoxylin-based stain) for the presence of microfilariae.

46. **D** The egg of *S. mansoni* is characterized by a large lateral spine; *S. haematobium* has the characteristic terminal spine.

47. **C** The request for blood films for malaria should always be considered a *stat* request. Any laboratory providing these services should be available 24 hours a day, 7 days a week. In cases of *P. falciparum* malaria, any delay in diagnosing the infection could be fatal for the patient.

48. **B** A latent infection with *S. stercoralis* acquired years before may cause severe symptoms in the immunosuppressed patient ("autoinfective" capability of life cycle and migratory route through the body).

49. **D** In a non-AIDS patient, the specimen of choice for the diagnosis of *P. carinii* pneumonia is the open lung biopsy. The lung is the site of the organisms and the optimal specimen for organism recovery.

50. **B** Eosinophilic meningoencephalitis is a form of larva migrans and is caused by *A. cantonensis*, the rat lungworm. This Pacific area infection is associated with CSF symptoms and sometimes eye involvement.

51. "Cultures of parasites are different from bacterial cultures; no quality control is needed." This statement is:
  A. True, if two tubes of media are set up for each patient
  B. True, if the media are checked every 24 hours
  C. False, unless two different types of media are used
  D. False, and organism and media controls need to be set up

Microbiology/Apply knowledge of diagnostic procedures/Parasitology/2

52. Protozoan cysts were seen in a concentrate sediment and tentatively identified as *Entamoeba coli*. However, the organisms were barely visible on the permanent stained smear because:
  A. The organisms were actually not present in the concentrate sediment
  B. There were too few cysts to allow identification on the stained smear
  C. *E. coli* cysts were present but poorly fixed
  D. The concentrate and permanent stained smear were not from the same patient

Microbiology/Apply knowledge of fixatives and diagnostic procedures/Parasitology/3

53. When humans have hydatid disease, the causative agent and host classification are:
  A. *Echinococcus granulosus*—accidental intermediate host
  B. *Echinococcus granulosus*—definitive host
  C. *Taenia solium*—accidental intermediate host
  D. *Taenia solium*—definitive host

Microbiology/Apply knowledge of life cycles/Parasitology/3

54. A 45-year-old hunter developed fever, myalgia, and periorbital edema. He has a history of bear meat consumption. The most likely causative agent is:
  A. *Toxoplasma gondii*
  B. *Taenia solium*
  C. *Hymenolepis nana*
  D. *Trichinella spiralis*

Microbiology/Apply knowledge of pathogenesis and life cycles/Parasitology/3

55. In a condition resulting from the accidental ingestion of eggs, the human becomes the intermediate rather than the definitive host. The correct answer is:
  A. Trichinosis
  B. Cysticercosis
  C. Ascariasis
  D. Strongyloidiasis

Microbiology/Apply knowledge of pathogenesis and life cycles/Parasitology/3

56. A transplant patient on immunosuppressive drugs developed increasing shortness of breath and cyanosis. The most likely combination of disease and diagnostic procedure is:
  A. Strongyloidiasis and trichrome stain
  B. Pneumocystosis and silver stain
  C. Toxoplasmosis and Gram stain
  D. Paragonimiasis and wet preparation

Microbiology/Apply knowledge of pathogenesis and diagnostic procedures/Parasitology/3

Answers to Questions 51–56

51. **D** Duplicate cultures should be set up, and specific American Type Culture Collection (ATCC) strains should be cultured along with the patient specimens to confirm that the culture system is operating properly. This approach is somewhat different from that used in diagnostic bacteriology and mycology.

52. **C** As *E. coli* cysts mature, the cyst wall becomes more impenetrable to fixatives. Consequently, the cysts may be visible in the concentrate sediment but appear very distorted or pale on the permanent stained smear.

53. **A** The cause of hydatid disease is *E. granulosus*, and the human is classified as the accidental intermediate host. Infection occurs when humans accidentally ingest the eggs of *E. granulosus* and the hydatid cysts develop in the liver, lung, and other organs of the human instead of sheep (normal cycle).

54. **D** Bear meat is another excellent source of *T. spiralis*. In this case, the patient had evidently consumed poorly cooked bear meat, thus ingesting the encysted larvae of *T. spiralis*.

55. **B** The accidental ingestion of *T. solium* eggs can result in the disease called cysticercosis. The cysticerci will develop in a number of different tissues, including the brain, and the human is the accidental intermediate host.

56. **B** The fact that the patient has received a transplant, is on immunosuppressive drugs, and has pulmonary symptoms suggests *Pneumocystis* pneumonia.

57. After returning from a 2-year stay in India, a patient has eosinophilia, an enlarged left spermatic cord, and bilateral inguinal lymphadenopathy. The most likely clinical specimen and organism match is:
- **A.** Thin blood films and *Leishmania*
- **B.** Urine and concentration for *Trichomonas vaginalis*
- **C.** Thin blood films and *Babesia*
- **D.** Thick blood films and microfilariae

Microbiology/Apply knowledge of pathogenesis and diagnostic procedures/Parasitology/3

58. Patients with severe diarrhea should use "enteric precautions" to prevent nosocomial infections with:
- **A.** *Giardia lamblia*
- **B.** *Ascaris lumbricoides*
- **C.** *Cryptosporidium parvum*
- **D.** *Isospora belli*

Microbiology/Apply knowledge of pathogenesis and life cycles/Parasitology/3

59. A 60-year-old Brazilian patient with cardiac irregularities and congestive heart failure suddenly dies. Examination of the myocardium revealed numerous amastigotes, an indication that the cause of death was most likely:
- **A.** Leishmaniasis with *Leishmania donovani*
- **B.** Leishmaniasis with *Leishmania braziliense*
- **C.** Trypanosomiasis with *Trypanosoma gambiense*
- **D.** Trypanosomiasis with *Trypanosoma cruzi*

Microbiology/Apply knowledge of pathogenesis and life cycles/Parasitology/3

60. When malaria smears are requested, what patient information should be obtained?
- **A.** Diet, age, sex
- **B.** Age, antimalarial medication, sex
- **C.** Travel history, antimalarial medication, date of return to United States
- **D.** Fever patterns, travel history, diet

Microbiology/Apply knowledge of pathogenesis and life cycle, and epidemiology/Parasitology/3

61. In an outbreak of diarrheal disease traced to a municipal water supply, the most likely causative agents are:
- **A.** *Cryptosporidium parvum* and *Giardia lamblia*
- **B.** *Giardia lamblia* and *Isospora belli*
- **C.** *Isospora belli* and *Entamoeba histolytica*
- **D.** *Entamoeba histolytica* and *Dientamoeba fragilis*

Microbiology/Apply knowledge of life cycles and epidemiology/Parasitology/2

62. Within the United States, sporadic mini-outbreaks of diarrheal disease have been associated with the ingestion of strawberries, raspberries, fresh basil, and mesclun (baby lettuce leaves). The most likely causative agent is:
- **A.** *Dientamoeba fragilis*
- **B.** *Cyclospora cayetanensis*
- **C.** *Schistosoma mansoni*
- **D.** *Isospora belli*

Microbiology/Apply knowledge of life cycles and epidemiology/Parasitology/2

Answers to Questions 57–62

57. **D** Based on the history, the most relevant procedure to perform is the preparation and examination of thick blood films for the recovery and identification of microfilariae. The symptoms suggest early filariasis.

58. **C** *C. parvum* oocysts (unlike those of *I. belli*) are immediately infective when passed in stool, and nosocomial infections have been well documented with this coccidian.

59. **D** *T. cruzi*, the cause of Chagas' disease, has two forms within the human, the trypomastigote in the blood and the amastigote in the striated muscle (usually cardiac muscle and intestinal tract muscle).

60. **C** Travel history (areas of drug resistance), the date of return to the United States (primary versus relapse case), and history of antimalarial medication and illness (severe illness, few organisms on smear) are very important questions to ask. Without this information, a malaria diagnosis can be missed or delayed with severe patient consequences.

61. **A** Both *C. parvum* oocysts and *G. lamblia* cysts can be transmitted through contaminated water. Such outbreaks have been well documented.

62. **B** The coccidian *C. cayetanensis* has been linked to mini-outbreaks of diarrheal disease. Epidemiological evidence strongly implicates various berries, basil, and mesclun as likely causes. These outbreaks are very sporadic and tend to occur primarily in March through May.

63. Which of the following statements is true regarding onchocerciasis?
   A. The adult worm is present in the blood
   B. The microfilariae are in the blood during the late evening hours
   C. The diagnostic test of choice is the skin snip
   D. The parasite resides in the deep lymphatics

   Microbiology/Apply knowledge of life cycles and diagnostic procedures/Parasitology/2

64. The most prevalent helminth to infect humans is:
   A. *Enterobius vermicularis*, the pinworm
   B. *Ascaris lumbricoides*, the large intestinal roundworm
   C. *Taenia saginata*, the beef tapeworm
   D. *Schistosoma mansoni*, one of the blood flukes

   Microbiology/Apply knowledge of life cycles and epidemiology/Parasitology/1

65. A helminth egg is described as having terminal polar plugs. The most likely helminth is:
   A. Hookworm
   B. *Trichuris trichiura*
   C. *Fasciola hepatica*
   D. *Diphyllobothrium caninum*

   Microbiology/Apply knowledge of organism morphology/Parasitology/1

66. Ingestion of which of the following eggs will result in infection?
   A. *Strongyloides stercoralis*
   B. *Schistosoma japonicum*
   C. *Toxocara canis*
   D. *Opisthorchis sinensis*

   Microbiology/Apply knowledge of life cycles/Parasitology/2

67. *Plasmodium vivax* and *Plasmodium ovale* are similar because they:
   A. Exhibit Schüffner's dots and have a true relapse in the life cycle
   B. Have no malarial pigment and multiple rings
   C. Commonly have appliqué forms in the red cells
   D. Have true stippling, do not have a relapse stage, and infect old red cells

   Microbiology/Apply knowledge of life cycles and morphology/Parasitology/2

68. The term internal *autoinfection* can be associated with the following parasites:
   A. *Cryptosporidium parvum* and *Giardia lamblia*
   B. *Isospora belli* and *Strongyloides stercoralis*
   C. *Cryptosporidium parvum* and *Strongyloides stercoralis*
   D. *Giardia lamblia* and *Isospora belli*

   Microbiology/Apply knowledge of life cycles/Parasitology/2

69. Microsporidia have been identified as causing severe diarrhea, disseminated disease in other body sites, and ocular infections. Routes of infection have been identified as:
   A. Ingestion
   B. Inhalation
   C. Direct contamination from the environment
   D. Ingestion, inhalation, and direct contamination

   Microbiology/Apply knowledge of life cycles/Parasitology/2

Answers to Questions 63–69

63. **C** The adult *O. volvulus* reside in subcutaneous nodules, and the microfilariae are found in the fluids right under the outer layers of skin; thus the appropriate diagnostic test is the microscopic examination of skin snips for the presence of microfilariae.

64. **A** The pinworm, *E. vermicularis*, is the most common parasitic infection throughout the world, and the eggs are infective within just a few hours. Some have said, "You either had the infection as a child, have it now, or will have it again when you have children."

65. **B** The eggs of *T. trichiura* (the whipworm) have been described as being barrel-shaped with a thick shell and two polar plugs.

66. **C** The eggs of *T. canis* are infectious for humans and cause visceral larva migrans. These ascarid eggs of the dog can infect humans; the eggs hatch and the larvae wander through the deep tissues, occasionally the eye. In this case, the human becomes the accidental intermediate host.

67. **A** Both *P. vivax* and *P. ovale* infect young red cells, have true stippling (Schüffner's dots), contain malarial pigment, and have a true relapse stage in the life cycle.

68. **C** Both *C. parvum* and *S. stercoralis* have an internal autoinfection capability in their life cycles. This means that the cycle and infection can continue even after the patient has left the endemic area. In the case of *C. parvum*, the cycle continues in patients who are immunocompromised and unable to self-cure.

69. **D** Infectious routes for microsporidial infections have been confirmed as ingestion and inhalation of the spores; direct transfer of infectious spores from environmental surfaces to the eyes has also been reported.

70. An immunocompromised patient continues to have diarrhea after repeated ova and parasites (O&P) examinations (sedimentation concentration, trichrome permanent stained smear) were reported as negative; organisms that might be responsible for the diarrhea include:

A. *Cryptosporidium parvum*, *Giardia lamblia*, and *Isospora belli*

B. *Giardia lamblia*, microsporidia, and *Endolimax nana*

C. *Taenia solium* and *Endolimax nana*

D. *Cryptosporidium parvum* and microsporidia

Microbiology/Apply knowledge of life cycles and diagnostic procedures/Parasitology/3

Answer to Question 70

70. **D** Routine O&P examinations usually do not allow the detection of *C. parvum* oocysts and microsporidial spores; special stains are required. Modified acid-fast stains for *C. parvum* and modified trichrome stains for the microsporidial spores are recommended.

PROBLEM SOLVING IN MICROBIOLOGY AND PARASITOLOGY

7.12

1. An emergency room physician ordered a culture and sensitivity test on a catheterized urine specimen obtained from a 24-year-old female patient. A colony count was done and gave the following results after 24 hours:

> Blood agar plate = >100,000 col/mL of gram-positive cocci resembling staphylococci
>
> MacConkey agar = No growth
> CNA plate = Inhibited growth
> Hemolysis = Neg   Catalase = Positive
> Novobiocin = Resistant

This isolate is:
A. *Staphylococcus saprophyticus*
B. *Micrococcus luteus*
C. *Staphylococcus aureus*
D. *Streptococcus pyogenes*

Microbiology/Select methods/Reagents/Media/Culture/3

2. An outbreak of *Staphylococcus aureus* in the Nursery Department prompted the Infection Control Committee to proceed with an environmental screening procedure. The best screening media to use for this purpose would be:
A. CNA agar
B. THIO broth
C. Mannitol salt agar
D. PEA agar

Microbiology/Select methods/Reagents/Media/Culture/3

3. A listless 12-month-old boy with a fever of 103°F was taken to the emergency room. He had been diagnosed with an ear infection 3 days earlier. A spinal tap was performed, but only one tube of CSF was obtained from the lumbar puncture. The single tube of CSF should be submitted first to which department?
A. Chemistry
B. Microbiology
C. Hematology
D. Cytology/Histology

Microbiology/Select methods/Reagents/Media/Culture/3

4. A 65-year-old female outpatient was requested by her physician to submit a 24-hour urine specimen for protein and creatinine tests. He also requested testing for mycobacteria in the urine. Should the microbiology laboratory accept this 24-hour specimen for culture?
A. Yes, if the specimen is kept on ice
B. Yes, if the specimen is for aerobic culture only
C. No, the specimen must be kept at room temperature
D. No, the specimen is unsuitable for the recovery of mycobacteria

Microbiology/Select methods/Reagents/Media/Culture/3

Answers to Questions 1–4

1. **A** CNA inhibits most strains of *S. saprophyticus*. Therefore, blood agar should be used when culturing catheterized urine samples from young female patients. Most *S. saprophyticus* isolates are obtained from female patients 20–30 years old.

2. **C** The high concentration of NaCl (7.5%) in mannitol salt agar allows for the recovery of *S. aureus* from heavily contaminated specimens while inhibiting other organisms. Also, *S. aureus* ferments mannitol, thus allowing for easy detection of yellow-haloed colonies of *S. aureus* on red mannitol salt agar.

3. **B** Generally, tube 2 or 3 is submitted to the microbiology laboratory for culture and Gram stain smear. To ensure recovery of any pathogens and correct diagnosis without other bacterial contamination, immediate centrifugation and inoculation to the appropriate media as well as a Gram stain smear should be performed prior to delivery of the specimen to the chemistry department for testing.

4. **D** In general, a 24-hour urine is unsuitable for culture; a first morning specimen is best for the recovery of mycobacteria in the urine.

5. A lymph node biopsy obtained from a 30-year-old male patient was submitted to the microbiology laboratory for a culture and AFB smear for mycobacteria. The specimen was fixed in formalin. This specimen should be:
A. Accepted for AFB smear and cultured
B. Rejected
C. Held at room temperature for 24 hours and then cultured
D. Cultured for anaerobes only

Microbiology/Select methods/Reagents/Media/Culture/3

6. A 49-year-old man who traveled to Mexico City returned with a bad case of dysentery. Along with a fever, abdominal cramping and bloody, mucoidal, frequent stools, many WBCs were seen on the Gram's stain smear. Stool culture gave the following results:

Gram stain: gram-negative rods Lactose = +

Indole = +   Lysine decarboxylase = Neg

Urease = Neg   Motility = Neg

What is the most likely organism?
A. *Salmonella* spp
B. *Proteus mirabilis*
C. *Escherichia coli*
D. Enteroinvasive *E. coli* (EIEC)

Microbiology/Evaluate laboratory data to make identification/Gram-negative bacilli/3

7. An 80-year-old male patient was admitted to the hospital with a fever of 102°F. A sputum culture revealed many gram-negative rods on MacConkey agar and blood agar. The patient was diagnosed with pneumonia. The following biochemical results were obtained from the culture:

H₂S = Neg   Lactose = +

Urease = +   Citrate = +

Indole = +   VP = + Motility = Neg

Resistance to ampicillin and carbenicillin

What is the most likely identification?
A. *Klebsiella oxytoca*
B. *Proteus mirabilis*
C. *Escherichia coli*
D. *Klebsiella pneumoniae*

Microbiology/Evaluate laboratory data to make identification/Gram-negative bacilli/3

8. An immunocompromised 58-year-old female chemotherapy patient received two units of packed RBCs. The patient died 3 days later, and the report from the autopsy revealed that her death was due to septic shock. The blood bags were cultured, and the following results were noted:

Growth of aerobic gram-negative rods on both MacConkey and blood agars		
Lactose = Neg	Sucrose = +	Citrate = Neg
Indole = Neg	VP = Neg	H₂S = Neg
Urease = +	Motility 22°C = +	Motility 37°C = Neg

What is the most likely identification?
A. *Escherichia coli*
B. *Yersinia enterocolitica*
C. *Enterobacter cloacae*
D. *Citrobacter freundii*

Microbiology/Evaluate laboratory data to make identification/Gram-negative bacilli/3

Answers to Questions 5–8

5. **B** Specimens submitted for culture and recovery of any bacteria should be submitted without fixatives.

6. **D** EIEC, or enteroinvasive *E. coli*, produces dysentery similar to that of *Shigella*, with invasion and destruction of the intestinal mucosal epithelium. Leukocytes are seen on the Gram's stain smear. Adults who are travelers to foreign countries, especially Mexico, are at greatest risk.

7. **A** *K. oxytoca* is similar to *K. pneumoniae* except that the indole test is positive for *K. oxytoca*.

8. **B** *Y. enterocolitica* has been associated with fatal bacteremia and septic shock from contaminated blood transfusion products. The motility at room temperature is a clue to this identification.

9. A pediatric patient with severe bloody diarrhea who had been camping with his parents was admitted to the hospital with complications of hemolytic uremic syndrome (HUS). Several stool specimens were cultured with the following results noted:

> Gram stain smear = many gram-negative rods with no WBCs seen
>
> Blood agar = Normal flora
> MacConkey agar = Normal flora
>
> MacConkey agar with sorbitol = Many clear colonies (sorbitol negative)
>
> Hektoen agar = Normal flora
> Campy agar = No growth

What is the most likely identification?
A. *Yersinia* spp
B. *E. coli* O157:H7
C. *Salmonella* spp
D. *Shigella* spp

Microbioloby/Evaluation laboratory data to make identification/Gram-negative bacilli/3

10. A 14-year-old emergency room patient had been to the doctor's office 2 days previously with abdominal pain, diarrhea, and a low-grade fever. He was diagnosed with pseudoappendicular syndrome. Cultures from the stool containing blood and WBCs showed the following results:

> Aerobic gram-negative rods on MacConkey agar (clear colonies)
>
> Campy agar = No growth

Lactose = Neg	Sucrose = +	Citrate = Neg
Indole = Neg	VP = Neg	H$_2$S = Neg
Motility 37°C = Neg	Motility 22°C = +	Hektoen agar = NF

What is the most likely identification?
A. *Yersina enterocolitica*
B. *Salmonella* spp
C. *Shigella* spp
D. *Escherichia coli*

Microbiology/Evaluate laboratory data to make identification/Gram-negative nonfermenter/3

11. A sputum culture from a 13-year-old cystic fibrosis patient grew a predominance of short, gram-negative rods that tested oxidase-negative. On MacConkey, chocolate, and blood agar plates, the organism appeared to have a lavender-green pigment. Further testing showed:

Motility = +	DNase = +
Glucose = + (oxidative)	Maltose = + (oxidative)
Lysine decarboxylase = +	Esculin hydrolysis = +

What is the most likely identification?
A. *Stenotrophomonas (Xanthomonas) maltophilia*
B. *Acinetobacter baumanii*
C. *Pseudomonas aeruginosa*
D. *Burkholderia (P.) cepacia*

Microbiology/Evaluate laboratory data to make identification/Gram-negative nonfermenter/3

Answers to Questions 9–11

9. **B** *E. coli* O157:H7 is usually the most common isolate from bloody stools of the enterohemorrhagic *E. coli* (EHEC) group, which results from undercooked beef. These strains are waterborne and foodborne, and the infections from *E. coli* O157:H7 are greatest during the summer months in temperate climates.

10. **A** *Y. enterocolitica* is responsible for diseases in younger persons. Blood and leukocytes can be present in stools. Patients (usually teens) exhibiting appendicitis-like symptoms with lactose-negative colonies growing on MacConkey agar (small colonies at 24 hours, but larger colonies at 48 hours if incubated at room temperature) should be tested for the growth of *Y. enterocolitica*.

11. **A** *S. (X.) maltophilia* is the third most frequently isolated nonfermentative gram-negative rod in the clinical laboratory. Cystic fibrosis patients are at greater risk for infections because of previous antimicrobial treatment and recurrent pneumonia and because some strains may be colonizers.

12. A patient with a human bite wound on the right forearm arrived at the clinic for treatment. The wound was inflicted 36 hours earlier, and a culture was taken by the physician on duty. After 48 hours, the culture results were:

> Gram-stain smear = gram-negative straight, slender rods
>
> Chocolate agar plate = "Pitting" of the agar by small, yellow, opaque colonies

Oxidase = +	Motility = Neg
Catalase = Neg	Glucose = +
Growth in increased CO_2 = +	Growth at 42°C = Neg

What is the most likely identification of this facultative anaerobe?
A. *Pseudomonas aeruginosa*
B. *Acinetobacter baumannii*
C. *Kingella kingae*
D. *Eikenella corrodens*

Microbiology/Evaluate laboratory data to make identification/Unusual gram-negative bacteria/3

13. A dog bite wound to the thumb of a 20-year-old male patient became infected. The culture grew a gram-negative, slender rod, which was a facultative anaerobe. The following results were noted:

> Oxidase = +
>
> Motility = Neg
>
> Catalase = +
>
> Capnophilic = +

"Gliding" on the agar was noted.
What is the most likely identification?
A. *Pseudomonas aeruginosa*
B. *Capnocytophaga canimorsus*
C. *Acinetobacter baumannii*
D. *Proteus mirabilis*

Microbiology/Evaluate laboratory data to make identification/Unusual gram-negative bacteria/3

14. A patient exhibits fever, chills, abdominal cramps, diarrhea, vomiting, and bloody stools 10–12 hours after eating. Which organisms will most likely grow from this patient's stool culture?
A. *Salmonella* or *Yersinia* spp
B. *E. coli* O157:H7 or *Shigella* spp
C. *Staphylococcus aureus* or *Clostridium perfringens*
D. *Salmonella* or *Staphylococcus* spp

Microbiology/Identification gram-negative bacteria/3

15. When testing for coagulase properties, staphylococci isolates from a 67-year-old male diabetic patient showed a positive tube test (free coagulase). The organism should be identified as:
A. *Staphylococcus aureus*
B. *Staphylococcus haemolyticus*
C. *Staphylococcus saprophyticus*
D. *Micrococcus luteus*

Microbiology/Identification gram-positive cocci/2

16. An isolate of *Staphylococcus aureus* was cultured from an ulcer obtained from the leg of a diabetic 79-year-old female patient. The organism showed resistance to methicillin. Additionally, this isolate should be tested for resistance or susceptibility to:
A. Erythromycin
B. Gentamicin
C. Vancomycin
D. Kanamycin

Microbiology/Select antibiotic/Identification/3

17. An isolate recovered from a vaginal culture obtained from a 25-year-old female patient who is 8 months pregnant is shown to be a gram-positive cocci, catalase-negative, and β-hemolytic on blood agar. Which tests are needed for further identification?
A. Optochin, bile solubility, PYR
B. Bacitracin, CAMP, PYR
C. Methicillin, PYR, trehalose
D. Coagulase, glucose, PYR

Microbiology/Evaluate data to make identification/Gram-positive cocci/3

Answers to Questions 12–17

12. **D** *E. corrodens* is part of the normal flora of the human mouth and typically "pits" the agar. This organism is capnophilic (needing increased CO_2).

13. **B** *C. carnimorsus* is associated with septicemia or meningitis following dog bites. All *Capnocytophaga* strains are capnophilic, facultative anaerobic, gram-negative slender or filamentous rods with tapered ends.

14. **B** Both *E. coli* O157:H7 and *Shigella* spp are invasive and cause bloody stools.

15. **A** *S. aureus* is an opportunistic human pathogen. A wound or ulcer infected with *S. aureus* that is left untreated is especially detrimental to a diabetic patient.

16. **C** MRSA isolates are usually tested for susceptibility or resistance to vancomycin, a glycopeptide.

17. **B** Group B streptococci (*S. agalactiae*) are important pathogens and can cause serious neonatal infections. Women who are found to be heavily colonized vaginally with *S. agalactiae* pose a threat to the newborn, especially within the first few days after delivery. The infection acquired by the infant is associated with pneumonia.

18. Which organism is the most often recovered gram-positive cocci (catalase-negative) from a series of blood cultures obtained from individuals with endocarditis?
  A. *Streptococcus agalactiae*
  B. *Clostridium perfringens*
  C. *Enterococcus faecalis*
  D. *Pediococcus* spp

  Microbiology/Evaluate data to make identification/Gram-positive cocci/3

19. A presumptive diagnosis of gonorrhea can be made from an exudate from a 20-year-old emergency room patient if which of the following criteria are present?
  A. Smear of urethral exudate (male only) shows typical gram-negative, intracellular diplococci; growth of oxidase-positive gram-negative diplococci on selective agar (modified Thayer-Martin)
  B. Smear from vaginal area shows gram-negative diplococci; growth of typical colonies on blood agar
  C. Smear from rectum shows typical gram-negative diplococci; no growth on chocolate agar
  D. Growth of gram-negative cocci on MacConkey agar and blood agar

  Microbiology/Select/Reagents/Media/Gram-negative cocci identification/3

20. "Clue cells" are seen on a smear of vaginal discharge obtained from an 18-year-old female emergency room patient. This finding, along with a fishy odor (amine) after the addition of 10% KOH, suggests bacterial vaginosis caused by which organism?
  A. *Staphylococcus epidermidis*
  B. *Streptococcus agalactiae*
  C. *Gardnerella vaginalis*
  D. *E. coli*

  Microbiology/Evaluate laboratory data for identification/Gram-variable coccobacilli/3

21. A 1-month-old infant underwent a spinal tap to rule out bacterial meningitis. The CSF was cloudy, and the smear showed many pus cells and short gram-positive rods. After 18 hours, many colonies appeared on blood agar that resembled *Streptococcus* spp or *L. monocytogenes*. Which of the following preliminary tests should be performed on the colonies to best differentiate *L. monocytogenes* from *Streptococcus* spp?
  A. Hanging-drop motility (25°C) and catalase
  B. PYR and bacitracin

  C. Oxidase and glucose
  D. Coagulase and catalase

  Microbiology/Select methods/Reagents/Media/Culture/3

22. Acid-fast positive bacilli were recovered from the sputum of a 79-year-old man who had been treated for pneumonia. Which of the following test reactions after 3 weeks of incubation on Löwenstein-Jensen agar are consistent with *Mycobacterium tuberculosis*?
  A. Niacin = +   Nitrate reduction = +   Photochromogenic = Neg
  B. Niacin = Neg   Optochin = +   Catalase = +
  C. PYR = +   Urease = +   Bacitracin = +
  D. Ampicillin = Resistant   Penicillin = Resistant

  Microbiology/Evaluate laboratory data to make identification/Acid-fast bacilli/3

Answers to Questions 18–22

18. **C** *Enterococcus* (*Streptococcus*) *faecalis* is the cause of up to 20% of the bacterial endocarditis cases and is the most commonly encountered species in this condition.

19. **A** *N. gonorrhoeae* can be presumptively identified from a male patient only from the Gram stain and growth on selective agar. In female patients, the normal flora from a urethral swab may appear to be *N. gonorrhoeae* (gram-negative diplococci) but may be part of the normal flora, such as *Veillonella* spp (an anaerobic gram-negative cocci resembling *N. gonorrhoeae*).

20. **C** *G. vaginalis*, a gram-negative or gram-variable pleomorphic coccobacillus, causes bacterial vaginosis but is also present as part of the normal vaginal flora of women of reproductive age with a normal vaginal examination. "Clue cells" are vaginal epithelial cells with gram-negative or gram-variable coccobacilli attached to them.

21. **A** *L. monocytogenes* is catalase-positive and displays a "tumbling" motility at room temperature. *Streptococcus* spp are catalase-negative and non-motile.

22. **A** *M. tuberculosis* is niacin-positive and nonphotochromogenic. This organism takes up to 3 weeks to grow on selective agar.

23. Which biochemical tests should be performed in order to identify colorless colonies growing on MacConkey agar (swarming colonies on blood agar) from a catheterized urine specimen?
   A. Indole, ornithine decarboxylase, and urease
   B. Glucose, oxidase, and lactose utilization
   C. Phenylalanine deaminase and bile solubility
   D. H_2S and catalase

Microbiology/Evaluate laboratory data to make identification/Gram-negative bacilli/3

24. A gram-negative nonfermenter was isolated from a culture taken from a burn patient. Which of the following is the best choice of tests to differentiate *Pseudomonas aeruginosa* from *Acinetobacter* spp?
   A. Growth on MacConkey agar, catalase, growth at 37°C
   B. Oxidase, motility, growth at 42°C
   C. Growth on blood agar, oxidase, growth at 35°C
   D. String test and coagulase test

Microbiology/Select methods/Reagent/Media/ Identification nonfermentative gram-negatives/3

25. A *Haemophilus* spp, recovered from a throat culture obtained from a 59-year-old male patient undergoing chemotherapy, required hemin (X factor) and NAD (V factor) for growth. This species also hemolyzed horse erythrocytes on blood agar. What is the most likely species?
   A. *H. ducreyi*
   B. *H. parahaemolyticus*
   C. *H. haemolyticus*
   D. *H. aegyptius*

Microbiology/Evaluate laboratory data to make identification/Gram-negative coccobacilli/3

26. Large gram-positive bacilli (boxcar-shaped) were recovered from a blood culture taken from a 70-year-old female diabetic patient. The following results were recorded:

Aerobic growth = Neg   Anaerobic growth = +
Spores = Neg   Motility = Neg
Lecithinase = +   Hemolysis = β (double-zone)
GLC (volatile acids) = acetic acid and butyric acid

What is the most likely identification?
   A. *Clostridium perfringens*
   B. *Fusobacterium* spp
   C. *Bacteroides* spp
   D. *Clostridium sporogenes*

Microbiology/Evaluate laboratory data to make identification/Anaerobic gram-positive bacilli/3

27. Anaerobic gram-negative rods were recovered from the blood of a patient after gallbladder surgery. The bacteria grew well on agar containing 20% bile but was resistant to kanamycin and vancomycin. What is the most likely identification?

   A. *Clostridium perfringens*
   B. *Bacteroides fragilis* group
   C. *Prevotella* spp
   D. *Porphyromonas* spp

Microbiology/Evaluate laboratory data to make identification/Anaerobic gram-negataive bacilli/3

28. In Breakpoint Antimicrobial Drug Testing, interpretation of susceptible (S), intermediate (I), and resistant (R) refers to testing antibiotics by using:
   A. The amount needed to cause bacteriostasis
   B. Only the specific concentrations necessary to report S, I, or R
   C. A MIC of 64 μg/mL
   D. A dilution of drug that is one tube less than the toxic level

Microbiology/Select methods/Reagents/Media/Antibiotic testing/2

Answers to Questions 23–28

23. **A** A swarmer on blood agar would most likely be a *Proteus* spp. A lactose nonfermenter and swarmer that is often isolated from urinary tract infections is *P. mirabilis*.

24. **B** *P. aeruginosa* has a distinctive grape odor. The best choice of tests is:

	42° C Growth	Oxidase	Motility
P. aeruginosa	+	+	+
Acinetobacter spp	+/Neg	Neg	Neg

25. **C** *H. haemolyticus* requires both X and V factors for growth and lyses horse erythrocytes.

26. **A** *C. perfringens* is an anaerobic gram-positive rod that is often isolated from the tissue of patients with gas gangrene (myonecrosis). Spore production is not usually seen with this organism, which may also stain gram-negative.

27. **B** *B. fragilis* is the most often isolated gram-negative anaerobic bacillus. It is resistant to many antibiotics. A good screening agar is a 20% bile plate that does not support the growth of *Prevotella* spp or *Porphyromonas* spp.

28. **B** Breakpoint susceptibility testing is done by selecting only two appropriate drug concentrations for testing. If the results show growth at both concentrations, then resistance is indicated; growth only at the lower concentration signifies an intermediate result; no growth at either concentration is interpreted as susceptible.

29. A CSF sample obtained from a 2-week-old infant with suspected bacterial meningitis grew gram-negative rods on blood and chocolate agars. The following results were noted:

MacConkey agar = No growth	ONPG = +
Glucose (open) OF = +	Urease = Neg
Glucose (closed) OF = Neg	Catalase = +
Indole = +	Oxidase = +
Motility = Neg	Pigment = Yellow
42° C growth = Neg	

What is the correct identification?
A. *Pseudomonas aeruginosa*
B. *Chryseobacterium meningosepticum*
C. *Acinetobacter baumannii*
D. *E. coli*

Microbiology/Evaluate laboratory data for identification/Gram-negative rods/3

30. During the summer break, several middle-aged elementary school teachers from the same school district attended a 3-day seminar in Chicago. Upon returning home, three female teachers from the group were hospitalized with pneumonia, flulike symptoms, and a nonproductive cough. Routine testing of sputum samples revealed normal flora. Further testing using buffered CYE agar with L-cysteine and α-ketoglutarate in 5% CO_2 produced growth of opaque colonies that stained faintly, showing thin gram-negative rods. What is the most likely identification?
A. *Legionella pneumophila*
B. *Haemophilus influenzae*
C. *Eikenella corrodens*
D. *Streptococcus pneumoniae*

Microbiology/Evaluate laboratory data for identification/Gram-negative rods/3

31. A vancomycin-resistant gram-positive coccobacillus resembling the streptococcus viridans group was isolated from the blood of a 42-year-old female patient undergoing a bone marrow transplant. The PYR and leucine aminopeptidase (LAP) tests were negative. The following results were noted:

Catalase = Neg	CAMP = Neg
Esculin hydrolysis = Neg	Gas from glucose = +
Hippurate hydrolysis = Neg	6.5% salt broth = Neg

What is the correct identification?
A. *Leuconostoc* spp
B. *Enterococcus* spp
C. *Staphylococcus* spp
D. *Micrococcus* spp

Microbiology/Evaluate laboratory data to make identification/Aerobic gram-positive coccobacilli/3

32. A catalase-negative, gram-positive coccus resembling staphylococci (clusters on the Gram-stained smear) was recovered from three different blood cultures obtained from a 60-year-old patient diagnosed with endocarditis. The following test results were noted:

PYR = Neg	LAP = Neg (V)
Esculin hydrolysis = Neg	6.5% Salt broth = Neg
Vancomycin = Sensitive	CAMP test = Neg

What is the correct identification?
A. *Leuconostoc* spp
B. *Gemella* spp
C. *Enterococcus* spp
D. *Micrococcus* spp

Microbiology/Evaluate laboratory data for identification/Gram-positive cocci/3

Answers to Questions 29–32

29. B *C. meningosepticum* is a well-known cause of neonatal meningitis. It will grow well on chocolate agar, producing yellow pigmented colonies.

30. A *L. pneumophila* is the cause of pneumonia and can occur as part of an epidemic sporadically or nosocomially or may be community acquired. The appearance of mottled, cut-glass colonies on buffered CYE agar under low power and the use of a direct immunofluorescence technique on sputum samples determine the presence of *L. pneumophila*. The most common environmental sites for recovery are shower heads, faucets, water tanks, and air-conditioning systems.

31. A *Leuconostoc* spp are vancomycin-resistant opportunistic pathogens and follow invasive procedures. They are often recovered from positive neonatal blood cultures resulting from colonization during delivery.

32. B *Gemella* spp are often recovered from patients with endocarditis and meningitis. On the Gram's stain, they resemble staphylococci morphologically but are catalase-negative.

33. An immunocompromised patient with prior antibiotic treatment grew aerobic gram-positive cocci from several clinical specimens that were cultured. The organism was vancomycin-resistant and catalase-negative. Additional testing proved negative for enterococci. What other groups of organisms might be responsible?

A. *Leuconostoc* spp and *Pediococcus* spp
B. *Streptococcus pyogenes* and *Streptococcus agalactiae*
C. *Micrococcus* spp and *Gemella* spp
D. *Clostridium* spp and *Streptococcus bovis*

Microbiology/Evaluate laboratory data for identification/Gram-positive cocci/3

34. A catalase-positive, gram-positive coccus (clusters on Gram's stain smear) grew pale yellow, creamy colonies on 5% sheep blood agar. The specimen was recovered from pustules on the face of a 5-year-old girl with impetigo. The following test reactions indicate which organism?

Glucose = + (Fermentation)
Oxidase = Neg

PYR = Neg   Bacitracin = Sensitive
Lysostaphin = Sensitive

A. *Micrococcus* spp
B. *Streptococcus* spp
C. *Enterococcus* spp
D. *Staphylococcus* spp

Microbiology/Evaluate laboratory data for identification/Gram-positive cocci/3

35. A wound (skin lesion) specimen obtained from a newborn grew predominantly β-hemolytic colonies of gram-positive cocci on 5% sheep blood agar. The newborn infant was covered with small skin eruptions that gave the appearance of a "scalding of the skin." The gram-positive cocci proved to be catalase-positive. Which tests should follow for the appropriate identification?

A. Optochin, bile solubility, PYR
B. Coagulase, glucose fermentation, DNase
C. Bacitracin, PYR, 6.5% salt broth
D. CAMP, bile-esculin, 6.5% salt broth

Microbiology/Evaluate laboratory data to make identification/Gram-positive cocci/3

36. A 20-year-old female patient entered the emergency clinic complaining of abdominal pain, fever, and a burning sensation during urination. An above normal WBC count along with pus cells and bacteria in the urine specimen prompted the emergency physician to order a urine culture. The colony count reported for this patient revealed >100,000 col/mL of a non-hemolytic, catalase-negative, gram-positive organism on 5% sheep blood agar. The following test results indicate which organism?

PYR = +   Bile Esculin = +
6.5% Salt Broth = + growth
Bacitracin = Neg   Optochin = Neg

A. *Enterococcus faecalis*
B. *Streptococcus pyogenes*
C. *Streptococcus agalactiae*
D. *Streptococcus bovis*

Microbiology/Evaluate laboratory data to make identification/Gram-positive cocci/3

Answers to Questions 33–36

33. **A** *Leuconostoc* spp and *Pediococcus* spp are vancomycin-resistant, catalase-negative, gram-positive aerobic organisms recovered from immunosuppressed patients.

34. **D** *S. aureus* is a usual cause of skin infections and a common cause of cellulitis, impetigo, postsurgical wounds, and scalded skin syndrome in infants.

35. **B** *S. aureus* is the cause of "scalded skin" syndrome in newborn infants. The production of a potent exotoxin (exfoliatin) causes the epidermis to slough off, leaving the newborn's skin with a red, raw texture or a burned, scalded look.

36. **A** *E. faecalis* gives a positive reaction to the PYR test and is often implicated in urinary tract infections (UTIs). It is part of the normal flora of the female genitourinary tract and the human gastrointestinal tract. On 5% sheep blood agar, *E. faecalis* colonies may appear as nonhemolytic, α-hemolytic or β-hemolytic colonies, depending on the strain.

37. A sputum specimen from an 89-year-old male patient with suspected bacterial pneumonia grew a predominance of gram-positive cocci displaying alpha-hemolysis on 5% sheep blood agar. The colonies appeared donut-shaped and mucoidy and tested negative for catalase. The most appropriate tests for a final identification are:
   A. Coagulase, glucose fermentation, lysostaphin
   B. Penicillin, bacitracin, CAMP
   C. Optochin, bile solubility, PYR
   D. Bile esculin, hippurate hydrolysis

Microbiology/Evaluate laboratory data to make identification/Gram-positive cocci/3

38. A tissue biopsy specimen of the stomach was obtained from a 38-year-old male patient diagnosed with gastric ulcers. The specimen was transported immediately and processed for culture and histology. At 5 days, the culture produced colonies of gram-negative (curved) bacilli on chocolate and *Brucella* agar with 5% sheep blood. The cultures were held at 35°–37°C in a microaerophilic atmosphere. The colonies tested positive for urease. The most likely identification is?
   A. *E. coli*
   B. *Helicobacter pylori*
   C. *Enterococcus faecalis*
   D. *Streptococcus bovis*

Microbiology/Evaluate data for identification/Gram-negative curved rods/3

39. A catalase-positive, gram-positive short rod was recovered from the blood of a prenatal patient. The organism appeared on 5% sheep blood as white colonies surrounded by a small zone of beta-hemolysis. The following tests were performed, indicating the patient was infected with which organism?

   Motility = + (tumbling on wet prep) room temperature

   Motility = + (umbrella-shape on semi-solid agar) room temperature

   Glucose = + (fermentation)

   Esculin = +

   Voges-Proskauer = +

   A. *Listeria monocytogenes*
   B. *Streptococcus agalactiae*
   C. *Streptococcus pyogenes*
   D. *Lactobacillus* spp

Microbiology/Evaluate data for identification/Gram-positive short rods/3

Answers to Questions 37–39

37. C *S. pneumoniae* colonies appear as α-hemolytic "donut" shaped colonies on 5% sheep blood agar. The mucoid colonies may appear "wet" or "watery" due to the capsule surrounding the organism. The Gram-stained smear reveals lancet-shaped gram-positive cocci in pairs surrounded by a clear area (the capsule). To differentiate the viridans streptococci from *S. pneumoniae*, the most appropriate test is the optochin disk test. *S. pneumoniae* on blood agar are susceptible to optochin but viridans streptococci are resistant.

38. B *H. pylori* is not easily cultured for growth and identification. Tissue samples should be transported in appropriate media and tested immediately. Other means of successful identification are rapid urease test on biopsy material; urea breath test; and serological tests for the detection of antibodies to *H. pylori* by ELISA and IFA procedures.

39. A *L. monocytogenes* colonies recovered from blood and CSF display a narrow zone of β-hemolysis on 5% sheep blood agar which often mimics group B β-hemolytic streptococci. A catalase test and a Gram stain will differentiate the two organisms. *L. monocytogenes* are catalase-positive and are motile (tumbling motility at room temperature) as well as rod-shaped instead of cocci-shaped.

40. An emergency room physician suspected *Coryne-bacterium diphtheriae* when examining the sore throat of an exchange student from South America. What is the appropriate media for the culture of the nasopharyngeal swab obtained from the patient?
  A. Chocolate agar
  B. Thayer-Martin agar
  C. Tinsdale medium
  D. MacConkey agar

Microbiology/Evaluate data for identification/ Gram–positive rods/2

41. A 25-year-old pregnant patient complained of vaginal irritation. Cultures taken for STDs proved negative. A Gram-stained vaginal smear revealed many epithelial cells with gram-variable short rods (coccobacilli) covering the margins. What is the most likely cause of the vaginosis?
  A. Group B streptococci spp
  B. *Gardnerella vaginalis*
  C. *Staphylococcus aureus*
  D. *Staphylococcus saprophyticus*

Microbiology/Evaluate data for identification/Gram-variable rods/3

42. A 50 year-old male transplant patient was experiencing neurological difficulties after a pulmonary infection. A spinal tap revealed a cloudy CSF with a Gram-stained smear revealing gram-positive long beaded bacilli. An acid-fast smear showed filamentous partially acid-fast bacilli. What is the most likely identification of the organism?
  A. *Nocardia asteroides*
  B. *Mycobacterium avium*
  C. *Mycobacterium bovis*
  D. *Legionella* spp.

Microbiology/Evaluate data for identification/Gram-positive bacilli/3

43. A 22-year-old pregnant woman (third trimester) entered the emergency room complaining of diarrhea, fever, and other flulike symptoms. Blood cultures were ordered along with a urine culture. After 24 hours, the urine culture was negative, but the blood cultures revealed a gram-positive short rod that grew aerobically on blood agar. The colonies were small and smooth, resembling a *Streptococcus* spp with a small narrow zone of β-hemolysis. The following test results indicate which organism?

> Motility = + (Wet mount = Tumbling)
>
> Catalase = +
>
> Glucose = + (Acid)   Esculin hydrolysis = +

  A. *Listeria monocytogenes*
  B. *Streptococcus pneumoniae*
  C. *Streptococcus agalactiae*
  D. *Corynebacterium* spp

Microbiology/Evaluate laboratory data for identification/Gram-positive rod/3

Answers to Questions 40–43

40. **C** *C. diphtheriae*, unlike other *Corynebacterium* spp, are not part of the normal flora of the human nasopharynx. Exposure through direct contact (respiratory or cutaneous lesions) is the most likely mode of transmission. Underdeveloped countries are the prime places for exposure to *C. diphtheriae*. The diagnosis is made more rapidly when the examining physician alerts the laboratory that diphtheria is suspected, so that Tinsdale agar or other media containing tellurite salts can be used for culture. *Corynebacterium* will grow on blood and chocolate agars, but Tinsdale agar is the preferred culture medium because the potassium tellurite in the agar causes *C. diphtheriae* to produce brown colonies surrounded by a brown halo. The halo effect is seen with *C. diphtheriae*, *C. ulcerans*, and *C. pseudotuberculosis* but not with other *Corynebacterium* or with other pigmented colonies growing on Tinsdale agar such as *Streptococcus* or *Staphylococcus* spp.

41. **B** *G. vaginalis* is part of the normal flora (anorectal) of adults and children. Clue cells (vaginal epithelial cells with gram-variable coccobacilli on the cell margins) are seen in vaginal washings and the organism grows slowly on chocolate agar, 5% sheep blood agar, and V-agar.

42. **A** *N. asteroides* is a gram-positive, beaded, long bacillus and is partially acid-fast. It is an intracellular pathogen that grows in human cells. Immunocompromised patients are susceptible to infections, especially pulmonary, which then disseminate to other organs, often proving fatal.

43. **A** Early detection in pregnant women is very important when dealing with *L. monocytogenes*. If it is not detected and treated, infection of the fetus, resulting in stillbirth, abortion, or premature birth may result. Detection can also be made postpartum by culturing the CSF, blood, amniotic fluid, and respiratory secretions of the neonate.

44. Anaerobic gram-positive, spore-forming bacilli were recovered from the feces of a chemotherapy patient with severe diarrhea. The patient had undergone antibiotic therapy 1 week prior. The fecal culture produced growth only on the CCFA plate. No aerobic growth of normal flora was seen after 48 hours. The following results were noted:

Kanamycin = Sensitive	Vancomycin = Sensitive	Colistin = Resistant
Lecithinase = Neg	Lipase = Neg	Nitrate = Neg
Indole = Neg	Urease = Neg	Catalase = Neg
Spores = +	CCFA agar = Growth of yellow, "ground-glass" colonies that fluoresce chartreuse (yellow-green)	

What is the correct identification?
A. *Clostridium perfringens*
B. *Clostridium tetani*
C. *Clostridium sordellii*
D. *Clostridium difficile*

Microbiology/Evaluate laboratory data for identification/ Anaerobic gram-positive rods/3

45. Anaerobic gram-positive diphtheroids (nonspore formers) were cultured from two separate blood culture bottles (at 5 days) obtained from a 25-year-old patient admitted to the hospital with dehydration, diarrhea, and other flulike symptoms. Four other blood culture bottles did not grow any organisms at 7 days and were discarded. The following results were obtained from the recovered anaerobe:

Indole = +	Nitrate = +
Catalase = +	Kanamycin = Sensitive
Vancomycin = Sensitive	Colistin = Resistant
Major acid from PYG broth by GLC = Propionic acid	

What is the correct identification?
A. *Eubacterium lentum*
B. *Propionibacterium acnes*
C. *Actinomyces* spp
D. *Peptostreptococcus* spp

Microbiology/Evaluate laboratory data for identification/ Anaerobic gram-positive rods/3

46. Anaerobic gram-positive bacilli with subterminal spores were recovered from several blood cultures obtained from a patient diagnosed with a malignancy of the colon. The following results were recorded:

Indole = Neg	Growth on blood agar = Swarming colonies
Urease = Neg	Lipase = Neg
Catalase = Neg	Lecithinase = Neg

What is the correct identification?
A. *Clostridium septicum*
B. *Clostridium perfringens*
C. *Clostridium sordellii*
D. *Proprionibacterium acnes*

Microbiology/Evaluate laboratory data for identification/Anaerobic gram-positive rods/3

Answers to Questions 44–46

44. **D** The overgrowth of *C. difficile* in the bowel is the cause of antimicrobial-associated colitis. Culturing for *C. difficile* is the least specific but the most sensitive method to detect possible disease related to *C. difficile*. A characteristic "horse-stable" odor is noted on CCFA growing *C. difficile*.

45. **B** *P. acnes* is a diphtheroid (pleomorphic rod) that may appear to branch on the Gram-stained smear. It is one of the most common organisms isolated from blood cultures and is often a contaminant. Abundant propionic acid is produced by GLC.

46. **A** *C. septicum* is often recovered from patients with malignancies or other diseases of the colon, especially the cecum. The following chart defines the swarming *Clostridium* spp.

	Indole	Urease	Spores
C. septicum	Neg	Neg	Subterminal
C. tetani	–/+	Neg	Terminal
C. sordellii	+	+	Subterminal

47. Anaerobic gram-negative bacilli were recovered from fluid obtained from drainage of a postsurgical abdominal wound. The following test results were recorded:

Kanamycin = Resistant	Vancomycin = Resistant	Colistin = Resistant
Growth on 20% bile plate = +	Pigment = Neg	Indole = V (Neg)
Nitrate = Neg	Urease = Neg	Lipase = Neg

What is the correct identification?

A. *Prevotella* spp
B. *Bacteroides fragilis* group
C. *Porphyromonas* spp
D. *Clostridium* spp

Microbiology/Evaluate laboratory data for identification/Anaerobic gram-negative rods/3

48. Anaerobic, nonpigmented, gram-negative rods were recovered from an anaerobic blood agar plate after 48 hours of incubation. The Gram-stained smear showed thin bacilli with pointed ends. The colonies on blood agar had the appearance of dry, irregular, white breadcrumb-like morphology with greening of the agar. The following reactions were noted:

Kanamycin = Sensitive	Vancomycin = Resistant	Colistin = Sensitive
Growth on 20% bile agar = Neg	Nitrate = Neg	Indole = +
Catalase = Neg	Lipase = Neg	Urease = Neg

What is the correct identification?

A. *Fusobacterium nucleatum*
B. *Bacteroides fragilis*
C. *Clostridium perfringens*
D. *Peptostreptococcus* spp

Microbiology/Evaluate laboratory data for identification/Anaerobic gram-negative rods/3

49. A 2-month-old infant in good health was scheduled for a checkup at the pediatrician's office. After arriving for the appointment, the mother noted white patches on the baby's tongue and in his mouth. The baby constantly used a pacifier. What is the most likely organism causing the white patches?

A. *Cryptococcus neoformans*
B. *Candida albicans*
C. *Aspergillus fumigatus*
D. None of the above

Microbiology/Evaluate laboratory data to make identification/Mycology/3

50. A 69-year-old male patient who was a cigarette smoker visited the doctor's office complaining of a cough and congestion of the lungs. Routine cultures of early morning sputum ($\times$ 3) for bacteria as well as for AFB revealed no pathogens. A fungal culture was also ordered that grew the following on Sabouraud dextrose agar after 3 days:

Hyphae = septate with dichotomous branching

Spores = produced by conidial heads with numerous conidia

Colonies = velvety or powdery, white at first, then turning dark greenish to gray (reverse = white to tan)

Vesicle = holding phialides usually on upper two thirds only

What is the most likely identification?
A. *Aspergillus niger*
B. *Absidia* spp
C. *Mucor* spp
D. *Aspergillus fumigatus*

Microbiology/Evaluate laboratory data to make identification/Mycology/3

Answers to Questions 47–50

47. **B** The *B. fragilis* group is a dominant part of the indigenous flora of the large bowel and is recovered most commonly from postoperative abdominal fluids. The *B. fragilis* group is more resistant to antibiotics and is not pigmented. *Prevotella* and *Porphyromonas* spp are pigmented.

48. **A** A slender gram-negative rod with pointed ends that does not grow on 20% bile agar rules out *B. fragilis* group and indicates *F. nucleatum*.

49. **B** *C. albicans* is the common cause of oral thrush involving the mucocutaneous membranes of the mouth. *C. albicans* is part of the normal flora of the skin, mucous membranes, and gastrointestinal tract.

50. **D** *A. fumigatus* is the cause of aspergillosis and involves the organism colonizing the mucous plugs in the lung. This is called allergic aspergillosis and is characterized by a high titer of IgE antibody to *Aspergillus*. Invasive aspergillosis seen in neutropenic patients exhibits sinusitis, and is disseminated throughout the body.

51. A young male patient with a fungus of the feet visited the podiatrist for relief from the itching. A culture was sent to the microbiology laboratory that grew after 8 days on Sabouraud dextrose agar. Colonies were powdery pink with concentric and radial folds, with the reverse side showing brownish-tan to red in color. Other observations were:

Hyphae = Septate	Macroconidia = Cigar-shaped, thin-walled with 1–6 cells
Urease = +	Microconidia = Round and clustered on branched conidiophores
Red pigment on cornmeal (1% dextrose) = Neg	In vitro hair perforation = +

The most likely identification is:
A. *Trichophyton mentagrophytes*
B. *Trichophyton rubrum*
C. *Candida albicans*
D. *Aspergillus niger*

Microbiology/Evaluate laboratory data to make identification/Mycology/3

52. A 79-year-old female nursing home patient was admitted to the hospital with a fever and central nervous system dysfunction. Routine blood work and blood cultures were ordered. After 48 hours, the blood cultures revealed a budding yeast. The following tests performed from Sabouraud dextrose agar (after 3 days of growth) showed:

Germ tube = Neg growth	Birdseed agar = Brown
Urease = +	Pseudohyphae = Neg
Blastospores = +	Chlamydospores = Neg
Arthrospores = Neg	Assimilation agar = + (dextrose, sucrose, maltose)

What is the most likely identification?
A. *Candida albicans*
B. *Cryptococcus laurentii*
C. *Cryptococcus neoformans*
D. *Candida tropicalis*

Microbiology/Evaluate laboratory data for identification/Mycology/3

53. A dehydrated 25-year-old male patient was admitted to the hospital with symptoms similar to those of chronic fatigue syndrome. Serological testing proved negative for recent streptococcal infection, Epstein-Barr virus, and hepatitis. Which of the following viral serological tests should help with a possible diagnosis?
A. CMV
B. Echovirus
C. Respiratory syncytial virus
D. Measles virus

Microbiology/Select tests for identification/Virology/3

54. A nursing student working in the emergency room accidentally stuck herself with a needle after removing it from an intravenous set taken from a suspected drug user. The best course of action, after reporting the incident to her supervisor, is to:
A. Test the student for HIV virus if flu-like symptoms develop in 2-4 weeks
B. Immediately test the patient and the student for HIV using an EIA or ELISA test
C. Perform a Western blot assay on the student's serum
D. Draw blood from the student only and freeze it for further testing

Microbiology/Evaluate testing for viral testing/Virology/3

Answers to Questions 51–54

51. A *T. mentagrophytes*, a common cause of athletes' foot, is sometimes confused with *T. rubrum*, the most common dermatophyte to infect humans. The differential tests are shown in the chart below.

	Urease	Hair Perforation	Red Pigment on Cornmeal (1% dextrose)
T. menta-grophytes	+	+	Neg
T. rubrum	Neg or W	Neg	+

52. C *C. neoformans* produces brown colonies on birdseed agar, is urease-positive, and produces only blastospores. Immunosuppressed patients are vulnerable to this organism.

53. A CMV infection in young adults causes a self-limited mononucleosis syndrome. CMV infections are common and usually self-limited, except in neonates and immunosuppressed patients, in whom they may cause a life-threatening situation.

54. B With the permission of the patient (state law may require him or her to sign a consent form) and counseling of the student nurse, the appropriate course of action is to test the patient for HIV using a screening test (EIA or ELISA). The student should also be baseline tested. If the test result is positive for the patient, the student is administered the appropriate antiviral drug(s) immediately or within 2 hours of the incident. Confirmatory testing is done on any positive HIV tests.

55. A 30-year-old female patient complained of vaginal irritation and symptoms (fever, dysuria, and inguinal lymphadenopathy) associated with sexually transmitted disease (STD). Examination showed extensive lesions in the genital area. *Chlamydia* spp testing, *Neisseria gonorrhoeae*, and *Gardnerella vaginalis* cultures were negative. Rapid plasma reagin (RPR) testing was also negative. What is the next line of testing?
  A. Darkfield examination
  B. Herpes simplex testing
  C. *Trichomonas* spp testing
  D. Group B streptococcal testing

Microbiology/Evaluate tesing for identification/ Virology/3

56. A patient is being seen in the emergency room for a low-grade fever, headache, and general malaise after returning from Africa on a photographic safari. The physician has requested blood for malaria; the laboratory would like to have patient information regarding:
  A. Specific travel history and body temperature every 4 hours
  B. Liver function tests and prophylactic medication history
  C. Transfusion history and body temperature every 4 hours
  D. Prophylactic medication history and specific travel history

Microbiology/Apply knowledge of life cycles, diagnostic techniques, and clinical presentation/Parasitology/3

57. Examination of a modified acid-fast stained fecal smear reveals round structures measuring approximately 8–10 μm, some of which are stained and some of which are not. They do not appear to show any internal morphology. The patient is symptomatic with diarrhea, and the cause may be:
  A. *Blastocystis hominis*
  B. Polymorphonuclear leukocytes
  C. *Cyclospora cayetanensis*
  D. Large yeast cells

Microbiology/Apply knowledge of the morphology of artifacts, organism life cycles, and diagnostic methods/ Parasitology/3

58. A patient has been diagnosed as having amebiasis but continues to be asymptomatic. The physician has asked for an explanation and recommendations regarding follow-up. Suggestions should include:
  A. Consideration of *Entamoeba histolytica* versus *Entamoeba dispar*
  B. A request for an additional three stools for culture

  C. Initiating therapy, regardless of the patient's asymptomatic status
  D. Performance of barium x-ray studies

Microbiology/Apply knowledge of the morphology of organisms and pathogenesis/Parasitology/3

Answers to Questions 55–58

55. **B** Herpes genitalis is an infection caused by HSV-2. Symptomatic primary herpes by HSV-2 is responsible for about 85% of herpes infections. HSV-1 (causing the other 15%) does not involve recurring infections of herpes and causes fever blisters. HSV-2 causes 99% of recurrent genital herpes.

56. **D** If the patient has malaria and has been taking prophylaxis (often sporadically), the number of parasites on the blood smear will be reduced and examination of routine thick and thin blood films should be more exhaustive. Also specific geographic travel history may help to determine whether chloroquine-resistant *Plasmodium falciparum* may be a factor.

57. **C** One of the newer coccidian parasites, *C. cayetanensis*, has been implicated in cases of human diarrhea. The recommended stains are modified acid-fast stains, and the organisms are quite variable in their staining characteristics. The oocysts are immature when passed (no internal morphology) and they measure about 8–10 μm.

58. **A** It is now well established that *E. histolytica* is being used to designate pathogenic zymodemes (strains of former "*E. histolytica*" based on isoenzyme analysis patterns), whereas *E. dispar* is now being used to designate nonpathogenic zymodemes. However, unless trophozoites containing ingested red blood cells (*E. histolytica*) are seen, the two organisms cannot be differentiated on the basis of morphology. Based on this information, there are now two separate species, only one of which (*E. histolytica*) is pathogenic. Because this patient is asymptomatic, the organisms seen in the fecal smears are probably *E. dispar* (nonpathogen); the laboratory report should have said "*Entamoeba histolytica/E. dispar*"—unable to differentiate on the basis of morphology unless trophozoites are seen to contain ingested RBCs (*E. histolytica*).

59. Although a patient is strongly suspected of having giardiasis and is still symptomatic, three routine stool examinations (O&P exam) have been performed correctly and reported as negative. Biopsy confirmed the patient had giardiasis. Reasons for these findings may include:

A. The patient was coinfected with several bacterial species

B. *Giardia lamblia* tends to adhere to the mucosal surface and more than three stool examinations may be required to confirm a suspected infection

C. The organisms present did not stain with trichrome stain and therefore the morphology is very atypical

D. Special diagnostic procedures such as the Knott concentration and nutrient-free agar cultures should have been used

Microbiology/Apply knowledge of life cycles, organism morphology, pathogenesis, and diagnostic procedures/ Parasitology/3

60. A transplant patient is currently receiving steroids. The patient is now complaining of abdominal pain and has symptoms of pneumonia and positive blood cultures with gram-negative rods. The individual has been living in the United States for 20 years but grew up in Central America. The most likely parasite causing these symptoms is:

A. *Trypanosoma brucei rhodesiense*

B. *Giardia lamblia*

C. *Strongyloides stercoralis*

D. *Schistosoma japonicum*

Microbiology/Apply knowledge of fundamental life cycles, pathogenesis, and immunosuppressives/ Parasitology/3

Answers to Questions 59–60

59. B It is well known that *G. lamblia* trophozoites adhere to the intestinal mucosal surface by means of the sucking disk. Although a patient may have giardiasis and be symptomatic, confirmation of the infection from stool examinations may require more than the routine three stools or may require the examination of duodenal contents.

60. C Although infection with *S. stercoralis* may have been acquired in Central America many years before, the patient may have remained asymptomatic while the infection was maintained at a low level in the body via the autoinfective portion of the life cycle. As the patient became more immunosuppressed (steroids), the life cycle began to reactivate with penetration of the larvae through the intestinal wall (abdominal pain) and through the lungs (pneumonia), and the patient may have presented with evidence of sepsis (often with gram-negative bacteria carried with the larvae as they penetrate the intestinal wall). Patients who become immunosuppressed may see the life cycle of *Strongyloides* reactivated with serious illness resulting; this can occur many years after the initial infection and after the patient has left the endemic area.

BIBLIOGRAPHY

1. Forbes, B.A., Sahm, D.F., Weissfeld, A.S., Trevino, E.: Bailey and Scott's Diagnostic Microbiology. CV Mosby, St. Louis, 2002.
2. Fisher, F., Cook, N.B.: Fundamentals of Diagnostic Microbiology. W.B. Saunders, Philadelphia, 1998.
3. Garcia, L.S.: Diagnostic Medical Parasitology, 5th ed. ASM Press, Washington, DC, 2007.
4. Koneman, E.W., Allen, S.D., Janda, W.M., et al: Color Atlas and Textbook of Diagnostic Microbiology. JB Lippincott, Philadelphia, 2005.
5. Larone, D.H.: Medically Important Fungi: A Guide to Identification. ASM Press, Washington, DC, 2002.
6. Mahon, C.R., Manuselis, G.: Textbook of Diagnostic Microbiology. W.B. Saunders, Philadelphia, 2000.
7. Murray, P.R., Baron, E.J., Jorgensen, J.H., Pfaller, M.A., Yolken, R.H.: Manual of Clinical Microbiology. ASM Press, Washington, D.C., 2003.

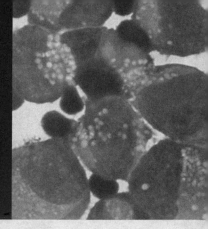

CHAPTER **8**

Molecular Diagnostics

8.1 MOLECULAR METHODS

8.2 MOLECULAR DIAGNOSTICS

1. Which double-stranded DNA molecule has the highest melting temperature?

    A. An oligonucleotide with a repeating sequence of A-A-A at the 5′ end

    B. A molecule of 5000 base pairs with a high number of A-T base pairs

    C. An oligonucleotide with a large number of repeating C-G-C codons

    D. A DNA polymer of 100,000 base pairs

Molecular/Apply knowledge of fundamental biological characteristics/DNA/2

2. Which base pair sequence is most likely to serve as a binding site for a restriction endonuclease?

    A. A-T-T-C-A
       T-A-A-G-T

    B. C-T-A-C-T-G
       G-A-T-G-A-C

    C. C-A-C
       G-T-G

    D. A-A-G-C-T-T
       T-T-C-G-A-A

Molecular/Apply knowledge of fundamental biological characteristics/DNA/2

Answers to Questions 1–2

1. C The melting temperature of DNA refers to the temperature required to separate the molecule into single strands. The T_m is the temperature required to convert half of the DNA from dsDNA to ssDNA. This is done by breaking the hydrogen bonds between base pairs. A-T base pairs have two hydrogen bonds while C-G base pairs have three. Therefore, molecules with a high proportion of C-G base pairs are more resistant to heat denaturation or melting.

2. D Restriction endonucleases are enzymes that cut double-stranded DNA into fragments and are important tools used in molecular diagnostics. Each restriction enzyme recognizes a specific oligonucleotide sequence, and the size and number of fragments it produces when DNA is digested depend upon the number of times that sequence is repeated in the DNA molecule. Restriction endonucleases recognize palindromic sequences (i.e., the base sequence of complementary strands reads the same from opposite directions). The sequence

A-A-G-C-T-T
T-T-C-G-A-A

is the recognition site for *HindIII*, a restriction endonuclease isolated from *Haemophilus influenzae*. If a disease gene produces a base pair substitution at the restriction site, the enzyme will not recognize it and not cut the DNA. This results in a longer fragment that can be recognized by electrophoresis. This process has been used to identify the hemoglobin S gene.

3. Cloning a human gene into a bacterium in order to make a large molecular probe requires which vector?

   A. Plasmid

   B. Bacterial microsome

   C. 30S bacterial ribosome

   D. Single-stranded DNA

Molecular/Apply principles of special procedures/DNA/1

4. What process can be used to make a DNA probe produce a fluorescent or chemiluminescent signal?

   A. Enzymatic attachment of acridinium esters to terminal ends of the probe

   B. Substitution of biotinylated or fluorescent nucleotides into the probe

   C. Splicing the gene for β-galactosidase into the probe

   D. Heat denaturation of the probe followed by acid treatment

Molecular/Apply principles of special procedures/DNA/1

Answers to Questions 3–4

3.   A A plasmid is a piece of circular double-stranded DNA located in the cytoplasm of a bacterium. Although not attached to a chromosome, the plasmid is replicated like chromosomal DNA. The plasmid is cut with the restriction endonuclease that is used to isolate the DNA fragment containing the gene of interest. The fragment anneals to the sticky ends of the plasmid DNA, and the cut is repaired by DNA ligase. The recombinant plasmid is added to a culture of bacteria that is disrupted to promote the uptake of plasmid DNA. Commercially available plasmids have promoter and reporter genes such as *lac* and *lacZ* that produce β-galactosidase. These can be used to identify colonies with successful recombinants and antibiotic resistance genes that allow the recombinants to be purified. Culture of the recombinant bacteria results in large amounts of the gene, which can be harvested using the restriction enzyme, denatured, and labeled to make the probe.

4.   B Fluorescent or enzyme labels are attached to probes by nick translation. A DNase is used to cut the probe at a few phosphodiester linkages. Pol I repairs the nicks by removing nucleotides from the 3′ end and replacing them with labeled nucleotides at the 5′ end of the nick. Alternatively, a primer containing labeled nucleotides can be added to the end of the probe with DNA polymerase. A common label used for probes consists of biotin conjugated to the bases of each nucleotide. After hybridization, strepavidin conjugated to an enzyme such as alkaline phosphatase is added. Strepavidin strongly binds to biotin, forming an enzyme-labeled complex with the DNA. After washing to remove unbound strepavidin, a colorimetric, fluorescent, or chemiluminescent substrate is added.

5. What term describes the products produced when DNA is digested by restriction endonucleases?

A. Mosaicisms

B. Chimeras

C. Amplicons

D. Restriction fragment length polymorphisms

Molecular/Apply principles of basic laboratory procedures/DNA/1

6. The following figure shows a DNA size standard (ladder) made by restriction enzyme digestion (*PstI*) of lambda phage DNA that his been separated by agarose gel electrophoresis. Which DNA band has the highest molecular weight?

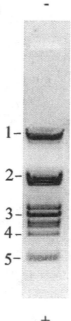

A. 1

B. 2

C. 3

D. 4

Molecular/Apply principles of basic laboratory procedures/DNA electrophoresis/2

7. What reagent is most commonly used to stain DNA separated by electrophoresis?

A. Silver nitrate

B. Nicotinamide adenine dinucleotide

C. Cationic dye

D. Ethidium bromide

Molecular/Apply principles of basic laboratory procedures/DNA electrophoresis/2

5. D Mosaicism occurs when cells within the same individual contain different numbers of chromosomes and results from nondisjunction during early embryonic development. Chimeras are molecules created when translocation occurs between genes (exons) on different chromosomes. Amplicons are copies of a DNA template produced by DNA amplification techniques such as the polymerase chain reaction (PCR). When a restriction enzyme cuts two DNA molecules, the size of the fragments differ if the base sequence at the restriction site is different and the restriction enzyme is not able to recognize it. Such fragments are termed RIF-LIPS for restriction fragment length polymorphisms (RFLPs). Analysis of RFLPs can be used to test for disease genes, study genetic linkage, and establish identity. It is used usually when PCR is impractical, such as when contamination occurs repeatedly or when the genes to be analyzed comprise a length of DNA too long for efficient amplification.

6. A Each phosphoric acid subunit with a phosphodiester bond to adjacent deoxyribose molecules has a single negative charge at an alkaline pH. Since the charge is distributed evenly, smaller fragments move more rapidly through the gel. When suspended in an alkaline buffer (pH 8) such as tris-borate-EDTA (TBE) or tris-acetate-EDTA (TAE), the DNA fragments migrate toward the anode at a rate that is inversely proportional to the log_{10} of molecular size. If the distance traveled is plotted against the log of molecular weight, the plot will be a straight line with a negative slope because the larger the molecule, the more slowly it moves through the pores of the gel. The plot can be calibrated with a DNA size ladder, and the molecular weight of DNA fragments can be determined from the calibration curve.

7. D When ethidium bromide inserts between the base pairs of double-stranded DNA, the dye becomes fluorescent, releasing 480 nm light when stimulated by long wavelength ultraviolet light. Ethidium bromide staining has a sensitivity of approximately 10 ng/mL (1.5 ng per band) DNA. It is frequently added to molten agarose or capillary electrophoresis buffer at a concentration of 0.5 μg/mL in order to visualize and quantify DNA. Its binding to single stranded DNA and RNA is not as efficient as that of more sensitive dyes such as SYBR gold, picoGreen, and YOYO-1.

8. Which technique is used to detect DNA containing a specific base sequence by applying a labeled probe to DNA bands immobilized onto nitrocellulose paper following electrophoresis?
   A. Southern blot
   B. Northern blot
   C. Dot blot
   D. Western blot

   Molecular/Apply principles of basic laboratory procedures/DNA blotting/2

9. Which of the following types of mutation causes the premature termination of protein synthesis?
   A. Missense
   B. Nonsense
   C. Insertion
   D. Frame shift

   Molecular/Apply knowledge of fundamental biological characteristics/DNA/1

10. In humans which component of a gene is translated into a protein?
    A. Intron
    B. Exon
    C. Promoter
    D. TATA box

    Molecular/Apply knowledge of fundamental biological characteristics/DNA/1

Answers to Questions 8–10

8. **A** Southern blot hybridization is a method commonly used to detect disease genes in both PCR products and RFLP testing. The DNA fragments are electrophoresed, and the DNA bands are transferred by suction to a nylon or nitrocellulose membrane. The bands are immobilized and denatured on the membrane, and a solution containing the labeled probe is added. Hybridization is the binding of the complementary base sequence of the probe to the target sequence. This process is highly dependent upon temperature, ionic strength, and the presence of reagents in the hybridization solution that influence stringency (the degree of exactness of base pairing). A Northern blot test follows the same process except that the sample is RNA. In a Western blot test the sample is a mixture of proteins, and the probes used are (labeled) antibodies to the proteins of interest. There is no procedure known as Eastern blot. A dot blot is a hybridization method in which samples of DNA are placed directly on the nitrocellulose membrane as a circular spot (or bar in the case of a slot blot), followed by the hybridization process.

9. **B** A nonsense mutation occurs when a nucleotide substitution within a codon changes the code from that for an amino acid to a stop sequence. For example, a change from TTC to GTC changes the mRNA transcript from AAG to UAG. AAG codes for lysine and UAG is a stop codon; therefore instead of lysine's being added to the protein during translation, protein synthesis is terminated. In the reverse situation the point mutation changes a termination codon into one for an amino acid and a longer protein is produced. A missense mutation occurs when a base substitution alters the codon so that a different amino acid is inserted during translation. A frame shift mutation occurs when there is a deletion or insertion of more or less than three bases. This changes the triplet order, altering the amino acid sequence of the protein.

10. **B** Exons are the components of genes that determine the amino acid sequence of the protein synthesized. Exons are separated by noncoding regions called introns that are transcribed and later removed from mRNA before translation. Promoters are sequences located near the gene at the 5′ end and facilitate binding of proteins that facilitate transcription. A TATA box is an oligonucleotide sequence often found in the promoter region. The AT base pairs have two hydrogen bonds that separate more easily than CG bonds, thus creating a point where the double helix is easier to open.

11. Which statement best describes a DNA polymorphism?
   A. A point mutation arising in a gene
   B. Any change in DNA that is associated with abnormal function
   C. A change in the base sequence of DNA that is translated into an abnormal protein
   D. An variation in DNA that occurs with a frequency of at least 1%

Molecular/Apply knowledge of fundamental biological characteristics/DNA/1

12. Which of the following is the most common type of polymorphism?
   A. Single nucleotide polymorphism (SNP)
   B. Variable number tandem repeat (VNTR)
   C. Short tandem repeat (STR)
   D. Short repetitive interspersed element (SINES)

Molecular/Apply knowledge of fundamental biological characteristics/DNA/1

Answers to Questions 11–12

11. **D** The human genome contains approximately 3 billion base pairs and approximately 25,000 genes. Post-transcription modification of mRNA enables production of about 100,000 proteins. However, approximately 99.9% of the DNA is homologous. The remaining 0.1% is variable and accounts for individual differences. A polymorphism is an individual difference in DNA sequence or length that occurs in at least 1% of the population. Polymorphisms arise from mutation and are transmitted to offspring. They are subject to selection pressures that cause genes to drift in the population. Over 350,000 such differences are present in the human genome, but very few are associated with human disease.

12. **A** Approximately 80% of polymorphisms result from single nucleotide substitutions and are called single nucleotide polymorphisms. Some SNPs are silent, whereas others cause a change in the codon within the gene. VNTRs, STRs, and SINES refer to polymorphisms involving differences in the length of as opposed to the sequence of bases. These are specific base sequences that occur throughout the genome that are repeated at a particular locus. The number of times the sequence repeats is an inherited trait. For example, the sequence AATG is a repeat that occurs within the tyrosine hydroxylase gene on chromosome 11. The sequence can repeat 3 to 14 times, resulting in 12 different alleles. Someone who inherits allele 6 (AATG repeats six times) on both chromosomes will have a DNA molecule that is four base pairs longer than someone who inherits allele 5 on both chromosomes (AATG repeats five times). This locus, called TH01, is used in forensic and parentage testing to establish identity.

13. Which of the following mechanisms facilitates DNA separation by capillary electrophoresis?
   A. Molecular sieving
   B. Partitioning
   C. Adsorption
   D. Deflection

   Molecular/Apply principles of special procedures/ Electrophoresis/1

14. The polymerase chain reaction (PCR) involves three processes. Select the order in which these occur.
   A. Extension ⟶ Annealing ⟶ Denaturation
   B. Annealing ⟶ Denaturation ⟶ Extension
   C. Denaturation ⟶ Annealing ⟶ Extension
   D. Denaturation ⟶ Extension ⟶ Annealing

   Molecular/Apply principles of special procedures/PCR/1

15. In the PCR method, how is denaturation accomplished?
   A. Heat
   B. Alkali treatment
   C. Addition of sulfonylurea
   D. Formamide

   Molecular/Apply principles of special procedures/PCR/1

Answers to Questions 13–15

13. **A** Capillary electrophoresis (CE) is a method commonly used to separate DNA fragments. Unlike conventional electrophoresis, a stationary support such as agarose is not used. Instead, a small-bore open tubular column is immersed in buffer solution at its ends and subjected to an electric field. Molecules such as proteins and DNA are injected by application of either pressure or high voltage (electrokinetic transfer). The negative nature of the glass capillary attracts cations that are pulled to the cathode when the voltage is applied. This creates an electro-osmotic force (EOF) that draws water and other molecules toward the cathode. An ultraviolet light detector or laser-induced fluorescence detector is located near the cathode and detects the molecules as they migrate. At an alkaline pH, DNA and protein molecules are negatively charged but are pulled toward the cathode by EOF at a rate inversely proportional to their size. More commonly, the column is coated with a gel such as acrylamide or a polymer that neutralizes the EOF, and the polarity of the power supply is reversed. DNA molecules are drawn toward the anode at a rate inversely related to the molecular size. DNA molecules such as PCR products of 100 to 1000 base pairs can be detected with a band resolution of approximately 5 to 15 base pairs and a sensitivity of approximately 1 ng/mL DNA. Such high resolution is possible because very high voltage can be used, since the heat produced is lost through the capillary wall.

14. **C** The PCR process results in identical copies of a piece of double-stranded DNA. The process involves three steps that are repeated to double the number of copies produced with each cycle. The first step is denaturation to separate the complementary strands. Annealing occurs when a primer binds upstream to the segment of interest on each strand, called the template. Extension involves the enzymatic addition of nucleotides to the primer to complete the new strand.

15. **A** In PCR the separation of dsDNA occurs by heating the sample to a temperature between 90°C and 94°C. This breaks the double bonds between the base pairs and is reversible by lowering the temperature. Alkali and high salt and formamide also denature dsDNA, but they are not used in PCR because they would have to be removed and added with every cycle.

16. **What is the composition of the primer used in PCR?**
    A. A cocktail of enzymes and nucleotide triphosphates that bind to the target
    B. An oligonucleotide complementary to bases at the beginning of the target
    C. A small piece of dsDNA that attaches to the template
    D. A probe made of mRNA that binds downstream from the target

    Molecular/Apply principles of special procedures/PCR/1

17. **The master mix solution used for PCR contains which of the following reagents?**
    A. Deoxyribonucleotide triphosphates
    B. Deoxyribonucleotide monophosphates
    C. Deoxyribonucleosides
    D. Ribonucleotide monophosphates

    Molecular/Apply principles of special procedures/PCR/1

18. **What is the unique characteristic of the DNA polymerase, *Taq* DNA polymerase, used in PCR?**
    A. It can be enzyme labeled
    B. It is more efficient than eukaryotic polymerases
    C. It is heat-stable
    D It works with DNA of any species

    Molecular/Apply principles of special procedures/PCR/1

19. **In real-time PCR methods, how can products of multiple loci be identified?**
    A. By following the increase in absorbance at 260 nm during melting
    B. By labeling the primers with specific fluors
    C. By simultaneous addition of hybridization probes to the master mix
    D. By analysis of adenosine tail signatures

    Molecular/Apply principles of special procedures/PCR/1

Answers to Questions 16–19

16. **B** PCR primers are small oligonucleotides, usually 12 to 36 bases, complementary to the base sequence at the $3'$ end of the target DNA. Two primers are used, one to the sense strand of DNA (the strand containing the gene) and the other to its complement (the antisense strand). Primers for PCR are made only for the $3'$ end of each target sequence (i.e., one primer is $5' \rightarrow 3'$ and the other is $3' \rightarrow 5'$) because the DNA polymerase that extends the primer does so only by addition of bases in the $5' \rightarrow 3'$ direction.

17. **A** Master mix solutions must contain all of the reagents needed to generate new dsDNA. This includes DNA polymerase, the enzyme needed to replicate the target sequence, primers to initiate replication, magnesium (a polymerase cofactor), buffers to maintain pH, and deoxyribonucleotide triphosphates that are the substrates for DNA polymerase (adenosine triphosphate, guanosine triphosphate, thymidine triphosphate, and cytosine triphosphate).

18. **C** Since heat is used to denature dsDNA with every cycle of PCR, the polymerase used must be heat-stable. *Taq* polymerase is obtained from *Thermus aquaticus,* a bacterium that lives in the hot springs of Yellowstone National Park. It retains its activity even after repeated heating at 95°C. The optimal temperature for extension by *Taq* is 64°C. A typical PCR cycle involves heating to 94°C for denaturation, cooling to 64°C for annealing, and heating to 72°C for extension.

19. **B** In PCR, several target sequences can be tested for simultaneously using multiple primers (multiplex PCR). Several methods exist for detection and quantitation of possible PCR products. The traditional method is Southern blotting, in which fluorescent-labeled probes to each template hybridize with their respective product after PCR. Alternatively, the primers can be labeled with different fluorescent labels. These can be detected after PCR by capillary electrophoresis or during PCR (in real-time) by counter labeling one member of each primer pair with a fluorescence-quenching molecule. When primers are in solution, fluorescence is inhibited by the quenching molecule. When PCR products are made, the primers are at opposite ends of the dsDNA, rendering the quenching molecule inoperative. A fluorometer built inside the thermocycler detects the increase in light of specific wavelengths emitted by the respective PCR products, and these signals identify and allow quantitation of each product that is made.

20. Which formula predicts the number of PCR products that can be produced?
   A. 2^n where n is the number of cycles
   B. N^4 where N is the number of cycles
   C. $p^2 + 2pq + q^2$ where p and q are the number of primers
   D. $N^2/2$ where N is the number of cycles

Molecular/Apply principles of special procedures/PCR/2

21. How can PCR be applied to the detection of human immunodeficiency and other RNA viruses?
   A. The virus must be inserted into human DNA by viral integrase prior to PCR
   B. Substituting deoxyuridine triphosphate in place of deoxythymidine triphosphate in the master mix
   C. Adding a heat-stable reverse transcriptase enzyme to the master mix
   D. Substituting ribonucleotide triphosphates for deoxyribonucleotide triphosphates in the master mix

Molecular/Apply principles of special procedures/PCR/2

22. Which statement best describes the method of branched DNA signal amplification?
   A. The DNA template is amplified directly using patented enzymes
   B. Multiple primers are used to create branches of the template DNA, permitting multiple extension sites
   C. The target DNA is denatured and hybridized to RNA, and the hybrid molecules are amplified by both DNA and RNA polymerases
   D. The target DNA is bound by multiple probes, and those are amplified instead of the target DNA

Molecular/Apply principles of special procedures/DNA amplification/1

23. A PCR reaction is performed, and the negative control demonstrates the presence of a detectable number of PCR products (amplicons). What is the most likely cause?
   A. False-positive post-PCR hybridization reaction due to low stringency
   B. Dimerization of PCR primers
   C. Contamination of sample with a trace amount of template DNA
   D. Background signal from gel fluorescence or inadequate removal of unbound probe

Molecular/Evaluate sources of error/PCR/3

Answers to Questions 20–23

20. **A** PCR has the potential to double the quantity of PCR products with every cycle. Therefore 2^n predicts the number of PCR products that can be produced from n cycles. For example, if 30 cycles are programmed, then 2^{30} predicts slightly over 1 billion PCR products. The formula $p^2 + 2pq + q^2 = 1$ describes the distribution of a two-allele gene in a population.

21. **C** Reverse transcriptase PCR (RT-PCR) is used to detect RNA viruses and to amplify RNA transcription products by converting the template to DNA. The master mix contains the same components needed for PCR with the addition of a heat-stable reverse transcriptase (enzyme that transcribes RNA to DNA, such as rTth DNA polymerase), manganese (a cofactor for this enzyme), and an mRNA primer. In addition to infectious testing for HIV, hepatitis C and hepatitis E, RT-PCR is used to identify translocations in leukemia where the crossover regions are too large for efficient PCR.

22. **D** PCR is a licensed technology, and other methods of nucleic acid amplification have since been developed. In branched DNA (bDNA) signal amplification, the target DNA is denatured and added to a well containing immobilized probes. One end of each probe hybridizes with the target DNA, capturing it, and the other contains multiple branches that hybridize with alkaline phosphatase–labeled probes. After washing to remove the unbound labeled probes, dioxetane is added, and chemiluminescence is measured. A thermocycler is not used and the target DNA is not amplified. Other nucleic acid amplification methods include nucleic acid sequence–based amplification (NASBA), transcription-mediated amplification (TMA), hybrid capture, and rolling circle amplification (RCA).

23. **C** PCR and other methods of DNA amplification have a great potential for error caused by contamination of sample or reagents with template DNA. This can derive from other samples, positive controls, or amplicons from preceding samples, but the most common source of contamination is by amplicons. Each run must contain a negative (as well as positive) control. The negative control contains all PCR reagents except the template DNA and should produce no detectable amplicons. However, PCR reactions that detect product by enzymatic, fluorescent, or chemiluminescent methods instead of gel or capillary electrophoresis will generate a signal for the negative control. This signal should be comparable to that for a substrate blank. Signals above a predetermined cutoff point will invalidate the test.

24. How can a false-negative PCR test caused by the presence of an inhibitor of the reaction in a patient's sample be detected?
  A. Using a positive control
  B. Using an internal control
  C. Performing each test in duplicate
  D. Performing serial dilutions of the sample

Molecular/Evaluate sources of error/PCR/3

25. All of the following are requirements for reducing contamination in DNA amplification methods *except*:
  A. Use of aerosol barrier pipette tips when transferring samples or reaction products
  B. Preparation of reagents in a dead air box or biological cabinet
  C. A separate area for performing preamplification, postamplification, and detection steps
  D. Pretreatment of samples with high-intensity ultraviolet light

Molecular/Apply knowledge to identify sources of error/ PCR/2

26. Which method has been used successfully to reduce contamination in the preamplification stage of PCR?
  A. Substitution of deoxyuridine triphosphate for deoxythymidine triphosphate in the master mix
  B. Use of low molecular size primers
  C. Use of a denaturation temperature above 95°C
  D. Pretreatment of samples with antisense RNA

Molecular/Apply knowledge to identify sources of error/ PCR/2

Answers to Questions 24–26

24. B Some samples may contain inhibitors of the PCR reaction. For example, a sample in which cDNA was extracted using a cation chelator to prevent DNA degradation may be contaminated with residual chelating reagent. Since DNA polymerase requires Mg^{+2}, this will inhibit amplicon production. An internal control can identify this problem. The sample is mixed with the internal control, a DNA molecule with the same primer binding region. The internal control should always be amplified, but the product can be distinguished from the target amplicons. Failure of a sample to demonstrate the internal control product in an assay where positive and negative control reactions are valid indicates the presence of an inhibitor in the sample.

25. D The laboratory area where DNA amplification methods are performed should be organized so that work flow moves from preamplification to amplification and detection. In addition to standard precautions, cotton plugged tips are used to prevent aerosol contamination of samples. As few as 10 copies of the template introduced by accident are likely to cause a false-positive reaction. Ultraviolet light causes cross-linking of thymine bases in dsDNA, which prevents replication. This has been used as a post-PCR method of reducing contamination.

26. A One method of preventing PCR products from previous assays from contaminating a sample or test in progress is to substitute the RNA base uracil for thymine in the PCR product. *Taq* polymerase will insert deoxyuridine phosphate instead of deoxythymidine phosphate during the primer extension phase of each cycle. The enzyme uracil N-glycosidase is added to the master mix along with deoxyuridine triphosphate, which replaces deoxythymidine triphosphate. Prior to the first denaturation the enzyme hydrolyzes the bond between uracil and deoxyribose. When the sample is heated to separate the strands, the enzyme becomes denatured and the PCR products fragment into small oligonucleotides that cannot be replicated.

27. How are PCR methods adapted to yield quantitative data?

   A. By comparing PCR product to an internal standard
   B. By applying a conversion factor to the PCR signal that converts it to copies per mL
   C. By determining the mass of PCR product using ultraviolet spectrophotometry
   D. By making serial dilutions of the sample

Molecular/Apply knowledge of special procedures/PCR/2

28 A PCR analysis of a vaginal sample for *Chlamydia trachomatis* gives a negative result (optical density of biotinylated reaction product below the cutoff point). The internal control result is also below the cutoff. Positive and negative controls produced acceptable results. What action should be taken?

   A. The test should be reported as negative
   B. The sample should be diluted and the test repeated
   C. The result should not be reported and the sample should be repeated
   D. A preliminary result of negative should be reported but should be confirmed by further testing using a different method of analysis

Molecular/Apply knowledge to identify sources of error/ PCR/3

29. Which statement accurately describes the process of fluorescent in situ hybridization (FISH)?

   A. Hybridization is performed on DNA extracted from cells
   B. Hybridization is performed directly on intact chromosomes
   C. Hybridization probes are attached to histones associated with the chromosomes
   D. Hybridization occurs by attachment to the probe only at the centromere

Molecular/Apply principles of special procedures/FISH/1

27. **A** Quantitative PCR can be used to measure viral load and gene expression. However, the PCR process is associated with a high run to run variance that can be reduced by simultaneously measuring the PCR products of an internal standard of known concentration (molecules per PCR). For example, in competitive PCR a DNA template having the same primer binding region but that is shorter than the native DNA is added to each sample. The signal used to determine concentration is derived from the ratio of the native DNA product to the competitive template product. This value is compared to the signal generated by adding a known amount of DNA from a reference gene (internal standard) and is reported as copies per mL or copies per molecule of reference gene. Some quantitative PCR methods use external standards. However, an advantage of the internal standard method is that the calibrator is subject to the same influences as the target DNA by being mixed with DNA from the patient's sample.

28. **C** The internal control in PCR is an oligonucleotide sequence different from that of the target but that binds the same primers. Its product is detected using a different probe than is used for the target sequence. If the internal control is not amplified, this indicates an invalid test. Causes include the presence of a PCR inhibitor, denaturation of the polymerase, hybridization failure, or error in the detection system (e.g., improper pH preventing enzyme-conjugated strepavidin from acting on the substrate). The assay of this sample must be repeated.

29. **B** FISH is used to detect abnormalities of chromosomes in cells and tissues by facilitating the direct attachment of a fluorescent-labeled oligonucleotide probe or probes to the chromosome. Hybridization of the oligonucleotide probe requires treatment of the cells with proteinase K and other agents such as nonionic detergent to increase permeability. Prehybridization may be required to decrease background fluorescence. Denaturation requires controlled temperatures at or near the melting point and the addition of a hybridization solution. This usually contains formamide, sodium chloride and sodium citrate, and EDTA to weaken the hydrogen bonds of the dsDNA target. Hybridization of the fluorescent-labeled probe(s) to the chromosomal DNA also requires controlled temperature incubation. After incubating with the cells, any unattached probe is removed by washing, and the cells are examined with a fluorescent microscope containing the appropriate filters to transmit the excited light from the specific probe(s).

30. Which type of specimen would be unsuitable for FISH analysis?
   A. Paraffin embedded tissue
   B. Cells with chromosomes in metaphase
   C. Cells with chromosomes in interphase
   D. A cell suspension containing maternal and fetal blood

Molecular/Apply knowledge to recognize sources of error/FISH/2

31. FISH can distinguish each of the following chromosomal abnormalities *except*
   A. Aneuploidy
   B. Translocation
   C. Deletion
   D. Trinucleotide repeats

Molecular/Apply principles of special procedures/FISH/1

32. In microarray and macroarray analysis, which molecules are labeled?
   A. The immobilized DNA molecules
   B. The sample DNA
   C. Both target and sample molecules
   D. The substrate matrix

Molecular/Apply principles of special procedures/DNA arrays/1

30.   D FISH can be used with almost any type of cell preparation, including frozen sections, formalin fixed tissues, embedded tissues, and cell suspensions such as those derived from amniotic fluid or chorionic villus sampling provided they are pure. Cells in suspension can be dropped onto glass slides or concentrated using a cytocentrifuge before processing. However, a mixture of cells from different individuals is inappropriate because the probe cannot distinguish between sources such as fetal and maternal cells.

31.   D FISH can detect conditions that are associated with structural chromosomal abnormalities and an abnormal number of chromosomes (aneuploidy). A screening test for aneuploidy employs probes labeled with different fluorescent dyes that simultaneously detect trisomy 21, 18, and 13 and the X and Y chromosomes. Deletions cause the absence of a fluorescent signal when expected, and microdeletions such as those that occur on the short arm of chromosome 5 in cri du chat syndrome can be detected by FISH. Translocations cause two different FISH probes to bind to the same chromosome. Such probes are used to identify *IgH* gene translocations such as t(11:14) in multiple myeloma that are of prognostic value. However, trinucleotide repeats, repetitive sequences of the same three base pairs, are not detected by FISH. This is associated with fragile X syndrome, myotonic dystrophy, Huntington's disease, and other genetic diseases and PCR or Southern blotting are used for detection of these repeats, depending upon their number.

32.   B An array is an organized arrangement of known molecules (either DNA or proteins for proteomic array analysis). DNA arrays are used primarily for studying gene expression and single nucleotide polymorphisms. Commercially prepared arrays use short synthetic oligonucleotides (12-36 bases) of single-stranded DNA immobilized onto a substrate, usually a glass or a silicon chip. These are usually called the targets, and a single array can contain hundreds to many thousands of targets. The sample DNA is usually derived by RT-PCR of test cells. This produces single-stranded complementary DNA (cDNA) representative of active genes within the cells. These are labeled with one or two fluorescent dyes and therefore are usually termed probes. However, some commercial systems refer to the immobilized (array) DNA as the probe and the labeled DNA as the target.

33. How can all of the mRNA within a sample be amplified to prepare microarray probes?
   A. A specific primer for each mRNA must be synthesized
   B. A primer is made to the polyA tail of mRNA
   C. Nonspecific attachment of T7 polymerase occurs when the cells are treated with detergent
   D. Random primer sets are used under low stringency conditions

Molecular/Apply principles of special procedures/DNA arrays/1

34. What is the difference between a microarray and a macroarray DNA assay?
   A. The number of targets is larger on a macroarray
   B. The molecular size of each target is larger on a macroarray
   C. The amount of each target is larger on a macroarray
   D. The substrate used for a macroarray is different from a microarray

Molecular/Apply principles of special procedures/DNA arrays 2

35. Protein microarray analysis requires the use of which of the following techniques to generate protein profile data?
   A. Electrophoresis
   B. Mass spectroscopy
   C. Thin layer chromatography
   D. Gas chromatography

Molecular/Apply principles of special procedures/DNA arrays/1

Answers to Questions 33–35

33. **B** When messenger RNA is transcribed, the enzyme polyA polymerase adds 50 to 250 adenine bases to the 3′ end of the molecule. This polyA tail protects the mRNA from enzymatic degradation and promotes its binding to the ribosome. Since almost all eukaryotic mRNA has a polyA tail, oligo dT primers are used to initiate reverse transcription, making cDNA copies of the mRNA, and oligo dA primers are used to initiate amplification of the cDNA product.

34. **C** The difference between a micro- and a macroarray assay is that the amount of DNA "printed" onto the substrate is larger in a macroarray assay, necessitating a larger spot. A microarray uses less than 200 μL of DNA and allows a larger number of targets to be applied. Commercially available microarrays are available that contain over 250,000 oligonucleotide spots. Short oligonucleotide targets can be synthesized on the substrate or applied by photolithography, inkjet spraying, or manually with print plates and tips that can be purchased.

35. **B** Protein microarray analysis uses immobilized bait to isolate proteins from serum, body fluids, or cell lysates. The array may contain antibodies, antigens, receptor molecules, or protein binding ligands (e.g., drugs). The proteins can be identified by fluorescent- or enzyme-labeled probes and can be analyzed by mass spectroscopy to produce a fingerprint of the proteins isolated on the array. This can be compared to a learning set, a combination of proteins that is associated with a specific disease such as ovarian cancer. If the pattern falls within specified parameters determined by the learning set, then cancer is identified. Analysis is based upon determining the time required for each protein to move through a mass filter. Two related instrument principles are used, matrix-assisted laser desorption/ionization — time of flight mass spectrometry (MALDI-TOF), and surface enhanced laser desorption/ionization — time of flight mass spectrometry (SELDI-TOF). Both use a laser to ionize the proteins and a mass filter to separate them based upon their mass/charge ratio. Since protein expression of cancer cells is altered before morphology changes, the analysis of protein patterns of serum and suspected cells provides an opportunity for diagnosis at an early stage of progression or at a premalignant state.

1. Which method is most useful for confirmation that a culture isolate is Group B streptococcus?
  A. Southern blotting
  B. Polymerase chain reaction
  C. Direct hybridization
  D. Probe capture assay

Molecular/Apply principles of special procedures/DNA hybridization/1

2. In situ hybridization (ISH) tests for human papilloma virus (HPV) using cervical smears differ from immunochemical staining of tissue in which regard?
  A. ISH has lower analytical sensitivity
  B. ISH has lower analytical specificity
  C. ISH differentiates subtypes more easily
  D. ISH differentiates cervical neoplasia from genital warts

Molecular/Apply principles of special procedures/ISH//2

Answers to Questions 1–2

1. **C** In direct hybridization a specific labeled probe reacts directly with the sample. Since a colony or pure broth culture of a primary isolate represents the progeny of a single bacterium there is no need for the use of Southern blotting. The quantity of DNA available for testing is sufficient, so that amplification methods such as PCR or probe capture hybridization are unnecessary. The colony or broth isolate is lysed, and a hybridization solution is used to promote denaturation. The sample is heated above the melting temperature, and a DNA probe is added that hybridizes with bacterial DNA or ribosomal RNA. The probe is conjugated to a chemiluminescent label. A reagent is added to neutralize the unbound probe, and H_2O_2 and NaOH are added to cause chemiluminescence. The signal is read in a luminometer and compared to a cutoff value. Such tests take approximately 1 hour to perform and most are 99%–100% sensitive and specific.

2. **C** In situ hybridization using probes that anneal with specific subtypes of HPV are able to distinguish the subtype of virus most commonly responsible for sexually transmitted warts and associated with neoplasia. Positive reactions can be detected by light microscopy using probes conjugated to biotin. After the hybridization reaction, the slides are washed to remove the unbound probe, and strepavidin conjugated to horseradish peroxidase is added. Addition of hydrogen peroxide and aminoethylcarbazole results in the formation of a reddish-brown precipitate. Sensitivity is approximately 88% and specificity 99%, which is higher than for histochemical immunoperoxidase staining. HPV is present in normal-appearing cells as well as those demonstrating intraepithelial neoplastic lesions. However, persons testing positive for HPV types associated with cervical cancer such as type 16 are at higher risk for the disease.

3. How can cell proliferation be explained by the *BCR/ABL* gene rearrangement that occurs in the 9:22 translocation that causes the Ph^1 chromosome of CML?

   A. It causes underexpression of *p53*

   B. A hybrid protein is made that up-regulates the cell cycle

   C. Translocation induces a point mutation in the *ABL* oncogene

   D. *ABL* activates *p23*

Molecular/Apply knowledge of fundamental biological characteristics/CML/2

4. Which statement accurately describes the clinical utility of translocation testing in leukemia?

   A. Relapse is predicted by any new translocation occurring after treatment

   B. Specific translocations associated with a type of leukemia will occur in all cases

   C. Translocation products for each leukemia subtype are always the same

   D. Translocation is a sensitive way to identify surviving leukemic cells following treatment

Molecular/Correlate clinical and laboratory data/ Translocation/2

5. How can cell proliferation be explained by the *BCL* 2 translocation t(14;18) that occurs in up to 90% of persons with follicular B-cell lymphoma?

   A. *p53* is underexpressed

   B. A hybrid protein is made that up-regulates the cell cycle

   C. Transcription of the *BCL* 2 oncogene is increased by the translocation

   D. The *BCL* 2 gene joins with the *p21* gene, making it inactive

Molecular/Apply knowledge of fundamental biological characteristics/Translocation/2

Answers to Questions 3–5

3. **B** Cancers are caused by genetic damage to cells that disrupt the cell cycle. Cell proliferation can be induced by underexpression of genes with tumor suppressor properties (e.g., *p53*) or overexpression of oncogenes (e.g., *p21*) that increases cell signaling, transcription, and mitosis. In CML, relocation of the *ABL* oncogene from chromosome 9 to the 3′ end of the *BCR* (breakpoint cluster region or area where recombination occurs) of chromosome 22 results in production of a hybrid *BCR/ABL* mRNA. This produces a chimeric protein with increased tyrosine kinase activity causing the cell to enter G1. FISH can be used to identify cells with the *BCR/ABL* translocation. DNA probes specific for *ABL* and *BCR* are labeled with two different fluorescent dyes. In normal cells, each dye produces two colored spots (e.g., red and green) on chromosome pairs 9 and 22. If a *BCR/ABL* translocation is present, the probes bind next to each other, producing a spot of a different color (e.g., yellow).

4. **D** Some translocations occurring after treatment are predictive of relapse. For example, a second translocation in a person with Philadelphia chromosome-positive CML occurs in the majority of persons preceding blast crisis. However, other translocations, such as the 15:22 translocation associated with M3 AML are seen during remission and not associated with relapse. Some translocations occur with 100% or near 100% frequency, such as 9:22 in CML and 15:17 in M3 AML. However, others occur only in some affected persons. Translocations associated with a type of leukemia are not identical in all cases. For example, the 9:22 translocation associated with CML can give rise to transcripts of different length. RT-PCR can detect as few as 1 per million cells containing the translocation, making translocations useful markers for detecting cells that have escaped destruction following treatment.

5. **C** In follicular B-cell lymphoma, relocation of the *BCL* oncogene next to the gene for the immunoglobulin heavy chain (*IgH*) occurs. The *BCL* oncogene product is a protein that inhibits apoptosis. When the cell transcribes the *IgH* gene it produces the *BCL* 2 protein as well, which protects the cell from apoptosis. This translocation occurs in all cases of follicular B-cell lymphoma, and can be identified using FISH with fluorescent-labeled DNA probes to *IgH* and *BCL* 2 genes.

6. **Which mechanism is responsible for retinoblastoma?**
   A. Mutation of a tumor suppressor gene
   B. Mutation of a tyrosine kinase gene
   C. Activation of an oncogene
   D. Deletion of a gene encoding a GTPase activator

   Molecular/Apply knowledge of fundamental biological characteristics/Malignancy/2

7. **Which oncogene is involved in the etiology of Burkitt's lymphoma?**
   A. *ABL*
   B. *Myc*
   C. *Ras*
   D. *HER/neu*

   Molecular/Apply knowledge of fundamental biological characteristics/Malignancy/2

8. **The majority of cases of Duchenne's muscular dystrophy are caused by which type of genetic damage?**
   A. Point mutation
   B. Insertion
   C. Deletion
   D. Trinucleotide repeats

   Molecular/Apply knowledge of fundamental biological characteristics/Muscular dystrophy/2

9. **How are cases of Duchenne's muscular dystrophy not detected by PCR usually confirmed?**
   A. DNA sequencing
   B. Linkage analysis
   C. Multiplex PCR
   D. Dystrophin protein staining

   Molecular/Apply knowledge of special procedures/ Muscular dystrophy/2

Answers to Questions 6–9

6. **A** A mutation or deletion of a tumor suppressor gene such as *p53, p14,* or *RB1* (the retinoblastoma gene) causes loss of a protein that inhibits mitosis and is associated with an increased risk of malignancy. Mutations of *p53* occur frequently in several cancers, including lung, breast, liver, and colon cancer. *RB1* mutations are associated primarily with retinoblastoma, a tumor of the retina occurring in young children. Although they may be inherited, both mutations usually arise in somatic cells. Mutations that produce more active proteins with tyrosine kinase activity such as *HER-2/neu* are oncogenic because they stimulate the signal transduction pathway for mitosis. Likewise, a deletion of a GTPase activator is also oncogenic, since it permits higher levels of intracellular GTP, which is involved in the same pathway.

7. **B** Burkitt's lymphoma is associated with a translocation involving the long arm of chromosome 8 on which the *c-myc* gene is located with one of three immunoglobulin genes. The translocation most often involves the *IgH* gene on chromosome 14. The result is a hybrid mRNA that produces the *c-myc* protein whenever the immunoglobulin gene is transcribed. The *c-myc* protein is an activator of genes involved in mitosis.

8. **C** The dystrophin gene is approximately 2.5 million bases and has extensive sites at which both large and small deletions, insertions, and point mutations can occur. Approximately 60% of cases are caused by deletions that can be detected by the absence of one or more PCR product produced by the normal gene. The remaining 40% can be caused by microdeletions, point mutations, or insertions that are not usually detected by available primer sets.

9. **B** The majority of gene deletions associated with Duchenne's muscular dystrophy are detected by PCR using multiple primers (multiplex PCR). The others are usually detected by indirect gene analysis. Since the gene is so large, sequencing is not cost-effective. An alternative to testing for these mutations is linkage analysis. This process follows other genetic markers located near the disease gene so that crossing over is improbable. Linkage analysis for an X-linked disease or an autosomal recessive disease such as cystic fibrosis requires DNA from at least one affected family member However, linkage analysis for an autosomal dominant disease such as Huntington's disease requires DNA from at least two family members.

10. Inheritance of *BRCA1* or *BRCA2* mutations increases the risk of breast and ovarian cancer by which mechanism?
A. Oncogene production
B. Transcription signaling by the mutant protein
C. Deficient tumor suppressor function
D. Chimeric protein production

Molecular/Apply knowledge of fundamental biological characteristics/BRAC/2

11. Polymorphisms of the cytochrome *p450* genes are important in identifying which condition?
A. Poor drug metabolism
B. Risk for primary biliary cirrhosis
C. Progression of hepatitis C to hepatic cirrhosis
D. Parentage in cases where HLA results are inconclusive

Molecular/Correlate clinical and laboratory data/ Pharmacogenomics/2

12. Approximately how may mutations have been identified in the gene coding for the cystic fibrosis *trans* membrane conductor regulator protein (*CFTR*)?
A. 10
B. 100
C. 1000
D. 10,000

Molecular/Apply knowledge of fundamental biological characteristics/CF/2

10. C *BRCA1* and *BRCA2* are mutations of genes that produce tumor suppressor proteins. These downregulate cell signaling events that lead to cell division. The mutations are inherited as autosomal dominant traits and are associated with >85% lifetime risk at age 70 of developing breast cancer if one is found in a person with a positive family history.

11. A Pharmacogenetics (sometimes called pharmacogenomics) is the study of the role inheritance plays in the metabolism of drugs. Individual differences in drug metabolism can be attributed in part to polymorphisms in the genes coding for enzymes comprising the cytochrome *p450* system. Of the hundred or so CYP genes, seven are principally involved in drug metabolism. Of these, *CYP2D6*, *CYP2C9*, *CYP2C19*, and *CYP2A6* are polymorphic genes that account for metabolism of approximately 40% of drugs. Phenotypical expression varies with the locus involved. For the *CYP2C19* locus that metabolizes several dozen drugs, including some tricyclic antidepressants, antiepileptics, and acid reflux inhibitors, persons who inherit one copy of the wild type gene metabolize normally, whereas homozygotes or double heterozygotes for any of the seven polymorphisms metabolize poorly. For *CYP2D6*, which metabolizes tricyclic antidepressants, antipsychotics, antihypertensives, and a host of other drugs, heterozygotes with one wild type gene have intermediate and those with no wild type gene have poor drug metabolism. Persons with poor metabolic efficiency are at a greater risk of drug toxicity. On the other hand, their response to some antibiotics may be more positive.

12. C The *CFTR* protein regulates the movement of chloride across the cell membrane, and a defect in this protein results in cystic fibrosis (CF). The *CFTR* gene is located on the long arm of chromosome 7 and consists of 27 exons spread over 230,000 bases. The most common mutation is a deletion of three base pairs that code for phenylalanine at position 508 of the protein, ΔF508. This mutation accounts for 70% of CF genes in whites. It causes a severe form of CF involving pancreatic insufficiency. No single test can detect all possible CF carriers and a core panel consisting of 25 probes is recommended for initial screening. The core panel is used to screen for carriers of the CF gene and can detect more than 85% of CF mutations. Since two mutations are required to produce CF, the core panel can detect approximately 80% of CF.

13. Which statement about CF is accurate?
   A. A sweat chloride test is abnormal in all forms of CF
   B. Immunoreactive trypsin is deficient in all persons with CF
   C. Some CF mutations can cause male infertility with no other symptoms
   D. The CF genotype always predicts the severity of the disease

Molecular/Correlate clinical and laboratory data/CF/3

14. Which of the following alleles has the highest frequency in the general population?
   A. ΔF508 (cystic fibrosis)
   B. Factor V-Leiden (hereditary thrombophilia)
   C. Prothrombin G20210A (hereditary thrombophilia)
   D. Methylene tetrahydrofolate reductase mutation C677T (homocysteinemia)

Molecular/Correlate clinical and laboratory data/ Mutations/2

13. **C** Serum immunoreactive trypsin is the recommended screening test for CF, but pancreatic insufficiency is not found in about 15% of CF cases. An abnormal result is confirmed by sweat chloride testing. Some infants may be too young for accurate sweat testing, and some mild forms of CF may give indeterminate results. DNA testing can be used in these cases. The CF genotype is not predictive of phenotype in most cases (an exception being ΔF508, which is almost always associated with pancreatic disease). CF mutations are responsible for about 75% of congenital bilateral absence of the vas deferens. Affected persons have at least one abnormal CF gene. Other than infertility they are asymptomatic and may or may not have a sweat chloride level above 65 mmol/L.

14. **D** Methylene tetrahydrofolate reductase (MTHFR) mutation is a point mutation in which thymidine replaces cytosine at nucleotide 677 in the gene. This results in a codon that substitutes valine for alanine and results in an enzyme that is more heat-sensitive. The enzyme converts 5,10 methylenetetrahydrofolate to 5-methyltetrahydrofolate (folate). The methyl group from the latter is transferred to homocysteine, forming methionine. In homozygotes (TT) with less than optimal dietary folate intake, deficiency of the enzyme reduces the availability of 5-methyltetrahydrofolate, causing the serum homocysteine to be increased. Such persons have an approximately threefold increased risk of coronary artery disease. In the general population the C677T allele of MTHFR has a frequency of 30%. All of the alleles above are of sufficiently high frequency to warrant screening of at risk populations. The prothrombin G20210A allele has a frequency of approximately 2%, factor V-Leiden 5%, and ΔF508 approximately 3% (in whites). Both factor V-Leiden and the prothrombin G20210A mutation result in proteins that increase the risk of thrombosis. The point mutation in factor V-Leiden results in a protein that is resistant to inactivation by protein C. The base substitution in G20210A (guanine for adenine at position 20210) results in increased transcription of the gene and overproduction of prothrombin.

15. HLA typing can be done by which molecular method?

   A. PCR analysis using 96 well microtrays with allele or groups specific primers in each.

   B. Restriction fragment length polymorphism testing

   C. Direct hybridization with WBCs on a peripheral blood film

   D. Fluorescent in situ hybridization reactions with peripheral blood lymphocytes

Molecular/Apply knowledge of special procedures/HLA/2

16. Which statement best describes the relationship between HLA DNA typing and serological haplotypes?

   A. One or two bands are seen for each locus correlating to reactivity with a specific antigen or group of antigens

   B. HLA alleles cannot be related to HLA antigens because antisera specificity is unrelated to genetic polymorphism

   C. A single antibody specificity always corresponds to a single allele

   D. Not all HLA genes produce antigens recognized by antibodies

Molecular/Apply knowledge of special procedures/HLA/2

17. Highest resolution HLA typing is needed for which of the following transplants?

   A. Heart

   B. Liver

   C. Kidney

   D. Bone marrow

Molecular/Correlate clinical and laboratory data/HLA/2

18. Which method of DNA analysis is used most often to detect the hemoglobin S gene?

   A. FISH

   B. PCR followed by RFLP

   C. Cytogenetic analysis of chromosome 11

   D. Labeled probe painting of chromosome 11

Molecular/Apply knowledge of special procedures/HLA/2

Answers to Questions 15–18

15. **A** The DNA is extracted from peripheral blood leukocytes, added to the master mix, and an aliquot is transferred to each well of a 96-well plate. Each well contains a primer to a specific base sequence of one allele or allele group. Gel electrophoresis is performed after PCR to identify those wells that contain amplified products. Each well also contains a primer to a second nucleotide sequence, such as a region of the growth hormone gene that serves as a PCR internal control. Bands are stained with ethidium bromide and can be visualized by direct observation with a near ultraviolet light source.

16. **A** Antibodies to HLA antigens recognize determinants that may be shared by several polymorphisms. However, it is possible to correlate primer specificities to gene products that react with commercial HLA typing seras. For example, DR103 correlates with the primer recognizing DRB1*0103. On the other hand, alleles DRB3*010101-10, DRB3*0101-14 and DRB3*030101-03 will all react with antisera to DR52.

17. **D** Solid organ transplants require medium resolution of alleles belonging to HLA class I and class II genes. Bone marrow transplants require high resolution typing. This involves identifying which allelic groups are present by medium resolution testing, then sequencing of the PCR products to determine the exact alleles present.

18. **B** The β-globin gene is located near the end of the short arm on chromosome 11 and consists of three exons and two introns constituting 1600 base pairs. The substitution of valine for glutamic acid at position 6 of the protein is the result of a single point mutation at position 6(A3) in exon 1, in which GAG is replaced by GTG. In hemoglobin C, the same codon is mutated but the substitution involves the preceding base at the 5′ end (GAG is changed to AAG). The hemoglobin S mutation alters the restriction site for *MstII*, preventing the enzyme from cutting the DNA. This causes production of a fragment that is 200 base pairs longer than seen for the normal β-gene. Most commonly PCR is used to amplify a portion of the exon containing the S mutation, and *MstII* is used to digest the PCR product. Heterozygotes produce one normal and one longer band, whereas homozygotes produce a single band that is 200 base pairs longer than the normal amplicon. Alternatively, PCR is performed followed by Southern blotting, using specific oligonucleotide probes for hemoglobin A and S.

19. Which of the following genetic diseases is caused by an expanded trinucleotide repeat?
  A. Prader-Willi syndrome
  B. Angelman's syndrome
  C. Fragile X syndrome
  D. Williams' syndrome

Molecular/Correlate clinical and laboratory data/Length polymorphism/2

20. Which is the most common method used for parent-age testing in the U.S.?
  A. Short tandem repeat analysis
  B. Nuclear DNA sequencing
  C. HLA DNA typing
  D. Mitochondrial DNA sequencing

Molecular/Apply knowledge of special procedures/ Paternity testing /2

19. C Prader-Willi and Angleman's syndromes are most often caused by microdeletion, and Williams' syndrome is caused by a microdeletion in the gene coding for elastin. Fragile X syndrome, Huntington's disease, and mytonic dystrophy are examples of diseases caused by an expansion of trinucleotide repeats. Fragile X is so named because when cells from an affected individual are cultured in folate-deficient medium, the long arm of the X chromosome appears to have a break caused by deficient staining. The Xq27 region contains a CGG tandem sequence that can repeat up to 50 times in normal individuals. In fragile X syndrome, the repeat is extended and its length determines whether the affected persons will show mental retardation. Repeats of 50 to 230 times are associated with a carrier (premutation) state. During meiosis in females, the CGG repeat can undergo further expansion. The probability of this expansion increases with each generation. As the size of the repeat increases, so does the chance that it will cause methylation of the promoter for the *FMR1* gene. The gene is needed for normal brain function and its underexpression results in mental retardation. Females in whom the premutation expands in size to a full mutation transmit the syndrome to all of their male and half of their female offspring.

20. A DNA testing is the primary method of determining parentage because it is 100% accurate in exclusion and >99.9 % accurate for inclusion of parentage. DNA testing is at least tenfold more conclusive than the combination of HLA, blood group, and protein markers, and DNA samples can be tested prenatally, neonatally, and post mortem. Testing is performed on nuclear DNA because mitochondrial DNA is inherited exclusively from the mother. Rather than testing for base sequence variations within genes, DNA is tested for length polymorphisms. These are short base sequences within the introns that repeat. The number of times the sequence repeats is inherited as a trait. Variable number tandem repeat sequences (VNTRs) are longer than short tandem repeats (STRs), and the repeat frequency is usually higher. Consequently they are spread over a larger section of DNA and can be analyzed by digestion with restriction enzymes and detection with Southern blotting using locus-specific probes. STRs are amplified by PCR and identified using specific oligonucleotide primers labeled with fluorescent dyes.

21. In order to prove exclusion in DNA paternity testing, why must two genes be identified that must come from the biological father and did not?
  A. A single exclusion can result from laboratory error
  B. A single exclusion can result from germ line mutation within one locus being tested
  C. The biological father may be a blood relative to the alleged father
  D. The biological mother may be different than the purported mother

Molecular/Apply knowledge of special procedures/ Paternity testing /3

22. Hereditary hemochromatosis is the result of which type of mutation?
  A. Nonsense mutation
  B. Microdeletion
  C. Translocation
  D. Single nucleotide substitution

Molecular/Correlate clinical and laboratory data/Point mutations/2

23. *p21* is a GTP binding protein produced by which oncogene?
  A. *RET*
  B. *RAS*
  C. *HER-2/neu*
  D. *N-myc*

Molecular/Apply knowledge of fundamental biological characteristics/p21/2

24. Which of the following thalassemias can be detected by PCR followed by blotting with a single specific oligonucleotide probe?
  A. α-Thalassemia
  B. Hemoglobin S/β-thalassemia
  C. β-Thalassemia
  D. Hemoglobin S/β-thalassemia

Molecular/Apply knowledge of special procedures/thalassemia /2

25. Which method is used to determine if the hemoglobin C gene is present in fetal cells?
  A. Chromosome painting
  B. FISH
  C. Restriction enzyme analysis
  D. PCR followed by blotting with a specific oligonucleotide probe

Molecular/Apply knowledge of special procedures/ Hemoglobin C/3

Answers to Questions 21–25

21. B Two exclusions are needed rather than one to be 100% certain of nonpaternity because of the rare possibility of a mutation's having occurred in one of the loci being tested. Loci used for DNA testing are sufficiently polymorphic that the mother's sample is not necessary to determine paternity. Exclusion is based on the premise that the biological father must have at least one allele in common with the child at each locus. In the case of identical twins, an exclusion would rule out both as possible parents.

22. D Hereditary hemochromatosis is an autosomal recessive disease with a frequency as high as 0.5% in the white population. The mutation occurs in the *HFE* gene on chromosome 6 and involves a single base that results in tyrosine substituting for cysteine in the *HFE* protein. The *HFE* protein binds to β-microglobulin on the intestinal epithelial membrane, down-regulating iron absorption. The mutant protein does not bind to β-microglobulin, and iron absorption increases by at least 100%. Homozygous *HFE* mutation *(C28Y)* accounts for approximately 80% of hereditary hemochromatosis. The remaining cases are caused by a single point mutation at position 63 on the protein *(H63D)*, which produces a milder increase in iron absorption. Genotype is determined by PCR using specific oligonucleotide probes to identify the products.

23. B All of the genes above are oncogenes. *RAS* is a group of three genes that produce GTP binding proteins, which activate transcription by up-regulating the signal transduction pathway of the cell. *RAS* is implicated in lung, breast, colon, and other carcinomas. It is measured by RT-PCR, which quantifies the amount of mRNA present in the malignant cells.

24. A α-Thalassemia carriers have a full or partial deletion of one or two of their four globin genes. Genotyping can determine whether two deletions are *cis* or *trans* and is performed by PCR using primers that are specific for the four most common deletions. β-Thalassemia may be caused by single base substitutions, deletions, or mutations in the flanking regions of the β-gene. Over 200 different mutations have been described, and 20 are relatively common. Microarray analysis is required to detect these.

25. D The base substitution of hemoglobin C does not affect the *MstII* restriction site and is not visible by FISH or other tests that detect damage to larger areas of the chromosome. PCR is used to amplify the gene region involved, and the product is tested by Southern blotting using a labeled-specific oligonucleotide probe.

26. In flow cytometry the term "gating" refers to:
    A. Selection of a subpopulation of cells to count
    B. Determining the fluorescent emission spectrum of cells of interest
    C. Interference caused by binding of more than a single antibody
    D. Selecting the appropriate counting aperture

    Molecular Diagnostics/Apply principles of special procedures/Flow cytometry/1

27. Which of the following parameters are used to gate cells processed by the flow cytometer?
    A. Font surface fluorescence versus incident laser intensity
    B. Forward light scatter versus side scatter
    C. The ratio of light emitted at two different wavelengths
    D. Impedance amplitude versus background conductance

    Molecular Diagnostics/Apply principles of special procedures/Flow cytometry/1

28. In general, which statement best characterizes the relationship between white blood cells and light scattering in flow cytometry?
    A. Forward scatter is related to cell size and side scatter to granularity
    B. Forward scatter is related to nuclear density and side scatter to size
    C. Forward scatter is inversely related to size and side scatter is directly related to size
    D. Forward scatter is related to shape and side scatter to size

    Molecular Diagnostics/Apply principles of special procedures/Flow cytometry/ 2

29. Fluorescent dyes most conjugated to antibodies used in flow cytometry are:
    A. Fluorescein isothiocyanate and Texas red
    B. Calcofluor white and Texas red
    C. Phycoerythrin and fluorescein isothiocyanate
    D. Acridine orange and rhodamine

    Molecular Diagnostics/Apply principles of special procedures/Flow cytometry/ 1

30. A cell population is positive for surface markers CD45, CD3, CD4, and Tdt. Which type of leukocytes are these?
    A. Lymphocytes
    B. Granulocytes
    C. Monocytes
    D. Early myeloid precursors

    Molecular Diagnostics/Apply principles of special procedures/Flow cytometry/3

Answers to Questions 26–30

26. **A** In flow cytometry cells can be divided into subpopulations based upon their light scattering properties. Cells to be interrogated by the laser(s) are selected by identifying the area in which they appear on a scatterplot.

27. **B** The gated population is selected by evaluating the scatterplot of forward light scattering (*x* axis) and right angular scatter (*x* axis). Cells falling within the specified limits are counted. For example, monocytes can be differentiated from neutrophils because the former have greater forward scatter and less side scatter.

28. **A** Forward scatter of light from a laser directed through the aperture of the cytometer is directly related to cell size. Right angular scatter (side scatter) is dependent upon the number of granules inside the cytoplasm. For example, small lymphocytes that are agranular have the lowest forward and side scatter and are easily identified as the cluster of cells closest to the bottom and left of the scatterplot.

29. **C** In flow cytometry, cells are mixed with a panel of specific antibodies that bind to surface antigens that characterize their lineage and maturation state. The antibodies are conjugated to fluorescent dyes that are excited by the laser. If light of the characteristic wavelength emitted by the fluorescent label is detected, then the cell bound the labeled antibody and is positive for the respective antigen. The two most frequently used dyes are fluorescein isothiocyanate (FITC) and phycoerythrin (PE). Since they emit green and red light, respectively, they can be differentiated in the same sample, allowing two antibodies to be tested simultaneously. Using more dyes allows for the simultaneous measurement of more markers. For example, different fluorescent dyes can be attached to latex beads in different proportions so that up to 100 combinations can be discriminated by the optics. This allows 100 different markers to be measured in the same sample simultaneously. Flow cytometry is used to measure specific plasma proteins and antibodies using fluorescent antibody–coated beads.

30. **A** CD45 is a panleukocyte marker and reacts with all white blood cells and precursors. CD3, CD4, and Tdt are markers for T lymphocytes. Typically, a panel of 12 or more antibodies is used to characterize the lineage and maturity of a cell population. The abbreviation CD stands for cluster of differentiation. Monoclonal antibodies with the same CD number recognize the same marker, although the specific moiety they react with may be different.

BIBLIOGRAPHY

1. Burtis, C.A., Ashwood, E.R., Bruns, D.E.: Tietz Textbook of Clinical Chemistry and Molecular Diagnostics, ed 4. Elsevier-Saunders, St. Louis, 2006.
2. Henry, J.B.: Clinical Diagnosis and Management by Laboratory Methods, ed 21. WB Saunders. Philadelphia, 2001.
3. Kaplan, L.A., Pesce, A.J., Kazmierczak, S.C.: Clinical Chemistry, Theory, Analysis, Correlation, ed 4. Mosby, St. Louis, 2003.
4. Lodish, H., Scott, M.P., Matsudaira, P., et al: Cell Biology, ed 5.. W. H. Freeman. NY, 2003.
5. Patrinos, G., Ansorge, W.: Molecular Diagnostics. Elsevier Press, Burlington, MA, 2005.
6. Persing, D.H., Tenover, F.C., Versalovic, J., et al: Molecular Microbiology: Diagnostic Principles and Practice. ASM Press, Washington, 2004.

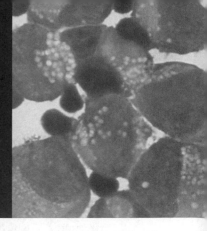

CHAPTER 9

Education and Management

1. A comparison of methods for the determination of alkaline phosphatase is categorized in which domain of educational objectives?
   A. Affective
   B. Psychomotor
   C. Cognitive
   D. Behavioral

   Education and management/Apply knowledge of educational methodology/1

2. Attitude, judgment, and interest refer to which domain of educational objectives?
   A. Cognitive
   B. Affective
   C. Psychomotor
   D. Competency

   Education and management/Apply knowledge of educational methodology/1

3. Criterion-referenced examinations are used in order to determine the:
   A. Competency of a student according to a predetermined standard
   B. Validity of a test
   C. Status of one student compared to the whole group
   D. Accuracy of a test

   Education and management/Apply knowledge of educational testing/1

4. An instructor "curved" a blood bank examination given to medical technology students. The highest grade was an 85% and the lowest grade was a 60%. What type of test is this?
   A. Subjective
   B. Objective
   C. Norm-referenced
   D. Criterion-referenced

   Education and management/Apply knowledge of educational testing/2

5. A stated competency requirement for a medical technology student is to perform calibration, plot data, and evaluate the acceptability of controls. This com-

petency requirement encompasses which educational objective?
   A. Cognitive
   B. Psychomotor
   C. Affective
   D. All of the above

   Education and management/Apply knowledge of educational methodology/3

Answers to Questions 1–5

1. **C** The cognitive domain of educational objectives deals with application, analysis, synthesis, and evaluation of information or knowledge learned to be utilized in problem solving.

2. **B** The affective domain of educational objectives includes those that emphasize values, attitudes, and interests that attach a worth to an activity, situation, or phenomenon.

3. **A** A criterion-referenced test is used to determine the mastery of predetermined competencies, whereas a norm-referenced test evaluates students by comparison to the group. Criterion-referenced examinations use questions of known difficulty and can be calibrated against established criteria in order to evaluate the examinee's performance.

4. **C** This type of test compares the students to each other rather than grading the students on a set of standards or criterion that must be met.

5. **D** The student will perform the actual calibration (psychomotor skills), utilize the cognitive domain of analysis to plot the standards, construct a best-fit calibration line, and determine the concentration of the controls. The affective domain describes the student's ability to value the results as acceptable or to repeat the calibration if an error is apparent.

6. A chemistry test result from a chemotherapy patient was within normal limits on Tuesday. The same test was reported as abnormal on Monday ("flagged" high and approaching a critical value). The technologist performing the test noted a delta-check error and remembered that both controls ran much higher on Monday, although they were within acceptable limits. The technologist's decision to follow-up on this discrepancy before reporting the results is an example of which domain of behavioral objectives?
   A. Cognitive
   B. Affective
   C. Psychomotor
   D. Organizational

Education and management/Apply knowledge of educational methodology/3

7. In general, academic evaluation of students depends on the ability of the instructor to create a test that reflects the stated objectives of the course material as well as making the test:
   A. Reliable and valid
   B. Normally distributed and practical
   C. Fair and short
   D. Written and oral

Education and management/Apply knowledge of educational testing/1

8. When dealing with the instruction of complex instrumentation, a demonstration by the instructor is necessary and should include the following:
   A. Detailed diagrams of the electrical system
   B. A blueprint of the optical system
   C. A step-by-step narrative with comparisons to a manual method
   D. A quiz as soon as the demonstration is complete

Education and management/Apply knowledge of educational methodology/1

9. One method of learning is by giving a small group of students a topic to discuss or a problem to solve rather than a formal lecture by the instructor. Each participant is given a portion of the topic to discuss or solve. This method of learning is popular and used easily with which of the following approaches?
   A. Case study
   B. Manual demonstration
   C. Implementing new equipment
   D. Histogram evaluation

Education and management/Apply knowledge of educational methodology/2

10. An instructor of clinical laboratory science was given the task of expanding the curriculum for the senior (baccalaureate degree) medical technology students. Which of the following courses should be included in the curriculum?
   A. Cytology—cytogenetics
   B. Histology—special stains
   C. Computer (laboratory information systems [LIS])
   D. Economics—budget analysis

Education and management/Education/Apply knowledge of entry level skills/1

Answers to Questions 6–10

6. **B** The technologist chose to investigate the situation in order to resolve a discrepancy. The responding, valuing, and characterization refer to the affective domain in dealing with the problem presented here. In doing so, a rule-based process is followed that includes evaluation of the specimen, instrument performance, potential sources of interference (such as the effects of drugs), and physiological variation before determining whether to report the result, repeat the test, or call for a new specimen.

7. **A** A test should be based on stated, measurable objectives and contain five attributes: reliability, validity, objectivity, fairness, and practicality.

8. **C** When a demonstration of a complex instrument is necessary, a small group of students should be assembled around the instrument to permit clear visibility. A diagram with the major functioning parts should be provided along with an assignment of a written summary or questions about the function, principle, testing done, and reagents needed.

9. **A** The case study approach allows a student to engage in problem solving and to utilize the input of all members of the group. This allows for interaction and use of higher cognitive levels in order to determine the cause of the patient's illness and various laboratory test results.

10. **C** The ever-changing role of the medical technologist in a clinical laboratory prompts the curriculum committee to re-evaluate the courses required by the students on a yearly basis. The heart of the laboratory, the LIS, is one of the first important areas to which students are introduced when entering the professional clinical training portion of their degree.

11. McGregor's X-Y theory advocates managing employees by stressing:
    A. Equal pay for equal work
    B. A pyramid of attainable goals for satisfaction at work
    C. Respect for the worker and acknowledgment of his/her ability to perform a task
    D. Collective bargaining

    Education and management/Apply knowledge of management theory/1

12. Maslow's theory of management is based upon:
    A. The premise that all workers are unmotivated
    B. A pyramid of goals for the satisfaction of employee needs
    C. Use of detractors and perks to keep employees happy
    D. The professional development of the employee

    Education and management/Apply knowledge of management theory/1

13. Herzberg's theory relies on motivators that are part of the job design in order to instill job satisfaction. These same motivators can become dissatisfiers if they are lacking in a job. Herzberg's motivators are:
    A. Opportunity for achievement and advancement
    B. Performance evaluations every 24 months
    C. Continuing education sessions requiring supervisory approval
    D. Punitive actions taken when improvement diminishes

    Education and management/Apply knowledge of management theory/1

14. Management by objective (MBO) is *LEAST* effective for managing employees in which situation?
    A. Employees must be creative in their work
    B. The laboratory is converting to a new computer system
    C. The laboratory is undergoing a renovation
    D. Employees jointly agree to institutional goals

    Education and management/Apply knowledge of management theory/2

15. The four essential functions of a manager are:
    A. Staffing, decision making, cost analysis, evaluating
    B. Directing, leading, forecasting, implementing
    C. Planning, organizing, directing, controlling
    D. Innovating, designing, coordinating, problem solving

    Education and management/Apply knowledge of management theory/1

16. Which of the following questions is allowable during a pre-employment interview?
    A. How many times have you been pregnant?
    B. Have you been convicted of any felonies?
    C. Does your husband belong to any religious societies?
    D. Are you planning to use the hospital day care center?

    Education and management/Labor law/3

Answers to Questions 11–16

11. **C** McGregor's theory deals with participatory management in which the employee is considered a valuable asset.

12. **B** Maslow's theory of managing people deals with six levels. As the basic needs of an employee are met, the next higher need is substituted. The needs, in ascending order, are physiological, safety, security, social, esteem and self-actualization. Unsatisfied needs are considered motivators.

13. **A** According to Frederick Herzberg, achievement, opportunity for advancement, recognition, challenging work, responsibility, and a chance for advancement and personal growth are motivators and should be included as part of a job design.

14. **A** MBO stresses teamwork and shared goals and objectives but stifles creativity.

15. **C** While managing may involve all of the functions listed, the four core processes for all managers are planning, organizing, directing, and controlling. Planning includes formulating of goals and objectives, organizing the tasks, and establishing schedules. Organizing includes establishing effective communication, relationships, job descriptions, and training. Directing involves oversight of the various steps and stages of the plan, including coordination and leadership. Controlling involves evaluating resource utilization and outcomes, managing costs, and modifying the process to improve quality.

16. **B** Title VII of the Civil Rights Act of 1964 states that questions are permissible during interviews if they are related to legitimate occupational qualifications. Inquiries concerning convictions for drug use or theft are legitimate questions when hiring a laboratory night supervisor or other individuals who will utilize controlled substances.

17. Direct laboratory costs for tests include which of the following?
   A. Equipment maintenance
   B. Insurance
   C. Depreciation
   D. Overtime pay

Education and management/Laboratory economics/1

18. Which of the following accounts for the largest portion of the direct cost of a laboratory test?
   A Reagents
   B. General supplies
   C. Technologist labor
   D. Instrument depreciation

Education and management/Laboratory economics/1

19. Using the surcharge/cost-plus method for determining test charges, determine the charge for an ova and parasite examination on fecal specimens, given the following information:

   Collection, handling, clerical, and so forth = $2.00

   Reference laboratory charge to laboratory = $20.00

   Lab "mark-up" = 100%

   A. $22.00
   B. $32.00
   C. $42.00
   D. $122.00

Education and management/Laboratory economics/2

20. In deciding whether to adopt a new test on the laboratory's automated chemistry analyzer, which parameters are needed to determine the number of tests that must be performed to break even?
   A. Test turnaround time
   B. Cost of labor per hour
   C. Number of other tests performed per month
   D. Total fixed laboratory costs

Education and management/Laboratory economics/2

21. Which statement best represents the relationship between test volume and revenue or costs for batch-run tests?
   A. As volume increases the fixed cost per test also increases
   B. As volume increases the revenue also increases
   C. Revenue is approximately equal for both high and low volume tests
   D. 90% of the revenue is generated by 5% of the tests offered

Education and management/Laboratory economics/2

22. A hospital submits a bill for $200.00 to the patient's insurance company for the cost of outpatient laboratory tests. The laboratory services rendered by the hospital are paid according to an agreed-upon fee schedule. The specific laboratory procedures are billed according to which system of coding?

   A. Diagnosis-related group (DRG)
   B. Current procedural terminology (CPT)
   C. Medicare
   D. Medicaid

Education and management/Laboratory economics/1

Answers to Questions 17–22

17. **D** All costs that are specifically linked to a test (e.g., personnel, overtime, chemicals, supplies) are direct costs.

18. **C** Labor accounts for 60%–70% of the direct cost per test in most laboratories. The cost of labor, reagents, and supplies are direct costs but instrument depreciation is not.

19. **C** The "mark-up" factor is used to establish part of the cost of a test in order to obtain the desired profit margin. Tests sent to reference laboratories or done in-house have the added cost that is referred to as the surcharge/cost-plus method of determining test charges.

20. **D** The formula for calculating the break-even point in test volume is:

Number of tests = total fixed costs ÷ (average reimbursement – variable cost per test)

The total fixed costs are the expenses that are not expected to change as the workload increases (e.g., cost of the instrument). The variable cost per test includes any costs that increase as the workload increases (e.g., cost of reagents). The average reimbursement represents the expected revenue generated per billable test result.

21. **B** As volume increases, costs should decrease and revenues should increase. The large fixed costs such as instrumentation, labor, and management do not change with the size of the batch. As volume increases, reagent and consumable costs per test often become lower, thus reducing the variable cost per test. In most laboratories, about 80% of the revenue is generated by the laboratory tests that constitute the top 20% of the test volume.

22. **B** The CPT code refers to Current Procedural Terminology. Codes are assigned to all medical procedures, which are grouped according to common disease characteristics. The insurance company or payer (e.g., Medicare) usually has agreed to a reimbursement amount per test or procedure. The American Medical Association publishes *Current Procedural Terminology,* or CPT, which is updated yearly.

23. A hospital has a contract with a major medical insurer that reimburses the laboratory at a rate of $1.00 per insured life per year. This type of reimbursement is termed:
A. A prospective payment system
B. A preferred provider discount
C. Capitation
D. DRG

Education and management/Laboratory economics/2

24. According to federal and state regulations, a hospital's capital budget should include which of the following before projects costing $150,000 can be submitted for approval?
A. A timetable of completion
B. A cost analysis
C. Salaries and wages for new employees
D. A certificate of need

Education and management/Laboratory economics/1

25. A rural hospital laboratory employs 8.25 FTEs (full-time equivalents). In order to budget for next year's salaries for these employees, the laboratory manager needs to submit which figures for the laboratory's projected annual budget?
A. Total (paid) hours
B. Productive (worked) hours
C. Total hours of full-time employees
D. Total hours of part-time employees

Education and management/Laboratory economics/1

26. A chemistry profile that includes electrolytes, glucose, blood urea nitrogen (BUN), and creatinine is ordered on an 80-year-old woman with symptoms of vomiting and dizziness. How should the laboratory submit the charge for these tests for reimbursement by Medicare?
A. Submit as one test
B. Submit each test separately
C. Submit Medicare-approved tests only
D. Submit as four individual tests

Education and management/Laboratory regulation and law/2

27. According to the Clinical Laboratory Improvement Act of 1988 (CLIA '88), control of laboratory test reliability is accomplished by all of the following requirements *except:*
A. Documentation of quality control results and corrective actions
B. Participation in proficiency testing for all nonwaived tests
C. Professional certification of all testing personnel
D. Demonstration that all quantitative tests meet the manufacturer's performance specifications

Education and management/Laboratory regulation and law/2

Answers to Questions 23–27

23. **C** Capitation plans provide the laboratory with a fixed (known) revenue based upon a negotiated per capita fee for the members of the group. In order to profit, the laboratory must manage its resources to provide covered laboratory tests to the group at a cost that does not equal or exceed its reimbursement. A prospective payment system is used by Medicare and Medicaid programs for outpatient reimbursements and is based upon projecting the cost of a laboratory test in a specific region. For inpatients the fees for laboratory tests are incorporated into the reimbursement covering the specific diagnosis-related group rather than the type or number of laboratory procedures performed.

24. **D** A certificate of need (CON) is an authorization to proceed with a needed project, such as a new obstetrics department or adding a new wing to the laboratory. There are specific federal guidelines (most states also require them) to follow, and the limit is set at $150,000. This is done to control duplication of services as well as to avoid creating oversupply of hospital beds.

25. **A** The total (paid) hours are the total number of hours for which employees are paid. This includes vacation time, sick time, and the actual time spent working in the laboratory. On the other hand, productive (worked) hours refer only to the actual hours worked, including overtime. A budget must include the total (paid) hours in order to give a clear picture of what is needed for the next year of wages and salaries.

26. **A** A chemistry profile that includes electrolytes, glucose, BUN, and creatinine is considered a billable procedure and has a single CPT code (currently this panel is called the Basic Metabolic Panel and is coded as CPT 80049). Splitting a profile into many individual tests for billing purposes may be prohibited by law. For example, a complete blood count (CBC) cannot be split into five parts with each component being charged separately.

27. **C** CLIA '88 requires that all clinical laboratories be certified, but the requirements differ for each of the three certification levels—waivered, moderate, or high complexity. For example, quality control must be practiced by all laboratories, but standards for testing personnel differ for all three levels and do not specify certification, only educational levels.

28. CLIA '88 specifies the minimum requirements for proficiency testing (PT) of analytes for which PT is required (excluding cytology) to be:
  A. One challenge per analyte and one testing event per year
  B. Ten challenges per analyte and five testing events per year
  C. Five challenges per analyte and at least three testing events per year
  D. Twelve challenges per analyte and one testing event per month

Education and management/Laboratory regulation and law/1

29. According to CLIA '88, satisfactory performance for ABO, Rh, and compatibility tests requires a score of:
  A. 100%
  B. 90%
  C. 80%
  D. 75%

Education and management/Laboratory regulation and law/1

30. In order to comply with CLIA '88, calibration materials must:
  A. Be purchased by an authorized agency such as the College of Pathology
  B. Have concentration values that cover the laboratory's reportable range
  C. Be traceable to the National Calibration Board
  D. Be identical in concentration to those sold by the reagent manufacturer

Education and management/Laboratory regulation and law/1

31. According to CLIA '88, calibration materials should be appropriate for the methodology and be:
  A. Of bovine origin
  B. Three times the normal range for the specific analyte
  C. Traceable to a reference method and reference material of known value
  D. Twice the laboratory's reference range for the analyte

Education and management/Laboratory regulation and law/1

32. Under CLIA '88, testing personnel with an associate degree and appropriate training in the clinical laboratory are authorized to perform:
  A. Waivered tests only
  B. Tests that are qualitative or waivered and some moderate-complexity tests
  C. Waivered and moderate-complexity tests
  D. Waivered, moderate-complexity, and high-complexity tests

Education and management/Laboratory regulation and law/1

33. Sexual harassment is a form of discrimination and therefore is prohibited by the:
  A. Occupational Safety and Health Administration (OSHA)
  B. Civil Rights Act of 1964 (Title VII)
  C. Right to Privacy Act of 1974
  D. Department of Health and Human Services

Education and management/Labor law/1

Answers to Questions 28–33

28. **C** Analytes for which proficiency testing is required are identified in section 493 subpart I of the CLIA rules. A minimum number of five challenges for each analyte and at least three testing events per year are required. The testing events are evenly spaced throughout the year. Unsatisfactory performance for the same analyte for two out of two events or two out of the three most recent events constitutes unsuccessful participation and may result in punitive action.

29. **A** Unsatisfactory performance occurs when any challenge for ABO, Rh, or compatibility testing is in error. For all other tests, a score below 80% is defined as unsatisfactory performance. Unsatisfactory performance for the same analyte for two out of two events or two out of the three most recent events constitutes unsuccessful participation.

30. **B** According to CLIA '88, the minimum requirement for calibration is every 6 months or more frequently if specified by the manufacturer. The calibrators must cover the reportable range of the method. A minimum of two levels of calibrant must be used (more if specified by the manufacturer).

31. **C** Calibrators must have an assigned concentration determined by assay using a reference method. The reference method should be calibrated using standards that are traceable to National Bureau of Standards material or acceptable primary standards.

32. **D** Testing personnel with an associate degree and approved laboratory training may perform high-complexity tests as well as waivered and moderate-complexity tests. However, the laboratory must be certified at all three levels.

33. **B** The Civil Rights Act of 1964 prohibits discrimination in employment by federal law because of race, color, religion, or gender. The law established the EEOC to hear complaints of discrimination by employees and initiate legal action as appropriate.

34. Which order of events should be followed at the conclusion of a laboratory worker's shift in order to prevent the spread of bloodborne pathogens?
A. Remove gloves, disinfect area, wash hands, remove laboratory coat
B. Disinfect area, remove gloves, remove laboratory coat, wash hands
C. Disinfect area, remove gloves, wash hands, remove laboratory coat
D. Remove gloves, wash hands, remove laboratory coat, disinfect area

Education and management/Laboratory safety and standard precautions/2

35. Records of a patient's laboratory test results may not be released without his or her consent to anyone outside the clinical laboratory except to the:
A. American Athletic Association
B. Church affiliate
C. American Automobile Association
D. Physician and nursing staff

Education and management/Laboratory regulation and law/2

36. Unethical behavior by a laboratory supervisor that results in a compromise of employee safety should be:
A. Reported to a higher authority
B. Directly confronted
C. Reported to the Equal Employment Opportunity Commission (EEOC)
D. All of the above

Education and management/Apply principles of laboratory management/Personnel/2

37. The most common deficiency cited during an onsite laboratory inspection by the College of American Pathologists (CAP) and the Joint Commission on Accreditation of Healthcare Organizations (JCAHO) is:
A. Improper documentation
B. Insufficient work space area
C. Improper reagent storage
D. Improper instrument calibration frequency

Education and management/Laboratory regulation and certification/2

38. Which of the following circumstances is considered a form a sexual harassment?
A. Unwelcome sexual advances by a supervisor
B. Requests for favors of a sexual nature from a fellow laboratory employee
C. Physical conduct of a sexual nature from an employee working in another department
D. All of the above

Education and management/Labor law/2

39. The material safety data sheets (MSDS) for hazardous chemicals address which of the following conditions?
A. Physical characteristics of the chemical
B. Safe handling and storage of the chemical
C. Specific health hazards associated with the chemical
D. All of the above

Education and management/Laboratory regulation and safety/1

Answers to Questions 34–39

34. **B** According to the OSHA (Occupational Safety and Health Administration) Bloodborne Pathogens Rule of 1992, gloves and laboratory coats are to be removed after disinfection of the work area.

35. **D** The Privacy Act of 1974 prohibits the release of medical records without the patient's consent except to the patient's attending physician, attorney, or next of kin if deceased unless solicited by a valid subpoena. HIPPA (Health Insurance Portability and Accountability Act, 1996) protects patient test confidentiality.

36. **D** Direct confrontation is in order, followed by reporting the behavior to a higher authority at the clinical site. Major violations that are a threat to the safety of employees, patients, and the facility in general should be reported to the EEOC or OSHA if the violations are not corrected in a timely fashion, and if all avenues of action have been exhausted.

37. **A** Improper documentation accounts for the majority of laboratory deficiencies, whereas outdated or inadequate procedure manuals are the second most frequently cited deficiency.

38. **D** Sexual harassment is a form of discrimination and it is prohibited by the Civil Rights Act of 1964 (Title VII). The suggestion that a sexual favor must be performed to avoid punitive action or receive a favorable performance evaluation constitutes sexual harassment. Additionally, offensive language and behavior with sexual connotations are a form of sexual harassment.

39. **D** The MSDS documents describe the chemical and physical characteristics, safe handling and storage, and potential health hazards of reagents used in the laboratory. These documents must be located in an easily accessible place so that all employees have access to them. They should be reviewed at least once per year during safety in-service training.

40. A new employee's performance is to be evaluated at the end of his or her probationary period and must relate to:
- **A.** The person's job description
- **B.** Verbal instructions given
- **C.** Wage and salary policies
- **D.** Recruitment practices

Education and management/Apply principles of laboratory management/Personnel/1

41. Which regulatory agency mandates the following requirements for protection of employees of clinical laboratories?

- Provide personal protective equipment (PPE)
- Require hepatitis B vaccinations at no cost
- Require specific biohazard materials labeling
- Provide training and updating yearly of safety standards

- **A.** Food and Drug Administration (FDA)
- **B.** Occupational Safety and Health Administration (OSHA)
- **C.** American Association of Blood Banks (AABB)
- **D.** American Society of Clinical Pathologists (ASCP)

Education and management/Apply knowledge of laboratory regulations/1

42. The Clinical Laboratory Improvement Act of 1988 (CLIA '88) was enacted to regulate the following:
- **A.** All clinical laboratories in the U.S.
- **B.** Independent laboratories not regulated by OSHA
- **C.** Environmental Protection Agency laboratories
- **D.** Industrial laboratories

Education and management/Apply knowledge of laboratory regulations/1

43. Records of a patient's laboratory test results may be released without the prior consent of the patient to all of the following *except:*
- **A.** Insurance provider
- **B.** Physician
- **C.** Nursing staff
- **D.** Mother-in-law

Education and management/Apply knowledge of laboratory regulations/2

44. The following is (are) successful indicator(s) of Quality Assurance (QA) and Quality Improvement (QI) programs in a clinical laboratory:
- **A.** A "log" of incident report and solutions attained
- **B.** Emergency department and *stat* "turn around times"
- **C.** Positive patient identification wristbands for blood bank operations
- **D.** All of the above

Education and management/Apply knowledge of Quality Performance/2

Answers to Questions 40–44

40. A The information used for the employee's performance review should reflect the job description used at the time of hire. An employee should receive a written job description that states the responsibilities and activities of the position. Job performance criteria and the rating system used should be clearly stated and available to the employee.

41. B The U.S. Department of Labor through OSHA mandates a workplace that is safe and healthy. Other agencies that inspect clinical laboratories (CLIA '88, CAP, JCAHO, etc.) also require safety guidelines for the health care workers in the clinical laboratory.

42. A The regulations for clinical laboratories (CLIA '88) were finally published in 1992 in the *Federal Register* (USDHHS, 1992). The federal mandate was designed to regulate a specific standard for each laboratory test as well as categorize the laboratories according to the level of testing and the lab personnel.

43. D HIPPA (Health Insurance Portability and Accountability Act, 1996) provides increased access to health care by making it easier for providers to send medical information to insurance companies electronically. The law requires health care providers to safeguard the confidentiality of patient medical information and to provide patients with a compliance statement that defines who is entitled to receive their health information. The physician ordering the tests as well as health care workers directly involved with the patient are allowed to see laboratory results. Laboratory results may also be released to the patient's insurance provider and to medical review officers and public health officials. They may also be released to the patient's family provided that the patient is notified of this policy beforehand and is given the right to approve or object.

44. D These policies, along with laboratory performances on proficiency surveys, are a part of QA, QI, and TQI (Total Quality Improvement), which are now included in the JCAHO accreditation process.

45. Continuous Quality Improvement (CQI) is a team effort approach for clinical laboratories to:
A. Identify potential problems and correct them
B. Set laboratory financial benchmarks for the year
C. Make up new CPT codes
D. Improve overall wages for laboratory employees

Education and management/Quality Improvement/2

46. Which of the following is *not* an appropriate guideline for phlebotomists to follow in order to prevent a malpractice lawsuit?
A. Use one form of patient ID, such as a last name
B. Keep patient confidentiality at all times
C. Use aseptic venipuncture technique at all times
D. Label specimens only after the blood has been drawn

Education and management/Malpractice law/2

47. According to CLIA '88, testing personnel performing high-complexity laboratory tests must have at least a:
A. Bachelor of Arts degree
B. Bachelor of Science degree in medical laboratory technology
C. Associate's degree in laboratory science or medical technology
D. High school diploma

Education and management/Regulation lab/2

48. During an interview, an employer may request the following from a prospective new employee:
A. Marital status
B. Age of children
C. Arrests for DUI
D. Professional certification

Education and management/Labor law/2

49. A new Laboratory Information System (LIS) will be evaluated by the laboratory staff. Which of the following points should be considered in the evaluation?
A. Cost of updating software
B. Interface ability with existing laboratory instruments
C. Tracking of uncrossmatched blood units in the Blood Bank
D. All of the above

Education and management/Laboratory economics/3

50. Point-of-Care Testing (POCT) refers to:
A. All testing done to the patient to save time
B. All laboratory testing done in the central lab
C. Any clinical laboratory testing done at the bedside of a patient
D. Satellite laboratory testing

Education and management/Laboratory economics/2

Answers to Questions 45–50

45. **A** The CQI team identifies problems by collecting data, analyzing it, and developing methods of correcting problems. By identifying potential problems and correcting existing problems, a high competency level is achieved and potential lawsuits are avoided.

46. **A** Outpatient identification through two means (name and date of birth) are standard procedures to avoid drawing the wrong patient. Other malpractice prevention measures include treating people equally; securing informed consent before testing; and listening to patient's concerns.

47. **C** CLIA '88 requires personnel who perform high-complexity tests to have earned at least an associate's degree in medical laboratory science or attained a level of college education and clinical laboratory training equivalent to an associate's degree in medical laboratory science.

48. **D** All of the questions are in violation of Title VII of the Civil Rights Act of 1964 except the request for certification. The certification is usually a requirement for job performance and is listed in the job description.

49. **D** Each laboratory has specific needs to determine the appropriate LIS. However, storage capacity, reliability, security, upgrade costs, instrument interface availability, inventory management, and quality control functions are common parameters that must be considered.

50. **C** Point-of-care testing saves time and is invaluable for patient care. When a device is used at the bedside of a patient to produce a laboratory result, it is considered a point-of-care instrument. Many such devices are often waived by CLIA, thus allowing them to be used by personnel without laboratory training. However, the institution must have a CLIA license to perform the testing, and appropriate quality control procedures must be followed. Some devices used for point-of-care testing utilize equivalent quality control, usually electronic simulation of the measurement that takes place with disposable unit-dose reagent packs.

BIBLIOGRAPHY

1. Harmening, D.M.: Laboratory Management. Prentice Hall, N. J., 2002.
2. McGregor, D.: The Human Side of Enterprise. McGraw-Hill, N.Y., 1985.
3. Regulations Implementing the Clinical Laboratory Improvement Amendments of 1988 (42 CFR Part 405). Federal Register, February 28, 57(40), 1992.
4. Varnadoe, L.A.: Medical Laboratory Management and Supervision. FA Davis, Philadelphia, 1996.
5. Wallace, M.A., Klosinski, D.D.: Clinical Laboratory Science Education and Management. W.B. Saunders, Philadelphia, 1998.

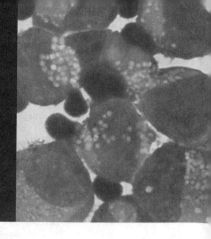

CHAPTER 10

Photomicrographs and Color Plates

Refer to the photomicrographs and color plates that follow p. 494.

1. Plate 1 is a photomicrograph of an antinuclear antibody test using human fibroblasts, fluorescein isothiocyanate (FITC)–conjugated antihuman serum, and transmitted fluorescence microscopy. Which pattern of immunofluorescence is demonstrated in this 400× field?
   A. Homogeneous
   B. Peripheral
   C. Nucleolar
   D. Speckled

   Immunology/Identify microscopic morphology/ Immunofluorescence/2

2. Plate 2 shows the electrophoresis of serum proteins on a high-resolution agarose gel at pH 8.6. Sample 1 (in lane 1) is a normal serum control. Which sample can be presumptively classified as a monoclonal gammopathy?
   A. Sample 2
   B. Sample 4
   C. Sample 6
   D. Sample 8

   Chemistry/Evaluate clinical and laboratory data/ Electrophoresis/3

3. Plate 3 shows a densitometric scan of a control serum for protein electrophoresis. The percentages of each fraction are shown below the scan. Given these results, what is the most appropriate initial corrective action?
   A. Repeat the electrophoresis run using fresh control serum
   B. Report the results provided that the previous run was in control
   C. Move the fourth fraction mark to the right and redraw the scan
   D. Calculate the concentration of each fraction in grams per deciliter

   Chemistry/Identify sources of error/Densitometry/3

Answers to Questions 1–3

1. **A** Using FITC-conjugated antihuman serum, diffuse apple green fluorescence seen over the entire nucleus characterizes the homogeneous pattern. At a significant titer, this pattern occurs in a variety of systemic autoimmune diseases, including systemic lupus erythematosus, rheumatoid arthritis, systemic sclerosis, and Sjögren's syndrome. The antibodies are directed against nucleoprotein; although they are mainly nonpathological, they are useful markers for active disease.

2. **C** A monoclonal gammopathy causes a band showing restricted electrophoretic mobility usually located in the γ or the β region. The band represents the accumulation of identical immunoglobulin molecules or fragments secreted by a malignant or benign clone of plasma cells. Confirmation of the band as immunoglobulin is required because other homogeneous proteins (such as fibrinogen or carcinoembryonic antigen) can occur in the same regions.

3. **C** The fraction marker between the α_2- and β-fractions is marked improperly. High-resolution gels produce individual peaks for haptoglobin and α_2-macroglobulin, which partially splits the α_2-band into two subfractions. In addition, the β-band may contain three subfractions corresponding to β-lipoprotein, transferrin, and complement. In this scan, the valley between the α_2-subfractions was selected incorrectly as the boundary between the α_2- and β-fractions. This fraction marker should be placed at the next valley to the right and the scan redrawn to determine the area under the α_2- and β-fractions correctly.

4. Plate 4 shows the electrophoresis of serum proteins on a high-resolution agarose gel at pH 8.6. Which band represents the β-lipoprotein?

- **A.** A
- **B.** B
- **C.** C
- **D.** D

Chemistry/Evaluate clinical and laboratory data/Protein electrophoresis/2

5. Plate 5 is a densitometric scan of a serum protein electrophoresis sample. The relative and absolute concentrations of each fraction and reference limits are shown below the scan. What is the correct classification of this densitometric pattern?

- **A.** Polyclonal gammopathy associated with chronic inflammation
- **B.** Nephrotic syndrome
- **C.** Acute inflammation
- **D.** Hepatic cirrhosis

Chemistry/Evaluate clinical and laboratory data/ Electrophoresis/3

6. Plate 6 shows an agarose gel on which immunofixation electrophoresis (IFE) was performed at pH 8.6. The gel contains the same serum sample as number 6 shown in Plate 2. What is the heavy and light chain type of the monoclonal protein present in this sample?

- **A.** IgA κ
- **B.** IgG κ
- **C.** IgG λ
- **D.** IgM λ

Chemistry/Evaluate clinical and laboratory data/ Electrophoresis/3

7. Plate 7 shows the electrophoresis of hemoglobin (Hgb) samples performed on agarose gel, pH 8.8. The control sample is located in lanes 2 and 10 and contains Hgb A, S, and C. Which sample(s) are from neonates?

- **A.** Samples 1 and 5
- **B.** Sample 3
- **C.** Sample 7
- **D.** Samples 8 and 9

Chemistry/Evaluate clinical and laboratory data/ Hemoglobin electrophoresis/2

4. **C** Using high current, β-lipoprotein can be separated from transferrin and complement (C3). β-lipoprotein migrates anodal to the transferrin (band labeled D) and appears as a thin wavy band. C3 migrates cathodal to the transferrin band. The band labeled A is α_1-antitrypsin, and the band labeled B contains α-2 macroglobulin and haptoglobin. The α-2 macroglobulin is usually anodal to the haptoglobin.

5. **C** This pattern is characterized by significant increases in the α_1- and α_2-fractions and a decrease in serum albumin concentration. This pattern is most often caused by increased production of acute phase reactants such as α_1-antitrypsin and haptoglobin that are associated with acute inflammation. This pattern is seen in myocardial infarction and other forms of acute tissue injury, the early stage of acute infection, and pregnancy.

6. **B** IFE is performed by placing the patient's sample in all six lanes and separating the proteins by electrophoresis. Following electrophoresis, the proteins in lane 1 are precipitated and fixed by overlaying sulfosalicylic acid onto the gel. Monospecific antiserum against each heavy or light chain is applied to the gel over the lanes as labeled and incubated to precipitate the immunoglobulins containing the corresponding chain. The gel is washed to remove unprecipitated proteins, then stained to visualize the precipitated bands. This IFE gel shows an insoluble immunoprecipitate restricted to a single band in lanes 2 and 5. The proteins in lane 2 reacted with anti-γ (anti-IgG), and the proteins in lane 5 reacted with anti-κ. Lane 5 also contains a small restricted band anodal to the IgG band. This band is not present in lane 2 (does not contain γ chains) and represents free κ light chains.

7. **A** Neonates and infants up to 6 months old have Hgb F levels between 8% and 40%. The Hgb F level falls to below 2% in children over 2 years old. Hgb F is more acidic than Hgb S and less acidic than Hgb A. Therefore, at an alkaline pH, Hgb F has a greater net negative charge than Hgb S but a lesser net negative charge than Hgb A, and it migrates between Hgb A and Hgb S.

8. Plate 8 shows the electrophoresis of Hgb samples on acid agar gel, pH 6.0. The sample order is the same as for plate 7 with the A, S, and C control hemolysate in lanes 2 and 10. Based upon the electrophoretic mobility of sample 7 as seen in both plates 7 and 8, what is the patient's Hgb phenotype?

A. SS

B. AS

C. AD

D. AG

Chemistry/Evaluate clinical and laboratory data/ Hemoglobin electrophoresis/3

9. Plate 9 is a photomicrograph of a fungal slide culture stained with lactophenol cotton blue, 400×. Which of the following fungi are present?

A. *Microsporum gypseum*

B. *Microsporum canis*

C. *Aspergillus niger*

D. *Aspergillus fumigatus*

Microbiology/Identify microscopic morphology/Fungi/2

10. Plate 10 is a photomicrograph of a fungal slide culture stained with lactophenol cotton blue, 400×. Which of the following fungi is present?

A. *M. gypseum*

B. *M. canis*

C. *Trichophyton schoenleinii*

D. *Epidermophyton floccosum*

Microbiology/Identify microscopic morphology/Fungi/2

11. Plate 11 is a photomicrograph of a fungal slide culture stained with lactophenol cotton blue, 400×. The morphology is most consistent with which fungus?

A. *Aspergillus* spp

B. *Penicillium* spp

C. *Scedosporium* spp

D. *Fusarium* spp

Microbiology/Identify microscopic morphology/ Mycology/2

Answers to Questions 8–11

8. **A** Sample 7 demonstrates one major band on plate 7 in the Hgb S position. Because Hgb A is not present, there is no normal β-gene, and the patient can be classified as a homozygote for Hgb S, D, or G, which migrate to the same position on agarose gel at a pH of between 8.4 and 9.2. Hgb S can be differentiated from Hgbs D and G by performing electrophoresis on agar gel at pH 6.0–6.2. On agar at acid pH, Hgb C migrates farthest toward the anode. Hgb S migrates toward the anode, but not as far as Hgb C. Hgb F migrates farthest toward the cathode, whereas Hgbs A, D, G, and E migrate to the same position, slightly cathodal to the point of application. On plate 8, sample 7 shows a single large band that migrated toward the anode at the same position as the S band in the control sample.

9. **D** *A. fumigatus* produces hyaline, septate hyphae and dome-shaped vesicles, the upper one half to two-thirds of which are covered with a row of phialides producing long chains of conidia. *A. niger* produces spherical vesicles that are completely covered with phialides. The phialides produce jet black conidia that obscure the vesicle surface, forming a radiated head. *M. gypseum* and *M. canis* produce septate macroconidia, not vesicles with phialides.

10. **A** *M. gypseum* produces enormous numbers of symmetric, rough macroconidia. These have thin walls with not more than six compartments and have rounded ends. *M. canis* produces spindle-shaped macroconidia with usually more than six compartments and pointed ends. *E. floccosum* forms macroconidia but not microconidia. The macroconidia are smooth and club-shaped with rounded ends. Each contains two to six cells and is found singly or in clusters. *T. schoenleinii* does not produce macroconidia or microconidia and is identified by its hyphae-forming characteristics. *T. schoenleinii* forms antler-like branching hyphae called *favic chandeliers*.

11. **A** This plate shows a fungus with thin, septate, branching hyphae. A conidiophore is present in the center that contains a double row of phialides producing round conidia. *Fusarium* spp produce canoe-shaped macroconidia. These are made by phialides attached to the hyphae in the absence of conidiophores. *Penicillium* spp produce conidia from a single row of phialides that resembles a brush or the skeleton of a hand. *Scedosporium* spp produce annellids on short conidiophores with oval conidia that are tapered at one end.

12. Plate 12 is a bronchoalveolar lavage sample concentrated by cytocentrifugation and stained with Wright's stain, 1000×. The sample was obtained from a patient with AIDS who resides in the midwestern United States. Which infectious agent is present?

   A. *Pneumocystis carinii*
   B. *Mycobacterium avium-intracellulare*
   C. *Histoplasma capsulatum*
   D. *Cryptococcus neoformans*

   Microbiology/Identify microscopic morphology/
   Mycology/2

13. Plate 13 is a fecal specimen seen under 400× using brightfield microscopy. The plate shows the ovum of which parasite?

   A. *Necator americanus*
   B. *Trichuris trichiura*
   C. *Ascaris lumbricoides*
   D. *Enterobius vermicularis*

   Microbiology/Identify microscopic morphology/
   Parasites/2

14. Plate 14 is a fecal specimen unstained seen under 400× using brightfield microscopy. The plate shows the ovum of which parasite?

   A. *N. americanus*
   B. *T. trichiura*
   C. *A. lumbricoides*
   D. *E. vermicularis*

   Microbiology/Identify microscopic morphology/
   Parasites/2

15. Plate 15 is an iodine-stained fecal specimen seen under 400× using brightfield microscopy. The plate shows the ovum of which parasite?

   A. Pinworm
   B. Threadworm
   C. Hookworm
   D. Whipworm

   Microbiology/Identify microscopic morphology/
   Parasites/2

16. Plate 16 is an unstained fecal specimen seen under 400× using brightfield microscopy. The plate shows the ovum of which parasite?

   A. *Clonorchis sinensis*
   B. *Fasciola hepatica*
   C. *Paragonimus westermani*
   D. *Fasciolopsis buski*

   Microbiology/Identify microscopic morphology/
   Parasites/2

12. **C** This plate shows abundant *Histoplasma capsulatum* (yeast phase) within the cytoplasm of both the macrophage and histiocyte. All of the organisms above may cause pulmonary pneumonia in immunodeficient patients. Small oval yeast cells, 2–5 μ in diameter, are seen.

13. **B** The ova of *T. trichiura* are brown and shaped like a football with mucus plugs at both ends. Ova have a thick wall and measure about 50 μ long by 20 μ wide. *Enterobius* ova are approximately the same size but have a clear (hyaline) shell, flat on one side with a visible larva within. *Necator* eggs are larger (approximately 65–75 μ long by 40 μ wide) and have a clear shell.

14. **C** *Ascaris* ova are large and oval, usually measuring 50–75 μ long by 35–50 μ wide. They are often bile-stained and may have a thick shell with a coarse covering (corticated). This egg demonstrates a contracted embryo, leaving space between the shell and the embryo at the opposing poles. This indicates that the egg is fertilized.

15. **C** Hookworm ova are approximately 60–75 μ in length and 35–40 μ in width. They have a thin outer shell usually containing an unembryonated or partly embryonated egg within. The ova of *Necator* and *Ancylostoma* cannot be differentiated from one another. Threadworm (*Strongyloides*) produces similar ova, but these hatch in the intestine, releasing the rhabditoid larvae that are found in the feces. Pinworm (*Enterobius*) ova are approximately the same size but are more elongated and flat on one side. Whipworm (*Trichuris*) ova are smaller and thick-walled with mucus plugs at both ends.

16. **A** *C. sinensis* produces small, bile-stained ova approximately 25–35 μ in length and 10–20 μ in width. Ova have a collar (shoulder) on both sides of the operculum and a knob at the end opposite the operculum. *Fasciola*, *Paragonimus*, and *Fasciolopsis* all produce large, yellow-brown operculated ova.

17. Plate 17 is an unstained fecal specimen seen under 400× using brightfield microscopy. The plate shows the ovum of which parasite?
A. *Fasciola hepatica*
B. *Paragonimus westermani*
C. *Metagonimus yokogawai*
D. *Opisthorchis viverrini*

Microbiology/Identify microscopic morphology/ Parasites/2

18. Plate 18 is a peripheral blood film stained with Giemsa's stain, 1000×. What condition is suspected from this field?
A. Macrocytic anemia
B. Agranulocytosis
C. Relapsing fever
D. Lead poisoning

Microbiology/Identify microscopic morphology/ Spirochete/2

19. Plate 19 shows an organism isolated from an eyewash of a patient with a corneal infection who had been wearing contact lenses for the past 2 years. What is the name of the causative agent?
A. *Naegleria* spp
B. *Acanthamoeba* spp
C. *Entamoeba histolytica*
D. *Trichomonas vaginalis*

Microbiology/Identify microscopic morphology/ Parasites/2

20. Plate 20 is a Wright's-stained peripheral blood film, 1000×. Which malarial stage is present in the RBC in the center of the plate?
A. Ring trophozoite of *Plasmodium vivax*
B. Mature trophozoite of *Plasmodium malariae*
C. Macrogametocyte stage of *Plasmodium falciparum*
D. Mature gametocyte stage of *Plasmodium ovale*

Microbiology/Identify microscopic morphology/ Parasites/3

21. Plate 21 is a modified acid-fast stain with malachite green counterstain of a stool specimen, 1000× magnification. The oocysts seen in this field are approximately 5μ in diameter. Which organism is present?
A. *Isospora belli*
B. *Cryptosporidium parvum*
C. *Cyclospora* spp
D. *Sarcocystis* spp

Microbiology/Identify microscopic morphology/ Parasites/2

17. **B** *P. westermani* produces large, operculated ova measuring approximately 80–100 μ in length and 50–70 μ in width. They are yellow-brown and non-embryonated. *Metagonimus* and *Opisthorchis* ova are small ova resembling *Clonorchis*. *Fasciola* produces ova that are also yellow-brown, operculated, and unembryonated. The ova are larger than those of *Paragonimus* and lack the small shoulders adjacent to the operculum of *Paragonimus* ova.

18. **C** This field shows long helical bacteria between red blood cells (RBCs) of normal size and color. These spirochetes are sometimes seen in the blood of patients suffering from the febrile septic phase of infection with *Borrelia* or *Leptospira* spp. The former are more commonly encountered in differential examinations, especially in patients infected with *Borrelia recurrentis* and other species that cause relapsing fever. *Borrelia burgdorferi*, the causative agent of Lyme disease, is rarely seen in Wright's stained blood films and is usually diagnosed by enzyme-linked immunosorbent assay (ELISA) and other serological methods.

19. **B** This is a large trophozoite with spiculated cytoplasm characteristic of *Acanthamoeba*. Eye infections caused by this organism have been documented in contact lens wearers who do not properly disinfect lenses. *Acanthamoeba* spp are large trophozoites measuring 25–50 μ. They may also cause primary amoebic meningoencephalitis, although they are isolated less often than *Naegleria* in the CSF of patients with this disease.

20. **A** The infected RBC demonstrates enlarged amoeba-like cytoplasm and Schüffner's dots, which are characteristic of *P. vivax* and *ovale*. The parasite is at the ring-form trophozoite stage.

21. **B** All of the organisms above are coccidian parasites that cause diarrhea, especially in immunodeficient patients such as those with AIDS. *Cryptosporidium* produces the smallest oocysts (half the size of *Cyclospora*, which is the next smallest) and is visible in stools using either the acid-fast or immunofluorescent staining techniques. The oocysts are round, about 5 μ in diameter, and deep pink.

22. Plate 22 is a gram-stained CSF concentrated by centrifugation, 1000×. Which organism is present?
   A. *Neisseria meningitidis*
   B. *Staphylococcus aureus*
   C. *Streptococcus pneumoniae*
   D. *Listeria monocytogenes*

   Microbiology/Identify microscopic morphology/CSF/2

23. Plate 23 is a urinary sediment viewed under 400× magnification using a brightfield microscope. What is the object located in the center of the field?
   A. *Schistosoma haematobium* ovum
   B. Oval fat body
   C. Glitter cell
   D. Fecal contaminant

   Body fluids/Identify microscopic morphology/Urine sediment/2

24. Plate 24 is a urinary sediment viewed under 400× magnification using a brightfield microscope. Which crystals are seen?
   A. Uric acid
   B. Calcium oxalate
   C. Ammonium magnesium phosphate
   D. Hippuric acid

   Body fluids/Identify microscopic morphology/Urine sediment/2

25. Plate 25 is a urinary sediment viewed under 400× magnification using a brightfield microscope. Which crystals are seen?
   A. Uric acid
   B. Calcium oxalate
   C. Ammonium magnesium phosphate
   D. Hippuric acid

   Body fluids/Identify microscopic morphology/Urine sediment/2

26. Plate 26 is a urinary sediment viewed under 400× magnification using a brightfield microscope. Which formed element is seen?
   A. Hyaline cast
   B. Broad cast
   C. Waxy cast
   D. Coarse granular cast

   Body fluids/Identify microscopic morphology/Urine sediment/2

Answers to Questions 22–26

22. **C** This field shows abundant gram-positive diplococci with the lancet shape that is characteristic of *S. pneumoniae*. Group B streptococci will also cause meningitis in infants. *Listeria* may cause bacterial meningitis in infants and elderly patients, whereas *S. pneumoniae* is most often encountered in middle-aged adults and older patients. *Staphylococcus, Streptococcus,* and *Listeria* spp are gram-positive. whereas *Neisseria* is gram-negative. *Listeria* is a small coccobacillus or rod. *Staphylococcus* is rarely isolated from CSF and appears as small grapelike cocci.

23. **B** Oval fat bodies are degenerated renal tubular epithelia that contain a high concentration of neutral fat, largely reabsorbed cholesterol droplets. These appear highly refractile under brightfield microscopy, and the fat globules produce a Maltese-cross effect under a polarizing microscope. Oval fat bodies occur in conditions associated with increased urinary lipoprotein excretion such as the nephrotic syndrome.

24. **A** Uric acid crystals are yellow to reddish brown in color and occur in acid or neutral urine. Common forms include whetstones and rhombic plates (as seen here) as well as thin needles and rosettes. Calcium oxalate crystals are usually colorless octahedrons. Ammonium magnesium phosphate crystals are long, colorless six-sided prisms, and hippuric acid crystals are colorless long, flat, hexagonal plates.

25. **C** Ammonium magnesium phosphate crystals (triple phosphate) occur in alkaline or neutral urine. They are long, colorless hexagonal prisms that often resemble a "coffin lid." They may also occur in a feathery form that resembles a fern leaf. Triple phosphate crystals may form calculi in the renal pelvis, appearing on an x-ray as an outline of the calyces and referred to as "stag-horn" calculi.

26. **D** Coarse granular casts often form from degeneration of cellular casts. The finding of more than a rare granular cast is significant and helps to identify the kidney as the source of urinary protein and cells. Coarse and fine granular casts have the same significance as cellular casts and point to glomerular damage.

COLOR PLATE SECTION

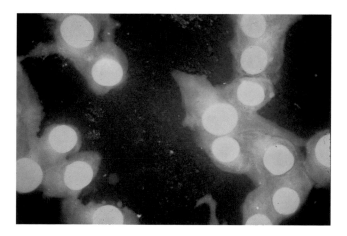

Plate 1

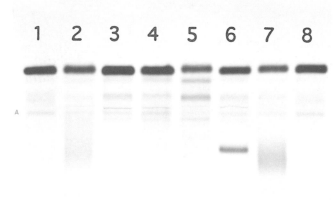

Plate 2

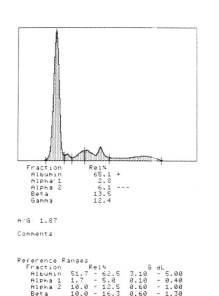

Plate 3

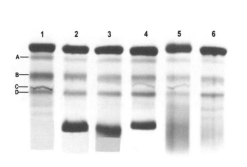

Plate 4

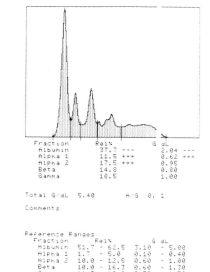

Plate 5

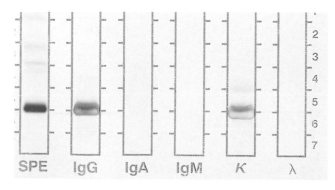

Plate 6

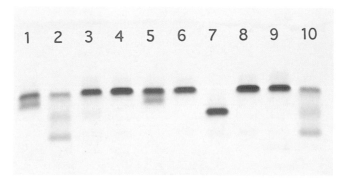

Plate 7

COLOR PLATE SECTION

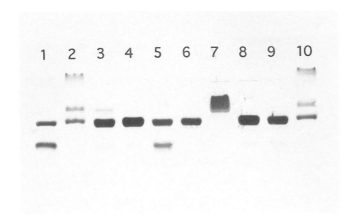

Plate 8

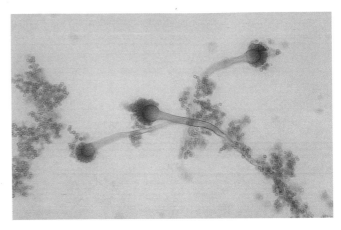

Plate 9

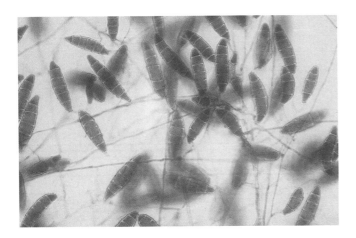

Plate 10

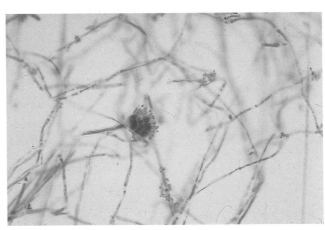

Plate 11

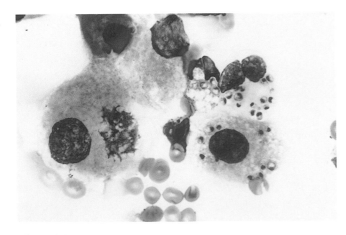

Plate 12

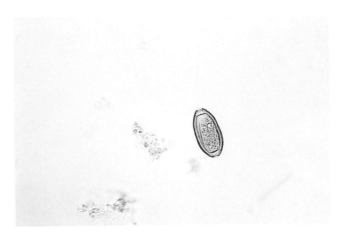

Plate 13

COLOR PLATE SECTION

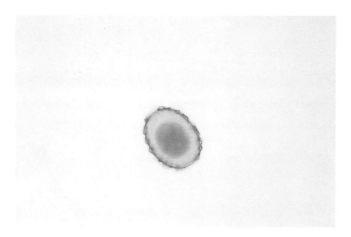

Plate 14

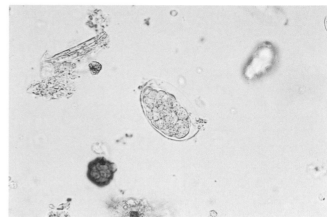

Plate 15

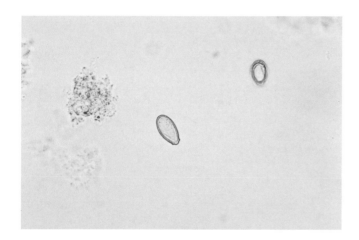

Plate 16

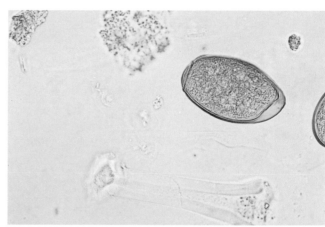

Plate 17

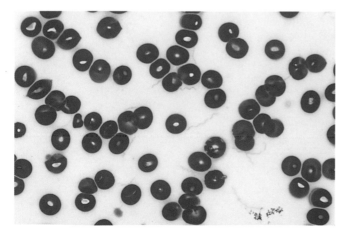

Plate 18

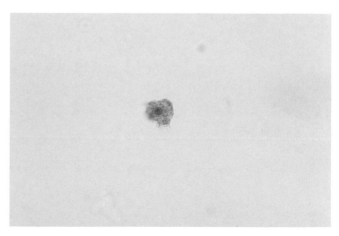

Plate 19

COLOR PLATE SECTION

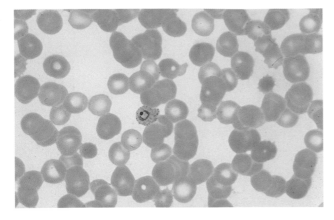

Plate 20

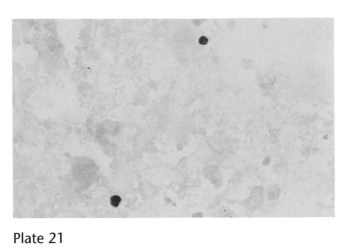

Plate 21

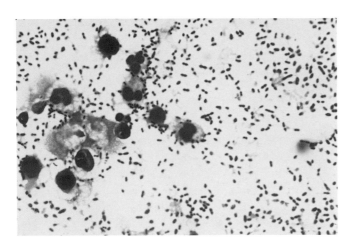

Plate 22

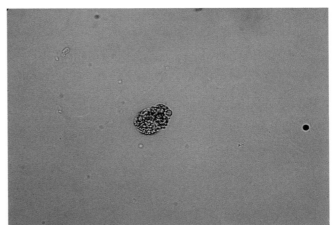

Plate 23

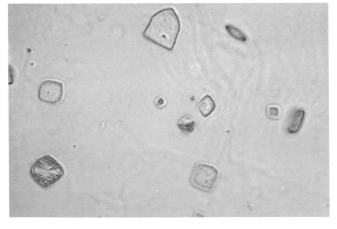

Plate 24

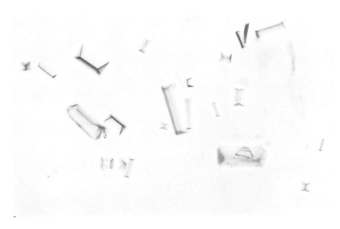

Plate 25

COLOR PLATE SECTION

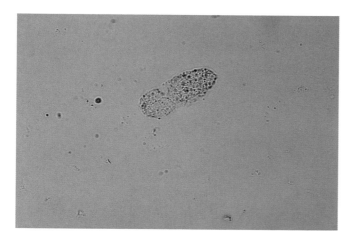

Plate 26

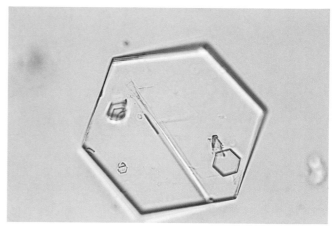

Plate 27

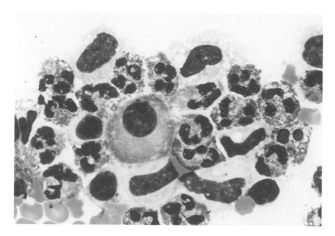

Plate 28

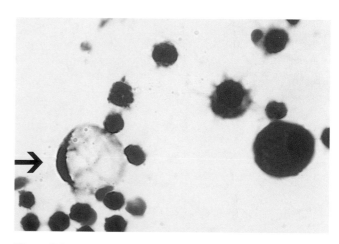

Plate 29

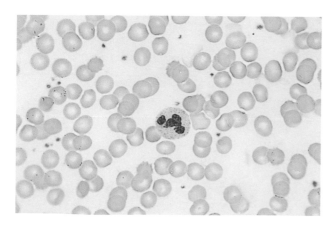

Plate 30

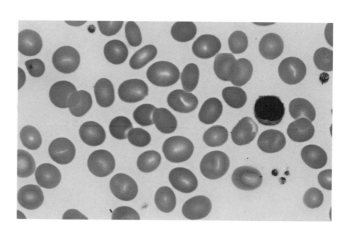

Plate 31

COLOR PLATE SECTION

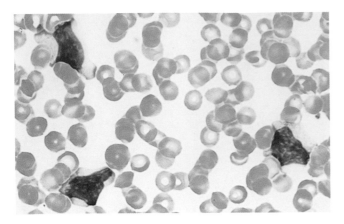

Plate 32

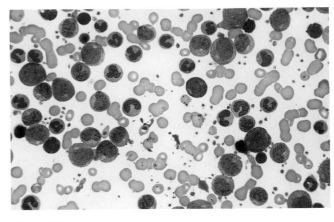

Plate 33

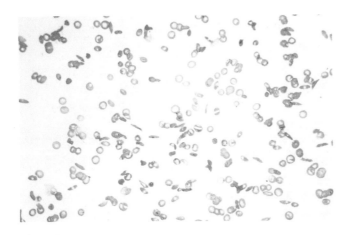

Plate 34

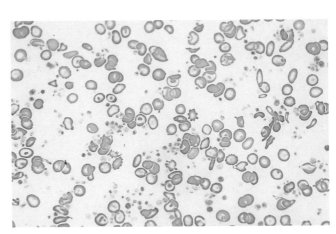

Plate 35

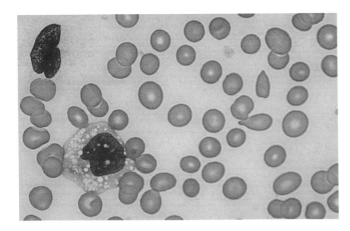

Plate 36

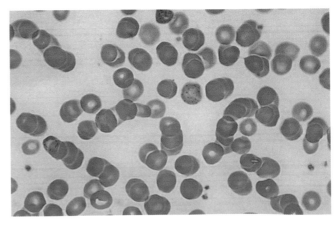

Plate 37

COLOR PLATE SECTION

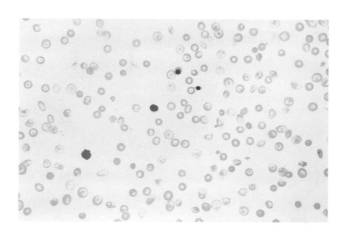

Plate 38

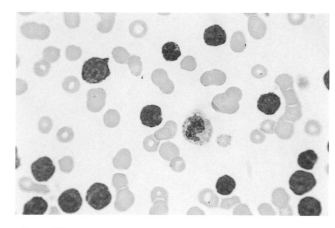

Plate 39

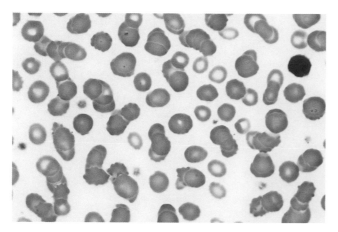

Plate 40

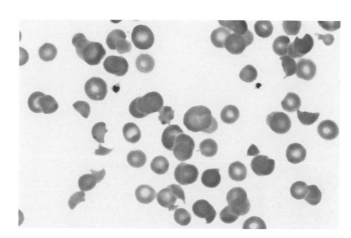

Plate 41

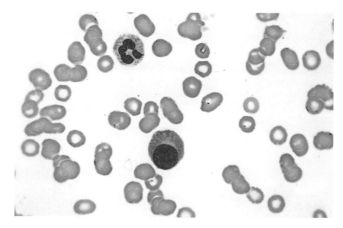

Plate 42

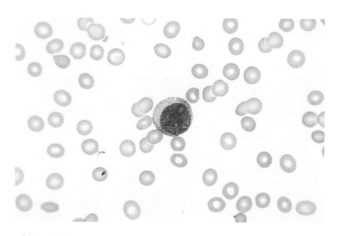

Plate 43

COLOR PLATE SECTION

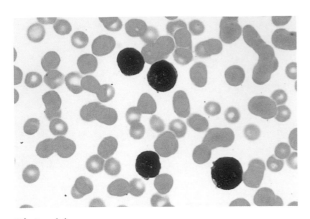

Plate 44

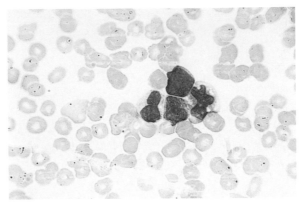

Plate 45

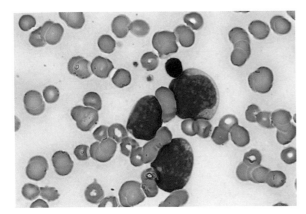

Plate 46

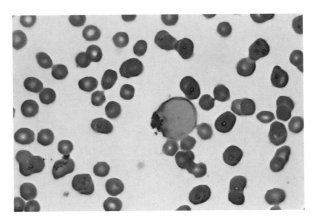

Plate 47A

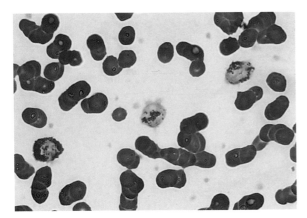

Plate 47B

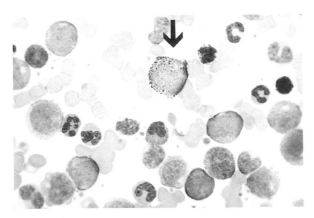

Plate 48

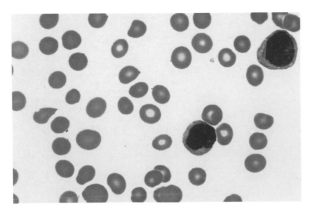

Plate 49

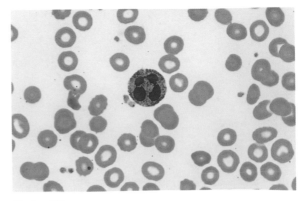

Plate 50

27. Plate 27 shows a urinary sediment viewed under 400× magnification using brightfield microscopy. This colorless crystal is presumptively identified as:
   A. Calcium phosphate
   B. Acetaminophen
   C. Cystine
   D. Hippuric acid
   Body fluids/Identify microscopic morphology/Urine sediment/2

28. Plate 28 is a Wright's-stained cytocentrifuge preparation of pleural fluid, 1000×. What is the correct classification of the largest mononuclear cell located in the center of the plate?
   A. Histiocyte
   B. Macrophage
   C. Lymphoblast
   D. Mesothelial cell
   Body fluids/Identify microscopic morphology/Pleural fluid/2

29. Plate 29 is a Wright's-stained smear of pleural fluid prepared by cytocentrifugation. The largest cell in this field (see arrow) is identified as a:
   A. Signet ring macrophage
   B. Reactive mesothelial cell
   C. Foam cell
   D. Metastatic cell from the breast
   Body fluids/Identify microscopic morphology/Pleural fluid/2

30. Plate 30 is from a Wright's-stained peripheral blood film, 1000×. Which of the following best describes the cells in this plate?
   A. Normal morphology
   B. Macrocytic red blood cells
   C. Hypersegmented neutrophil present
   D. Reduced platelets
   Hematology/Identify microscopic morphology/RBCs/2

31. Plate 31 is a Wright's-stained peripheral blood film, 1000×. What is the most appropriate classification of the red cell morphology seen in this field?
   A. Microcytic, hypochromic
   B. Microcytic, normochromic
   C. Normocytic, normochromic
   D. Macrocytic, normochromic
   Hematology/Identify microscopic morphology/RBCs/3

Answers to Questions 27–31

27. **C** Cystine crystals form in acid urine and appear as colorless uniform six-sided hexagonal plates in urinary sediment. Calcium phosphate crystals form in neutral to alkaline urine and appear as thin amorphous crystals resembling a sheet of ice or as flat needles that form a rosette. Acetaminophen crystals are cylinder-shaped with round edges. Hippuric acid crystals form long six-sided prisms in acid urine. Cystine crystals must be differentiated from uric acid on the basis of solubility, polarized microscopy, or biochemical testing. Cystine crystals are less anisotropic than uric acid. They are soluble in dilute hydrochloric acid (HCl), but uric acid is not. Cystine causes a positive cyanide-nitroprusside test and uric acid does not.

28. **D** Mesothelial cells are specialized epithelium that line the serous membranes, and they may be seen in small numbers in normal pleural, pericardial, and ascites fluids. They are often seen in increased numbers when there is an inflammatory injury involving the serous membranes. They are large mononuclear or binucleate cells with an open chromatin pattern and abundant agranular cytoplasm. Mesothelial cells may transform into phagocytic cells and undergo morphological changes that cause them to resemble malignant cells.

29. **A** Macrophages are frequently seen in serous fluids. They are present in increased numbers in exudative conditions. Signet ring forms result from compression of the nucleus against the cell wall, usually caused by large vacuoles that form after phagocytosis of erythrocytes or fat.

30. **A** The size, shape, and central pallor of the red cells in this plate are normal. The morphology of the neutrophil is typical in appearance. Platelets of normal size and shape are present. On average, there should be less than three platelets per oil immersion (100×) field when thrombocytopenia is present.

31. **D** Many of the RBCs in this field are larger than the nucleus of the small lymphocyte, indicating that they are macrocytic. Several of the RBCs are elliptical in shape and are classified as ovalocytes. The region of central pallor of most of the cells is normal. Macrocytic anemia (anemia with an increased mean cell volume [MCV]) is commonly seen in patients with chronic liver disease, vitamin B_{12} or folate deficiency, hypothyroidism, or alcoholism.

32. Plate 32 is a Wright's-stained peripheral blood film, 1000×. What is the most appropriate classification of the white blood cells (WBCs) present in this field?
   A. Reactive (atypical) lymphocytes
   B. Large lymphoblasts exhibiting L2 morphology
   C. The M4 subtype of acute granulocytic leukemia
   D. Monocytes

   Hematology/Identify microscopic morphology/WBCs/3

33. Plate 33 is from a Wright's-stained peripheral blood film, 400×. Which of the following tests may be performed to enable an accurate diagnosis?
   A. Leukocyte alkaline phosphatase (LAP) stain
   B. Myeloid marker study by flow cytometry
   C. Myeloperoxidase stain
   D. Periodic acid–Schiff (PAS) stain

   Hematology/Identify microscopic morphology/WBCs/3

34. Plate 34 is from a Wright's-stained peripheral blood film, 400×. The cells seen are diagnostic of which condition?
   A. Intravascular hemolytic anemia
   B. Sickle cell disease
   C. Myelofibrosis
   D. Erythroleukemia

   Hematology/Identify microscopic morphology/RBCs/3

35. Plate 35 is from a Wright's-stained peripheral blood film, 1000×. Which description of the RBC morphology and platelets is correct?
   A. Microcytic, hypochromic with marked poikilocytosis and increased platelets
   B. Macrocytic, hypochromic with marked anisocytosis and normal platelets
   C. Normocytic, normochromic with mild poikilocytosis and increased platelets
   D. Microcytic, hypochromic, with mild anisocytosis and normal platelets

   Hematology/Identify microscopic morphology/RBCs/2

36. Plate 36 is a Wright's-stained peripheral blood film, 1000×. The RBCs in this plate are characteristic of:
   A. Hemolytic anemia
   B. Myelofibrosis
   C. Hgb C disease
   D. Sideroblastic anemia

   Hematology/Identify microscopic morphology/RBCs/3

Answers to Questions 32–36

32. **A** These cells are lymphocytes characteristic of those found in viral infections such as infectious mononucleosis. In these conditions, the WBC count is increased (usually $15–25 \times 10^3/\mu L$), and lymphocytes account for the majority of the WBCs. Reactive lymphocytes are larger than normal. The cytoplasm is increased in volume and may be vacuolated, and the edges of the cell are often scalloped and basophilic. The nuclear chromatin pattern is open and reticular.

33. **A** This plate shows marked granulocytosis demonstrating cells at all stages of maturity and marked thrombocytosis. These characteristics suggest chronic granulocytic leukemia (CGL), but they also occur in the leukemoid response, which is a severe granulocytosis in response to infection, inflammation, tissue damage, or malignancy. The LAP test is performed to distinguish the two conditions. In CGL the LAP score is markedly reduced, usually 10 or below. In the leukemoid response (and leuko-erythroblastosis) the LAP score is elevated (reference range 20–100). In addition to the LAP stain, cytogenetic evaluation is another important diagnostic marker for CGL. Ninety-five percent of patients with CGL display the Philadelphia (Ph[1]) chromosome in their granulocytes.

34. **B** This plate displays polychromasia, abundant target cells (leptocytes), and well-defined sickle cells (drepanocytes) characteristic of sickle cell disease. Sickle cells are elongated with pointed ends, and the Hgb is concentrated in the center of the cell. They may also be encountered in a few other hemoglobinopathies, such as Hgb SC disease, but they are rarely seen in patients with sickle cell trait.

35. **A** These RBCs demonstrate extreme central pallor characteristic of cells that are microcytic and hypochromic. Target cells, ovalocytes, burr cells, and cell fragments are present. On average, when more than 20 platelets are seen per oil immersion field, the platelet count is elevated.

36. **B** The peripheral blood in myelofibrosis is leuko-erythroblastic and is characterized by teardrop cells (dacrocytes), ovalocytes, nucleated RBCs, basophilic stippling, poikilocytosis, leukocytosis, and (often) micromegakaryocytes. Hgb C disease produces normocytic or slightly microcytic anemia with many target cells. Sideroblastic anemia produces both microcytic, hypochromic RBCs, and normocytic RBCs in the blood (dimorphic RBC morphology). Hemolytic anemias are usually normocytic, normochronic, or macrocytic with polychromasia, but morphology varies with the cause of hemolysis.

37. Plate 37 is a Wright's-stained peripheral blood film, 1000×. The cells seen in this plate are associated with:
  A. Lead poisoning
  B. Aplastic anemia
  C. Iron deficiency anemia
  D. Intravascular hemolysis

Hematology/Identify microscopic morphology/RBCs/3

38. Plate 38 is from a Wright's-stained peripheral blood film, 400×. Which of the following conditions is consistent with this RBC morphology?
  A. Erythroleukemia
  B. β-Thalassemia major
  C. Folate deficiency anemia
  D. Autoimmune hemolytic anemia

Hematology/Identify microscopic morphology/RBCs/3

39. Plate 39 is from a Wright's-stained smear of peripheral blood, 1000× from a patient with a WBC count of 35×10^9/L. The patient is 60 years old with firm, enlarged lymph nodes and hepatosplenomegaly. These same cells comprise 50% of the bone marrow WBCs and are PAS-positive and myeloperoxidase and nonspecific esterase–negative. What is the most likely diagnosis?
  A. Epstein-Barr virus infection
  B. Infectious mononucleosis
  C. Chronic lymphocytic leukemia
  D. Waldenström's macroglobulinemia

Hematology/Evaluate clinical and laboratory data/Leukemia/3

40. Plate 40 is from a Wright's-stained peripheral blood film, 400×. The RBC morphology is most consistent with which of the following anemias?
  A. Folate deficiency
  B. Iron deficiency
  C. Hemolytic
  D. Sideroblastic

Hematology/Identify microscopic morphology/RBCs/3

Answers to Questions 37–40

37. **A** Several RBCs in this plate show coarse basophilic stippling. Basophilic stippling results from unstable RNA within the cell and is associated with defects in Hgb synthesis. This is most often associated with lead poisoning, hemoglobinopathies, myelofibrosis, and megaloblastic anemias.

38. **B** This plate shows severe microcytic, hypochromic RBCs with numerous target cells and marked anisocytosis. A polychromatophilic normoblast is present. In addition, thalassemia is also associated with poikilocytes, Howell-Jolly bodies, ovalocytes, and siderocytes. Folate deficiency produces a macrocytic anemia, and autoimmune hemolytic anemia is usually normocytic and normochromic. The peripheral blood in erythroleukemia contains many nucleated RBC precursors, demonstrating bizarre shapes.

39. **C** The WBCs in this plate (with the exception of one granulocyte) are small lymphocytes. Chronic lymphocytic leukemia is rare in patients under the age of 30. The peripheral blood demonstrates a predominance of small lymphocytes, usually $20–200 \times 10^9$/L, which constitutes at least 40% of the bone marrow WBCs. Flow cytometry indicates these cells to be B cells in approximately 95% of cases. The bone marrow in Waldenström's macroglobulinemia is infiltrated by plasmacytoid lymphocytes, plasma cells, and mast cells as well as small lymphocytes; however, a severe peripheral lymphocytosis is not seen. Lymphadenopathy and hepatosplenomegaly occur in infectious mononucleosis. The lymphocyte count is usually $15–25 \times 10^9$/L, but the cells are atypical, being characterized by reactive features. The bone marrow is usually hyperplastic but not infiltrated by small lymphocytes.

40. **D** The RBC morphology of this field is characterized by the presence of both microcytic, hypochromic, and normocytic, normochromic cells. This dimorphic appearance is a characteristic of sideroblastic anemias. Folate deficiency causes a megaloblastic anemia, producing a macrocytic, normochromic appearance. Iron deficiency is associated with a microcytic, hypochromic RBC morphology. Hemolytic anemias are often normocytic and normochromic.

41. An Italian immigrant has been hospitalized with tachycardia, a rapidly decreasing hematocrit, and blood in his urine. Twenty-four hours prior to admission he had taken his first dose of a sulfonamide prescribed for a urinary tract infection. Plate 41 is from a Wright's-stained smear of his peripheral blood, 1000×. Which laboratory test would be helpful in establishing a diagnosis of the patient's hematological problem?
   A. Heinz body preparation
   B. Hgb H preparation
   C. Iron stain
   D. New methylene blue stain

Hematology/Identify microscopic morphology/RBCs/3

42. Plate 42 is from a Wright's-stained smear of peripheral blood, 1000×. The bone marrow aspirate of this patient demonstrated an abundance of cells with this morphology. Which of the following conditions is most likely to be associated with this sample?
   A. Sézary's syndrome
   B. Hodgkin's disease
   C. Burkitt's lymphoma
   D. Multiple myeloma

Hematology/Identify microscopic morphology/WBCs/3

43. Plate 43 is from a Wright's-stained peripheral blood film, 1000×. The WBC appearing in this plate is most likely a:
   A. Myeloblast
   B. Promyelocyte
   C. Myelocyte
   D. Monoblast

Hematology/Identify microscopic morphology/WBCs/2

Answers to Questions 41–43

41. **A** The RBC morphology seen in this plate shows both anisocytosis and poikilocytosis with prominent schistocytes that indicate a hemolytic anemia. The patient's ethnic background, clinical findings, and sulfonamide therapy point to a hemolytic episode of glucose-6-phosphate dehydrogenase (G6PD) deficiency as the cause. This can be substantiated by an assay of erythrocyte G6PD. The enzyme deficiency results in oxidative damage to RBCs, causing formation of Heinz bodies (precipitated Hgb). Heinz bodies are demonstrated by staining with crystal violet and are pitted from the RBCs by the spleen, resulting in RBC fragments sometimes called *bite* or *helmet* cells.

42. **D** The cell in the center of the plate is a plasma cell. Such cells have a dense, eccentric nucleus that is surrounded by a clear perinuclear area that represents the Golgi apparatus. The cytoplasm is basophilic and more abundant than is seen in small lymphocytes. Plasma cells are not normally seen in peripheral blood. They may be found in cases of viral and chronic infections and connective tissue diseases as well as in myeloma and other plasma cell dyscrasias. The RBCs in this plate demonstrate rouleaux, which is a characteristic seen in multiple myeloma. The peripheral blood in Hodgkin's disease is characterized by neutrophilia and lymphopenia. Burkitt's lymphoma produces very large, intensely basophilic lymphoblasts (L3 morphology). Abnormal lymphocytes appearing in peripheral blood in Sézary's syndrome are large with a convoluted nucleus of fine chromatin and almost no cytoplasm.

43. **A** Blasts are usually 15–20 μ in diameter with a large nucleus containing fine chromatin. The cytoplasm is usually agranular and basophilic. Lymphoblasts are differentiated from myeloblasts by cytochemical staining and flow cytometry. The blast in this plate contains uniform, unclumped chromatin, multiple nucleoli, the absence of azurophilic granules, and is from a patient with acute myelogenous leukemia, FAB M1. Lymphoblasts often display irregular clumping of the chromatin and azurophilic granules. They usually lack prominent nucleoli.

44. Plate 44 is a Wright's-stained peripheral blood film, 1000×. The white blood cells in this field are peroxidase, chloroacetate esterase, and Sudan B–negative. The cells are positive for terminal deoxynucleotidyl transferase (Tdt) and PAS. On the basis of these findings, what is the most appropriate classification of these cells?
   A. Lymphoblasts with L1 morphology
   B. Lymphoblasts with L2 morphology
   C. Lymphoblasts with L3 morphology
   D. Chronic lymphocytic leukemia cells

Hematology/Identify microscopic morphology/WBCs/3

45. Plate 45 is from a Wright's-stained peripheral blood film, 1000×. Sixty percent of the WBCs are positive for naphthol AS-D chloroacetate esterase (specific esterase), and 70% are positive for α-naphthyl acetate esterase (nonspecific esterase). The WBCs in this plate are characteristic of which FAB subtype of acute nonlymphocytic leukemia?
   A. M1
   B. M2
   C. M3
   D. M4

Hematology/Identify microscopic morphology/WBCs/3

46. Plate 46 is from a Wright's-stained peripheral blood film, 1000×. The WBCs shown in this field are classified as:
   A. Blasts
   B. Prolymphocytes
   C. Plasma cells
   D. Myelocytes

Hematology/Identify microscopic morphology/WBCs/3

47. Plate 47A shows cells from the same sample as plate 46 after peroxidase staining, 1000×. Plate 47B is a normal peroxidase-stained peripheral blood film, 1000×, which is used as a control. The blast cell shown in 47A is classified as:
   A. Peroxidase-positive
   B. Weakly peroxidase-positive
   C. Peroxidase-negative
   D. Invalid because of an improper control reaction

Hematology/Identify microscopic morphology/Special stains/3

44. **A** The cytochemistry of these cells is characteristic of lymphoblasts, and they exhibit morphology that is characteristic of the L1 subtype of acute lymphocytic leukemia. L1 cells have scarce cytoplasm that is moderately basophilic. The cells are small and uniform in size and shape. They either lack a nucleolus or have one or two small nucleoli. L2 cells are large and irregular in size and often contain one or more prominent nucleoli. L3 cells are large and uniform in size with deeply blue cytoplasm. The have multiple prominent nucleoli.

45. **D** These WBCs are large blasts containing a convoluted nucleus, large nucleoli, lacy nuclear chromatin, and abundant cytoplasm. These are characteristics of monoblasts. M1 is myeloblastic leukemia without maturation. M2 is myeloblastic leukemia with maturation. M3 is promyelocytic leukemia, and M4 is myelomonocytic leukemia. Acute myelomonocytic leukemia constitutes 20%–30% of acute myelogenous leukemias in adults and usually occurs in persons over 50 years old. More than 30% of nucleated cells in the bone marrow are blasts, and 20% or more of the nucleated bone marrow cells are monoblasts or monocytes.

46. **A** The nucleated cells shown in this photomicrograph have a large nucleus with open, unclumped chromatin and scant agranular blue cytoplasm. Chromatin is reticular and nucleoli are prominent. Although nuclear folding is present, Auer rods are not seen and, therefore, the origin of the blasts must be determined by cytochemical and immunological characteristics.

47. **A** The control slide shows peroxidase staining of the granules in three mature neutrophils and indicates that the stain is functioning properly. The cytoplasm of the blast in Plate 47A is strongly positive for peroxidase, indicating that it is a myeloblast. When at least 3% of blasts stain positive, the test is considered positive. Acute myeloblastic leukemia (AML) with minimal differentiation, M0, is negative with peroxidase stain. M1 through M4 classes of AML are peroxidase-positive. M5 may be weakly positive, and myeloblasts in M6 are positive. Lymphoblasts, hairy cells, erythroid cells, megakaryocytes, and platelets are negative. Reactions for Sudan black B stain parallel those of peroxidase.

48. Plate 48 is from a Wright's-stained peripheral blood film, 1000×. The WBC shown in the center of the field (see arrow) is classified as a:
   A. Blast
   B. Promyelocyte
   C. Myelocyte
   D. Prolymphocyte

Hematology/Identify microscopic morphology/WBCs/2

49. Plate 49 is a Wright's-stained peripheral blood film, 1000×. What is the most appropriate classification of the WBCs seen in this field?
   A. Lymphoblasts
   B. Myeloblasts
   C. Promyelocytes
   D. Prolymphocytes

Hematology/Identify microscopic morphology/WBCs/3

50. Plate 50 is a Wright's-stained peripheral blood film, 1000×. Which description best characterizes the morphology of the neutrophil shown in this plate?
   A. Normal morphology
   B. Döhle bodies
   C. Toxic granulation
   D. Hypersegmentation

Hematology/Identify microscopic morphology/WBCs/2

Answers to Questions 48–50

48. **B** Promyelocytes are often larger than myeloblasts, and the cytoplasm is more abundant than in the myeloblast. The nuclear chromatin is open but usually is slightly condensed, and one or more nucleoli may be present. The cytoplasm is blue and contains large azurophilic (primary) granules but no secondary granules. In contrast, the myelocyte has a round nucleus that is smaller, the chromatin is more condensed, and nucleoli are absent. The cytoplasm of the myelocyte is more orange-purple, and secondary granules predominate.

49. **B** The nucleated cells shown in this field are blasts. The large blast seen in the corner of the plate contains a prominent Auer rod. Auer rods are linear projections of azurophilic granules and are seen only in acute myelocytic leukemia. Auer rods are usually found in myeloblasts or promyelocytes and are most often seen in M1, M2, and M3 subtypes of AML.

50. **C** This neutrophil displays an abundance of large purple azurophilic granules characteristic of toxic granulation. The granules contain peroxidase and acid hydrolyases that result in increased basophilia. Toxic granulation is found in severe infections and inflammatory conditions and is often present in band cells and metamyelocytes, which are usually increased in these conditions. Döhle bodies and vacuolated neutrophils may be seen in association with toxic granulation.

BIBLIOGRAPHY

1. Garcia, L.S.: Diagnostic Medical Parasitology. 5th ed. ASM Press, Washington, DC, 2007.
2. Harmening, D.: Clinical Hematology and Fundamentals of Hemostasis. 4th ed. F.A. Davis, Philadelphia, 2002.
3. Henry, J.B. (ed.): Clinical Diagnosis and Management by Laboratory Methods. 20th ed. W.B. Saunders, Philadelphia, 2001.
4. Murray, P.R., Baron, E.J., Jorgensen, J.H., et al.: Manual of Clinical Microbiology. ASM Press, Washington, D.C., 2003.

CHAPTER 11

Sample Certification (Self-Assessment) Examination

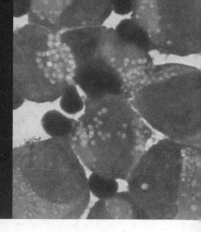

DIRECTIONS: Each question is followed by four answers, labeled A through D. Choose the best answer and write the corresponding letter in the space to the left of the question number. An answer key is provided on the page following the examination. Use the key to score your examination; a score below 70% correct on any section indicates the need for further study.

Chemistry

_____ 1. Which instrument requires a primary and secondary monochromator?
   A. Spectrophotometer
   B. Atomic absorption spectrophotometer
   C. Fluorometer
   D. Nephelometer

_____ 2. The term RT/nF in the Nernst equation defines the:
   A. Potential at the ion selective membrane
   B. Slope of the electrode
   C. Decomposition potential
   D. Isopotential point of the electrode

_____ 3. Which glucose method is subject to falsely low results caused by ascorbate?
   A. Hexokinase
   B. Glucose dehydrogenase
   C. Trinder glucose oxidase
   D. Polarography

_____ 4. Which condition is caused by deficient secretion of bilirubin into the bile canaliculi?
   A. Gilbert's disease
   B. Neonatal hyperbilirubinemia
   C. Dubin-Johnson syndrome
   D. Crigler-Najjar syndrome

_____ 5. Which of the following 2-hour glucose challenge results would be classified as impaired glucose tolerance (IGT)?
   A. 130 mg/dL
   B. 135 mg/dL
   C. 150 mg/dL
   D. 204 mg/dL

_____ 6. A patient's blood gas results are: pH 7.50; P_{CO_2} 55 mm Hg; HCO_3^- 40 mmol/L
   These results indicate:
   A. Respiratory acidosis
   B. Metabolic alkalosis
   C. Respiratory alkalosis
   D. Metabolic acidosis

_____ 7. A blood sample is left on a phlebotomy tray for 4 hours before it is delivered to the laboratory. Which group of tests could be performed?
   A. Glucose, Na, K, Cl, T_{CO_2}
   B. Uric acid, blood urea nitrogen (BUN), creatinine
   C. Total and direct bilirubin
   D. Creatine kinase, alanine aminotransferase, alkaline phosphatase, acid phosphatase

_____ 8. A patient's BUN is 60 mg/dL and serum creatinine is 3.0 mg/dL. These results suggest:
   A. Laboratory error measuring BUN
   B. Renal failure
   C. Prerenal failure
   D. Patient was not fasting

_____ 9. Which condition produces the highest elevation of serum lactate dehydrogenase?
   A. Pernicious anemia
   B. Myocardial infarction (MI)
   C. Acute hepatitis
   D. Muscular dystrophy

501

_____ **10.** Which substrate is used in the Bowers-McComb method for alkaline phosphatase?
  A. p-Nitrophenylphosphate
  B. β-Glycerophosphate
  C. Phenylphosphate
  D. α-Naphthylphosphate

_____ **11.** Which of the following liver diseases produces the highest levels of transaminases?
  A. Hepatic cirrhosis
  B. Obstructive jaundice
  C. Chronic hepatitis
  D. Alcoholic hepatitis

_____ **12.** Zollinger-Ellison syndrome is characterized by great (e.g., 20-fold) elevation of:
  A. Gastrin
  B. Cholecystokinin
  C. Pepsin
  D. Glucagon

_____ **13.** Which of the following hormones is often decreased by approximately 25% in the serum of pregnant women who have a fetus with Down's syndrome?
  A. Estriol
  B. Human chorionic gonadotropin (hCG)
  C. Progesterone
  D. Estradiol

_____ **14.** **SITUATION:** A peak blood level for orally administered theophylline (therapeutic range 8–20 mg/L) measured at 8 a.m. is 5.0 mg/L. The preceding trough level was 4.6 mg/L. What is the most likely explanation of these results?
  A. Laboratory made an error on peak measurement
  B. Specimen for peak level was collected from wrong patient
  C. Blood for peak level was drawn too soon
  D. Elimination rate has reached maximum

_____ **15.** Select the hormone that is associated with galactorrhea, pituitary adenoma, and amenorrhea.
  A. Estradiol
  B. Progesterone
  C. Follicle-stimulating hormone
  D. Prolactin

_____ **16.** In the Oliver-Rosalki method, the reverse reaction is used to measure creatine kinase activity. The enzyme(s) used in the coupling reactions are:
  A. Hexokinase and glucose-6-phosphate dehydrogenase
  B. Pyruvate kinase and lactate dehydrogenase
  C. Luciferase
  D. Adenylate kinase

_____ **17.** The following results are reported on an adult male patient being evaluated for chest pain:

	Myoglobin (Cutoff = 100 μg/L)	Troponin I (Cutoff = 0.04 μg/L)	CK-MB (Cutoff = 8 μg/L)
Admission	12 μg/L	1.1 μg/L	18 μg/L
3 hours postadmission	360 μg/L	1.8 μg/L	30 μg/L
6 hours postadmission	300 μg/L	2.4 μg/L	40 μg/L

What is the most likely cause of these results?
  A. The wrong sample was assayed for the first myoglobin
  B. The patient did not suffer an MI until after admission
  C. Hemolysis caused interference with the 3-hour and 6-hour myoglobin result
  D. The patient is suffering from unstable angina

Hematology

_____ **18.** Which of the following electrophoretic results is consistent with a diagnosis of sickle cell trait?
  A. Hgb A: 40% Hgb S: 35% Hgb F: 5%
  B. Hgb A: 60% Hgb S: 40% Hgb A$_2$: 2%
  C. Hgb A: 0% Hgb A$_2$: 5% Hgb F: 95%
  D. Hgb A: 80% Hgb S: 10% Hgb A$_2$: 10%

_____ **19.** Which ratio of anticoagulant to blood is correct for coagulation procedures?
  A. 1:4
  B. 1:5
  C. 1:9
  D. 1:10

_____ **20.** A patient's peripheral smear reveals numerous NRBCs, marked variation of red cell morphology, and pronounced polychromasia. In addition to decreased Hgb and Hct values, what other CBC parameters may be anticipated?
  A. Reduced platelets
  B. Increased MCHC
  C. Increased MCV
  D. Decreased RDW

_____ 21. In a vitamin K-deficient patient, which of the following coagulation tests would be abnormal?
  A. Prothrombin time and activated partial thromboplastin time
  B. Bleeding time
  C. Fibrinogen level
  D. Thrombin time

_____ 22. A manual white blood cell (WBC) count gave a total of 36 cells counted in all 9 mm² of a Neubauer ruled hemacytometer. A 1:10 dilution was used; what is the WBC count?
  A. 0.4×10^9/L
  B. 2.5×10^9/L
  C. 4.0×10^9/L
  D. 8.0×10^9/L

_____ 23. If a patient has a reticulocyte count of 7% and an Hct of 20%, what is the corrected reticulocyte count?
  A. 1.4%
  B. 3.1%
  C. 3.5%
  D. 14%

_____ 24. A decreased osmotic fragility test would be associated with which of the following conditions?
  A. Sickle cell anemia
  B. Hereditary spherocytosis
  C. Hemolytic disease of the newborn
  D. Acquired hemolytic anemia

_____ 25. Given the following values, which set of red blood cell (RBC) indices suggests spherocytosis?

A.	MCV 76 µm³	MCH 19.9 pg	MCHC 28.5%
B.	MCV 90 µm³	MCH 30.5 pg	MCHC 32.5%
C.	MCV 76 µm³	MCH 36.5 pg	MCHC 39.0%
D.	MCV 76 µm³	MCH 29.0 pg	MCHC 34.8%

_____ 26. Which anemia has red cell morphology similar to that seen in iron deficiency anemia?
  A. Sickle cell anemia
  B. Thalassemia syndrome
  C. Pernicious anemia
  D. Hereditary spherocytosis

_____ 27. In myelofibrosis, the characteristic abnormal red cell morphology is that of:
  A. Target cells
  B. Schistocytes
  C. Teardrop cells
  D. Ovalocytes

_____ 28. Which type of anemia is usually present in a patient with acute leukemia?
  A. Microcytic, hyperchromic
  B. Microcytic, hypochromic
  C. Normocytic, normochromic
  D. Macrocytic, normochromic

_____ 29. **SITUATION:** A peripheral smear shows 75% blasts. These stain positive for both Sudan black B (SBB) and peroxidase (Px). Given these values, which of the following disorders is most likely?
  A. Acute myelocytic leukemia (AML)
  B. Chronic myelocytic leukemia (CML)
  C. Acute undifferentiated leukemia (AUL)
  D. Acute lymphocytic leukemia(ALL)

_____ 30. A 50-year-old white man has been on heparin for the past 7 days. Which combination of the following tests is expected to be abnormal?
  A. Prothrombin time and activated partial thromboplastin time
  B. Activated partial thromboplastin time, thrombin time
  C. Activated partial thromboplastin time, thrombin time, fibrinogen assay
  D. Prothrombin time, activated partial thromboplastin time, thrombin time

_____ 31. Which of the following are most characteristic of the red cell indices associated with megaloblastic anemias?

A.	MCV 99 fL	MCH 28 pg	MCHC 31%
B.	MCV 62 fL	MCH 27 pg	MCHC 30%
C.	MCV 125 fL	MCH 36 pg	MCHC 34%
D.	MCV 78 fL	MCH 23 pg	MCHC 30%

_____ 32. Disseminated intravascular coagulation (DIC) is most often associated with which of the following types of acute leukemia?
  A. Acute myeloid leukemia without maturation
  B. Acute promyelocytic leukemia
  C. Acute myelomonocytic leukemia
  D. Acute monocytic leukemia

_____ 33. A patient's peripheral blood smear and bone marrow both show 70% blasts. These cells are negative for Sudan black B. Given these data, which of the following is the most likely diagnosis?
  A. Acute myeloid leukemia
  B. Chronic lymphocytic leukemia
  C. Acute promyelocytic leukemia
  D. Acute lymphocytic leukemia

_____ 34. When performing platelet aggregation studies, which set of platelet aggregation responses would most likely occur in a patient with Bernard-Soulier syndrome?
A. Normal platelet aggregation in response to collagen, adenosine diphosphate (ADP), and ristocetin
B. Normal platelet aggregation in response to collagen, ADP, and epinephrine; decreased in response to ristocetin
C. Normal platelet aggregation in response to epinephrine and ristocetin; decreased in response to collagen and ADP

D. Normal platelet aggregation in response to epinephrine, ristocetin, and collagen; decreased in response to ADP

_____ 35. **SITUATION:** The following laboratory values are seen in the chart below:

Which test helps most to establish a diagnosis?
A. Leukocyte alkaline phosphatase (LAP) stain
B. Nonspecific esterase stain
C. Acid phosphatase
D. Sudan black B stain

WBC DIFFERENTIAL

WBCs 76 × 10⁹/L	55% PMNs	RBC morphology normocytic, normochromic
RBCs 4.20 × 10¹²/L	15% bands	Occasional Döhle body
Platelets 398 × 10⁹/L	12% lymphocytes	
Hgb 12.5 g/dL	7% monocytes	
Hct 26.7%	2% eosinophils	
	1% basophils	
	8% metamyelocytes	

Immunology

_____ 36. Which disease is likely to show a rim (peripheral) pattern in an immunofluorescence (IF) microscopy test for ANA?
A. Mixed connective tissue disease (MCTD)
B. Rheumatoid arthritis
C. Systemic lupus erythematosus
D. Scleroderma

_____ 37. Interpret the following quantitative RPR test results. RPR titer: weakly reactive 1:8; reactive 1:8–1:64
A. Excess antibody, prozone effect
B. Excess antigen, postzone effect
C. Equivalence of antigen and antibody
D. Impossible to interpret; testing error

_____ 38. Which T- helper-to-T-suppressor ratio (T_h:T_s) is most likely in a patient with acquired immunodeficiency syndrome (AIDS)?
A. 2:1
B. 3:1
C. 2:3
D. 1:2

_____ 39. Which hepatitis B marker is the best indicator of early acute infection?
A. Hepatitis B surface antigen (HBsAg)
B. HBeAg

C. Antibody to hepatitis B core antigen (anti-HBc)
D. Anti-HBs

_____ 40. What is the most likely interpretation of the following syphilis serological results?

RPR: reactive; VDRL: reactive; MHA-TP: nonreactive

A. Neurosyphilis
B. Secondary syphilis
C. Syphilis that has been successfully treated
D. Biological false-positive syphilis

_____ 41. Interpret the following results for Epstein-Barr virus (EBV) infection: IgG and IgM antibodies to viral capsid antigen (VCA): positive
A. Infection in the past
B. Infection with a mutual enhancer virus such as human immunodeficiency virus (HIV)
C. Current infection
D. Impossible to interpret; need more information

_____ **42.** What type of disorders would show a decrease in C3, C4, and CH_{50}?
  A. Autoimmune disorders such as SLE and rheumatoid arthritis (RA)
  B. Immunodeficiency disorders such as common variable immunodeficiency
  C. Tumors
  D. Bacterial, viral, fungal, or parasitic infections

_____ **43.** Blood products are tested for which virus before being transfused to newborns?
  A. EBV
  B. Human T-lymphotropic virus II (HTLV-II)
  C. CMV
  D. Hepatitis D virus

_____ **44.** A 12-year-old female patient has symptoms of fatigue and presents with a localized lymphadenopathy. Laboratory tests reveal a peripheral blood lymphocytosis, a positive RPR, and a positive spot test for infectious mononucleosis. What test should be performed next?
  A. HIV test by enzyme-linked immunosorbent assay (ELISA)
  B. Venereal Disease Research Laboratory (VDRL)
  C. EBV specific antigen test
  D. Microhemagglutinin assay–_Treponema pallidum_ (MHA-TP)

_____ **45.** Which increase in antibody titer (dilution) best indicates an acute infection?
  A. From 1:2 to 1:8
  B. From 1:4 to 1:8
  C. From 1:16 to 1:256
  D. From 1:64 to 1:128

_____ **46.** Which of the following is used in rapid slide tests for detection of rheumatoid factors?
  A. Whole IgM molecules
  B. Fc portion of the IgG molecule
  C. Fab portion of the IgG molecule
  D. Fc portion of the IgM molecule

_____ **47.** Which MHC class of antigens is necessary for antigen recognition by CD4-positive T cells?
  A. Class I
  B. Class II
  C. Class III
  D. No MHC molecule is necessary for antigen recognition.

_____ **48.** Interpret the following results for HIV infection. ELISA: positive; repeat ELISA: negative; Western blot: no bands
  A. Positive for HIV
  B. Negative for HIV
  C. Indeterminate
  D. Further testing needed

_____ **49.** Interpret the following description of an immunofixation electrophoresis assay of urine. Dense wide bands in both the κ and λ lanes. No bands present in the heavy chain lanes.
  A. Normal
  B. Light chain disease
  C. Increased polyclonal Fab fragments
  D. Multiple myeloma

_____ **50.** What is the titer in tube 8 if tube 1 is undiluted and dilutions are doubled?
  A. 64
  B. 128
  C. 256
  D. 512

Blood Banking

_____ **51.** Which donor unit is selected for a recipient with anti-c?
  A. $r'r$
  B. R^oR^1
  C. R^2r''
  D. $r'r^y$

_____ **52.** Which of the following patients would be a candidate for RhIg?
  A. B-positive mother; B-negative baby; first pregnancy; no anti-D in mother
  B. O-negative mother; A-positive baby; second pregnancy; no anti-D in mother

  C. A-negative mother; O-negative baby; fourth pregnancy; anti-D in mother
  D. AB-negative mother; B-positive baby; second pregnancy; anti-D in mother

_____ **53.** Can crossmatching be performed on October 14 using a patient sample drawn on October 12?
  A. Yes, a new sample would not be needed
  B. Yes, but only if the previous sample has no alloantibodies
  C. No, a new sample is needed because the 2-day limit has expired
  D. No, a new sample is needed for each testing

_____ **54.** Which of the following distinguishes between the blood groups A_1 and A_2?

    A. A_2 antigen will not react with anti-A; A_1 will react strongly (4+)

    B. An A_2 person may form anti-A_1; an A_1 person will not form anti-A_1

    C. An A_1 person may form anti-A_2; an A_2 person will not form anti-A_1

    D. A_2 antigen will not react with anti-A from a nonimmunized donor; A_1 will react with any anti-A

_____ **55.** What should be done if all forward and reverse ABO results and the autocontrol are positive?

    A. Wash the cells with warm saline; autoadsorb the serum at 4°C

    B. Retype the sample using a different lot number of reagents

    C. Use polyclonal typing reagents

    D. Report the sample as group AB

_____ **56.** What antibodies could an R^1R^1 individual make if exposed to R^2R^2 blood?

    A. Anti-e and anti-C

    B. Anti-E and anti-c

    C. Anti-E and anti-C

    D. Anti-e and anti-c

_____ **57.** Which typing results characterize a secretor who is group O?

    A. Anti-A + saliva + A cells = positive; anti-B + saliva + B cells = negative; anti-H + saliva + O cells = negative

    B. Anti-A + saliva + A cells = positive; anti-B + saliva + B cells = positive; anti-H + saliva + O cells = positive

    C. Anti-A + saliva + A cells = positive; anti-B + saliva + B cells = positive; anti-H + saliva + O cells = negative

    D. Anti-A + saliva + A cells = negative; anti-B + saliva + B cells = negative; anti-H + saliva + O cells = negative

_____ **58.** What procedure would help to distinguish between an anti-e and anti-Fy^a in an antibody mixture?

    A. Lower pH of test serum

    B. Run an enzyme panel

    C. Use a thiol reagent

    D. Run a regular panel

_____ **59.** Which of the following individuals is acceptable as a blood donor?

    A. A 29-year-old man who received the hepatitis B vaccine last week

    B. A 21-year-old woman who has had her nose pierced last week

    C. A 30-year-old man who lived in Zambia for 3 years and returned last month

    D. A 54-year-old man who tested positive for hepatitis C (HCV) last year but has no active symptoms of the disease

_____ **60.** A patient's serum contains a mixture of antibodies. One of the antibodies is identified as anti-D. Anti-Jk^a or anti-Fy^a and possibly another antibody are present. What technique(s) may be helpful to identify the other antibody(ies)?

    A. Enzyme panel; select panel cell

    B. Thiol reagents

    C. Lowering the pH and increasing the incubation time

    D. Using albumin as an enhancement media in combination with selective adsorption

_____ **61.** A unit of whole blood is collected at 10:00 a.m. and stored at 20°C–24°C. What is the last hour platelet concentrates may be made from this unit?

    A. 4:00 p.m.

    B. 6:00 p.m.

    C. 7:00 p.m.

    D. 8:00 p.m.

_____ **62.** What corrective action should be taken when rouleaux causes positive test results?

    A. Perform a saline replacement procedure

    B. Perform an autoadsorption

    C. Run a panel

    D. Perform an elution

_____ **63.** Six units are crossmatched. Five units are compatible, one unit is incompatible, and the recipient's antibody screen is negative. Identify the problem.

    A. The patient may have a high frequency alloantibody

    B. The patient may have an abnormal protein

    C. The donor unit may have a positive direct antiglobulin test (DAT)

    D. The donor may have high-frequency antigens

_____ **64.** What is the disposition of a donor unit that contains an antibody?

    A. The unit must be discarded

    B. Only the plasma may be used to make components

    C. The antibody must be adsorbed from the unit

    D. The red cell unit may be labeled, indicating it contains antibody, and released into inventory

_____ 65. Given a situation where screen cells, cross-match, autocontrol, and DAT (anti-IgG) are all positive, what procedure should be performed next?
   A. Adsorption using rabbit stroma
   B. Antigen type the patient's cells
   C. Elution followed by a cell panel on the eluate
   D. Selected cell panel

_____ 66. Which physical examination result is cause for rejecting a blood donor?
   A. Weight of 105 pounds
   B. Pulse of 75
   C. Temperature of 99.3°F
   D. Diastolic pressure of 110 mm Hg

_____ 67. John comes into donate a unit of whole blood for the local blood supplier. The EIA screen is reactive for anti-HIV-1/2. The test is repeated in duplicate and is nonreactive. John is:
   A. Cleared for donation
   B. Deferred for 6 months
   C. Status is dependent on confirmatory test
   D. Deferred for 12 months

_____ 68. A unit of packed RBCs is split using the open system. One of the half units is used. What may be done with the second half unit?
   A. Must be issued within 24 hours
   B. Must be issued within 48 hours
   C. Must be discarded
   D. Retains the original expiration date

_____ 69. **SITUATION:** A cancer patient recently developed a severe infection. The patient's hemoglobin is 8 g/dL due to chemotherapy with a drug known to cause bone marrow depression and immunodeficiency. Which blood products are indicated for this patient?
   A. Liquid plasma and cryoprecipitate
   B. Crossmatched platelets and washed RBCs
   C. Factor IX concentrate and fresh frozen plasma
   D. Irradiated RBCs, platelets, and granulocytes

_____ 70. Which immunization has the longest deferral period?
   A. Hepatitis B immune globulin (HBIG) injection
   B. Rubella vaccine
   C. Influenza vaccine
   D. Yellow fever vaccine

Body Fluids

_____ 71. Urine that is dark red or port wine in color may be caused by:
   A. Lead poisoning
   B. Porphyria cutanea tarda
   C. Alkaptonuria
   D. Hemolytic anemia

_____ 72. The presence of tyrosine and leucine crystals together in a urine sediment usually indicates:
   A. Renal failure
   B. Chronic liver disease
   C. Hemolytic anemia
   D. Hartnup's disease

_____ 73. Urine with a specific gravity (SG) consistently between 1.002 and 1.003 indicates:
   A. Acute glomerulonephritis
   B. Renal tubular failure
   C. Diabetes insipidus
   D. Addison's disease

_____ 74. **SITUATION:** What is the most likely cause of the following CSF results? CSF glucose = 20 mg/dL; CSF protein = 100 mg/dL; CSF lactate = 50 mg/dL
   A. Viral meningitis
   B. Viral encephalitis

   C. Cryptococcal meningitis
   D. Acute bacterial meningitis

_____ 75. Given the following data, calculate the creatinine clearance. Serum creatinine = 1.5 mg/dL; urine creatinine = 102 mg/dL; urine volume = 1.7 mL/min; body surface area = 1.73 m^2
   A. 47 mL/min
   B. 97 mL/ min
   C. 100 mL/ min
   D. 116 mL/ min

_____ 76. Given the urinalysis below, select the most appropriate course of action.

pH 6.5	Protein, Neg
Glucose, Neg	Ketone, Tr
Blood, Neg	Bilirubin, Neg
Mucus, Sm	Ammonium biurate crystals, Lg

   A. Recheck urine pH
   B. Report these results, assuming acceptable quality control
   C. Repeat the dry reagent strip tests to confirm the ketone result
   D. Request a new sample and repeat the urinalysis

_____ 77. What is the principle of the colorimetric reagent strip determination of SG in urine?
  A. Ionic strength alters the *pKa* of a polyelectrolyte
  B. Sodium and other cations are chelated by a ligand that changes color
  C. Anions displace a pH indicator from a mordant, making it water-soluble
  D. Ionized solutes catalyze oxidation of an azo dye

_____ 78. Which of the following semen analysis results is abnormal?
  A. Volume 1.0 mL
  B. Liquefaction 40 min
  C. pH 7.6
  D. Motility 50% rapid progressive movement

_____ 79. Which condition below is associated with the greatest proteinuria?
  A. Acute glomerulonephritis
  B. Chronic glomerulonephritis
  C. Nephrotic syndrome
  D. Acute pyelonephritis

_____ 80. Which of the following results on a serous fluid is most likely to be caused by a traumatic tap?
  A. An RBC count of 8000/μL
  B. A WBC count of 6000/μL
  C. An Hct of 35%
  D. A neutrophil count of 45%

_____ 81. Which statement best describes the clinical utility of tests for microalbuminuria?
  A. Testing may detect early renal involvement in diabetes mellitus
  B. Microalbuminuria refers to a specific subfraction of albumin found only in persons with diabetic nephropathy
  C. A positive test result indicates the presence of orthostatic albuminuria
  D. Testing should be part of the routine urinalysis

_____ 82. Which of the following results are discrepant?
  A. Small blood but negative protein
  B. Moderate blood but no RBCs in microscopic examination
  C. Negative blood but 6–10 RBCs/high power field
  D. Negative blood, positive protein

Microbiology

_____ 83. The ortho-nitrophenyl-β-galactopyranoside (ONPG) test is most useful when differentiating:
  A. *Salmonella* spp from *Pseudomonas* spp
  B. *Shigella* spp from some strains of *Escherichia coli*
  C. *Klebsiella* spp from *Enterobacter* spp
  D. *Proteus vulgaris* from *Salmonella* spp

_____ 84. Lysostaphin is used to differentiate *Staphylococcus* from which other genus?
  A. Streptococcus
  B. Stomatococcus
  C. Micrococcus
  D. Planococcus

_____ 85. Which of the following tests best differentiate *Shigella* spp from *E. coli*?
  A. Hydrogen sulfide, Voges-Proskauer (VP), citrate, and urea
  B. Lactose, indole, ONPG, and motility
  C. Hydrogen sulfide, methyl red, citrate, and urea
  D. Gas, citrate, and VP

_____ 86. A gram-negative rod is recovered from a catheterized urine specimen from a nursing home patient. The lactose-negative isolate tested positive for indole, urease, potassium cyanide (KCN), ornithine decarboxylase, and phenylalanine deaminase. The most probable identification is:
  A. *Ewardsiella* spp
  B. *Morganella* spp
  C. *Ewingella* spp
  D. *Shigella* spp

_____ 87. A helminth egg is described as having terminal polar plugs. The most likely helminth is:
  A. Hookworm
  B. *Trichuris trichiura*
  C. *Fasciola hepatica*
  D. *Dipylidium caninum*

_____ 88. A leg culture from a nursing home patient grew gram-negative rods on MacConkey's agar as pink to dark pink oxidase-negative colonies. Given the following results, which is the most likely organism?

TSI = A/A   Indole = Neg

Methyl red = Neg   VP = +

Citrate = +   H$_2$S = Neg

Urease = +   Motility = Neg

Antibiotic susceptibility: resistant to carbenicillin and ampicillin

A. *Serratia marcescens*

B. *Proteus vulgaris*

C. *Enterobacter cloacae*

D. *Klebsiella pneumoniae*

_____ 89. A curved gram-negative rod producing oxidase-positive colonies on blood agar was recovered from a stool culture. Given the following results, what is the most likely identification?

Lysine decar-boxylase = +	Arginine decar-boxylase = Neg	Indole = +
KIA = Alk/Acid	VP = Neg	Lactose = Neg
Urease = ±	String test = Neg	TCBS agar = Green colonies

A. *Vibrio cholerae*

B. Vibrio *parahaemolyticus*

C. *Shigella* spp

D. *Salmonella* spp

_____ 90. Which test group best differentiates *Acinetobacter* spp from *Pseudomonas aeruginosa?*

A. Oxidase, motility, 42°C growth

B. MacConkey's growth, 37°C growth, catalase

C. Blood agar growth, oxidase, catalase

D. Oxidase, triple sugar iron (TSI), MacConkey's growth

_____ 91. A gram-negative S-shaped rod recovered from selective media for *Campylobacter* species gave the following results:

Catalase = +	Oxidase = +
Motility = +	Hippurate hydrolysis = +
Growth at 42°C = +	Nalidixic acid = Susceptible
Pigment = Neg	Grape odor = Neg
Cephalothin = Resistant	

The most likely identification is:

A. *Pseudomonas aeruginosa*

B. *Campylobacter jejuni*

C. *Campylobacter fetus*

D. *Pseudomonas putida*

_____ 92. Which media is best for recovery of *Legionella pneumophila* from clinical specimens?

A. Chocolate agar

B. Bordet-Gengou agar

C. New yeast extract agar

D. Buffered charcoal-yeast extract (CYE) agar

_____ 93. A small, gram-negative coccobacillus recovered from CSF of a 2-year-old gave the following results:

Indole = +	Glucose = + (acid)
X requirement = +	V requirement = +
Urease = +	Lactose = Neg
Sucrose = Neg	Hemolysis = Neg

Which is the most likely identification?

A. *Haemophilus parainfluenzae*

B. *Haemophilus influenzae*

C. *Haemophilus ducreyi*

D. *Haemophilus aphrophilus*

_____ 94. Urine cultured from the catheter of an 18-year-old female patient produced more than 100,000 col/mL on a CNA plate. Colonies were catalase-positive and coagulase-negative by the latex agglutination slide method as well as the tube coagulase test. The best single test for identification is:

A. Lactose fermentation

B. Urease

C. Catalase

D. Novobiocin susceptibility

_____ 95. A gram-positive spore-forming bacillus growing on sheep blood agar anaerobically produces a double zone of β-hemolysis and is positive for lecithinase. What is the presumptive identification?

A. *Bacteroides ureolyticus*

B. *Bacteroides fragilis*

C. *Clostridium perfringens*

D. *Clostridium difficile*

_____ 96. β-Hemolytic streptococci, not of group A or B, usually exhibit which of the following reactions?

	Trimethoprim-sulfamethoxazole	Bacitracin
A.	Susceptible	Resistant
B.	Resistant	Resistant
C.	Resistant	Susceptible
D.	Susceptible	Indeterminate

_____ **97.** A *Mycobacterium* species recovered from a patient with AIDS gave the following results:

Niacin = Neg	T$_2$H = +
Tween 80 hydrolysis = Neg	Nitrate reduction = Neg
Heat stable catalase (68°C) = ±	Nonphotochromogen

What is the most likely identification?
A. *M. gordonae*
B. *M. bovis*
C. *M. avium-intracellulare* complex
D. *M. kansasii*

_____ **98.** A germ tube–negative, pink yeast isolate was recovered from the respiratory secretions and urine of a patient with AIDS. Given the following results, what is the most likely identification?

Cornmeal Tween 80 Agar

Blastospores = +	Pseudohyphae = +
Arthrospores = Neg	Urease = +

A. *Candida albicans*
B. *Rhodotorula* spp
C. *Cryptococcus* spp
D. *Trichosporon* spp

_____ **99.** Upon examination of stool material for *Isospora belli*, one would expect to see:
A. Cysts containing sporozoites
B. Precysts containing chromatoidal bars
C. Oocysts that are acid-fast
D. Sporozoites that are hematoxylin-positive

_____ **100.** Which of the following viruses is implicated along with Epstein-Barr virus as a cause of infectious mononucleosis?
A. CMV
B. Coxsackie A virus
C. Coxsackie B virus
D. Hepatitis B virus

Table of Specifications

Section	Taxonomy 1	Taxonomy 2	Taxonomy 3	Number of Questions
Clinical Chemistry	2	10	5	17
Hematology	4	7	7	18
Immunology	4	9	2	15
Blood banking	7	6	7	20
Body fluids	2	8	2	12
Microbiology	4	7	7	18
Totals	23	47	30	100

Answer Key

Chemistry	Hematology	Immunology
1. **C**	18. **B**	36. **C**
2. **B**	19. **C**	37. **A**
3. **C**	20. **C**	38. **D**
4. **C**	21. **A**	39. **A**
5. **C**	22. **A**	40. **D**
6. **B**	23. **B**	41. **C**
7. **B**	24. **A**	42. **A**
8. **C**	25. **C**	43. **C**
9. **A**	26. **B**	44. **D**
10. **A**	27. **C**	45. **C**
11. **C**	28. **C**	46. **B**
12. **A**	29. **A**	47. **B**
13. **A**	30. **D**	48. **B**
14. **C**	31. **C**	49. **C**
15. **D**	32. **B**	50. **B**
16. **A**	33. **D**	
17. **A**	34. **B**	
	35. **A**	

Answer Key

Blood Banking	Body Fluids	Microbiology
51. **D**	71. **B**	83. **B**
52. **B**	72. **B**	84. **C**
53. **A**	73. **C**	85. **B**
54. **B**	74. **D**	86. **B**
55. **A**	75. **D**	87. **B**
56. **B**	76. **A**	88. **D**
57. **C**	77. **A**	89. **B**
58. **B**	78. **A**	90. **A**
59. **A**	79. **C**	91. **B**
60. **A**	80. **A**	92. **D**
61. **B**	81. **A**	93. **B**
62. **A**	82. **C**	94. **D**
63. **C**		95. **C**
64. **D**		96. **C**
65. **C**		97. **C**
66. **D**		98. **B**
67. **A**		99. **C**
68. **A**		100. **A**
69. **D**		
70. **A**